Clinical Manual of Emergency Pediatrics

Fifth Edition

Clinical Manual of Emergency Pediatrics

Fifth Edition

Editors

Ellen F. Crain

Jeffrey C. Gershel

Associate Editor

Sandra J. Cunningham

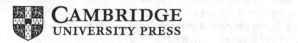

CAMBRIDGE
UNIVERSITY PRESS

University Printing House, Cambridge CB2 8BS, United Kingdom

One Liberty Plaza, 20th Floor, New York, NY 10006, USA

477 Williamstown Road, Port Melbourne, VIC 3207, Australia

4843/24, 2nd Floor, Ansari Road, Daryaganj, Delhi - 110002, India

79 Anson Road, #06-04/06, Singapore 079906

Cambridge University Press is part of the University of Cambridge.

It furthers the University's mission by disseminating knowledge in the pursuit of education, learning and research at the highest international levels of excellence.

www.cambridge.org
Information on this title: www.cambridge.org/9780521736879

© Cambridge University Press 2010

First published 2010
Reprinted with correction 2011
3rd printing 2012

A catalogue record for this publication is available from the British Library

Library of Congress Cataloging in Publication data
Clinical manual of emergency pediatrics / [edited by] Ellen Crain,
Jeffrey C. Gershel. – 5th ed.
      p. ; cm.
   Other title: Emergency pediatrics
   Includes bibliographical references and index.
   ISBN 978-0-521-73687-9 (Paperback)
   1. Pediatric emergencies–Handbooks, manuals, etc.
I. Crain, Ellen F.   II. Gershel, Jeffrey C.   III. Title: Emergency
pediatrics.
   [DNLM: 1. Emergencies–Handbooks.   2. Child.
3. Emergency Medicine–methods–Handbooks.   4. Infant.
5. Pediatrics–methods–Handbooks. WS 39 C641 2010]
   RJ370.C55 2010
   618.920025–dc22   2010016794

ISBN 978-0-521-73687-9 Paperback

Additional resources for this publication at www.cambridge.org/delange

....

Contents

List of contributors   x
Preface   xv

1. **Resuscitation**   1
   Waseem Hafeez
   Cardiopulmonary resuscitation
   overview   1
   Emergency department priorities   1
   Initial management   5
   Foreign-body airway obstruction   6
   Oxygenation, ventilation, and
   intubation   8
   Rapid-sequence intubation   14
   Circulation   16
   Medications and electrical therapy in
   resuscitation   20
   Cardioversion and defibrillation   22
   Shock   23

2. **Allergic emergencies**   30
   Stephanie R. Lichten
   Anaphylaxis   30
   Angioedema   34
   Urticaria   36

3. **Cardiac emergencies**   39
   Michael H. Gewitz and Paul K. Woolf
   Arrhythmias   39
   Atrial fibrillation   39
   Atrial flutter   40
   Sinus tachycardia   41
   Supraventricular tachycardia   42
   Ventricular premature
   contractions   47
   Ventricular tachycardia   48
   Ventricular fibrillation   50
   Heart block   50
   Pacemaker and defibrillator
   assessment   53
   Chest pain   54

   Congestive heart failure   56
   Cyanosis   60
   Cyanotic (Tet) spells   61
   Heart murmurs   62
   Infective endocarditis   64
   Pericardial disease   66
   Syncope   68

4. **Dental emergencies**   72
   Nancy Dougherty
   Dental anatomy   72
   Dental eruption   72
   Dental caries and odontogenic
   infections   74
   Oral trauma   77
   Tooth discoloration   80
   Oral soft tissue lesions   82

5. **Dermatologic emergencies**   87
   Alexandra D. McCollum and
   Sheila F. Friedlander
   Definition of terms   87
   Acne   91
   Alopecia   93
   Atopic dermatitis   96
   Bacterial skin infections   98
   Candida   100
   Contact dermatitis   102
   Diaper dermatitis   103
   Drug eruptions and severe drug
   reactions   107
   Erythema annulare   111
   Erythema marginatum   111
   Erythema multiforme   111
   Erythema nodosum   112
   Granuloma annulare   113
   Herpes simplex   115

Hypopigmented lesions 118
Infestations: lice 120
Infestations: scabies 122
Neonatal rashes 123
Palpable purpura 126
Pityriasis rosea 127
Psoriasis 128
Tinea 129
Verrucae and molluscum 132

6. **ENT emergencies** 135
Jeffrey Keller and Stephanie R. Lichten
Acute otitis media 135
Cervical lymphadenopathy 138
Epistaxis 142
Foreign bodies 144
Mastoiditis 146
Neck masses 147
Otitis externa 149
Parotitis 150
Periorbital and orbital cellulitis 151
Peritonsillar abscess 153
Pharyngotonsillitis 154
Retropharyngeal abscess 156
Serous otitis media 157
Sinusitis 157
Upper respiratory infections 159

7. **Endocrine emergencies** 161
Joan Di Martino-Nardi
Adrenal insufficiency 161
Diabetes insipidus 165
Diabetic ketoacidosis: Ellen F. Crain
and Sandra J. Cunningham 168
Hypercalcemia: Morri Markowitz 174
Hyperkalemia 176
Hypernatremia 177
Hypocalcemia: Morri Markowitz 180
Hypoglycemia 183
Hyponatremia 186
Thyroid disorders 189

8. **Environmental emergencies** 194
Anthony J. Ciorciari
Burns 194
Drowning 199

Electrical injuries 200
Frostbite 203
Heat-excess syndromes 205
Hyperbaric oxygen therapy:
Katherine J. Chou 207
Hypothermia 210
Inhalation injury 212
Lead poisoning 215
Lightning injuries 217

9. **Gastrointestinal emergencies** 219
Teresa McCann and Julie Lin
Abdominal pain 219
Acute pancreatitis 223
Appendicitis 225
Assessment and management of
dehydration: Ellen F. Crain and
Sandra J. Cunningham 228
Colic 234
Constipation 235
Diarrhea 239
Gallbladder and gallstone disease 244
Hepatomegaly 247
Intussusception 248
Jaundice 249
Liver failure 253
Lower gastrointestinal bleeding 256
Upper gastrointestinal bleeding 259
Meckel's diverticulum 262
Pyloric stenosis 263
Rectal prolapse 265
Umbilical lesions 266
Viral hepatitis 268
Vomiting 273

10. **Emergencies associated with genetic syndromes** 278
Robert W. Marion and Joy Samanich
Congenital malformations 278

11. **Genitourinary emergencies** 283
Sandra J. Cunningham
Balanoposthitis 283
Renal and genitourinary trauma 284
Meatal stenosis 288
Paraphimosis 288

Phimosis   289
Priapism   290
Scrotal swellings   291
Undescended testis   295
Urinary retention   296
Urethritis   297

12. **Gynecologic emergencies**   300
Dominic Hollman, Elizabeth M.
Alderman, and Anthony J. Ciorciari
Breast disorders   300
Dysfunctional uterine bleeding   304
Dysmenorrhea   308
Pregnancy and complications   310
Sexually transmitted diseases   314
Vaginal discharge and
vulvovaginitis   325

13. **Hematologic emergencies**   332
Mark Weinblatt
Anemia   332
Hemostatic disorders   336
Thrombophilia   340
Transfusion therapy   341
The abnormal CBC   342
Infection and the immunocompromised
host   343
Leukemia and lymphoma   345
Lymphadenopathy   347
Oncologic emergencies   350
Sickle cell disease   354
Splenomegaly   359

14. **Infectious disease emergencies**   362
Glenn Fennelly and Michael Rosenberg
Botulism   362
Cat scratch disease   363
Dengue viruses   365
Encephalitis   366
Evaluation of the febrile child:
Ellen F. Crain   370
HIV-related emergencies   374
Infectious mononucleosis and
mononucleosis-like illnesses   386
Infectious disease associated
with exanthems   388

Kawasaki syndrome   395
Leptospirosis   396
Lyme disease   398
Meningitis   401
Mycoplasma pneumoniae
infections   405
Nontuberculous mycobacteria
diseases   407
Parasitic infections: *Christina
M. Coyle*   408
Pertussis   414
Rickettsial diseases   416
Toxic shock syndrome   420
Tuberculosis   423
Diseases transmitted by exposure to
animals (zoonoses) or arthropod
vectors   428

15. **Ingestions**   433
Stephen M. Blumberg and Carl Kaplan
Evaluation of the poisoned
patient   433
Acetaminophen   448
ADHD medications   450
Anticholinergics   451
Antidepressants   453
Antipsychotics   454
Beta agonists   456
Beta blockers   456
Caffeine   458
Calcium channel blockers   459
Carbon monoxide: *Katherine
J. Chou*   460
Caustics   461
Cholinergics   462
Clonidine   464
Cough and cold medications   465
Diabetic agents   466
Digoxin and cardiac glycosides   467
Drugs of abuse   469
Ethanol   471
Foreign-body ingestion   473
Hydrocarbons   474
Inhalants   475
Iron   476

Mothballs   478
Nonsteroidal anti-inflammatory
drugs   479
Rat poison   480
Salicylates   481
Toxic alcohols (ethylene glycol,
methanol, and isopropanol)   483
Tricyclic antidepressants   485

16. **Neurologic emergencies**   487
Soe Mar
Acute ataxia   487
Acute hemiparesis and stroke   491
Acute weakness   494
Breathholding   498
Coma   499
Facial weakness   502
Headache   504
Head trauma   509
Implantable devices   515
Increased intracranial pressure   516
Seizures   518
Sleep disorders   524
Ventriculoperitoneal shunts   525

17. **Ophthalmologic emergencies**   528
Carolyn Lederman and Martin
Lederman
Anatomy   528
Evaluation   528
Decreased vision   529
Excessive tearing   530
Eyelid inflammation   533
Ocular trauma   535
The red eye   541
The white pupil (leukocoria)   545

18. **Orthopedic emergencies**   547
Sergey Kunkov and James Meltzer
Back pain   547
Fractures, dislocations, and
sprains   552
Common orthopedic injuries   557
Limp   566
Osteomyelitis   571
Splinting: *Katherine J. Chou*   573

19. **Physical and sexual abuse**   580
Stephen Ludwig, Mary Mehlman
and Scott Miller
Physical abuse   580
Sexual abuse   583
Chart documentation in child abuse:
Olga Jimenez   587
Medical testimony and court
preparation: *Olga Jimenez*   591
Abandonment and physical neglect   594

20. **Psychological and social
emergencies**   596
Stephen Ludwig, Mary Mehlman,
and Scott Miller
Death in the emergency
department   596
Psychiatric emergencies: *Daniel
Mason*   597
Sudden infant death syndrome   599
Suicide: *Daniel Mason*   601
Munchausen syndrome by proxy   602
Interpersonal violence   603

21. **Pulmonary emergencies**   606
Ellen F. Crain and Sergey Kunkov
Asthma   606
Bacterial tracheitis   613
Bronchiolitis   614
Cough   616
Croup   620
Epiglottitis   622
Foreign body in the airway   624
Hemoptysis   626
Pneumonia   629
Pulse oximetry: *Sandra
J. Cunningham*   633
Respiratory distress and failure   634

22. **Radiology**   638
Dan Barlev, with Robert Acosta
Ordering radiologic examinations   638

23. **Renal emergencies**   644
Sandra J. Cunningham and Preeti
Venkataraman, with Beatrice Goilav
Acute glomerulonephritis   644

Acute kidney injury 647
Hematuria 651
Hemolytic uremic syndrome 653
Henoch-Schönlein purpura 655
Hypertension 656
Nephrolithiasis 660
Proteinuria 662
Urinary tract infections 664

24. **Rheumatologic emergencies** 668
Michael Gorn and Svetlana Lvovich
Acute rheumatic fever 668
Arthritis 671
Henoch-Schönlein purpura 675
Juvenile dermatomyositis 677
Systemic lupus erythematosus 679

25. **Sedation and analgesia** 682
Sandra J. Cunningham
Procedural sedation and
analgesia 682
PSA medications 685
Local anesthesia 691
Topical anesthesia 692
Regional anesthesia: *Katherine J. Chou* 693

26. **Trauma** 702
Anthony J. Ciorciari
Cervical spine injuries 702
Hand injuries 705
Multiple trauma 710

Pericardial tamponade 719
Pneumothorax 720

27. **Wound care and minor trauma** 723
Anthony J. Ciorciari
Abscesses 723
Bite wounds 724
Foreign-body removal 726
Insect bites and stings 728
Marine stings and
envenomations 729
Rabies 731
Scorpion stings 733
Snakebites 734
Spider bites 736
Wound management 738

28. **Special considerations in pediatric emergency care** 745
The crying infant: *David P. Sole* 745
The critically ill infant: *Frank A. Maffei* 747
Children with special healthcare needs: *Joshua Vova* 753
Failure to thrive: *Kirsten Roberts* 764
Telephone triage: *Loren Yellin* 768

Index 771

Code Card: Waseem Hafeez

'Available online at
www.cambridge.org/9780521736879'

Contributors

Robert Acosta, MD
Assistant Professor of Pediatrics,
Albert Einstein College of Medicine,
Jacobi Medical Center,
Bronx, NY, USA

Elizabeth M. Alderman, MD
Professor of Clinical Pediatrics,
Albert Einstein College of Medicine,
Children's Hospital at Montefiore,
Bronx, NY, USA

Dan Barlev, MD
Assistant Professor of Radiology,
State University of New York at Stony Brook,
Winthrop University Hospital,
Mineola, NY, USA

Stephen M. Blumberg, MD
Assistant Professor of Pediatrics,
Albert Einstein College of Medicine,
Jacobi Medical Center,
Bronx, NY, USA

Katherine J. Chou, MD
Associate Professor of Clinical Pediatrics
and Clinical Emergency Medicine,
Albert Einstein College of Medicine,
Jacobi Medical Center,
Bronx, NY, USA

Anthony J. Ciorciari, MD
Associate Professor of Clinical Emergency
Medicine,
Albert Einstein College of Medicine,
Jacobi Medical Center,
Bronx, NY, USA

Christina M. Coyle, MD
Professor of Clinical Medicine,
Albert Einstein College of Medicine,
Jacobi Medical Center, Bronx, NY, USA

Ellen F. Crain, MD, PhD
Professor of Pediatrics and Emergency
Medicine,
Albert Einstein College of Medicine,
Jacobi Medical Center,
Bronx, NY, USA

Sandra J. Cunningham, MD
Associate Professor of Clinical Pediatrics
and Clinical Emergency Medicine,
Albert Einstein College of Medicine,
Jacobi Medical Center,
Bronx, NY, USA

Joan Di Martino-Nardi, MD
Professor of Clinical Pediatrics,
Albert Einstein College of Medicine,
Northern Westchester Hospital Center,
Mt Kisco, NY, USA

Nancy Dougherty, DMD, MPH
Clinical Associate Professor of Pediatric
Dentistry,
New York University College of Dentistry,
New York, NY, USA

Glenn Fennelly, MD
Associate Professor of Clinical Pediatrics,
Albert Einstein College of Medicine,
Jacobi Medical Center,
Bronx, NY, USA

Sheila Fallon Friedlander, MD
Clinical Professor of Pediatrics and
Medicine,
University of California San Diego School
of Medicine,
Rady Children's Hospital,
San Diego, CA, USA

Jeffrey C. Gershel, MD
Professor of Clinical Pediatrics,
Albert Einstein College of Medicine,

Jacobi Medical Center,
Bronx, NY, USA

Michael H. Gewitz, MD
Professor of Pediatrics,
New York Medical College,
Maria Fareri Children's Hospital at
Westchester Medical Center,
Valhalla, NY, USA

Beatrice Goilav, MD
Assistant Professor of Pediatrics,
Albert Einstein College of Medicine,
The Children's Hospital at Montefiore,
Bronx, NY, USA

Michael Gorn, MD
Pediatric Emergency Medicine,
St. Joseph's Regional Medical Center,
Paterson, NJ, USA

Waseem Hafeez, MBBS
Associate Professor of Clinical Pediatrics,
Albert Einstein College of Medicine,
The Children's Hospital at Montefiore,
Bronx, NY, USA

Dominic Hollman, MD
Assistant Professor of Pediatrics,
Mount Sinai Medical Center,
New York, NY, USA

Olga Jimenez, MD
Assistant Professor of Pediatrics,
Albert Einstein College of Medicine,
Jacobi Medical Center,
Bronx, NY, USA

Carl Kaplan, MD
Clinical Assistant Professor of Emergency
Medicine and Pediatrics,
Stony Brook University School of Medicine,
Stony Brook, NY, USA

Jeffrey Keller, MD
Assistant Professor of Otolaryngology/Head
and Neck Surgery,
Mount Sinai Medical Center,

Mt Kisco Medical Group,
Mt Kisco, NY, USA

Sergey Kunkov, MD, MS
Associate Professor of Pediatrics,
Stony Brook University School of Medicine,
Stony Brook, NY, USA

Carolyn Lederman, MD
Assistant Clinical Professor,
Columbia University, Edward. S. Harkness
Eye Institute of New York Presbyterian
Hospital,
New York, NY, USA

Martin Lederman, MD
Associate Clinical Professor,
Columbia University, Edward. S. Harkness
Eye Institute of New York Presbyterian
Hospital, New York, NY, USA

Stephanie R. Lichten, MD
Assistant Professor of Pediatrics,
Albert Einstein College of Medicine,
Jacobi Medical Center,
Bronx, NY, USA

Julie Lin, MD
Instructor of Pediatrics,
Albert Einstein College of Medicine,
Jacobi Medical Center,
Bronx, NY, USA

Stephen Ludwig, MD
Professor of Pediatrics and Emergency
Medicine,
University of Pennsylvania School of
Medicine,
Philadelphia, PA, USA

Svetlana Lvovich, MD
Assistant Professor of Pediatrics,
Drexel University College of Medicine,
Philadelphia, PA, USA

Frank A. Maffei, MD
Associate Professor of Pediatrics,
Temple University School of Medicine,

Janet Weis Children's Hospital at Geisinger,
Danville, PA, USA

Soe Mar, MD
Assistant Professor in Neurology and
Pediatrics,
Washington University School of Medicine,
St. Louis, MO, USA

Robert W. Marion, MD
Professor, Pediatrics and Obstetrics and
Gynecology and Women's Health,
Albert Einstein College of Medicine,
The Children's Hospital at Montefiore,
Bronx, NY, USA

Morri Markowitz, MD
Professor of Pediatrics,
Albert Einstein College of Medicine,
Children's Hospital at Montefiore,
Bronx, NY, USA

Daniel Mason, MD
Department of Psychiatry,
Northern Westchester Hospital Center,
Mt Kisco, NY, USA

Teresa McCann, MD
Assistant Professor of Pediatrics,
Albert Einstein College of Medicine,
Jacobi Medical Center,
Bronx, NY, USA

Alexandra D. McCollum, MD
Clinical Research Fellow,
Pediatric and Adolescent Dermatology,
Rady Children's Hospital,
San Diego, CA, USA

Mary Mehlman, MD
Chief Resident in Pediatrics,
Albert Einstein College of Medicine,
Jacobi Medical Center,
Bronx, NY, USA

James Meltzer, MD
Assistant Professor of Pediatrics,
Albert Einstein College of Medicine,

Jacobi Medical Center,
Bronx, NY, USA

Scott Miller, MD
Instructor in Pediatrics,
Albert Einstein College of Medicine,
Jacobi Medical Center,
Bronx, NY, USA

Kirsten Roberts, MD
Assistant Professor of Pediatrics,
Albert Einstein College of Medicine,
Jacobi Medical Center,
Bronx, NY, USA

Michael Rosenberg, MD
Associate Professor of Clinical Pediatrics,
Albert Einstein College of Medicine,
Jacobi Medical Center,
Bronx, NY, USA

Joy Samanich, MD
Assistant Professor, Pediatrics and Obstetrics and Gynecology and Women's Health,
Albert Einstein College of Medicine,
The Children's Hospital at Montefiore,
Bronx, NY, USA

David P. Sole, DO
Clinical Assistant Professor of Emergency
Medicine,
Temple University,
School of Medicine,
Philadelphia, PA, USA

Preeti Venkataraman, MD
Attending Pediatrician,
Jacobi Medical Center,
Bronx, NY, USA

Joshua Vova, MD
Assistant Professor of Physical Medicine
and Rehabilitation,
Emory University School of Medicine,
Atlanta, GA, USA

Mark Weinblatt, MD
Professor of Clinical Pediatrics,
Stony Brook University School of Medicine,

Winthrop University Hospital,
Mineola, NY, USA

Paul K. Woolf, MD
Associate Professor of Pediatrics,
New York Medical College,
Maria Fareri Children's Hospital at
Westchester Medical Center,
Valhalla, NY, USA

Loren Yellin, MD
Assistant Professor of Pediatrics,
Albert Einstein College of Medicine,
Jacobi Medical Center,
Bronx, NY, USA

Preface

In this fifth edition of the *Clinical Manual of Emergency Pediatrics*, we have endeavored to remain true to our original intention: to provide a dependable, comprehensive, portable handbook that offers concise advice regarding the approach to the majority of conditions seen in a pediatric emergency department. For each topic, we have included essential points and priorities for diagnosis, management, and follow-up care, as well as indications for hospitalization and a bibliography to guide further reading.

Traditionally, manuals such as this one were written for trainees, as well as experienced pediatric emergency and emergency medicine physicians, who needed a summary of the myriad conditions that present to the emergency department and a guide as to how to differentiate among them. Now, however, primary care providers are expected to manage acute illnesses in ambulatory settings. Ill children are hospitalized less often, and they tend to be discharged back to their primary care providers sooner than ever before. In addition, increasing numbers of chronically ill and medically fragile children are receiving care in ambulatory sites. As a result of these shifting practices, physicians working in settings such as private offices and clinics may be faced with potential, or real, pediatric emergencies. These caregivers, as well as emergency physicians, can benefit from a practical handbook.

Since the publication of the first edition of this manual, on-line and portable resources have become readily available. However, many are not geared to pediatric conditions or presentations. It is our observation that there is a lack of detail, particularly when discussing differential diagnoses. Our hope is that this manual, which gathers the necessary facts and management recommendations in a user-friendly, easily accessible manual, will facilitate decision-making and safe care.

In the fifth edition, we have maintained the book's unique features while making many changes that increase its utility. Because the scope of childhood illnesses and injuries seen in acute care settings is constantly increasing, we have revised and updated every chapter. We have added new sections on several infectious and rheumatic diseases that had been overlooked in previous editions, along with sections on regional anesthesia, hyperkalemia, and nephrolithiasis. The ingestion and orthopedic sections have been completely revised and updated, and there is specific attention paid to MRSA, where relevant.

A word of caution is in order. Although a manual for emergency care can be very useful, it may tempt physicians, particularly those still in training, to look for automatic solutions. It is not our intent that this text be used as a protocol book. We urge students and housestaff not to use this manual as a substitute for their own critical thinking and sensitivity when caring for children and their families.

We owe special thanks to our associate editor, Sandra J. Cunningham, MD, for her contributions and diligent editing. Her careful attention to detail greatly improved the quality of the book. Katherine J. Chou, MD, and Anthony Ciorciari, MD, our colleagues in pediatric emergency medicine and the Department of Emergency Medicine, respectively, reviewed much of the text to ensure that recommendations were updated and evidence-based. Although the quality of this fifth edition reflects the hard work of all the contributors, the final manuscript reflects our approach to any given illness or problem, and we are responsible for the book's content.

By what they have taught us and by their example we are especially grateful to the pediatric emergency department nurses, attendings, and nurse practitioners at the Jacobi Medical Center. We have become better teachers and caregivers by observing them and their interactions with patients and families.

We are particularly indebted to the pediatric and emergency medicine house staffs and the pediatric emergency medicine fellows at the Jacobi Medical Center, and the medical students of the Albert Einstein College of Medicine whom we have had the privilege of teaching and learning from over the years. Their thoughtful questions provided the impetus for this manual.

This book is dedicated to the memory of Dr. Lewis M. Fraad, our beloved mentor, whose name has been memorialized in the name of our department, the Lewis M. Fraad Department of Pediatrics at Jacobi Medical Center. Day in and day out he set an example for all of us by combining intellectual rigor with a deep respect for children and their families. He will always be with us when we are at our best.

Ellen F. Crain and Jeffrey C. Gershel

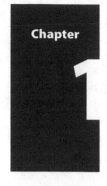

Chapter 1

Resuscitation

Waseem Hafeez

Cardiopulmonary resuscitation overview

Cardiopulmonary arrest in infants and children is rarely a sudden event. The usual progression of arrest is respiratory failure, caused by hypoxia and hypercarbia, which eventually leads to asystolic cardiac arrest. Common etiologies that may lead to cardiopulmonary arrest include sudden infant death syndrome (SIDS), respiratory disease, sepsis, major trauma, submersion, poisoning, and metabolic/electrolyte imbalance. In contrast, primary cardiac arrest is relatively rare in the pediatric age group and is most frequently caused by congenital heart disease, myocarditis, and chest trauma with myocardial injury. Although asystole and pulseless electrical activity (PEA) are the primary rhythms in pediatric cardiac arrest, the patient may also have ventricular tachycardia (VT) or ventricular fibrillation (VF).

The outcome of unwitnessed cardiopulmonary arrest in infants and children is poor. Only 8.4% of pediatric patients who have out-of-hospital cardiac arrests survive to discharge and most are neurologically impaired, while the in-hospital survival rate is 24%, with a better neurological outcome. The best reported outcomes have been in children who receive immediate high-quality cardiopulmonary resuscitation (resulting in adequate ventilation and coronary artery perfusion), and in those with witnessed sudden arrest (presenting with ventricular rhythm disturbance) that responds to early defibrillation.

Emergency department priorities

To optimize outcome, it is essential to recognize early signs and symptoms of impending respiratory failure and circulatory shock prior to the development of full cardiopulmonary arrest. All equipment, supplies, and drugs must be available and organized for easy access. It is imperative that the staff have training in Pediatric Advanced Life Support (PALS), and routinely practice mock pediatric resuscitations.

Pre-calculated drug sheets or the Broselow tape and a comprehensive plan to organize the resuscitation team (Table 1-1) will optimize care in a high-stress situation. Assign a role to each team member: team leader, airway management, chest compressions, vascular access, obtaining a history, medication administration, recorder, and runner. Identify a team leader early whose sole responsibility is to oversee the resuscitation and give instructions. Ideally, a respiratory therapist will assist the team, and a clock must be available to facilitate record keeping. Prepare in advance the essential equipment needed for resuscitation, using the mnemonic IMSOAPP. (Table 1-2).

Rapid cardiopulmonary assessment

Quickly perform a primary evaluation, which focuses on the Appearance, Airway, Breathing and Circulatory (ABCs) status of the patient. This initial examination provides assessment

Table 1-1. Resuscitation team roles and preparation

Roles

Team leader

Airway management

Chest compressions

Vascular access

Medication administration

Obtaining a history

Recorder

Runner

Preparation

IV-IO/monitors/suction/O_2/airway equipment/medications

Assess weight (in kg) = 2 × (age in years + 4)

Airway (C-collar): head tilt–chin lift; jaw thrust; oxygen; suction

Breathing: rate; air; retractions; O_2 saturation (oximetry); R/O pneumothorax

Circulation: pulse rate; BP; capillary refill; peripheral pulses

IV/IO Access: NS 20 mL/kg × 3; pressors; packed RBCs

Disability: AVPU; pupils; neurologic examination; GCS

Dextrose: $D_{25}W$ = 2 mL/kg ; < 3 mo: $D_{10}W$ = 5 mL/kg

Exposure: log roll; rectal and guaiac

Evaluation: secondary head-to-toe examination

Fever: maintain normal temperature

Fast (trauma): RUQ, sub-xiphoid, cardiac, LUQ, suprapubic

Foley: contraindicated for high prostate; blood in meatus or scrotum

Gastric tube (NGT): not if there is a midface injury (use orogastric tube)

History: allergies; usual medications; PMH; last meal time

of the patient's acuity, and prioritizes the urgency and aggressiveness of intervention in response to the degree of physiologic compromise. Following stabilization of the ABCs, the secondary assessment includes a complete examination of the patient, while maintaining normothermia and normoglycemia.

Appearance

Assess the general appearance of the patient. Evaluate the activity level of the child, reaction to painful or unfamiliar stimuli, interaction with the caretaker, consolability, and strength of the cry, relative to the patient's age.

Table 1-2. IMSOAPP. mnemonic for resuscitation

I   IV fluids/IV catheter/intraosseous needle

M   Monitors: cardiorespiratory; pulse oximeter; blood pressure

S   Suction: tonsil tipped (Yankauer) and flexible catheters

O   100% Oxygen source

A   Airway equipment

    Bag-mask: different size masks

    Oral airway: nasopharyngeal and oral

    Laryngoscope with assorted blades: Miller, Macintosh

    Tracheal tube: cuffed and uncuffed, multiple sizes

    Stylet

P   Pharmacy: medications, either a pre-calculated drug sheet or Broselow tape

P   Personnel: call a code, have resuscitation team available

Airway

Airway patency is particularly prone to early compromise in pediatric patients, as the airway diameter and length are smaller than in adults. Determine whether the airway is clear (no intervention required), maintainable with noninvasive intervention (positioning, oropharyngeal or nasopharyngeal airway placement, suctioning, bag-mask ventilation) or not maintainable without intubation.

Breathing

Ventilation and oxygenation are reflected in the work of breathing and can be quickly assessed by the mnemonic RACE:

- Rate: age-dependent (Table 1-3). Tachypnea is often the first sign of respiratory distress.
- Air entry
  - Listen to breath sounds in all areas: anterior and posterior chest, axillae
  - Must rule out pneumothorax: absent breath sounds, tracheal deviation
  - Abnormal sounds: rales, rhonchi, wheezing
- Color
  - Pink, pallid, cyanotic, or mottled
  - Pulse oximetry: use the O_2 saturation as the fifth vital sign
- Effort/mechanics
  - "Tripod" position, nasal flaring, grunting, stridor, head bobbing
  - Accessory muscle use: sternocleidomastoid prominence
  - Retractions: suprasternal, subcostal, and/or intercostal

The presence of abnormal clinical signs of breathing such as grunting, severe retractions, mottled color, use of accessory muscles, and cyanosis are precursors to impending respiratory failure.

Table 1-3. Normal vital signs

Age	Weight (kg)	Respiratory Rate/min	Pulse Rate/min	Systolic BP 10th–90th	Diastolic BP 10th/90th
<1 month	3–4	35–55	95–180	65–90	35–55
1–11 months	5–8	25–40	110–170	85–105	45–65
1–3 years	10–15	20–30	90–150	90–105	45–65
4–6 years	15–20	20–25	65–135	95–110	50–70
7–9 years	20–30	18–25	60–130	100–115	50–70
10–12 years	30–40	16–22	60–110	100–120	50–70
13–15 years	40–60	15–22	60–110	105–125	55–70
16–18 years	60–70	15–20	60–100	110–130	55–75
>18 years	>70	12–20	60–100	110–135	65–85

Circulation

The circulatory status reflects the effectiveness of cardiac output as well as end-organ perfusion. The rapid assessment includes:

- Cardiovascular function
  - Heart rate: age-dependent (Table 1-3)
  - Central and peripheral pulses: compare the femoral, brachial, and radial pulses
  - Blood pressure: age-dependent. Use the following guidelines to estimate the lowest acceptable (5th percentile) systolic BP:

    - Newborn – 1 month = 60 mmHg
    - 1 month – 1 year = 70 mmHg
    - 1–10 years = 70 mmHg + (2 × age in years)
    - > 10 years = 90 mmHg

- End-organ perfusion (systemic circulation)
  - Skin perfusion: capillary refill (<2 sec normal), color, extremity temperature (relative to ambient temperature)
  - Renal perfusion: urinary output = 1 mL/kg per h (about 30 mL/h for an adolescent)
  - CNS perfusion: mental status, level of consciousness, irritability, consolability

    A awake
    V responsive to voice
    P responsive to pain
    U unresponsive

Tachycardia and tachypnea are early signs of cardiorespiratory compromise. Observe for central or peripheral cyanosis and feel the skin temperature and moisture. With the fingers at the level of the heart, apply pressure to the nail bed until it blanches, then release, timing the interval until the fingertip "pinks up." Delayed capillary refill (>2 sec), and cool, clammy extremities are clinical indicators of poor perfusion. A systolic blood pressure <5th percentile (measured with an appropriate-size cuff), loss of central pulses, oliguria, and altered level of consciousness are ominous signs of impending decompensated circulatory shock.

Initial management

Airway management

For patients requiring CPR, the sequence of ABC has changed to CAB for adolescents, children and infants, but not for newborns. For patients with a heart rate above 60, airway management is the first priority. Immediate goals in the ED include reversing hypoxemia, supporting ventilation, maintaining airway patency, and protecting the airway from secretions and vomitus. To open the airway, first use simple maneuvers such as repositioning the head, suctioning secretions from the mouth, and placing an oropharyngeal or nasopharyngeal airway.

Head tilt–chin lift

Open the airway using the head tilt–chin lift technique or jaw thrust maneuver. In an unresponsive child, perform the head tilt–chin lift maneuver by placing one hand on the patient's forehead and gently tilting the head back into a neutral position. Curl the fingers of the other hand gently under the jaw, and lift the mandible upward to open the airway.

Jaw thrust

In known or suspected trauma victims, use the jaw thrust maneuver without head extension. Protect the cervical spine by providing manual inline traction. Perform the jaw thrust by keeping the head midline, placing the fingers at the angle of the jaw on both sides, and lifting the mandible upward and forward without extending the neck.

Suction catheters

Suction secretions and blood from the nasal passages, oropharynx, and trachea with flexible suction catheters. These must be available in sizes small enough to pass through the smallest endotracheal tube (ETT). A 5 Fr catheter will pass through a 2.5 mm ETT (usually 2 × the ETT size). Large rigid tonsil tip catheters (Yankauer) have rounded tips which are less likely to injure the tonsils and are useful for clearing blood and particulate matter from the mouth and hypopharynx. Limit suctioning to about 10 seconds, while monitoring the pulse oximeter and heart rate, as vigorous suctioning may cause vagal stimulation resulting in bradycardia and hypoxia.

Oropharyngeal airway

The oropharyngeal airway is an adjunct for ventilating an unresponsive patient with an absent gag reflex. It will keep the base of the tongue away from the posterior pharyngeal wall, maintaining airway patency. Do not use it in an awake or obtunded patient as it can precipitate vomiting and laryngospasm.

An appropriately sized oral airway extends from the corner of the patient's mouth to the angle of the jaw. Depress the tongue with a blade, and insert the oropharyngeal airway with its curvature along the hard palate. In infants and children, avoid inserting an airway that is too large. Do not attempt to insert the airway in an inverted position and then rotate it 180°, as this technique may damage the palate and push the base of the tongue posteriorly, occluding the airway. The proximal part of the oral airway is firm and flat and is designed to be placed between the teeth to prevent biting (the tracheal tube or your finger). Tape the flange to the lips to prevent it from being dislodged.

Nasopharyngeal airway

Use an NP airway in an obtunded patient with an intact gag reflex who has upper airway obstruction secondary to a floppy tongue. Estimate the size by measuring the distance from the tip of the nose to the tragus of the ear; the appropriately sized airway extends from the nostril to the base of the tongue without compressing the epiglottis. Lubricate the device and gently insert it along the floor of the nostril to avoid injuring the nasal mucosa or adenoids. A nasopharyngeal airway is contraindicated in a patient with a possible basilar skull fracture.

Foreign-body airway obstruction

If choking or airway obstruction from a foreign body is suspected and the patient is awake and can speak, make no attempts to remove the object. Allow the patient to cough and clear the airway while observing for signs of complete obstruction (i.e. the victim is unable to make a sound). Remove the foreign body from the mouth only if it is visible. Do not perform blind finger sweeps in any age because the obstructing object may be pushed further into the pharynx and cause complete airway obstruction. If the patient deteriorates, use the procedures as summarized in Table 1-4.

Infants <1 year of age

Lay the infant prone over your thighs, with the head supported in a dependent position. Alternatively, hold the infant over your arm, in the prone position, supporting the head in your hand. Deliver five sharp back slaps, in rapid succession, between the baby's scapulae. Turn the infant over and give five chest thrusts using two fingers on the mid-sternum. Look into the mouth to see whether the foreign body is dislodged. Repeat these maneuvers until the object is expelled or the infant becomes unconscious. Do not perform abdominal thrusts in infants as there is risk of injury to the abdominal organs.

Unconscious infant

First open the mouth wide by grasping the tongue and jaw, and look for the foreign body in the oral cavity. If an object is seen, remove it, but do not perform a blind sweep. If there is no improvement, begin cardiopulmonary resuscitation (CPR) providing five cycles (30 compressions and two breaths per cycle) over 2 minutes. If breaths cannot be delivered, reposition the head and try again, or proceed with advanced airway maneuvers until respirations have been restored.

Children >1 year of age to adolescent

Use the Heimlich abdominal thrust maneuver in this age group. Place the child in a supine position and kneel at his or her feet. Position the heel of the hand in the midline of the epigastrium with the other hand on top of the first, then give a rapid series of separate and distinct upward thrusts. With each thrust use sufficient force to dislodge the foreign body. For a small child, the heel of one hand is sufficient, as overly vigorous abdominal thrusts may cause damage to internal organs. If the patient loses consciousness, reposition the head

Table 1-4. Summary of BLS maneuvers for infants, children, and adolescents

Maneuver	Infant <1 year	Child 1–8 years of age	Adolescent
Activate emergency response (lone rescuer)	Witnessed: Activate EMS and call for AED, if available, after checking for responsiveness and scanning chest for breathing Unwittnessed: Provide 2 min CPR before activating EMS		Activate EMS after checking for responsiveness and scanning the chest for breathing
C: Circulation			
Pulse check (5–10 sec)	Brachial	Femoral or carotid	Carotid
Compression landmarks	Just below nipple line One rescuer: 2 fingers Two rescuers: both thumbs with hands encircling the chest	Center of chest, mid sternum between nipples One hand: heel of one hand only Two hands: heel of one hand with second on top	
Compression rate	100/minute (30 compressions in 18 seconds)		
Compression depth	Approximately one-third the depth of the chest		2 inches
Compression ventilation ratio	One rescuer = 30:2 Two rescuers = 15:2		One or two rescuers = 30:2
Defibrillation (provide CPR until defibrillator ready)	Manual defibrillator or AED preferably with pediatric dose attenuator	Use child pads (if available, otherwise use adult pads)	Use adult pads only
A: Airway	Head tilt–chin lift; for suspected trauma, use jaw thrust.		
B: Breathing			
Rescue breathing without chest compressions	12–20 breaths/min (1 breath every 3–5 seconds)		10–12 breaths/min (approximately 1 breath every 5–6 sec)
Rescue breaths with advanced airway	8–10 breaths/min (approximately 1 breath every 6–8 sec)		
Foreign-body airway obstruction If unresponsive: remove visible object or start CPR	Five back slaps alternate with 5 chest thrusts until effective breaths or unresponsive. No abdominal thrusts or blind finger sweep. Remove visible FB. Activate EMS.	Five abdominal thrusts until effective or patient becomes unresponsive Unresponsive: begin CPR for 5 cycles/2 minutes Remove visible foreign body Activate EMS	

Source: Adapted with permission from: 2005AHA Guidelines for CPR and ECC, Part 3: Overview of CPR. Circulation 2005;112:IV–15; revisions from Hazinski MF (ed) BLS for Healthcare Providers, Amer Heart Assn, 2011.

and attempt to visualize the object. If not visible, begin CPR, providing five cycles for 2 minutes.

A foreign body may also be removed under direct visualization with a laryngoscope and Magill forceps. On rare occasions, if there is total obstruction of the proximal upper airway, cricothyrotomy may be needed. Consult an otolaryngologist to remove more distal tracheal or laryngeal foreign bodies via flexible bronchoscopy.

Oxygenation, ventilation, and intubation

Once the airway has been stabilized and the breathing assessed, the need for oxygenation and ventilation takes priority. Place patients with mild to moderate respiratory distress on supplemental oxygen. Reassess breathing effort by physical examination and pulse oximetry. The equipment for airway support is described below.

Nasal cannula

The actual oxygen concentration delivered by nasal cannula is unpredictable, so this method is appropriate only for patients who require minimal O_2 supplementation. Flow rates of 1-4 L/min deliver O_2 concentrations of 25-40%. However, flow rates >3 L/min are usually poorly tolerated by children, while flow rates >1-2 L/min may inadvertently administer positive airway pressure to newborns and infants.

Simple O_2 mask

This is the most frequently used method for oxygen delivery in spontaneously breathing patients and it is more easily tolerated than nasal cannula. The actual O_2 concentration that the patient receives is dependent on the flow rate and the patient's ventilatory pattern, as room air enters through the ventilation holes on the sides of the mask. Oxygen flow rates of 6-10 L/min will deliver O_2 concentrations of 35-60% and prevent rebreathing of exhaled CO_2.

O_2 mask with reservoir

This system consists of a simple mask attached to a reservoir bag that is connected to an O_2 source. Some models contain one-way valves at the exhalation ports to prevent the entrainment of room air, and a second valve at the reservoir bag to prevent the entry of exhaled gas back into the reservoir bag. The reservoir bag must be larger than the patient's tidal volume (5-7 mL/kg) and remain inflated during inspiration. Oxygen concentrations up to 60% can be achieved in partial rebreathing systems, and >90% is possible if the oxygen flow rate is 10-15 L/min, and there is a good seal around the face mask.

Ventilation

For patients with respiratory failure, ventilate with a bag-mask apparatus, until all the appropriate equipment and personnel for intubation are assembled. For optimum airway alignment, position the patient so that the auditory meatus is in line with the top of the anterior shoulder. Use the "sniffing" position in an older child by placing a folded towel under the head and elevating it. In an infant, keep the head midline and neck slightly extended with a pad under the shoulder. Flexing or overextending the neck may inadvertently obstruct the airway.

Adequate ventilation results in symmetric movement of the chest wall with good breath sounds heard on auscultation. If the patient is making any respiratory effort, synchronize the delivered breaths with his or her efforts. If positive-pressure ventilation causes distention of the stomach, use gentle pressure on the cricoid cartilage (Sellick maneuver) to occlude the proximal esophagus and prevent air from entering the stomach. However, excessive cricoid pressure may kink the trachea and prevent air from entering the lungs.

Bag mask

The most common system used to ventilate an apneic patient consists of a self-inflating bag (Ambu Bag), an O_2 reservoir (corrugated tubing), and mask with a valve. These bags do not need a constant flow of O_2 to refill; they entrain room air. Using a reservoir with a supplemental oxygen flow rate of 10–15 L/min delivers 60–95% oxygen to the patient. If the bag has a pop-off valve set at 35–45 cmH$_2$O, there must be a way to override it, since ventilatory pressure may be inadequate in patients with increased airway resistance or poor lung compliance.

Adequate ventilation requires an appropriate-size face mask, one that extends from the bridge of the nose to the cleft of the chin. The minimum volume for the bag in newborns, infants, and small children is 450–500 mL; use an adult bag for adolescents. If the only bags available are larger than the recommended size, ventilate infants and children by using the larger bag with a proper-size face mask and administering only enough volume to cause the chest to rise.

Use the E-C clamp technique to achieve proper ventilation with a bag-mask device. Hold the mask snugly to the face with the left thumb and index finger forming a "C". Apply downward pressure over the mask to achieve a good seal, while avoiding pressure to the eyes. Place the remaining three fingers of the left hand, which form an "E", on the mandible to lift the jaw, avoiding compression of the soft tissues of the neck.

Use a rate of 12–20 breaths per minute for an infant or child (Table 1-4) (approximately one breath every 3–5 seconds). Observe the chest rise, listen for breath sounds, and monitor the O_2 saturation. Bagging too rapidly or using excessive pressure causes inflation of the stomach and barotrauma to the airways. If ventilation is difficult or breath sounds are unequal, reposition the head, suction the airway, and consider foreign-body aspiration or pneumothorax. An oral or nasopharyngeal airway may help to maintain a patent airway during bag-mask resuscitation, and if the patient is ventilated for more than a few minutes, place a nasogastric tube to decompress air from the stomach to minimize the risk of aspiration.

Intubation

Tracheal intubation is the best way to manage the airway during cardiopulmonary resuscitation. The indications for tracheal intubation include:

- Apnea
- Excessive work of breathing leading to fatigue
- Lack of airway protective reflexes (gag, cough)
- Complete airway obstruction unrelieved by foreign-body airway obstruction maneuvers
- CNS disorder (increased intracranial pressure, inadequate control of ventilation)

Table 1-5. Laryngoscope blade size

Premature – newborn	Miller 0
One month – toddler	Miller 1
18 months – 8 years	Miller 2, Macintosh 2
>8 years	Macintosh 3

Table 1-6. Tracheal tube (ETT) size and depth

Age	Uncuffed ETT	Cuffed ETT	Depth
Premature	2.5 mm	—	6–7 mm
Newborn	3.0–3.5	—	8–10 mm
1 month – 1 year	3.5–4.0 mm	3.0 mm	10–11 mm
Older	4 + [(age in years)/4]	3+ [(age in years)/4]	3× ETT size

Before attempting intubation ensure that all necessary supplies (Table 1-2), medications, and personnel are available. All equipment must be available in various sizes along with spare laryngoscope handles, bulbs, and batteries. A Broselow tape, which accurately correlates weight with length (for patients ≤35 kg), gives precise sizes of airway equipment, as well as appropriate drug doses. "Straight blades" (Miller) are often easier to use than "curved blades" (Macintosh) in infants and young children. Estimate laryngoscope blade size by the distance from the incisors to the angle of the mandible. See Table 1-5 for the most popular age-appropriate blade sizes.

ETT tubes

Estimate the tracheal tube size by matching the diameter of the ETT to the width of the nail of the patient's fifth finger or the diameter of the nares. Tracheal tube sizes for different age groups are listed in Table 1-6. Alternatively, use the following formulae, but always have available tracheal tubes 0.5 mm larger and smaller than the calculated size:

uncuffed ETT size = 4 + (age in years/4)
cuffed ETT size = 3 + (age in years/4).

Previously, cuffed tracheal tubes were indicated only in children >8 years of age. Now there are high-volume, low-pressure cuffed tracheal tubes that may be used in all ages (except newborns), provided the cuff inflation pressure is kept <20 cmH$_2$O. However, cuffed tubes have smaller internal diameters than non-cuffed tubes, resulting in increased airflow resistance. In some patients in whom high mean airway pressures are expected (e.g., status asthmaticus), an alternate approach is to use a cuffed tube with the cuff initially deflated, and inflate only when necessary.

Prepare the tracheal tube with a stylet tip placed 1 cm from the distal end of the tube and bent in a gradual curve of the distal third. The tip and cuff of the tube may be lubricated with viscous lidocaine or a water-soluble gel for easy passage.

Intubation procedure

In emergency situations perform oral intubations, which are easier than nasal intubations. In general, use a straight Miller laryngoscope blade for pediatric intubations. Routine use of cricoid pressure (Sellick maneuver) to prevent aspiration during intubation is no longer recommended. Have a tonsil tipped suction (Yankauer) and an appropriate-size flexible suction catheter readily available. To intubate the patient, keep the head midline in the "sniffing" position. If cervical spine trauma is a concern, have an assistant maintain manual in-line stabilization during the intubation, avoiding traction or movement of the neck. Continuously monitor the heart rate and pulse oximeter throughout the procedure. Calculate and prepare all of the medications before beginning rapid sequence intubation (RSI, see below).

Place the thumb and index finger of the (gloved) right hand into the right side of the patient's mouth. Place the index finger on the patient's upper teeth and the thumb on the lower teeth, using the scissor technique to open the mouth as wide as possible. Hold the laryngoscope in the left hand and introduce the blade into the right edge of the mouth, sweeping the tongue towards the left and out of the line of vision. Place a straight blade under the epiglottis to elevate it, but insert a curved blade into the vallecula and pull the epiglottis upwards. An assistant providing cricoid pressure or retracting the right corner of the mouth laterally may improve visualization of the glottic opening. Pull the handle of the laryngoscope up and away at a 45° angle to the floor, in the direction of the long axis of the handle. If the blade is in too deep, slowly withdraw it until the glottis pops into view. Be careful not to tilt the handle or blade, which may risk damaging the teeth.

Once the glottis is exposed, take care to introduce the tracheal tube from the right side of the mouth (not down the barrel of the blade). Advance the ETT until the cuff just passes beyond the vocal cords. Uncuffed tubes often have a mark at the distal end of the tube, which when placed at the level of the cords will position the distal tip in the mid trachea. This mark is only useful if the tube is the appropriate size and the patient has a normal-sized trachea. A proper-size tracheal tube easily passes through the cords. If it meets resistance in the subglottic area, replace it with a smaller tube. Hold the tube securely against the upper teeth (or gums) and carefully withdraw the laryngoscope first, and then remove the stylet from the ETT.

Confirming position

Verify proper tube placement by listening for equal breath sounds and observing symmetrical rise of the chest. Confirm the presence of exhaled CO_2 from the tracheal tube with either a colorimetric CO_2 detector or a CO_2 analyzer, and use a pulse oximeter to monitor oxygen saturation. Colorimetric devices are inaccurate if the patient does not have a perfusing rhythm (even with appropriate chest compressions) or is <2 kg. If breath sounds are louder over the stomach than the chest, or if it is unclear that the tube is in the trachea, remove the tracheal tube and ventilate by bag mask. An audible air leak is expected, but if there is a large air leak or none at all, the tube size may be inadequate; replace it with an appropriately sized tracheal tube. On chest radiograph, confirm that the tip of the tube is opposite T2 (one fingerbreadth above the carina). Neck extension or head movement brings the tube higher while neck flexion pushes the ETT deeper. Once the tube position is verified, inflate the cuff to a pressure <20 cmH$_2$O, and secure it to the patient's face with tape or use a tracheal tube holder.

Complications

If the patient deteriorates after endotracheal intubation, use the mnemonic *DOPE* to reassess: *D*isplacement of the tube into the esophagus or down the right mainstem bronchus, *O*bstruction of the tube with blood or secretions, *P*neumothorax, or *E*quipment malfunction.

Alternate/adjunctive ventilation techniques

Alternate ventilation techniques are useful for securing a difficult airway when intubation is not feasible or unsuccessful. The presence of certain congenital anomalies (Pierre-Robin, Beckwith-Wiedemann, Down syndrome), anatomical defects (neck mass, laryngeal hemangioma, subglottic stenosis), or disease states (epiglottitis, angioedema, facial/neck trauma) may necessitate the use of advanced airway techniques. These include noninvasive positive-pressure ventilation (NIPPV), heliox, and laryngeal mask airways (LMAs). Other advanced airway techniques, such as fiberoptic laryngoscopy, a lighted stylet, needle cricothyrotomy, or surgical cricothyrotomy, require training and experience to perform successfully.

Noninvasive positive-pressure ventilation (NIPPV)

NIPPV provides short-term mechanical ventilation without placement of a tracheal tube in stable, spontaneously breathing, alert, and cooperative patients. Although tracheal intubation is often a life-saving procedure, NIPPV functions to bridge the gap between maximal medical management and intubation. Benefits include decreasing the work of breathing, improving oxygenation, and avoiding common complications of intubation. It is important to note that NIPPV is not a replacement for tracheal intubation in patients who have life-threatening respiratory failure or require airway protection. It is contraindicated in patients who are hemodynamically unstable, lethargic, vomiting, or have cardiac dysrhythmias. The decision to use NIPPV is dependent on the patient (conscious and cooperative), specific disease (status asthmaticus, bronchiolitis, acute pulmonary edema, and neuromuscular disease), and whether airway protection is required.

The two common methods of NIPPV are continuous positive airway pressure (CPAP) and bilevel positive airway pressure (BiPAP). These are delivered via a nasal or full-face mask in children and by nasal prongs in infants. Straps hold the BiPAP face mask firmly to the patient's face to create a tight seal. Neonates, who are obligate nose breathers, generally do not tolerate BiPAP and may benefit more from nasal prong CPAP. Typical initial settings include an inspiratory positive airway pressure (IPAP) of 8–10 cmH$_2$O, and an expiratory positive airway pressure (EPAP) of 3–5 cmH$_2$O. Titrate these settings upwards in 2 cmH$_2$O increments until the desired effects are achieved. Monitor the patient closely for worsening respiratory failure with serial lung exams, vital signs measurements, and oxygen saturation. If the patient's respiratory status worsens or does not improve, discontinue NIPPV and perform tracheal intubation.

Heliox

Helium is a biologically inert gas that decreases turbulent gas flow when mixed with oxygen. Heliox improves delivery of oxygen and aerosolized medications to constricted peripheral airways, thus reducing the work of breathing. It has been used in conditions that are refractory to medical measures, such as status asthmaticus, moderate to severe

Table 1-7. Laryngeal mask airway sizes (reproduced with permission from LMA North America, Inc.)

Mask size	Patient size	Maximum cuff volume
1	Neonates/infants up to 5 kg	up to 4 mL
1½	Infants 5–10 kg	up to 7 mL
2	Infants/children 10–20 kg	up to 10 mL
2½	Children 20–30 kg	up to 14 mL
3	Children 30–50 kg	up to 20 mL
4	Adults 50–70 kg	up to 30 mL
5	Adults 70–100 kg	up to 40 mL
6	Adults >100 kg	up to 50 mL

bronchiolitis, and severe croup. Heliox is delivered in mixtures of 80% helium and 20% oxygen (80/20 heliox) or 70% helium and 30% oxygen (70/30 heliox). It is administered to spontaneously breathing patients by using a face mask and reservoir bag. An in-line attachment can be placed to add a nebulizer for concurrent beta-agonist administration. Improvement of oxygenation and reduction of respiratory distress generally occurs within 1 hour of heliox initiation. If there is no improvement or a worsening of the patient's clinical status, change to an alternate means of ventilation.

Laryngeal mask airway (LMA)

The LMA is indicated for patients who require an airway but cannot be tracheally intubated or ventilated with a bag mask and it can be used in patients with decreased airway reflexes (i.e. obtunded or comatose). The LMA consists of a tube attached to a mask, rimmed with a soft, inflatable cuff. When properly placed, the LMA sits in the hypopharynx around the glottic opening and directs air into the trachea. Unlike a tracheal tube, it will not prevent aspiration of gastric contents into the trachea.

Select the appropriate-size LMA and check for possible air leaks by inflating the cuff. Hold the LMA like a pen, with the index finger of the dominant hand placed at the junction of the tube and proximal aspect of the mask. Lubricate the posterior surface of the deflated mask, and orient it so that the opening is directed towards the tongue. With one smooth motion, insert the mask firmly along the hard palate and advance until resistance is encountered. With the tip of the mask placed in the hypopharynx, inflate the cuff according to the cuff size (Table 1-7). Auscultate the lungs to confirm correct placement. If endo-tracheal intubation is subsequently necessary, insert the ETT blindly through the properly placed LMA as it will be directed into the trachea.

There are newer LMAs available for specific situations. One version (Proseal LMA) has a parallel drainage tube attached to the airway tube to allow passage of a nasogastric tube, potentially decreasing the risk of aspiration. Another variation, the intubating LMA (Fas-trach LMA) is designed to facilitate blind tracheal intubation while allowing for continuous positive-pressure ventilation.

Rapid-sequence intubation (RSI)

The goals of RSI are to create ideal intubating conditions by attenuating airway reflexes while minimizing elevations of intracranial pressure and maintaining adequate blood pressure. Rapid-sequence intubation is indicated for patients who require emergency tracheal intubation but are at high risk for pulmonary aspiration of gastric contents. In patients who are critically ill, hemodynamically unstable, uncooperative, or with increased intracranial pressure, attempting tracheal intubation without sedation is likely to cause significant agitation. This can then worsen the symptoms and increase the risk of vomiting and pulmonary aspiration. Patients in cardiac arrest, moribund patients, or babies within a few hours after delivery rarely require medications to facilitate intubation.

Anticipate the possibility of an unsuccessful intubation and prepare for alternate airway techniques before initiating sedation. Also, expect a difficult intubation and request help for patients with significant facial trauma, restricted neck extension, or if the tip of the uvula is not visible when the mouth is opened. Do not use sedation or muscle relaxation if there is any concern that bag-mask ventilation will be inadequate.

> NEVER sedate or paralyze a patient whom you may not be able to ventilate!

Procedure

RSI involves the use of premedications to minimize adverse events, preselected sedative/hypnotic agents with rapid onset and short duration of activity, neuromuscular blocking agents, the application of cricoid pressure to prevent aspiration, and gaining immediate control of the airway, all done in rapid sequence in the above order.

Preoxygenation

While preparing for RSI, have the patient breathe 100% oxygen via a nonrebreather face mask for at least 3 minutes. If the patient is apneic or has inadequate respiratory effort, deliver 4–5 breaths by bag mask in 30 seconds, while applying cricoid pressure. This will establish an oxygen reserve that will last up to 4 minutes in an infant and longer in older children and adolescents. During the period of preoxygenation, determine the likelihood of a difficult intubation, establish intravenous access, place the patient on cardiac and pulse oximeter monitors, and assemble all necessary equipment and personnel for tracheal intubation.

History and physical examination

No single feature on physical examination accurately predicts a difficult intubation. Therefore, perform a detailed pre-sedation assessment, including the SAMPLE history and a focused physical examination.

SAMPLE history:

Signs and symptoms

Allergy: allergy to drugs, latex, foods

Medications: current prescription and non-prescription drugs

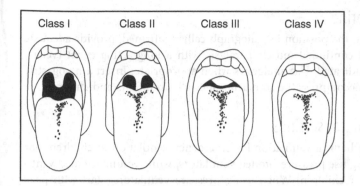

Class I   Class II   Class III   Class IV

Figure 1-1. Mallampati Classification. With permission from: Mallampati SR, et al: A clinical sign to predict difficult tracheal intubation: a prospective study. *Can Anaesth Soc J* 1985;32:429.

Past medical history: significant past medical and surgical history
Last meal time: last oral intake and type of food
Event: recent events or history of present illness

Upper airway examination

Ask a cooperative patient to open the mouth as wide as possible, with the tongue fully protruded. The Mallampati airway class I and II (visible faucial pillars and uvula) indicates relatively easier airway management (Figure 1-1). Use the "3–3–2 rule," which is a predictor of difficult intubation in adults. The patient should be able to place three fingers between the open incisors, three fingers from the mental tubercle of the mandible to the thyroid (two fingers in children, one finger in infants), and two fingers from the laryngeal prominence to the floor of the mouth.

For pre-medications, sedative/hypnotics and paralytics, see Table 1-8.

Cricoid pressure, BURP maneuver

Cricoid pressure to improve visualization of the larynx is no longer recommended. Take care not to move the cervical spine. After the patient loses consciousness, and as soon as the patient is paralyzed, intubate the trachea. Confirm correct placement of the ETT by auscultation of breath sounds, observation of chest rise, use of an exhaled CO_2 detector, and pulse oximetry.

If the laryngoscopic view is less than adequate, try the BURP maneuver – firm Backward, Upward, Rightward Pressure on the thyroid cartilage. This will improve the laryngeal view, especially in children, in whom the glottic opening is higher and more anterior compared to adults. Once the vocal cords are exposed, have the assistant maintain this view without releasing the cricoid pressure. If the intubation cannot be performed within 20 seconds, ventilate the patient with a bag mask. Change the laryngoscope blade, ETT size, patient's position, or laryngoscopist before attempting another intubation. Repeated intubation attempts will cause edema and bleeding and make visualization more difficult. If the patient cannot be intubated or ventilated by mask, insert a laryngeal mask airway or call for help with an advanced airway technique.

Post-intubation monitoring

Once the ETT is secured and the position is radiographically confirmed, provide adequate sedation and analgesia, and continued muscle paralysis with a long-acting agent (vecuronium or rocuronium), if indicated. Use analgesics when appropriate. Insert a nasogastric tube as soon as possible to decompress the stomach, especially in infants and children.

Initial mechanical ventilator settings

There are two modes of mechanical ventilation for emergency ventilation in children. For newborns and infants <10 kg use pressure-limited ventilators, while volume-limited ventilators are indicated for older children. When using pressure ventilators, start with peak inspiratory pressures (PIP) of 15–25 cmH$_2$O for newborns and 20–25 cmH$_2$O for infants <1 year of age. Set the respiratory rate appropriate for age (20–40/min) and the positive end-expiratory pressure (PEEP) at 3–5 cmH$_2$O.

For volume control ventilation, begin with tidal volumes of 8–10 mL/kg for children and 6–8 mL/kg for adolescents. Set an initial PEEP of 5 cmH$_2$O, unless contraindicated, with respiratory rates of 20–30/min in children, and 12–20/min in adolescents. For both types of ventilators, initially use 100% O$_2$, an inspiratory time of 0.8–1 sec, and the I/E ratio set at 1:2. Once the initial settings have been established, make repeated clinical assessments, monitoring continuously, making appropriate adjustments as dictated by the patient's clinical condition.

Circulation

For infants, children, and adolescents requiring CPR, start compressions immediately while a second health care provider prepares to provide ventilations. Give 15 compressions followed by 2 ventilations. For single rescuers, give one full cycle of 30 compressions in approximately 18 seconds followed by opening the airway and providing 2 ventilations of approximately 1 second each. For newborns, the recommended compression-ventilation ratio remains 3:1. In a real-life scenario, the code team, with assigned roles (Table 1-1), will be performing all tasks simultaneously. Begin chest compressions in patients with cardiac arrest or a heart rate <60 bpm associated with signs of poor perfusion (unresponsive, altered mental status, hypotension). For one rescuer CPR, provide 30 chest compressions followed by two breaths, repeating five cycles over 2 minutes. If there are two providers available and the child has not reached puberty, give 15 compressions and two breaths per cycle, repeating 10 cycles over 2 minutes. Instruct providers to switch roles after 2 minutes to prevent exhaustion. Deliver compressions by pushing hard and fast in a smooth motion, allowing complete chest recoil, and ensuring that each compression and relaxation phase is of equal time. Keep the fingers or hands on the chest during the relaxation phase of compressions to minimize interruptions. Coordinate compressions and ventilation to avoid simultaneous delivery. However, once the airway is secured by tracheal intubation, compressions and ventilation may be asynchronous and still be effective.

Chest compressions

Infant

Use the two-thumb hand encircling technique. Place two thumbs in the midline just below the nipple line and encircle the chest with the hands. Be sure not to compress the lateral walls of the chest with the hands. If the infant is too large for this technique, place

Table 1-8. Sedative agents for rapid-sequence intubation

Clinical status	Agents
Normotensive	Etomidate 0.3 mg/kg
	or midazolam 0.1–0.2 mg/kg
	or propofol 2–3 mg/kg (40 mg maximum)
Mild hypotension/no head injury	Etomidate 0.3 mg/kg
	or ketamine 1–2 mg/kg
	or fentanyl 1–5–4 mcg/kg
Severe hypotension/no head injury	None
	or etomidate 0.3 mg/kg
Head injury/no hypotension	Thiopental 3–5 mg/kg
	or etomidate 0.3 mg/kg
Head injury with mild hypotension	Etomidate 0.3 mg/kg
	or thiopental 1–3 mg/kg
	or midazolam 0.1 mg/kg
Status asthmaticus	Ketamine 1–2 mg/kg
Status epilepticus	Midazolam 0.1–0.2 mg/kg
	or thiopental 1–3 mg/kg

two or three fingers below the intermammary line. Compress the sternum to a relative depth of approximately one-third to one-half the anterior-posterior diameter of the chest, at a rate of at least 100 compressions per minute. Adequate compressions usually generate a pulse.

Child

Place the heel of one hand at the mid-sternum between the nipples. Compress to a relative depth of approximately one-third to one-half the anterior-posterior diameter of the chest, at a rate of 100 compressions per minute.

Adolescent

Use two hands, with the heel of one hand placed on top of the second hand interlocking the fingers. Place the hands at the mid-sternum between the nipples, avoiding pressure to the xiphoid process. With the arms straight and elbows locked, compress the sternum to a relative depth of approximately 1½–2 inches, at a rate of at least 100 compressions per minute.

Vascular access

Spend no more than 1–2 minutes attempting peripheral vascular access in cardiac arrest or other emergency situations.

Intraosseous approach

The intraosseous (IO) approach allows for rapid vascular access for patients of all ages. Any drug or fluid normally given through the IV route, including blood products, can be given via the IO needle, although high flow rates are not possible without using an infusion pump. Dilute hyperosmolar solutions, such as 50% dextrose and sodium bicarbonate, before infusion into the marrow cavity. The IO needle is an emergency access device only. Replace it with another secure intravascular catheter as soon as possible to prevent complications, such as infection, or compartment syndrome from fluid extravasation.

Intraosseous technique

The primary site for IO insertion is the proximal tibia. Locate the tibial tuberosity and palpate approximately two fingerbreadths (one fingerbreadth in infants) distally on the medial flat portion of the tibia. Contraindications to IO needle placement include a fracture or overlying skin infection at the site.

Intraosseous needle

The Jamshidi IO needle is available in 18G for infants and 15G for all others, while the Cook IO needle is available in 16G and 18G sizes. Select the appropriate site and direct the IO needle perpendicular to the bone. Use steady pressure with a screwing motion until a sudden loss of resistance is felt, indicating that the needle has entered the marrow cavity. If placed correctly, the needle will stand freely and upright without support. Inability to aspirate blood does not indicate improper placement; infusion of fluid easily without extravasation or resistance confirms proper placement. If fluid does extravasate (the calf expands or feels cold), remove the needle and make an attempt on the other side. Do not attempt more than once in the same bone. After proper placement is determined, tape the needle in place to prevent accidental dislodgement.

Automated IO infusion

There are various automated IO infusion devices on the market designed for use in children and adolescents. If your emergency department stocks one of these automated devices, become familiar with it and follow the specific product directions. Two of the most commonly used automated IO systems are the EZ-IO® and the FAST1®.

Fluid resuscitation

Shock and circulatory collapse may be the primary cause of cardiopulmonary arrest, and restoration of the circulating blood volume by fluid therapy is a mainstay of shock resuscitation. Once vascular access (peripheral, IO, central) is established, give an initial fluid bolus of 20 mL/kg of an isotonic crystalloid solution. In patients who are critically ill or in cardiopulmonary arrest, use a 60 mL syringe to infuse the fluid rapidly over a few minutes. However, the rapid infusion of dextrose-containing solutions results in an osmotic diuresis and is contraindicated in the initial phase of fluid resuscitation. Fluid resuscitation is particularly challenging in patients with cardiac disease or head injuries, as restoring and maintaining adequate tissue perfusion must be balanced with the risk of worsening cardiac output or cerebral edema.

Base the decision to give additional intravenous fluids on reassessment of perfusion: mental status, quality of pulses, blood pressure, heart rate, capillary refill, and urine output.

In severe shock, give additional fluid boluses of 20 mL/kg, up to a total of 60 mL/kg, until the vital signs and perfusion are restored. If further fluid is required, consider adding inotropic agents (see below) to maintain adequate vascular tone. If the patient is in septic shock, there may be significant capillary leakage. Large fluid volumes >60 mL/kg may be required and 5% albumin may also be given in 10 mL/kg doses. Infusion of multiple fluid boluses requires frequent and careful reassessment of the patient to prevent circulatory overload.

Vasoactive infusions

Inotropic agents are the drugs of choice for improving myocardial contractility and cardiac output in patients with shock. Because of their short half-life and potency, they are given as an infusion. In patients who remain hypotensive despite adequate fluid resuscitation, dopamine is the drug of choice to improve cardiac function and splanchnic circulation. Dopamine-resistant shock commonly responds to norepinephrine or high-dose epinephrine. Norepinephrine is the agent of choice for fluid-refractory warm septic shock (hyperdynamic cardiac output, bounding pulses, vasodilatation and wide pulse pressure). Use epinephrine for patients in hypodynamic cold shock (low cardiac output states). Dobutamine improves systolic function and decreases systemic vascular resistance without significantly increasing heart rate, and it is very effective in patients with cardiomyopathy and congestive heart failure. If the desired effect is not achieved with one agent, combinations of several agents may be necessary.

Dopamine (2–20 mcg/kg per min)

Dopamine is an endogenous catecholamine with complex effects on the heart and circulation. At low doses (2 mcg/kg per min) dopamine has relatively little chronotropic effects, and the primary result is an increase in renal and splanchnic perfusion. At high infusion rates, it has positive inotropic and chronotropic effects and tends to increase cardiac output and systemic vascular resistance (SVR). Infuse at an initial rate of 5–10 mcg/kg per min and titrate to the desired effect.

Dobutamine (2–20 mcg/kg per min)

Dobutamine has selective action on beta-adrenergic receptors with chronotropic and inotropic actions. It is an effective inotrope for the normotensive post-arrest patient with poor perfusion. Dobutamine is particularly useful for patients with congestive heart failure or cardiogenic shock, since it increases cardiac output without significantly increasing heart rate. At a dose >10 mcg/kg per min, dobutamine tends to produce hypotension due to afterload reduction and decreased SVR. The hypotension may then require dopamine or epinephrine to increase the SVR. An alternate approach is to start the patient on dopamine initially to stabilize the blood pressure and then switch to dobutamine. If dobutamine fails, use epinephrine. Infuse dobutamine at an initial rate of 2–10 mcg/kg per min, and titrate to the desired effect.

Epinephrine (0.1–1 mcg/kg per min)

Epinephrine is a potent inotropic agent that effectively increases myocardial perfusion pressure. Low-dose epinephrine (< 0.2 mcg/kg per min) stimulates both beta-1 cardiac and beta-2 peripheral vascular receptors, which results in increased heart rate, decreased

SVR, and decreased diastolic blood pressure. At doses >0.3 mcg/kg per min, alpha-adrenergic effects result in increased blood pressure. Epinephrine causes increased myocardial oxygen demand and may lead to myocardial ischemia; however, this is rare in children. An epinephrine infusion is useful for persistent hypotension after cardiopulmonary resuscitation, dopamine-resistant shock, and low-output septic shock. Infants can be less responsive to dopamine and dobutamine, so epinephrine may be better in maintaining blood pressure and cardiac output. Infuse at an initial rate of 0.1 mcg/kg per min, and titrate to the desired effect.

Norepinephrine (0.1–1 mcg/kg per min)

Norepinephrine acts on both alpha- and beta-adrenergic receptors, producing potent inotropic effects and peripheral vasoconstriction, significantly increasing mean arterial pressure. The increased blood pressure also improves renal perfusion in patients with septic shock. Norepinephrine is effective in dopamine-resistant shock, and maintains adequate perfusion pressure in children with warm shock. Infuse at an initial rate of 0.1 mcg/kg per min, and titrate to the desired effect.

Medications and electrical therapy in resuscitation

IV and IO are the preferred routes of drug administration. However, if an endotracheal tube is placed prior to IV or IO insertion, administer lipid-soluble medications (lidocaine, epinephrine, atropine, and naloxone, [LEAN]) via the ETT. Instill the drug directly into the ETT or through a 5F feeding tube that extends beyond the tip of the ETT and follow with 5 mL of normal saline.

Provide five manual positive-pressure ventilations after drug administration. Drug absorption via the ETT route is unpredictable so higher doses are required to achieve appropriate therapeutic levels. For epinephrine, use 0.1 mL/kg of the 1:1000 concentration; for other drugs, administer 2–3 times the usual IV dose.

Epinephrine

Epinephrine is indicated in cardiac arrest (asystole and pulseless electric activity), and in patients with symptomatic bradycardia and hypotension. It increases heart rate, myocardial contractility, systemic vascular resistance, and cardiac automaticity, although it also increases myocardial oxygen demand. Epinephrine can cause ventricular arrhythmias and is therefore contraindicated for symptomatic AV block secondary to intrinsic disease, such as myocarditis, cardiomyopathy, or post-operative cardiac conditions.

The IV/IO dose is 0.01 mg/kg (0.1 mL/kg) 1:10,000 concentration every 3–5 minutes (maximum 1 mg; 10 mL). The ETT dose is 0.01 mg/kg (0.1 mL/kg) 1:1000 concentration every 3–5 minutes. Use high-dose epinephrine for overdoses with specific toxins such as β-blockers (pp. 456–457) or calcium channel blockers (pp. 458–460) if there is no response after the usual IV/IO dose.

Atropine

Atropine is a parasympatholytic drug that inhibits vagal activity, accelerates sinoatrial pacemakers, and enhances atrioventricular conduction. Atropine is indicated for symptomatic bradycardia due to increased vagal tone, cholinergic drug toxicity, or AV heart block, with evidence of poor perfusion or hypotension. However, since hypoxia is commonly the underlying cause for bradycardia, particularly in small infants, efforts to improve oxygenation and perfusion must precede the administration of atropine. If the patient does not respond to atropine despite adequate oxygenation and ventilation, use epinephrine.

The dose is 0.02 mg/kg IV/IO (maximum single dose: 0.5 mg in children, 1 mg in adolescents). Atropine may be repeated once in 5 minutes.

Glucose

Check the blood glucose concentration at the bedside with a glucometer, during and after an arrest. Promptly give dextrose if the glucose level is <45 mg/dL in a neonate or <60 mg/dL in an infant or child. Recheck the blood glucose concentration after each administration, and try to avoid hyperglycemia.

The dose is 0.5 gm/kg. In neonates use 5 mL/kg of a 10% dextrose solution prepared by diluting $D_{50}W$ 1:4 with sterile water. For infants and children use 2 mL/kg of a 25% dextrose solution.

Calcium chloride 10%

Routine administration of calcium does not improve outcome of cardiac arrest, and can antagonize the action of epinephrine and other adrenergic agents. However, calcium is indicated for documented hypocalcemia, hyperkalemia, and hypermagnesemia, as well as calcium channel blocker overdose. Use the measured ionized calcium concentration to determine the need for subsequent doses. Avoid rapid calcium administration, which can cause bradycardia or sinus arrest. Due to the risk of sclerosis or extravasation with a peripheral venous line, administer calcium chloride via a central venous catheter, if possible. The dose is 20 mg/kg (0.2 mL/kg) IV (slow); this dose may be repeated once in 10 minutes.

Sodium bicarbonate

Do not use sodium bicarbonate routinely during cardiopulmonary resuscitation, as it may further depress cardiac contractility and inactivate simultaneously administered catecholamines. Sodium bicarbonate is recommended for symptomatic hyperkalemia, tricyclic antidepressant, or sodium channel blocker overdose or for severe metabolic acidosis or prolonged cardiopulmonary arrest after appropriate ventilation and restoration of volume are provided. The dose is 1 mEq/kg *slowly* IV. Use a 4.2% solution in infants.

Adenosine

Adenosine is the drug of choice for the treatment of stable supraventricular tachycardia (pp. 42–46) or unstable SVT while preparations are being made for cardioversion. Administer adenosine rapidly and follow with a rapid push of normal saline using a three-way stop cock. After a brief period (15–30 sec) of asystole or heart block, the rhythm either converts to sinus or reverts to SVT. If the patient deteriorates, immediately attempt synchronized cardioversion. The first dose is 0.1 mg/kg IV/IO (rapid) to a maximum of 6 mg. Follow with rapid push of 5–10 mL normal saline. If needed the second dose is 0.2 mg/kg IV/IO to a maximum of 12 mg. This dose may be repeated once for a total of three doses.

Amiodarone

Amiodarone (p. 41) is indicated for shock-refractory VF or pulseless VT, hemodynamically unstable VT, and stable SVT refractory to adenosine. Avoid administering amiodarone with any other drug that causes QT prolongation (procainamide), which may then precipitate polymorphic VT. The loading dose for SVT or VT (with pulses) is 5 mg/kg IV (300 mg maximum) over 20–60 minutes.

For VF or pulseless VT the loading dose is 5 mg/kg IV (300 mg maximum). Repeat this dose every 10 minutes to a maximum total dose of 15 mg/kg per day (2.2 g/day).

Lidocaine

Lidocaine (p. 41) is a second line alternative to amiodarone for VT with pulses and shock-resistant VF or pulseless VT. The initial IV/IO dose is 1 mg/kg. This dose may be repeated in 10–15 minutes. The ETT dose is 2–3 mg/kg. If maintenance infusion is required, prepare by mixing 1 g lidocaine in 250 mL of D_5W and infuse at 20–50 mcg/kg per min.

Procainamide

Procainamide is effective in the treatment of atrial fibrillation, flutter and adenosine-refractory stable SVT (including WPW syndrome) and can be used as an alternative therapy for refractory or recurrent stable VT with pulses. Infuse medication slowly to avoid heart block, myocardial depression, hypotension, or prolongation of the QT interval. Monitor blood pressure and the ECG continuously. If the QRS widens by more than 50% or hypotension develops, stop the infusion. Do not administer concurrently with other medications that prolong the QT interval (amiodarone). The dose is 15 mg/kg IV/IO (20 mg/min maximum) over 30–60 minutes.

Cardioversion and defibrillation

Cardioversion is synchronized electrical conversion of a rhythm disturbance. Synchronized cardioversion is timed with the QRS complex to avoid delivery during the relative refractory period of the cardiac cycle, during which a shock could induce potentially lethal VF. It is indicated for unstable SVT and monomorphic VT when the patient shows clinical signs of shock. The first dose is 0.5–1 J/kg (maximum 50–100 J). Increase subsequent doses to 2 J/kg if the initial dose is ineffective.

Defibrillation is indicated for VF or pulseless VT. Defibrillators are either manual or automated (AED), and deliver monophasic or newer biphasic waveforms.

Place the paddles or self-adhering electrodes on the chest wall, leaving about two fingerbreadths between the paddles. Use infant paddles for children <1 year of age or those weighing <10 kg. Place one paddle over the right side of the upper chest and the other to the left of the nipple on the left lower ribs. Alternatively, apply one electrode on the front of the chest just to the left of the sternum and the other over the upper back below the scapula. Immediately after the shock resume high-quality CPR for 2 minutes or five cycles, beginning with chest compressions. Try to limit interruption of CPR for rhythm checks to <10 seconds. If one shock does not convert the rhythm to normal, repeat the process. If VF or VT persists despite delivery of one shock followed by 2 minutes of CPR, give epinephrine as soon as IV or IO access is available.

The first dose is 2 J/kg. Deliver subsequent doses at 4 J/kg. In children, dosing is the same whether using a monophasic or biphasic system.

An automatic external defibrillator (AED) can accurately detect VF in children and can be safely and effectively used in patients >1 year of age or weighing >10 kg. In infants and children 1–8 years of age (weight 10–25 kg; length <50 inches), use an AED with a pediatric

Table 1-9. Classification and etiologies of shock

Type of shock	Etiology
Hypovolemic: Pump is empty	Dehydration (vomiting, diarrhea, poor intake, heat stroke)
	Hemorrhage (trauma, GI bleed)
	Metabolic disease (diabetes, adrenal insufficiency)
	Plasma losses (burns, peritonitis, hypoproteinemia)
Cardiogenic: Weak/sick pump	Rhythm disturbances
	Congestive heart failure
	Cardiomyopathy
	Post-resuscitation
Distributive: Fluid distribution	Sepsis
	Anaphylaxis
	Neurogenic shock (head trauma, spinal cord injury)
Obstructive: Obstruction of outflow	Tension pneumothorax
	Cardiac tamponade
	Pulmonary embolism

attenuator system. Use a standard adult AED if a pediatric system is unavailable in this age group, as well as for patients >8 years (>25 kg).

Shock

Shock is a clinical condition that results from the inadequate delivery of oxygen and nutrients needed to meet the metabolic demands of the tissues. Shock is categorized as hypovolemic, distributive, cardiogenic, and obstructive (Table 1-9). It can be further categorized by severity as compensated or hypotensive (previously known as decompensated) shock.

In the early phases of shock, multiple compensatory physiologic mechanisms act to maintain blood pressure and perfusion of vital organs (brain, heart, kidneys). In infants and children, cardiac output is primarily maintained by changes in heart rate. Poor tissue perfusion leads to metabolic acidosis, so that the respiratory rate is increased to promote the excretion of CO_2. Therefore, unexplained tachycardia and tachypnea, without other signs of shock, may be the earliest signs of cardiorespiratory compromise. When the cardiac output falls by 25%, rapid decompensation ensues; therefore, do not be reassured by a normal blood pressure if there is other evidence of circulatory compromise. Bradycardia and hypotension are ominous, and are present in advanced stages of hypotensive shock, which can rapidly progress to irreversible organ damage and cardiorespiratory arrest.

Hypovolemic shock

Hypovolemia is the most common etiology of shock in infants and children and diarrhea is the most common cause of hypovolemia. Other causes include hemorrhage, third spacing, vomiting, inadequate intake, or excessive diuresis as seen in DKA. A child's normal blood volume is about 80 mL/kg, and what may appear to be a minor hemorrhage can represent a significant loss of blood volume. Compensatory mechanisms in response to hypovolemia include an increase in heart rate, contractility, and SVR, with a redistribution of intravascular perfusion to the heart, brain, and kidneys. The shunting of blood flow away from the skin causes the changes in skin color, temperature, and moisture seen in compensated shock. However, compensatory mechanisms cannot be maintained indefinitely, and bradycardia, myocardial ischemia and subsequent cardiopulmonary arrest will occur without timely intervention.

Distributive shock

Distributive shock occurs when there is vasodilatation and inappropriate distribution of fluid within the vascular space. The most common causes are sepsis, anaphylaxis and neurologic injury.

Septic shock

Sepsis is the most common cause of distributive shock. Septic shock can evolve over a few hours (particularly in young infants) or days. The cardiac output may be high, normal, or low. Early phases of "warm"septic shock may not be clinically apparent since the skin may be warm and dry without an increase in capillary refill time. This is due to low SVR and cutaneous vasodilatation, which result in hyperdynamic cardiac output. Pulses will be rapid, full, and bounding, and the pulse pressure is wide. Normal or low-output "cold" septic shock is characterized by high SVR and peripheral vasoconstriction, resulting in cold extremities, with weak pulses and poor capillary refill time.

Anaphylaxis

Anaphylaxis (pp. 30–34) is a systemic reaction to an allergen involving two or more body systems (cutaneous, respiratory, cardiovascular, neurologic, or gastrointestinal). The shorter the interval between exposure and reaction, the more severe the reaction is likely to be. Common triggers include antibiotics, radiographic contrast agents, peanuts, shellfish, and latex (especially in healthcare workers and children with spina bifida). Initial symptoms of anaphylactic shock include urticaria, angioedema, upper airway edema (manifested by stridor) and dyspnea, which may rapidly progress to cardiovascular collapse and death.

Neurogenic shock

Neurogenic shock is a result of cervical or high thoracic (above T6) spinal cord injury with loss of sympathetic vascular tone. The patient has warm, dry skin, normal capillary refill, hypotension with wide pulse pressure, and paradoxical bradycardia. There is no compensatory tachycardia in response to hypotension. A careful assessment is necessary to differentiate neurogenic shock from other causes of shock. Hypovolemic shock classically presents with tachycardia, narrow pulse pressure, cool, moist skin, and delayed capillary refill. In warm septic shock, fever and tachycardia may be important distinguishing features, while neurogenic shock may present with flaccid paralysis and loss of bladder and rectal tone. Although patients in neurogenic shock may be warm with well-perfused skin, they may not respond to either fluid boluses or inotropic support.

Cardiogenic shock

Cardiogenic shock occurs when there is compromised cardiac output secondary to myocardial dysfunction. This is most often seen with congenital heart disease, viral myocarditis, dysrrhythmias (idiopathic or secondary to drug ingestions), cardiomyopathy, or postoperative complications of cardiac surgery. Occasionally, infants within the first 3 months of life with undiagnosed congenital heart disease present to the ED in congestive heart failure and shock due to closure of the ductus arteriosus. However, cardiogenic shock is a terminal complication of virtually all types of shock as a result of high myocardial oxygen requirement and decreased cardiac contractility. Cardiogenic shock can usually be distinguished from other forms of shock by signs of congestive heart failure, including tachycardia with a gallop rhythm, tachypnea with rales, and hepatomegaly. A 12-lead ECG may show low-voltage tachycardia or ST changes, and a chest radiograph reveals cardiomegaly and pulmonary edema. An urgent echocardiogram will demonstrate cardiac function as well as any underlying anatomic defects that may be contributing to the condition.

Obstructive shock

Obstructive shock occurs when mechanical pressure to the heart results in ventricular outflow tract obstruction. Causes include pericardial tamponade, tension pneumothorax, and pulmonary embolism. In pericardial tamponade (pp. 66–68), fluid accumulates within the pericardial sac, resulting in increased pericardial pressure, and decreased cardiac compliance and cardiac output. The classic signs are described as Beck's triad: hypotension, muffled heart sounds, and distended neck veins. In tension pneumothorax (pp. 720–722) free air accumulates within the pleural cavity causing a mediastinal shift toward the opposite side, collapsing the lung and compromising cardiac output. Patients present with severe respiratory distress, decreased breath sounds on the ipsilateral side, tracheal deviation, tachycardia and a shift in the apical cardiac impulse. Pulmonary embolism (PE) is rare in pediatrics, and may present with pleuritic chest pain (which may radiate to the shoulders), cough, hemoptysis, dyspnea, palpitations, and hypoxemia.

Clinical presentation

The clinical presentation of patients in compensated shock depends on the cardiac output relative to end-organ demand. Initially, the blood pressure is normal, although there may be tachycardia and irritability. Once 20–30% of the effective circulating blood volume is lost, the patient will decompensate into hypotensive shock. As the process continues untreated, there is multiple organ failure and death from irreversible shock. The signs of shock are summarized in Table 1-10.

Diagnosis

Perform an initial assessment of the patient, including the general appearance, mental status, and ABCs (see pp. 1–5). Rapid cardiopulmonary assessment). Obtain a SAMPLE history, and a complete set of vital signs (see pp. 14–15). During the initial assessment, do

Table 1-10. Signs of shock

Early	Late
Tachycardia	Hypotension
Orthostatic changes (adolescent)	Altered mental status
Delayed capillary filling >2 sec	Markedly delayed capillary filling >4 sec
Adequate central pulse	Weak or absent peripheral pulse
Tachypnea	Cold, pale mottled skin
Normal blood pressure	Oliguria

not delay providing critical interventions; properly position the head, provide supplemental oxygen, and establish vascular or IO access.

Since the signs of early shock are subtle, maintain a high index of suspicion. Be alert to tachycardia, mild tachypnea, slightly delayed capillary refill (>2 sec), orthostatic changes in blood pressure or pulse, and mild irritability. Patients with septic shock may have hypothermia or hyperthermia, altered mental status, irritability or lethargy; and peripheral vasodilatation with bounding pulses (warm shock) or mottled cool extremities with thready pulses (cold shock).

ED management

The most common error in treating shock is underestimating the severity of the condition. If compensated shock is suspected, treat promptly and aggressively to prevent progression to hypovolemic shock. All patients require a secure vascular access, oxygen therapy, and cardiopulmonary monitoring. The goals of initial management are to restore normal mental status, heart rate and blood pressure, good peripheral perfusion, and adequate urine output.

1. Position: allow a conscious patient to assume a position of comfort.
2. Oxygen: give 100% supplemental oxygen by nonrebreather mask to spontaneously breathing patients. Consider the use of noninvasive positive-pressure ventilation (BiPAP, CPAP) as an alternative to intubation in selected cases (awake and cooperative patients).
3. Assisted ventilation: if there is evidence of airway compromise, assist ventilation with either a bag-mask device or tracheal intubation.
4. Intravenous access: establish two large-bore peripheral IV lines or place a central catheter. If venous access is not possible or delayed, use an IO needle. In critically ill or injured patients, do not spend more than 1–2 minutes attempting to establish peripheral vascular access. The effort may be resumed after the IO line is secured.
5. Fluid: infuse a fluid bolus of 20 mL/kg of isotonic crystalloid (lactated Ringer's or normal saline) as rapidly as possible. Several boluses may be required; large volumes of fluid for resuscitation in previously healthy children do not increase the risk of developing acute respiratory distress syndrome or cerebral edema. Trauma victims may require blood (10 mL/kg) to replace ongoing losses; use cross-matched, type-specific or O-negative blood. Trauma patients who remain hypotensive after fluid resuscitation may require immediate operative intervention.

6. Reassess: after each intervention, look for improvement in vital signs, skin perfusion, and level of consciousness. Insert a Foley catheter and monitor urine output; the goal is 1–2 mL/kg/h or 30 mL/h in adolescents.

7. Inotropic infusion: if the patient remains hypotensive after initial fluid resuscitation of 40–60 mL/kg, an inotropic agent, or a combination of several agents, may be necessary to stabilize blood pressure (pp. 19–20). Titrate the dose to the desired effect. Monitor the patient carefully and switch to a less potent agent once the blood pressure has improved.

8. Septic shock: administer antibiotic therapy as soon as possible. Send the appropriate cultures, but do not delay therapy if cultures are not readily obtained. Empiric antibiotics include vancomycin plus cefotaxime or ceftriaxone for the possibility of resistant *Streptococcus pneumoniae* and methicillin-resistant *Staphylococcus aureus*. Consider adding acyclovir for HSV in neonates and cefepime for *Pseudomonas aeruginosa* in immunocompromised patients.

9. Anaphylactic shock: management involves early recognition of symptoms of anaphylaxis and anticipating need for advanced airway techniques (pp. 30–34).

10. Cardiogenic shock: give fluid boluses judiciously, at volumes of 5–10 mL/kg, to patients with a history of cardiomyopathy or congenital heart disease. Reassess frequently for signs of cardiac failure. Give patients in congestive heart failure supplemental oxygen, diuretics (furosemide 1 mg/kg), and inotropic agents (dobutamine, dopamine), and consult with a pediatric cardiologist. Treat pediatric dysrhythmias according to the PALS Guidelines (pp. 39–47).

   a. Asystole and PEA: epinephrine
   b. Symptomatic bradycardia: epinephrine and atropine
   c. Supraventricular tachycardia

      i. Stable: adenosine
      ii. Unstable: synchronized cardioversion (0.5–1 J/kg)

   d. Ventricular tachycardia (with pulses)

      i. Stable: amiodarone or procainamide (not concurrently) or lidocaine
      ii. Unstable: synchronized cardioversion (0.5–1 J/kg)

   e. Ventricular fibrillation and pulseless ventricular tachycardia: CPR followed by defibrillation, one shock, (2 J/kg) and immediate resumption of CPR, epinephrine, and/or amiodarone, and/or lidocaine. Alternate drugs with defibrillation (4 J/kg: single shock each time). Always resume CPR immediately after shock for 2 minutes or 5 cycles of 30:2 or 10 cycles of 15:2, then reassess rhythm. Once defibrillation is successful, many patients will required additional CPR before they regain a perfusing rhythm.

11. Obstructive shock: see pp. 66–68 for the treatment of pericardial tamponade and pp. 720–722 for the treatment of a tension pneumothorax. Therapy for pulmonary embolism includes supplemental oxygen and anticoagulation with IV heparin.

Post-resuscitation care

The goals of post-resuscitation care are to preserve brain function, avoid secondary organ injury, and to diagnose and treat the cause of illness. After successful initial resuscitation, patients require continuous reassessment to monitor signs of potential hypoxic-ischemic insult to vital organs. Post-resuscitation patients are often poorly perfused, hypotensive from arrest-associated myocardial ischemia, and have poor lung compliance. Continuously monitor heart rate, blood pressure, and oxygen saturation.

Monitor urine output with an indwelling catheter (>1 mL/kg per h in children or >30 mL/h in adolescents). Maintain normal temperature; treat fever with antipyretics, while infants, who are usually hypothermic, may need warming devices. For intubated patients, verify tube position, obtain ABGs, and adjust ventilatory settings as necessary. Control pain and discomfort with analgesics (fentanyl or morphine) and sedatives (lorazepam or midazolam). Infants and chronically ill children can easily become hypoglycemic, so check glucose early and treat as needed. Avoid hyperglycemia, targeting glucose levels <150 mg/dL. Patients usually have metabolic acidosis, which responds to adequate fluid therapy. The routine administration of sodium bicarbonate has not been shown to improve the outcome of resuscitation.

Family presence during resuscitation

Family presence during cardiopulmonary resuscitation has been a topic of debate in recent years, but it appears to be associated with beneficial outcomes for both family members and patients. Most family members who were present during resuscitation reported that being at the side of a loved one and saying goodbye during the final moments of life was comforting, and helped in their adjustment. Have a member of the resuscitation team offer the family the opportunity to be present, and if they decline, ensure that a team member is available to be with the family to inform them of the progress of resuscitation efforts. Gently ask family members who are disruptive to the resuscitation team efforts to leave. Assign one member of the team to remain with the family when they are present during the resuscitation in order to offer an explanation of events and answer questions.

Termination of resuscitation

Currently, there are no reliable predictors of outcome during resuscitation to guide when to terminate in-hospital resuscitation efforts. Bystander CPR for witnessed collapse, and a short interval from collapse to arrival of EMS, improve the chances of survival. Children with prolonged resuscitation efforts without return of spontaneous circulation after two doses of epinephrine are unlikely to survive, although survival after unusually prolonged in-hospital resuscitation has been documented in children with VF or VT, drug toxicity, or a primary hypothermic insult.

When resuscitation efforts are terminated, arrange for the team leader to meet with family members, in order to comfort and appraise them of the resuscitation efforts. Afterwards, organize a debriefing of the resuscitation team by the senior members, in order to acknowledge the contributions of the team and discuss how and why their efforts did not succeed.

Bibliography

www.sfparamedics.org/pages/pdfs/courses/ PALS2010comparison.pdf for 2010 Pediatric Advanced Life Support interim materials supplement.

Berg MD, Nadkarni VM: In-hospital pediatric cardiac arrest. *Pediatr Clin North Am* 2008;55:589–604.

Gerein RB, Osmond MH, Stiell IG, Nesbitt LP, Burns S: OPALS Study Group. What are the etiology and epidemiology of out-of-hospital pediatric cardiopulmonary arrest in Ontario, Canada? *Acad Emerg Med* 2006;13:653–8.

Mathers LH, Frankel LR: Pediatric emergencies and resuscitation. In Kliegman RM, Behrman RE, Jenson HB, Stanton BF (eds), *Nelson Textbook Of Pediatrics*, 18th ed. Philadelphia: Saunders Elsevier, 2007, pp. 387–405.

Sagarin MJ, Chiang V, Sakles JC, et al: National Emergency Airway Registry (NEAR) investigators: rapid sequence intubation for pediatric emergency airway management. *Pediatr Emerg Care* 2002;18:417–23.

Samson RA, Nadkarni VM, Meaney PA, et al: American Heart Association National Registry of CPR Investigators: outcomes of in-hospital ventricular fibrillation in children. *N Engl J Med* 2006;354:2328–39.

Topjian AA, Berg RA, Nadkarni VM: Pediatric cardiopulmonary resuscitation: advances in science, techniques, and outcomes. *Pediatrics* 2008;122:1086–98.

2 Allergic emergencies

Stephanie R. Lichten

Anaphylaxis

Anaphylaxis is a potentially life-threatening multi-system allergic reaction that can be triggered by a variety of agents (Table 2-1). The mechanism may be either IgE-mediated (anaphylactic reaction) or non-IgE-mediated (anaphylactoid reaction). However, each process leads to the release of immune mediators from mast cells and basophils, so that the clinical presentation and treatment is similar and the term "anaphylaxis" is often applied to both.

Clinical presentation

Anaphylaxis can present with a variety of signs and symptoms (Table 2-2). It involves at least two organ systems, most commonly cutaneous, respiratory, gastrointestinal, and/or cardiovascular. A reaction can occur as rapidly as seconds after exposure or it may be delayed for hours. Up to 20% of patients with a severe allergic reaction will have a biphasic response, and 30% of children with severe food allergies will do so. With a late-phase response, symptoms can recur 1–72 hours (average 8 hours) after the initial reaction has remitted. In protracted anaphylaxis, symptoms persist for 5–32 hours.

Diagnosis

The diagnosis of anaphylaxis is based on clinical manifestations fulfilling one of the following three criteria:

1. Acute onset with involvement of skin and/or mucosal tissues and at least one of the following: respiratory compromise, hypotension, evidence of end-organ dysfunction.
2. Rapid onset after exposure to an allergen of at least two of the following: skin or mucosal involvement, respiratory compromise, hypotension, persistent gastrointestinal symptoms.
3. Hypotension after exposure to a known allergen.

The differential diagnosis of anaphylaxis is summarized in Table 2-3.

ED management

Anaphylaxis is a medical emergency requiring immediate attention. Institute the ABCs of emergency care. Limit any continued exposure and discontinue any intravenous agents immediately. Avoid using latex products when caring for a latex-allergic patient. If the affected patient is taking beta-blocking medication, be prepared for a difficult recovery;

Table 2-1. Agents that can trigger anaphylaxis

Anaphylactic (IgE-dependent)

Hymenoptera sting (yellow jacket, hornet, wasp, honeybee, fire ant)

Antibiotics: beta-lactams, sulfonamides

Foods: shellfish (crustaceans, mollusks), peanuts, tree nuts (pecans, pistachios, walnuts), egg whites, fish, wheat, milk, soy, sesame

Latex

Animal dander

Colorants (carmine dye)

Hormones (estrogen, progesterone)

Anaphylactoid (IgE-independent)

Medications: opioids, muscle relaxants, nonsteroidal anti-inflammatories, aspirin

Physiologic factors: exercise, cold temperature, heat, pressure, sunlight

Immune aggregates

Transfusion reaction

IV immunoglobulin

Radiocontrast material (any)

Idiopathic

Table 2-2. Clinical manifestations of anaphylaxis

Organ system	Signs and symptoms	Frequency (%)
Cutaneous	Urticaria, angioedema	88
Cutaneous	Flushing	46
Cutaneous	Pruritus (no rash)	5
Respiratory	Wheezing, dyspnea, stridor	50
Gastrointestinal	Nausea, vomiting, diarrhea, abdominal pain	30
Cardiovascular	Syncope, hypotension, arrhythmias	30
Miscellaneous	Sense of impending doom, seizure, diaphoresis, rhinitis, headache, metallic taste	1–20

sometimes extraordinary efforts are required to overcome beta-blockade associated with anaphylaxis.

The first priority is to maintain airway patency. Allow the patient to assume a position of comfort. If adequate ventilation and oxygenation are documented by pulse oximetry, do not change the patient's position, but administer 100% oxygen as tolerated. Place a hypotensive patient in the recumbent position and elevate the lower extremities. If stridor is present, prepare to intubate the patient if initial therapy with epinephrine (see below) is

Table 2-3. Differential diagnosis of anaphylaxis

Diagnosis	Differentiating features
Airway foreign body	Aspiration history
	Auscultatory findings may be localized
Angioedema	No respiratory symptoms
Asthma	Involves only the respiratory system
Cardiac tamponade	Muffled heart sounds, pericardial rub, pulsus paradoxus
Croup	Barking cough
Food poisoning	Flushing 2° to ciguatera/scromboid
Flushing syndromes	Catecholamine excreting tumors; carcinoid
Globus hystericus	Sensation of a lump in the throat
Hereditary angioedema	May have a history of previous similar episodes
Panic attack	Precipitating event
	No cutaneous findings
Pulmonary embolism	Pleuritic pain, fourth heart sound
	Jugular venous distension
Red man syndrome	History of vancomycin exposure
Serum sickness	Fever, lymphadenopathy, arthralgias/arthritis
Urticaria	Skin is sole organ system involved
Vasovagal episode	Gradual onset after precipitating event
Vocal cord dysfunction	Onset is not acute

not effective. Monitor the ECG and oxygen saturation continuously, establish IV access and give a 20 mL/kg normal saline bolus. Make a rapid assessment of the rate of progression and the extent of the reaction.

Epinephrine

Epinephrine is the mainstay of treatment of anaphylaxis. The alpha-adrenergic effects reverse peripheral vasodilatation, decreasing hypotension and reducing angioedema and urticaria; the beta-adrenergic effects cause bronchodilatation, increase myocardial contractility, and suppress further release of mast cells and basophils.

If the patient is not hypotensive, give 0.01 mL/kg (0.5 mL maximum) of 1:1000 epinephrine intramuscularly. Repeat the dose every 5–15 minutes, as needed. As an alternative, use an EpiPen (>30 kg, 0.3 mg) or EpiPen Jr (<30 kg, 0.15 mg), also intramuscularly.

If the patient is hypotensive, give 0.01 mg/kg (0.1 mL/kg, 10 mL maximum) of 1:10,000 epinephrine intravenously. Repeat every 3–5 minutes. If venous access is not available, administer epinephrine (0.1 mL/kg of 1:1000) via the endotracheal tube. If the initial response to epinephrine is inadequate, use an intravenous drip, starting with 0.1 mcg/kg per min (1.5 mcg/kg per min maximum).

Vasopressor infusion

A vasopressor infusion is indicated for hypotension refractory to epinephrine and volume repletion. Give dopamine at 2–20 mcg/kg per min.

Antihistamines

H_1 and H_2 antihistamines block the effect of circulating histamines but do not decrease mediator release. H_2 blockers may also inhibit the histamine effects on peripheral vasculature and myocardial tissues. The onset of action of antihistamines is delayed, so epinephrine is still necessary. Give diphenhydramine (H_1), 1–2 mg/kg (50 mg/dose maximum, 400 mg/day maximum) IV or PO q 4–6 h and ranitidine (H_2), 2 mg/kg (50 mg/dose maximum) q 6–8 h IV or PO.

Albuterol

Treat bronchospasm resistant to epinephrine with nebulized albuterol, 0.15 mL/kg (2.5 mg minimum, 10 mg maximum) diluted in 3.0 mL of saline, either q 1 h or continuously. See Asthma (pp. 606–612) for the treatment of bronchospasm not responsive to albuterol.

Corticosteroids

Give systemic corticosteroids to patients with a history of asthma, idiopathic anaphylaxis, or severe or prolonged symptoms. Steroids may also reduce the risk of recurrent or protracted anaphylaxis. Use methylprednisolone 1–2 mg/kg per day (60 mg/day maximum) div q 6 h IV or prednisone 0.5–1 mg/kg per day (60 mg/day maximum) PO, for 5–7 days.

Glucagon

Anaphylaxis may be very difficult to treat in a patient taking beta-adrenergic blockers, which blunt the response to epinephrine. The patient is at increased risk for bronchospasm, hypotension, and paradoxical bradycardia. Glucagon has both inotropic and chronotropic effects that are mediated independently of α- and β-receptors and therefore can reverse refractory hypotension and bradycardia. Give a loading dose of 20–30 mcg/kg (1 mg maximum) IV over 5 minutes, followed by a continuous infusion of 5–15 mcg/min, titrating the dose to the desired blood pressure.

Discharge considerations

1. Observe for 6–8 hours. Most late-phase reactions occur within this time period
2. Give prednisone 0.5–1 mg/kg per day (60 mg/day maximum) for 5–7 days
3. Give diphenhydramine (5 mg/kg per day div q 6 h, 50 mg/dose maximum) for 2–3 days to treat urticaria
4. Give an H_2 antihistamine, ranitidine (2 mg/kg q 6–8 h, 50 mg/dose maximum) for 2–3 days
5. Prescribe injectable epinephrine (EpiPen Jr <30 kg, EpiPen >30 kg) and instruct the parent and/or child to administer it in the anterolateral aspect of thigh, through the clothing, while avoiding placing the thumb over tip
6. Educate the family regarding avoidance of the trigger(s)

7. Inform the family about MedicAlert bracelets (1–888–633–4298 or www.medicalert.org)
8. Refer all patients with an episode of anaphylaxis to an allergist

Indications for admission

- Severe anaphylaxis
- Hypotension
- Persistent bronchospasm or hypoxia
- Patient resides some distance from medical facilities

Bibliography

Joint Task Force on Practice Parameters; American Academy of Allergy, Asthma and Immunology; American College of Allergy, Asthma and Immunology; Joint Council of Allergy, Asthma and Immunology: The diagnosis and management of anaphylaxis: an updated practice parameter. *J Allergy Clin Immunol* 2005;115(3 Suppl 2): S483–523.

Oswalt ML, Kemp SF: Anaphylaxis: office management and prevention. *Immunol Allergy Clin North Am* 2007;27:177–91.

Sicherer SH, Leung DY: Advances in allergic skin disease, anaphylaxis, and hypersensitivity reactions to foods, drugs, and insects in 2007. *J Allergy Clin Immunol* 2008;121:1351–8.

Angioedema

Angioedema is swelling of the deeper layers of skin and/or submucosal tissue. It often occurs simultaneously with urticaria.

Clinical presentation

The face, neck, and extremities are most commonly affected, although angioedema may occur anywhere on the body. The swelling is most evident where the skin is loose, such as the scrotum, lips, and eyelids. There is usually accompanying erythema, warmth, and a sensation of pressure or pain, but pruritus is rare. Angioedema may also present as unexplained abdominal pain secondary to the swelling of any portion of the gastrointestinal tract.

The etiologies of angioedema are the same as for urticaria (pp. 36–38). In addition, hereditary angioedema (HAE) is an autosomal dominant condition that affects the gene for the plasma protein C1 inhibitor, leading to uncontrolled generation of bradykinin. The patient will have recurrent episodes of angioedema, usually beginning in childhood and worsening during puberty. Attacks of HAE are often sporadic, although about one-third are triggered by injury or trauma. Most episodes are of 1–2 day duration and are preceded by a prodrome of numbness, tingling, and pressure. The edema of HAE most commonly involves the hands and feet, although other sites can be affected, as well. In addition, life-threatening swelling of the airway can occur.

Diagnosis

Angioedema is most often confused with edema. However, angioedema is non-pitting and is not limited to dependent areas. It may be also difficult to distinguish angioedema from anaphylaxis, especially since angioedema can be the primary manifestation of anaphylaxis.

Table 2-4. Differential diagnosis of angioedema

Diagnosis	Differentiating features
Anaphylaxis	Other organ systems involved (respiratory, GI, etc.)
Edema	Occurs in dependent areas, may be pitting
Cellulitis	Usually localized, on exposed areas of skin
	May have fever, chills
Erysipelas	Raised above the level of the skin
	Sharply demarcated borders
Vasculitis	Fever, weight loss
	Paresthesias, joint/muscle pain
Lymphedema	Usually involves one extremity including digits

However, anaphylaxis involves at least two organ systems, while angioedema is solely an edema of the deeper tissues. Angioedema can present as abdominal pain from swelling in the GI tract as well, but again this can be differentiated from anaphylaxis by the absence of other system involvement. The differential diagnosis is summarized in Table 2-4.

Once it is clear that the patient has angioedema, and not anaphylaxis, obtain a complete history, seeking a possible offending agent, as well as a family history of similar episodes. Obtain blood for a CBC with differential, ESR, total serum IgE, thyroid function tests and C_1-inhibitor level (low in 85% of cases). A more extensive evaluation is indicated for severe or recurrent cases of angioedema, although this can be deferred to a primary care setting.

ED management

The priority is to ensure an adequate airway, as laryngeal edema can be rapidly progressive (see Anaphylaxis, pp. 30–34 for the treatment of airway edema). If the patient is known to have hereditary angioedema, give C_1-inhibitor concentrate as soon as possible for significant edematous attacks (i.e., laryngeal edema, extensive facial edema, and severe abdominal attacks). Use 10–20 units/kg (500 units maximum <50 kg; 1000 units maximum 50–100 kg) and repeat if needed in 1 hour.

The best treatment is prevention and education of the family and patient. Remove the offending agent, if identified. Advise the patient to avoid dry skin or harsh soaps/cream, as well as aspirin and oral contraceptives, which can precipitate an attack.

If the etiology is unknown, prescribe an H_1 antihistamine, such as diphenhydramine (5 mg/kg per day div q 6 h) or hydroxyzine (2 mg/kg per day div q 8 h). Reserve corticosteroids for severe cases (prednisone or prednisolone, 2 mg/kg per day, 60 mg/day maximum, for 5–7 days).

Follow-up

• Primary care follow-up in 1–2 weeks; dermatology or allergy follow-up in 2–4 weeks

Bibliography

Farkas H, Varga L, Széplaki G, et al:
Management of hereditary angioedema
in pediatric patients. *Pediatrics* 2007;
120:e713–22.

Ferdman R: Urticaria and angioedema.
Clin Ped Emerg Med 2007;8:72–80.

Frigas E, Park M: Idiopathic recurrent
angioedema. *Immunol Allergy Clin North Am*
2006;26:739–51.

Urticaria

Urticaria, or hives, is a common cutaneous reaction caused by release of chemical mediators, especially histamine, from mast cells or basophils. Urticaria may occur at any age and up to 25% of the population will have at least one episode in their lifetime.

Acute urticaria lasts less than 6–8 weeks in duration, while chronic urticaria is defined as hives persisting beyond this time frame. In 80% of cases the etiology is unknown, although chronic urticaria can be associated with systemic illnesses such as JRA, SLE, viral hepatitis, lymphomas, and thyroid disease. The most common causes are listed in Table 2-5.

Clinical presentation

A hive is a pruritic, well-circumscribed, raised, evanescent area of skin edema on an erythematous base. They are usually circular or annular in shape, found most commonly on the trunk and extremities, and vary in size from a few millimeters to centimeters (giant urticaria). Acute urticaria usually develops within minutes of exposure to the causative agent and is virtually always pruritic. Simple hives tend to come and go in crops, with individual lesions usually lasting for less than one day, although new lesions tend to evolve as older ones resolve. On rare occasions a hive will persist for up to 48 hours.

Diagnosis

The key feature in making the diagnosis of urticaria is the duration of the lesions. Hives that remain fixed in place for longer than 24–48 hours are not typical. A violet hue within the lesions, or the absence of pruritus, also suggests alternative etiologies. Obtain a history looking for a possible offending agent. Determine the time of onset, site, duration, and frequency of the lesions. Inquire about recent medication use, injections, insect bites, illness, and other triggers or provoking factors. Examine the distribution of lesions to check for temperature-exposed regions or contact etiologies. Stroke the skin to assess for dermatographism, which is caused by histamine release from mast cells. The differential diagnosis of urticaria is summarized in Table 2-6.

For patients with chronic urticaria, ascertain whether there are any related symptoms, such as fever, joint pain, abdominal pain, weight loss, or poor circulation in the hands or feet.

A priority is to assess for signs of associated respiratory, cardiovascular, or gastrointestinal involvement, which would imply that the urticaria is a manifestation of an anaphylactic episode. Similarly, look for the presence of associated angioedema on physical examination.

In general, for acute urticaria, no laboratory testing is required and it is not necessary to identify the trigger for a patient who is otherwise well, and in whom the history and physical examination do not suggest a cause. However, if the patient presents with chronic urticaria, and the history and physical examination do not suggest an etiology, obtain a CBC with differential, ESR and/or CRP, liver function tests, urinalysis, antinuclear antibody, thyroid function, anti-thyroid antibodies, and possibly a chest X-ray.

Table 2-5. Causes of urticaria

Acute urticaria

Hypersensitivity

    Foods: eggs, milk, wheat, soy, peanuts

    Antibiotics: beta-lactam, sulfa

    Stings and bites: bees, wasps, scorpions, spiders, jellyfish

Pseudoallergic reactions: medications, radiocontrast, foods

Toxin-mediated

Infectious: viral, bacterial (strep), parasitic, fungal

Contact urticaria: latex, animal saliva

Immune-complex-mediated: serum sickness, post-transfusion, post-viral

Idiopathic

Chronic urticaria

Autoimmune

Idiopathic

Exercise-induced

Cold/solar

Dermographism

Cholinergic

Adrenergic

Presumed immune-complex-mediated

    Thyroid disease

    Urticarial vasculitis

    Malignancy

    Collagen vascular disease: SLE, JRA, rheumatic fever, dermatomyositis

    Inflammatory bowel disease

    Behçet's disease

Hypersensitivity reactions

ED management

The priority for all patients with urticaria is to rule out anaphylaxis (pp. 30–34).

Acute urticaria

Remove or avoid the offending agent, if it can be identified. If there is airway involvement, give epinephrine as for anaphylaxis. Treat severe pruritus with 1:1000 epinephrine subQ (0.01 mL/kg, 0.5 mL maximum). Otherwise, oral H_1 antihistamines are the treatment of choice. Prescribe a non-sedating antihistamine for 3–4 days. Choices include loratadine

Table 2-6. Differential diagnosis of urticaria

Diagnosis	Differentiating features
Anaphylaxis	Involves more than one organ system
Erythema multiforme	Symmetrical target lesions
	Mucosal involvement with erythema multiforme major
Guttate psoriasis	Small salmon-pink drop-like papules
Henoch-Schönlein purpura	Abdominal pain, hematochezia, joint pain, purpura
Mastocytosis	Widespread symmetric lesion
	Macules, papules, nodules, plaques, bullae, and vesicles
	Darier sign (wheal develops after rubbing), hepatosplenomegaly
Pityriasis rosea	Herald patch precedes general eruption
	Christmas tree pattern of pruritic lesions on the back

(2–5 years old: 5 mg/day; >6 years old: 10 mg/day), cetirizine (6 months – 2 years old: 2.5 mg/day; 2–5 years old: 2.5 mg/day [may increase to 5 mg/day, if needed]; >6 years old: 5–10 mg/day), or fexofenadine (6–11 years old: 30 mg bid; >12 years old: 60 mg bid). Also prescribe an H_2 antihistamine, such as ranitidine (2 mg/kg per day div q 12 h, 300 mg/day maximum), cimetidine (20–40 mg/kg per day div q 6 h, 800 mg/day maximum), or famotidine (0.5–1 mg/kg q 12 h). For breakthrough itching, prescribe either diphenhydramine (5 mg/kg per day div q 6 h) *or* hydroxyzine (2 mg/kg per day div q 8 h).

Chronic urticaria

In addition to the treatment listed for acute urticaria, in severe cases, add an antileukotriene, montelukast (2–5 years old: 4 mg/day; 6–14 years old: 5 mg/day; >15 years old: 10 mg/day) in combination with the antihistamines. Refer patients with chronic urticaria to either an allergist or primary care provider for further evaluation.

Follow-up

- Acute urticaria: if no improvement; primary care in 3–5 days
- Allergy referral in 1–2 weeks: peanut- or latex-induced urticaria, urticarial vasculitis, urticaria with systemic manifestations, urticaria with angioedema, urticaria that responds poorly to therapy, or if the results of the ED evaluation do not suggest an etiology for chronic urticaria

Bibliography

Amar SM, Dreskin SC: Urticaria. *Prim Care* 2008;**35**:141–57.

Dibbern DA Jr.: Urticaria: selected highlights and recent advances. *Med Clin North Am* 2006;**90**:187–209.

Ferdman R: Urticaria and angioedema. *Clin Ped Emerg Med* 2007;**8**:72–80.

Cardiac emergencies

Michael H. Gewitz and Paul K. Woolf

Arrhythmias

Pediatric arrhythmias are increasing in prevalence secondary to improved patient survival following cardiac surgery and more extensive use of ECG monitoring. Proper management includes accurate electrocardiographic diagnosis, careful clinical evaluation, and initiation of appropriate therapy. With all rhythm disturbances, the approach to the patient begins with a 12-lead ECG, but, if there is hemodynamic instability, a single-lead ECG will suffice.

Cardiac arrhythmias requiring emergency therapy can be classified simply into tachy-cardias and bradycardias. The tachycardias can be further divided into narrow and wide QRS complex groups. Rhythms in the narrow complex group include atrial fibrillation, atrial flutter, and supraventricular tachycardia, although the most common is sinus tachycardia.

Atrial fibrillation

Atrial fibrillation is usually associated with dilatation of the right or left atrium. It most commonly occurs in patients with mitral valve disease, chronic atrioventricular (AV) valve insufficiency, Wolff-Parkinson-White syndrome, or following the Fontan procedure in patients with only one functional ventricle. Other associations include hyperthyroidism, Ebstein's anomaly, atrial septal defect, or atrial tumor. Atrial fibrillation suggests significant atrial conduction system disease and is usually a chronic problem. "Lone" atrial fibrillation, in the absence of other cardiac abnormalities, is rare in children.

Clinical presentation and diagnosis

Suspect atrial fibrillation when the pulse is "irregularly irregular." Heart sounds may vary in intensity, a pulse deficit may be present, and the cardiac impulse is markedly variable. The ECG shows chaotic fibrillatory waves of varying amplitude, morphology, and duration, causing variation of the baseline. The RR interval is irregularly irregular. The atrial rate is generally >350 bpm, while the ventricular rate varies between 100 and 200 bpm (Figure 3-1). Sporadic aberrant ventricular conduction can result in random wide QRS complexes.

ED management

Treatment can usually be delayed until the patient is admitted to an intensive care setting, where therapy is aimed at control of ventricular rate, conversion to sinus rhythm, and prevention of stroke. However, in the ED, treat acute atrial fibrillation associated with a

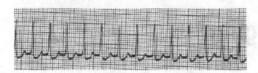

Figure 3-1. Atrial fibrillation.

rapid ventricular rate and signs of hemodynamic compromise with synchronized cardio-version (0.5–1 J/kg).

If the patient is hemodynamically stable, consult a pediatric cardiologist before initiating pharmacologic cardioversion, which can most frequently be accomplished with ibutilide. Rate control is best accomplished with diltiazem or digitalis. However, digitalis and verapamil are contraindicated if the patient is known to have Wolff-Parkinson-White syndrome, since they may facilitate conduction through an accessory AV connection, leading to ventricular fibrillation.

Although atrial thrombus is uncommon in children with atrial fibrillation, give anti-coagulation prior to cardioversion if there is chronic (>48 hours) atrial fibrillation. Obtain an echocardiogram in order to document the presence of a thrombus.

Indications for admission

* Acute onset of atrial fibrillation
* Chronic atrial fibrillation with an increase in ventricular rate requiring treatment with a new anti-arrhythmic medication

Bibliography

Doniger SJ, Sharieff GQ: Pediatric dysrhythmias. *Pediatr Clin North Am* 2006;53:85–105.

Fazio G, Visconti C, D'Angelo L, et al: Pharmacological therapy in children with atrial fibrillation and atrial flutter. *Curr Pharm Des* 2008;14:770–5.

Kannakeril PJ, Fish FA: Disorders of cardiac rhythm and conduction In Allen HD, Driscoll DJ, Shaddy RE, Feltes TF (eds), *Moss and Adams' Heart Disease in Infants, Children, and Adolescents: Including the Fetus and Young Adult*, 7th ed. Philadelphia: Lippincott, Williams & Wilkins, 2008, pp. 293–342.

Atrial flutter

Atrial flutter can be a manifestation of pre- or postoperative structural cardiac disease, cardiomyopathy, or primary electrical disease. Atrial flutter is relatively rare in childhood, although the incidence is increasing as more patients survive complex atrial surgery, such as the Fontan procedure.

Clinical presentation and diagnosis

Atrial flutter is characterized by an atrial tachycardia with a rate between 300 and 480 bpm. The atrial rhythm is extremely regular, and flutter waves are usually present. These form a continuous sawtooth undulation of the baseline P waves (Figure 3-2). The ventricular rate is dependent on AV conduction, which is most commonly 2:1. When 1:1 conduction is present, the flutter waves may not be apparent.

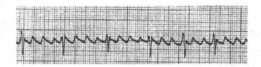

Figure 3-2. Atrial flutter.

When the diagnosis is in doubt, use vagal maneuvers or adenosine to increase the degree of AV block and slow the ventricular rate. This will make the flutter waves more apparent, but will not convert the rhythm to sinus.

ED management

Hemodynamically unstable patient

If the patient is hemodynamically unstable, presenting with hypotension or congestive heart failure, cardiovert using 0.5–1.0 J/kg, in the synchronized mode, as the initial dose. If the patient is taking digoxin, give 1 mg/kg of lidocaine IV prior to cardioversion to prevent ventricular arrhythmias. If initial cardioversion is unsuccessful, increase the dose to 2 J/kg.

Hemodynamically stable patient

If the patient is hemodynamically stable, first attempt pharmacologic treatment. Use IV digoxin (total digitalizing dose [TDD] = 30 mcg/kg; give ½ TDD initially, followed by ¼ TDD q 6–8 h × 2), IV amiodarone (5 mg/kg over 10–15 min), or IV ibutilide (0.01 mg/kg over 10 min), in order to slow the ventricular rate or convert to sinus rhythm. If these are unsuccessful, elective electrical cardioversion may be required in a critical care unit.

Indications for admission

- New onset atrial flutter
- Difficult to control atrial flutter for observation, or electrical or drug therapy

Bibliography

Doniger SJ, Sharieff GQ: Pediatric dysrhythmias. *Pediatr Clin North Am* 2006;53:85–105.

Fazio G, Visconti C, D'Angelo L, et al: Pharmacological therapy in children with atrial fibrillation and atrial flutter. *Curr Pharm Des* 2008;14:770–5.

Kannakeril PJ, Fish FA: Disorders of cardiac rhythm and conduction. In Allen HD, Driscoll DJ, Shaddy RE, Feltes TF (eds), *Moss and Adams Heart Disease in Infants, Children, and Adolescents: Including the Fetus and Young Adult*, 7th ed. Philadelphia: Lippincott, Williams & Wilkins, 2008, pp. 293–342.

Sinus tachycardia

Sinus tachycardia (ST) is an increased heart rate for age originating from the sinus node. The most common causes of ST are anxiety, fever, pain, hypovolemia, anemia, congestive heart failure, exercise, hyperthyroidism, emotional upset, and medications (stimulants, bronchodilators, decongestants).

Clinical presentation and diagnosis

Since normal hemodynamics are generally maintained, ST is usually an incidental finding in a patient with a non-cardiac disease process. The rate is generally between 100 and 180 bpm, although in infants the rate may reach 240 bpm.

Sinus tachycardia must be differentiated from supraventricular tachycardia (SVT), in which the rate can be as rapid as 340 bpm and the QRS complexes may not be preceded by recognizable P waves of sinus origin. In some cases of SVT, the QRS complexes may follow abnormally directed P waves which are negative in leads I and AVF. Also, in ST the rate may vary, while in SVT the RR interval is consistent. Increasing the ECG paper speed to 50 mm/sec may help to identify normal P waves.

ED management

Most often, ST is encountered in the settings mentioned above, so therapy is directed toward identifying and treating these conditions.

Bibliography

Doniger SJ, Sharieff GQ: Pediatric dysrhythmias. *Pediatr Clin North Am* 2006;53:85–105.

Vignati G, Annoni G: Characterization of supraventricular tachycardia in infants: clinical and instrumental diagnosis. *Curr Pharm Des* 2008;14:729–35.

Supraventricular tachycardia

Supraventricular tachycardia is the most common significant pediatric cardiac arrhythmia. The mechanism of SVT is usually reentry, sometimes secondary to microreentrant circuits, as in atrioventricular node reentry utilizing dual AV nodal pathways. In other cases there are macroreentrant circuits involving an atrioventricular bypass tract, sometimes manifest as Wolff-Parkinson-White (WPW) syndrome. In 20% of patients there is a trigger, such as infection or the use of cold remedies containing sympathomimetics (Table 3-1). Congenital heart disease, such as Ebstein's anomaly or corrected transposition, occurs in approximately 20% of patients.

Clinical presentation

The presentation depends on the age of the patient, the rate and duration of the tachycardia, and whether there is associated heart disease. Common clinical findings include palpitations, shortness of breath, chest pain, respiratory distress, dizziness, syncope, irritability, pallor, and poor feeding in infants. The heart rate is usually between 150 and 300 bpm. Heart failure is uncommon in patients >1 year of age and is usually associated with congenital heart disease, SVT for >24 hours, and heart rates >200 bpm.

Diagnosis

The electrocardiogram in SVT typically reveals a narrow complex tachycardia at a rate of 150–300 bpm with 1:1 AV conduction and a fixed RR interval (Figure 3-3). The P wave may not be seen; it may be inverted just after the QRS complex; or it may precede the QRS, but have an abnormal axis (negative in leads I or AVF). The ventricular complexes are usually normal in contour, although aberrant rate-dependent conduction can cause slight widening. In supraventricular tachycardia the atrial rate is 180–240 bpm.

Table 3-1. Factors predisposing to supraventricular tachycardia

Primary electrical disease	Mitral valve prolapse
Atrioventricular bypass tract (WPW)	Sepsis
Dual AV nodal pathways	Hyperthyroidism
Myocarditis	Fever
Cardiomyopathy	Drugs
Ebstein's anomaly	Epinephrine
Previous cardiac surgery	Decongestants
(Mustard or Senning procedure for	Ephedrine
TPGV; Fontan; TAPVR repair)	Methylphenidate

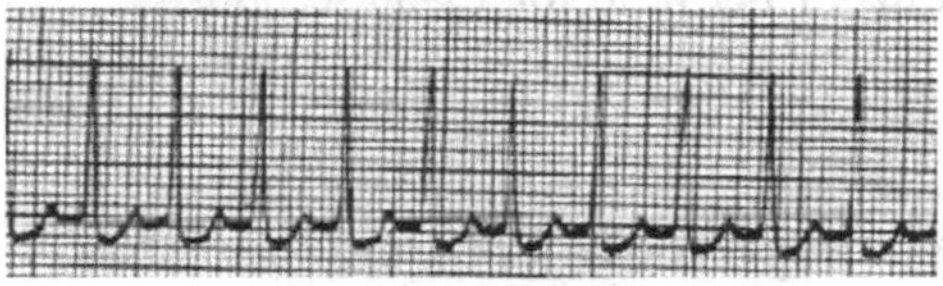

Figure 3-3. Supraventricular tachycardia.

Supraventricular tachycardia must be differentiated from sinus tachycardia. In the latter, the rate is usually <180 bpm (240 bpm in infants), a P wave with normal axis precedes the QRS complex, and some variation in the RR interval may be present.

Supraventricular tachycardia with wide QRS complexes due to aberrant conduction may be difficult to differentiate from ventricular tachycardia. Ventricular tachycardia is suggested by the presence of atrioventricular dissociation, a sicker patient, slower rate of the tachycardia, and isolated premature ventricular contractions elsewhere on the ECG. Assume that all wide complex tachycardias in children are ventricular tachycardia unless the diagnosis of SVT is absolutely certain.

ED management

Perform a history and physical examination, carefully evaluate the patient's hemodynamic status, and continuously monitor the ECG and blood pressure. Congestive heart failure or hemodynamic compromise are indications for rapid termination of the arrhythmia with synchronous cardioversion. After successful conversion to a sinus rhythm, obtain a complete ECG looking for WPW and refer the patient to a pediatric cardiologist.

Vagal maneuvers

Vagal nerve stimulation increases the effective refractory period of the AV node, thus interrupting the reentrant circuit. Continuously monitor the ECG when vagal maneuvers are attempted. If successful, the tachycardia breaks abruptly and is replaced by a normal sinus rhythm (Figure 3-4). Transient slowing of the ventricular rate suggests that either sinus tachycardia or atrial flutter was misdiagnosed as SVT. Eyeball pressure is not recommended, as retinal detachment can occur. Gagging and inducing vomiting can be effective, but may lead to aspiration in infants or agitated patients. Commonly employed vagal techniques include the following.

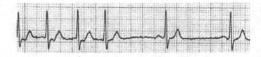

Figure 3-4. SVT: response to treatment.

Eliciting the diving reflex

Submerge the face of an older child in ice-cold water or place an ice bag with equal volumes of ice and water over the face for 10–20 seconds.

Unilateral carotid massage

Perform the massage at the junction of the carotid artery and the mandible. This is much more likely to be successful in the older child or adolescent.

Valsalva maneuver

Ask the patient to "bear down," or "strain," as if attempting to move his or her bowels. If this is unsuccessful, have the patient stand on his or her head for 15–30 seconds.

Pharmacotherapy

Adenosine

Adenosine, an endogenous purine metabolite, is the drug of choice for the treatment of SVT. It terminates SVT by blocking conduction in the AV node and thus breaks the reentry circuit. Give an initial dose of 0.1 mg/kg (6 mg maximum) as a rapid IV bolus, preferably at a proximal IV site. If ineffective in 2–3 minutes, double the dose (12 mg maximum). The onset of action is within 10–15 seconds and the half-life is about 15 seconds. Bradycardia or transient asystole may occur after termination of the arrhythmia; flushing, wheezing, and cough are transient side effects.

Verapamil

Verapamil is a calcium slow channel blocker which is extremely effective in treating SVT. The dose is 0.075–0.15 mg/kg, slowly IV. This can be repeated twice at 15-minute intervals. Verapamil is contraindicated <1 year of age because of possible cardiovascular collapse; other contraindications include congestive heart failure and beta-blocker (propranolol) use. Side effects may include bradycardia and hypotension; treat with atropine (0.01–0.04 mg/kg), isoproterenol (0.1 mcg/kg per min infusion), and calcium chloride (5–7 mg/kg of elemental calcium = 0.2–0.25 mL/kg of calcium chloride).

Digoxin

Digoxin terminates SVT through its vagal effect. While digoxin remains the mainstay of treatment for chronic SVT, it has been replaced by adenosine for acute SVT. The major drawback of digoxin is the delayed onset of action; SVT may not be terminated for 6–24 hours after beginning therapy. The IV total digitalizing dose (TDD) is 30 mcg/kg. Give one-half of the TDD initially, then one quarter of the TDD at 6–8 hour intervals. Digoxin is contraindicated in patients with WPW, as it shortens the refractory period of a bypass tract in up to one-third of these patients.

Cardioversion

Synchronous cardioversion is indicated when there is hemodynamic compromise (heart failure, shock, acidosis) or if other treatment modalities have failed. The dose is 0.5–1 J/kg,

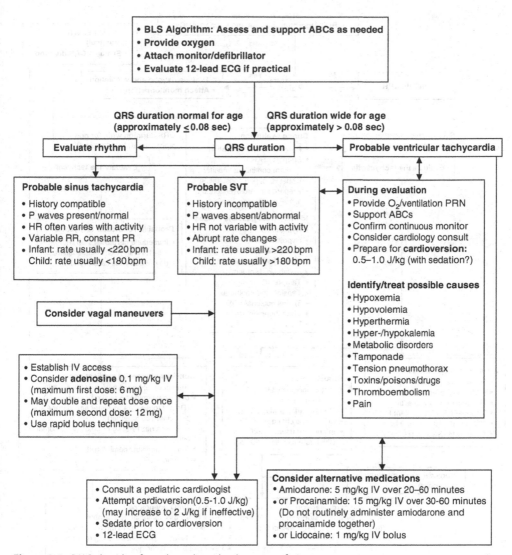

BLS Algorithm: Assess and support ABCs as needed
- Provide oxygen
- Attach monitor/defibrillator
- Evaluate 12-lead ECG if practical

QRS duration normal for age (approximately ≤ 0.08 sec)

QRS duration wide for age (approximately > 0.08 sec)

Evaluate rhythm ← **QRS duration** → **Probable ventricular tachycardia**

Probable sinus tachycardia
- History compatible
- P waves present/normal
- HR often varies with activity
- Variable RR, constant PR
- Infant: rate usually <220 bpm
  Child: rate usually <180 bpm

Probable SVT
- History incompatible
- P waves absent/abnormal
- HR not variable with activity
- Abrupt rate changes
- Infant: rate usually >220 bpm
  Child: rate usually >180 bpm

During evaluation
- Provide O₂/ventilation PRN
- Support ABCs
- Confirm continuous monitor
- Consider cardiology consult
- Prepare for **cardioversion:** 0.5–1.0 J/kg (with sedation?)

Identify/treat possible causes
- Hypoxemia
- Hypovolemia
- Hyperthermia
- Hyper-/hypokalemia
- Metabolic disorders
- Tamponade
- Tension pneumothorax
- Toxins/poisons/drugs
- Thromboembolism
- Pain

Consider vagal maneuvers

- Establish IV access
- Consider **adenosine** 0.1 mg/kg IV (maximum first dose: 6 mg)
- May double and repeat dose once (maximum second dose: 12 mg)
- Use rapid bolus technique

- Consult a pediatric cardiologist
- Attempt cardioversion(0.5-1.0 J/kg) (may increase to 2 J/kg if ineffective)
- Sedate prior to cardioversion
- 12-lead ECG

Consider alternative medications
- Amiodarone: 5 mg/kg IV over 20–60 minutes
- or Procainamide: 15 mg/kg IV over 30-60 minutes (Do not routinely administer amiodarone and procainamide together)
- or Lidocaine: 1 mg/kg IV bolus

Figure 3-5. PALS algorithm for tachycardia with adequate perfusion.

which can be repeated, doubling the dose to a maximum of 2 J/kg. Sedate older patients with midazolam (0.1 mg/kg IV) prior to cardioversion. To prevent ventricular dysrhythmias, give lidocaine (1 mg/kg IV) to digitalized patients prior to attempting cardioversion. Prior to cardioversion, be certain of synchronized mode setting, to avoid potentially lethal ventricular arrhythmias.

Conversion to sinus rhythm using vagal maneuvers, adenosine, verapamil, and/or cardioversion is within the realm of the ED physician. However, consult a pediatric cardiologist in cases when the SVT is refractory or after conversion is accomplished to arrange appropriate evaluation and follow-up. The Pediatric Advanced Life Support algorithms for tachycardia with adequate and poor perfusion are summarized in Figures 3-5 and 3-6.

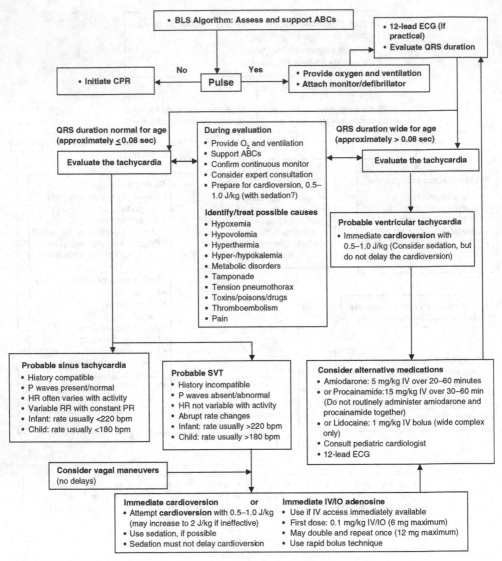

Figure 3-6. PALS algorithm for tachycardia with poor perfusion.

Follow-up
- SVT without hemodynamic compromise, terminated in ED: 2–3 days
- SVT with WPW: consult a pediatric cardiologist to determine appropriate follow-up

Indications for admission
- First episode of SVT with parental anxiety or need for parental education
- SVT causing hemodynamic compromise.
- Initiation of a medication with proarrhythmia potential (flecainide, sotalol, amiodarone)

Bibliography

Kannakeril PJ, Fish FA: Disorders of cardiac rhythm and conduction. In Allen HD, Driscoll DJ, Shaddy RE, Feltes TF (eds), *Moss and Adams' Heart Disease in Infants, Children, and Adolescents: Including the Fetus and Young Adult*, 7th ed. Philadelphia: Lippincott, Williams & Wilkins, 2008, pp. 293–342.

Manole MD, Saladino RA: Emergency department management of the pediatric patient with supraventricular tachycardia. *Pediatr Emerg Care* 2007;23:176–85.

Vignati G, Annoni G: Characterization of supraventricular tachycardia in infants: clinical and instrumental diagnosis. *Curr Pharm Des* 2008;14:729–35.

Ventricular premature contractions

Ventricular premature contractions (VPCs) most commonly occur due to primary electrical disease in asymptomatic adolescents without structural heart disease. Other etiologies include ingestions (tobacco, sympathomimetic agents, tricyclic antidepressants, digoxin, caffeine), electrolyte imbalances (hypokalemia, hypocalcemia), anesthesia, and underlying heart disease (mitral valve prolapse, myocarditis, hypertrophic or dilated cardiomyopathy, coronary artery malformation, status-post ventricular surgery).

Clinical presentation

Most cases are discovered during the routine examination of an asymptomatic patient, when an irregular heart beat is noted. However, some patients complain of chest discomfort, palpitations, chest pain, or syncope.

Diagnosis

Ventricular premature contractions are characterized by bizarre, widened QRS complexes which are not preceded by a P wave (Figure 3-7). They may occur in a fixed ratio with normal beats (bigeminy 1:1; trigeminy 2:1) (Figure 3-8). VPCs can be uniform (identical electrocardiographic appearance with consistent interval from the preceding QRS) or multiform (dissimilar ECG appearances with varying coupling intervals with the preceding QRS). It is possible for the VPC to fall on the T wave of the preceding normal complex (R-on-T phenomenon) and initiate ventricular tachycardia.

VPCs can also be divided into benign and ominous categories. Benign VPCs are asymptomatic, uniform, single, infrequent, with a normal resting ECG, including the QTc interval (<0.45), and not associated with an R-on-T phenomenon or structural heart disease. Benign VPCs can be suppressed by exercise, such as 20 seconds of jumping jacks.

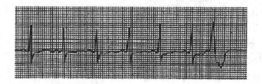

Figure 3-7. Ventricular premature contraction.

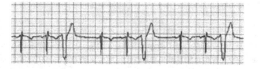

Figure 3-8. VPC in trigeminal pattern.

Ominous VPCs may be symptomatic, multiform, paired, associated with a prolonged QTc interval, an R-on-T phenomenon, or structural heart disease. Exercise either has no effect or increases the VPC frequency. Ominous VPCs indicate an increased risk of ventricular tachycardia (three or more consecutive VPCs).

ED management
Benign VPCs
No treatment is necessary. However, for reassurance, elective referral to a pediatric cardiologist may be indicated.

Ominous VPCs
Consult with a pediatric cardiologist, who may recommend admission and/or treatment.

Follow-up
• Benign VPCs: primary care follow-up in 1–2 weeks

Indication for admission
• Ominous VPCs

Bibliography
Doniger SJ, Sharieff GQ: Pediatric dysrhythmias. *Pediatr Clin North Am* 2006;53:85–105.

Kannakeril PJ, Fish FA: Disorders of cardiac rhythm and conduction. In Allen HD,

Driscoll DJ, Shaddy RE, Feltes TF (eds), *Moss and Adams' Heart Disease in Infants, Children, and Adolescents: Including the Fetus and Young Adult*, 7th ed. Philadelphia: Lippincott, Williams & Wilkins, 2008, pp. 293–342.

Ventricular tachycardia
Wide complex tachycardias are uncommon in children, but they are often difficult to diagnose and potentially more dangerous than narrow complex tachycardias. Wide complex tachycardias may be ventricular or supraventricular (with aberrancy secondary to a bundle branch block or WPW syndrome) in origin. However, in the ED, assume that a wide complex tachycardia is ventricular tachycardia and treat accordingly. Erroneously treating ventricular tachycardia as SVT can be devastating.

Nonetheless, it is important to remember that the upper limit of normal QRS duration varies with age. For example, a tachycardia with a QRS duration of 0.10 seconds is wide complex in a newborn, but narrow complex in a 10-year-old.

Ventricular tachycardia (VT) is defined as a series of three or more consecutive ectopic beats. Etiologies include primary electrical disease (long QTc syndrome), hypoxemia, arrhythmogenic right ventricular dysplasia, electrolyte imbalance (hyperkalemia), and ingestions (tricyclics, digoxin). Ventricular tachycardia can degenerate into ventricular fibrillation, either as a terminal event or in the setting of a prolonged QT interval.

Clinical presentation
The symptomatology depends on the rate and duration of the tachycardia and the presence or absence of underlying structural heart disease. Occasional patients are asymptomatic,

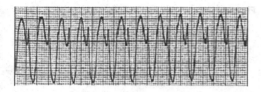

Figure 3-9. Ventricular tachycardia.

although chest pain, syncope, and palpitations are common, and lethargy, disorientation, hypotension, and sudden death with hemodynamic collapse can occur.

Diagnosis

Ventricular tachycardia is a wide QRS complex tachycardia. The rate of ventricular tachycardia (Figure 3-9) is 120–200 bpm, which is slower than supraventricular tachycardia with aberrant conduction. Ventricular tachycardia is suggested by AV dissociation or if the QRS morphology resembles that of a single VPC appearing during sinus rhythm elsewhere on the ECG.

ED management

Regardless of the patient's status, consult a pediatric cardiologist.

Hemodynamically stable

Give intravenous amiodarone (5 mg/kg over 10–15 min) and consult a pediatric cardiologist for further management in an intensive care setting. Bretylium is contraindicated in VT as its use may precipitate ventricular fibrillation.

Hemodynamically compromised with palpable pulses

The treatment of choice is synchronized cardioversion at an initial dose of 0.5 J/kg; double the dose and repeat if not successful. If the rhythm does not convert, give an IV lidocaine bolus (1 mg/kg), followed by a third attempt at cardioversion. Ventricular pacing by a cardiologist may be required. The treatment is summarized in Figure 3-5.

Hemodynamically compromised without pulses

Defibrillate with 2 J/kg, double to 4 J/kg for a maximum of three consecutive defibrillations or until conversion to sinus rhythm. The treatment is summarized in Figure 3-6.

Indications for admission

- Newly diagnosed or difficult to control ventricular tachycardia
- Presumed or documented ventricular tachycardia with long QT syndrome

Bibliography

Denjoy I, Lupoglazoff JM, Guicheney P, Leenhardt A: Arrhythmic sudden death in children. *Arch Cardiovasc Dis* 2008;**101**:121–5.

Doniger SJ, Sharieff GQ: Pediatric dysrhythmias. *Pediatr Clin North Am* 2006;**53**:85–105.

Kannakeril PJ, Fish FA: Disorders of cardiac rhythm and conduction. In Allen HD, Driscoll DJ, Shaddy RE, Feltes TF (eds), *Moss and Adams' Heart Disease in Infants, Children, and Adolescents: Including the Fetus and Young Adult*, 7th ed. Philadelphia: Lippincott, Williams & Wilkins, 2008, pp. 293–342.

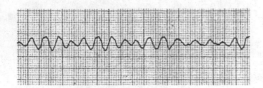

Figure 3-10. Ventricular fibrillation.

Ventricular fibrillation

Ventricular tachycardia can degenerate into ventricular fibrillation, either as a terminal event or when there is a prolonged QT interval or R-on-T phenomenon.

Clinical presentation

Patients with ventricular fibrillation are generally unresponsive and pulseless.

Diagnosis

In ventricular fibrillation (Figure 3-10) there is a wavy, sinusoidal line, without any true QRS complexes.

ED management

If the ventricular tachycardia degenerates into ventricular fibrillation, immediately defibrillate using 2 J/kg. If unsuccessful, double to 4 J/kg for three consecutive defibrillations. If unsuccessful, also give IV lidocaine (1 mg/kg) alternating with epinephrine (0.01 mg/kg of 1:10,000 IV or 0.1 mL/kg of 1:1000 ET). If fibrillation recurs, start a lidocaine continuous infusion (20–50 mcg/kg per min).

Indication for admission

• Any patient who survives after treatment for ventricular fibrillation

Bibliography

Denjoy I, Lupoglazoff JM, Guicheney P, Leenhardt A: Arrhythmic sudden death in children. *Arch Cardiovasc Dis* 2008;**101**:121–5.

Doniger SJ, Sharieff GQ: Pediatric dysrhythmias. *Pediatr Clin North Am* 2006;**53**:85–105.

Kannakeril PJ, Fish FA: Disorders of cardiac rhythm and conduction. In Allen HD, Driscoll DJ, Shaddy RE, Feltes TF (eds), *Moss and Adams' Heart Disease in Infants, Children, and Adolescents: Including the Fetus and Young Adult*, 7th ed. Philadelphia: Lippincott, Williams & Wilkins, 2008, pp. 293–342.

Heart block (atrioventricular [AV] block)

Heart block is secondary to abnormal atrioventricular conduction. It can be primary, as in patients with congenital complete heart block, or secondary, as with myocarditis or Lyme disease.

Clinical presentation and diagnosis

First-degree AV block

First-degree block is defined as prolongation of the PR interval (Figure 3-11). Patients are asymptomatic. It may be seen with increased vagal tone, digoxin administration, myocarditis, acute rheumatic fever, or diphtheria, or it may be a primary electrical phenomenon.

Second-degree AV block

Second-degree block may be secondary to acute or chronic heart disease, or it may occasionally occur in otherwise normal children. With Mobitz type I (Wenckebach) there is progressive lengthening of the PR interval, until the impulse is not conducted and a ventricular beat is dropped (Figure 3-12). Mobitz type I is thought to occur at the AV node and it can occur in normal patients. In Mobitz type II ventricular beats are dropped without prior prolongation of the PR interval (Figure 3-13). The site of block is in the more distal AV conduction system. Therefore, with Type II there is a greater chance of progression to complete (third-degree) heart block, while Type I is more likely to be benign.

Third-degree AV block

Third-degree AV block represents complete failure of conduction of the atrial impulses to the ventricles. There is AV dissociation; the atria and ventricles beat completely independently (Figure 3-14) and the atrial rate is faster than the ventricular rate. Generally, the lower the location of the pacemaker within the ventricular conduction system, the slower the rate and the wider the QRS complexes. The etiology may be congenital (isolated or associated with congenital heart disease) or acquired (postoperative, acute rheumatic fever, Lyme disease, streptococcal infection, digoxin toxicity, or hyper- and hypocalcemia).

Many patients with congenital third-degree heart block are asymptomatic. However, a patient may exhibit decreased exercise tolerance, congestive heart failure, dizziness, or syncope. Acquired complete heart block is usually symptomatic, with syncope, congestive

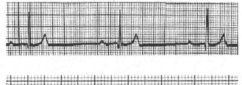

Figure 3-11. First-degree heart block.

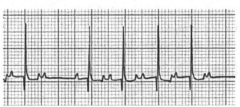

Figure 3-12. Mobitz I second-degree heart block.

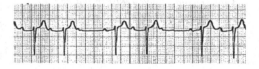

Figure 3-13. Mobitz II second-degree heart block.

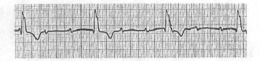

Figure 3-14. Third-degree heart block.

heart failure, shock, or sudden death. These are more likely in a patient with an awake pulse <50 bpm, VPCs, structural heart disease, and cardiomegaly.

ED management

First-degree AV block

No treatment is required other than determining the etiology of the disturbance.

Second-degree AV block

No intervention is needed for Type 1 block. For Type 2, in addition to determining the etiology, an ambulatory 24 hour Holter ECG is indicated. Admit symptomatic patients (dizzy spells or syncope) and consult a pediatric cardiologist to evaluate for possible pacemaker implantation.

Third-degree AV block

Congenital complete heart block usually requires pacemaker insertion eventually. Infants with congestive heart failure, hydrops, rates <50 bpm, or premature ventricular contractions require pacing. Older children or adolescents with congenital complete AV block and dizziness, syncope, exercise intolerance, or VPCs require pacing. Patients with acquired third-degree block require temporary or permanent pacing. The ventricular rate may occasionally be increased by β-adrenergic agents (isoproterenol) or vagolytics (atropine) in patients with reversible AV block (Lyme disease or ingestion) or while awaiting permanent pacemaker placement. Consult a pediatric cardiologist prior to instituting pharmacotherapy.

Follow-up

- Cardiology follow-up of newly diagnosed first- or second-degree AV block within one week

Indications for admission

- First degree: marked PR interval prolongation
- Second degree: newly diagnosed, postoperative, or symptomatic
- Third degree: newly diagnosed, congestive failure, or syncope

Bibliography

Denjoy I, Lupoglazoff JM, Guicheney P, Leenhardt A: Arrhythmic sudden death in children. *Arch Cardiovasc Dis* 2008; 101:121–5.

Doniger SJ, Sharieff GQ: Pediatric dysrhythmias. *Pediatr Clin North Am* 2006;53:85–105.

Kannakeril PJ, Fish FA: Disorders of cardiac rhythm and conduction. In Allen HD, Driscoll DJ, Shaddy RE, Feltes TF (eds), *Moss and Adams' Heart Disease in Infants, Children, and Adolescents: Including the Fetus and Young Adult*, 7th ed. Philadelphia: Lippincott, Williams & Wilkins, 2008, pp. 293–342.

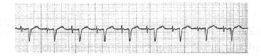

Figure 3-15. Pacemaker spikes.

Pacemaker and defibrillator assessment

An increasing number of children have permanent pacemakers or implanted defibrillators. These patients may have congenital complete heart block, cardiac channelopathy, or congenital or acquired cardiomyopathy, or may have had cardiac surgery.

Clinical presentation and diagnosis

Patients may present with palpitations, dizziness, syncope, or collapse, and may report the sensation of receiving a therapeutic shock. Obtain an ECG or place the patient on a monitor to determine the cardiac rhythm, but interrogation of the implanted device using a manufacturer-specific interrogation/programming device is also necessary for the accurate diagnosis of device function.

ED management

Pacemaker
Assess the ECG for pacemaker activity, rhythm, and rate (Figure 3-15). If heart rate is inadequate for cardiac output, emergency external pacing may be necessary. Contact a pediatric cardiologist or the local manufacturer's representative for interrogation of pacemaker parameters. Some pacemaker issues can be solved with reprogramming, while others will require change of lead and/or device.

Defibrillator
If the patient is stable, consult a pediatric cardiologist to assess the urgency of interrogation of the device and advisability of adjustments in medical therapy.

Follow-up

- As per the pediatric cardiologist, based upon the nature of the device problem and whether it can be solved by reprogramming

Indications for admission

- Significant problem with pacemaker, defibrillator, or lead that cannot be solved with reprogramming
- Ongoing symptoms that indicate either continuous or intermittent hemodynamic instability or the potential for life-threatening dysrhythmia

Bibliography

Silka MJ, Bar-Cohen Y: Pacemakers and implantable cardioverter-defibrillators in pediatric patients. *Heart Rhythm* 2006;3:1360–6.

Silvetti MS: Pacemaker and implantable cardioverter defibrillator implantation in pediatric patients. *Minerva Cardioangiol* 2007;55:803–13.

Chest pain

Chest pain is a common complaint in late childhood and adolescence. While it is often a manifestation of underlying cardiac disease in the adult population, this association is relatively infrequent in younger patients. In children chest pain is commonly associated with asthma and musculoskeletal conditions. However, at times, it is important to rule out a cardiac etiology.

Clinical presentation and diagnosis

Note the characteristics of the pain, including the subjective quality (e.g., sharp, dull, aching), the position in which it is greatest, radiation, duration, and alleviating or exacerbating factors. Cardiac pain is typically associated with exercise and improves with rest. Associated symptoms may be especially useful in determining the etiology of the pain. Also ask about a family history of sudden death (particularly during exercise), cardiomyopathy, or "heart attacks" at early ages.

Noncardiac etiologies

Musculoskeletal problems

Musculoskeletal problems are common causes of chest pain in the pediatric population. Tietze's syndrome (costochondritis) is characterized by anterior chest pain and tenderness to palpation over the sternocostal or costochondral junctions. Reproduction of the patient's pain on palpation is the most helpful sign. Intercostal muscle cramping (precordial catch syndrome) in the left substernal area may mimic this condition.

Psychogenic causes

Although psychogenic causes are the second most frequent, always consider them to be diagnoses of exclusion. Adolescents with hyperventilation or anxiety can present with chest pain. The history may reveal repeated episodes of hysterical behavior, recent personal or family stresses, or a relative with heart disease. Typical complaints include shortness of breath, palpitations, or tingling of the extremities. The pain often mimics one or more organic conditions, but usually it suggests several conditions in the differential diagnosis.

Pulmonary chest pain

Chest pain can be pleuritic in nature, exacerbated by deep inspiration, swallowing, and coughing. It is caused by inflammation or irritation of the pleura, and is seen most commonly in pneumonia, pleurodynia (Coxsackie virus), or pneumothorax. Pulmonary embolism or infarction can present similarly. Bronchospasm may be the most common pulmonary cause of chest pain. A careful history of associated symptoms (fever, cough, preceding upper respiratory infection), oral contraceptive use, and underlying chronic disease (sickle cell anemia, cystic fibrosis, asthma, lupus) is useful for differentiating among these etiologies.

Gastroesophageal disease

Gastrointestinal reflux (GERD), esophagitis, gastritis, and gastrointestinal spasm can all cause precordial pain. While upper esophageal pain is usually well localized, mid- and lower esophageal pain may be noted from the epigastrium to the suprasternal notch and radiate to the back or arms. The heart and esophagus have similar segmental innervation, so the substernal "burning" pain of GERD may mimic angina pectoris, which is distinctly uncommon in the pediatric age group. The discomfort may be associated with eating (postprandially or in the early morning before breakfast), accentuated in the recumbent position and with straining, and relieved with antacids or cold milk.

Cardiac etiologies

Pericarditis

Pericarditis can present with pleuritic-type chest pain that is relieved by sitting up. Patients are often unable to assume the supine position, and the pain is frequently referred to the neck, shoulders, and abdomen. On physical examination a pericardial friction rub may be noted in the midprecordial area with the patient supine or in the left lateral decubitus position. The ECG typically shows ST-segment elevation, and a chest X-ray may reveal cardiomegaly if there is a moderately large pericardial effusion. An echocardiogram is diagnostic in excluding a significant pericardial effusion, but may not be definitive in pericarditis without effusion.

Arrhythmias

Inadequate coronary blood flow secondary to an arrhythmia can cause chest pain.

Prolapse of the mitral valve

Vague anterior chest pain has been described in patients found to have prolapse of the mitral valve, although this occurs much less frequently than previously thought. Rarely, it may be part of a constellation of symptoms in this condition (dyspnea, palpitations, near syncope, and fatigue). The diagnosis is suggested by auscultation (mid-systolic click or clicks and late systolic murmur) and confirmed by two-dimensional echocardiography.

Aortic dissection

Although aortic dissection is extremely rare in childhood, consider it in patients with connective tissue disorders (Marfan's syndrome, Ehlers-Danlos syndrome). The severe pain is typically sudden in onset and "tearing" in quality. Radiation is from the anterior chest to the neck and back.

Coronary artery disease

Coronary artery disease (myocardial ischemia, angina pectoris, myocardial infarction) is extremely rare in the pediatric population. Arteritis and cocaine use may present with the pain of myocardial ischemia or infarction. Severe persistent irritability has been noted in infants with aberrant origin of the left coronary artery from the pulmonary artery; only very rarely do older children present with recurrent episodes of chest pain after exercise. Patients with a history of Kawasaki disease, who can be at risk for coronary artery thrombosis and aneurysm, may present with pallor, diaphoresis, or irritability. Coronary artery spasm leading to myocardial ischemia can also be seen, most commonly in teenagers.

ED management

Most cases of chest pain are either musculoskeletal, gastroesophageal, pulmonary, or psychogenic in origin. Therefore, a careful history, palpation of the chest wall, and pulmonary and cardiac auscultation usually suffice to determine the etiology and initiate appropriate therapy. Ask an adolescent about the possibility of recent cocaine use. Treat costochondritis with ibuprofen 10 mg/kg q 6 h.

If a cardiac etiology is suspected (irregular pulse, auscultation of an organic murmur, a systolic click, or a friction rub) obtain an ECG and check for ST- or T-wave abnormalities, chamber enlargement or hypertrophy, conduction abnormality, or arrhythmia. Many patients with noncardiac chest pain are concerned about the possibility of heart disease and are reassured by a normal ECG.

Further evaluation is dictated by the history and physical findings. A chest X-ray is indicated for patients with pleuritic chest pain, dyspnea, tachycardia, or cyanosis. Obtain a CBC, ESR, CRP, and ECG if acute pericarditis or myocarditis is suspected, and serial troponins if myocardial infarction is a possibility. An echocardiogram, while usually not required for assessment of chest pain in children, can be helpful if these specific conditions are being considered. If mitral valve prolapse or intermittent arrhythmia is suspected, refer the patient to a cardiologist for a nonemergent evaluation.

Follow-up

- Stable patient with noncardiac chest pain: primary care follow-up in 1–2 weeks

Indications for admission

- Suspected coronary artery disease, pleural effusion, myocarditis, pericarditis, or aortic dissection
- Severe chest pain of unknown etiology

Bibliography

Cava JR, Sayger PL: Chest pain in children and adolescents. *Pediatr Clin North Am* 2004;51:1553–68.

Ringstrom E, Freedman J: Approach to undifferentiated chest pain in the emergency department: a review of recent medical literature and published practice guidelines. *Mt Sinai J Med* 2006;73:499–505.

Singh AM, McGregor RS: Differential diagnosis of chest symptoms in the athlete. *Clin Rev Allergy Immunol* 2005;29:87–96.

Congestive heart failure

By definition, congestive heart failure (CHF) occurs when the heart cannot maintain adequate tissue perfusion to meet the body's basal metabolic requirements, which in children includes growth.

Four principal factors determine cardiac function: preload (ventricular end diastolic volume), contractility (force of ventricular contraction), afterload (force opposing ventricular ejection or intramyocardial tension during ejection), and heart rate. Changes in heart rate or stroke volume directly affect cardiac output, which, in turn, is a major determinant of blood pressure.

Table 3-2. Etiologies of congestive heart failure

Congenital heart disease	*Extracardiac diseases*
Structural problems	Metabolic-endocrine diseases
Left ventricular outflow obstruction	Hypoglycemia
Coarctation of the aorta	Hypocalcemia
Critical aortic stenosis	Electrolyte disorders
Large shunt lesions	Hypothyroidism and thyroid storm
Severe valvular regurgitation	Sepsis
Rhythm disorders	Lipid disorders
Postoperative cardiac problems	
Ischemic cardiomyopathy	*Toxins*
AV valve regurgitation	Primary cardiac medicines
	Cancer chemotherapy (adriamycin)
Acquired heart diseases	Digoxin
Inflammatory conditions	Antiarrhythmics
Myocarditis	Cocaine
Kawasaki disease	Cardiac depressants
Rheumatic fever	Phenytoin
Cardiomyopathy	Lidocaine
Endocarditis	

In general, physiologic problems include excessive pressure loads, excessive volume loads, inotropic depression from impaired muscle, and rhythm disturbances. Either congenital structural heart defects or acquired diseases affecting the strength of the heart muscle, or both, can lead to CHF (Table 3-2).

Clinical presentation

The clinical manifestations of CHF reflect physiologic adjustments to reduced cardiac function. These include mechanical (hypertrophy and dilatation), biochemical (cardiac cellular energetic changes), neurohumoral (adrenergic nervous system), hematologic (oxygen transport effects), and pulmonary (tachypnea) responses.

On examination, the patient is usually tachycardic and tachypneic. Pulmonary congestion causes rales, rhonchi, and wheezing which may be confused with primary pulmonary disease. In infants, rales may be absent despite considerable tachypnea, while in older children dyspnea on exertion or orthopnea may be present. A chronic cough may also be associated with the pulmonary congestion.

On cardiac auscultation, there may be a third heart sound (S_3), the ventricular gallop, which is a sign of poor ventricular compliance and increased resistance to filling. A fourth heart sound (S_4), the atrial gallop, can also be heard, particularly in older children, although sometimes both of these can be present with otherwise normal cardiac findings. Not infrequently, a holosystolic, blowing murmur associated with mitral regurgitation can be heard, associated with left ventricular dilatation.

There may also be central and peripheral edema, although this is unusual in infants. Liver enlargement, jugular venous distension, and other signs of tissue fluid accumulation may be seen. The extremities may be pale and cool secondary to compensatory vasoconstriction. Pulsus alternans (beat-to-beat variability in pulse strength) may also be a palpable sign of poor myocardial strength. With chronic CHF, growth failure, especially in young infants, reflects increased caloric expenditure as well as undernutrition associated with feeding difficulties. CHF can also be associated with tachypnea and diaphoresis, particularly during feeding in the infant.

Cardiac enlargement results from ventricular dilatation and is usually readily apparent, along with pulmonary congestion, on the chest X-ray. Often, cardiomegaly can also be detected by palpation of a laterally displaced cardiac impulse. Cardiac hypertrophy is usually easily noted on an ECG (left or combined ventricular hypertrophy).

Diagnosis

Obtain a thorough history, as the presence of preexisting cardiac disease or of conditions related to myocardial dysfunction can be important indicators of the possibility of CHF. Ask about a history of thalassemia or other chronic anemia; systemic infections such as HIV; systemic illnesses such as collagen vascular disease or metabolic diseases; or other acquired diseases such as rheumatic fever or Kawasaki disease.

Often, an older child with overt CHF presents with a combination of wheezing, respiratory distress, bibasilar rales, and hepatomegaly. In general, however, wheezing is most often secondary to asthma. There may be a history of asthma and allergies, or a family history of allergies, or the patient may have eczema. Bronchiolitis also causes similar findings during seasonal epidemics. The patient may have fever, rhonchi, and rales in addition to wheezing.

Other causes of tachypnea, respiratory distress, and cough are pneumonia (fever, localized fine end-inspiratory rales, no hepatomegaly), croup (fever, inspiratory stridor), and foreign-body aspiration (sudden onset of inspiratory stridor). Most etiologies of hepatomegaly (pp. 248–249) are not associated with tachypnea or respiratory distress. When the diagnosis is in doubt, obtain a chest X-ray to look for cardiomegaly and pulmonary vascular congestion.

ED management

Although the etiology dictates the specific therapy, begin with general treatment. Give supplemental humidified oxygen and elevate the head and shoulders. Start an IV and obtain blood for an ABG, electrolytes, and a CBC. Obtain an ECG early in the course, as therapy for an underlying arrhythmia may be necessary. Inquire about the chronic use of cardiac medications. Consult with a cardiologist to help confirm the diagnosis and develop a specific treatment strategy. The patient may be discharged once the CHF is compensated and the vital signs are stable, as long as appropriate cardiac follow-up is arranged.

Give IV diuretics (furosemide 1–2 mg/kg), unless pericardial tamponade (pp. 719–720) is suspected. Give morphine sulfate (0.05–0.1 mg/kg subcutaneously) if there is pulmonary edema and consequent air hunger and restlessness. A slow transfusion of packed RBCs (10 mL/kg) is indicated for severe anemia (hematocrit <28%). Give sodium bicarbonate

Table 3-3. Treatment of congestive heart failure

Preload reduction (diuretics)	
Furosemide	1 mg/kg PO or IV, up to qid
Hydochlorthiazide	2 mg/kg PO, up to bid
Metalozone	0.2 mg/kg PO, up to bid
Afterload reduction	
Captopril	0.1–0.5 mg/kg PO q 8 h
Enalapril	0.1 mg/kg PO, up to bid (0.5 mg/kg per day maximum)
Milrinone	0.5–1 mcg/kg per min IV
Nitroprusside	0.5–10 mcg/kg per min IV
Inotropic agents	
Dopamine	5–25 mcg/kg per min IV
Dobutamine	5–25 mcg/kg per min IV
Digoxin (IV doses are 75% of PO)	
Premature babies	0.005 mg/kg per day div bid
0–10 years	0.10 mg/kg per day PO div bid
>10 years	0.005 mg/kg per day PO per day

(1–2 mEq/kg) only for severe acidosis (pH <7.2); the airway must be secure since respiratory decompensation may elevate the pCO_2 and cerebral edema can develop.

Occasionally, respiratory support including intubation and mechanical ventilation may be required; inotropic support is then usually needed, also. In the acute setting, dobutamine or dopamine (3–5 mcg/kg per min) is preferred. Digoxin may also be given, but its onset of action is longer and specific control over dosage is less precise. In severe cases, addition of afterload-reducing agents (nitroprusside or enalapril) may be required, once indwelling pressure monitoring has been secured and a cardiologist is present (Table 3-3).

Two-dimensional echocardiography may help identify the cause of the CHF and document the magnitude of the decrease in ventricular function (ejection fraction), as well as the extent of cardiac chamber enlargement and valvar regurgitation. Long-term management usually includes an ACE inhibitor or beta-blocker.

Follow-up
- CHF successfully treated in the ED: 1–2 days

Indications for admission
- Newly diagnosed or worsening CHF
- New arrhythmia or a newly acquired complication, such as endocarditis, which requires urgent attention

Bibliography

Schweigmann U, Meierhofer C: Strategies for the treatment of acute heart failure in children. *Minerva Cardioangiol* 2008; 56:321–33.

Shaddy RE, Tani LY: Chronic congestive heart failure. In Allen HD, Driscoll DJ, Shaddy RE, Feltes TF (eds), *Moss and Adams' Heart Disease in Infants, Children, and Adolescents: Including the Fetus and Young Adult*, 7th ed. Philadelphia: Lippincott, Williams & Wilkins, 2008, pp. 1495–1504.

Shaddy RE, Wernovsky, G: *Pediatric Heart Failure*. New York: Marcel Dekker, 2005.

Cyanosis

Cyanosis specifically refers to a bluish tone visible in the mucous membranes and skin when desaturated or abnormal hemoglobin is present in the peripheral circulation. At least 5 g/dL of reduced hemoglobin is required for cyanosis to be visible. Thus, systemic desaturation may be substantial but inapparent to the eye if there is an associated anemia. Conversely, abnormal hemoglobins may be fully saturated with oxygen, yet unable to release it to the tissues, so cyanosis will also be visible. Methemoglobinemia is the classic example of this situation.

Central cyanosis occurs when poorly oxygenated blood enters the systemic circulation. This usually occurs through a cardiac defect allowing systemic venous blood to bypass the pulmonary capillary bed. This is termed a "right-to-left" shunt and may occur within the heart or in the pulmonary circulation itself. When there is primary parenchymal lung disease or neurologic disease causing alveolar hypoventilation, an "intrapulmonary" right-to-left shunt can occur.

Typical cyanotic lesions are the "five Ts" of congenital heart disease (tetralogy of Fallot, transposition of the great vessels, total anomalous pulmonary venous return, tricuspid atresia, and truncus arteriosus), but others may also be present. Pulmonary diseases causing cyanosis can occur anywhere along the airway, from upper airway obstructive problems (croup, epiglottitis) to lower airway diseases (asthma, cystic fibrosis, pneumonia with lobar consolidation).

Peripheral cyanosis, on the other hand, usually does not reflect reduced systemic arterial oxygenation but is typically found in otherwise healthy patients who are exposed to cold or who have a vasoconstrictor response to fever. Peripheral cyanosis, visible particularly in the nail beds but absent from the perioral mucous membranes or conjunctivae, can also occur as a result of circulatory insufficiency or chronic neuromuscular disease with changes in peripheral vasomotor tone.

Clinical presentation and diagnosis

Observation for the presence of cyanosis requires proper ambient conditions. Neon lighting, for example, may cause a false bluish tint, while cyanosis may be difficult to discern in a dark-skinned patient unless there is a strong light source.

Respiratory findings are of vital importance and may help to differentiate among the possible causes of cyanosis. Tachypnea may be present with most pulmonary diseases or with cardiac conditions associated with excess pulmonary blood flow. Shallow respirations, not necessarily associated with an increase in rate, may indicate a neurologic problem. Hyperpnea, or deep breathing with only a mild increase in rate, is more characteristic of a primary cardiac disorder where alveolar ventilation is maximized but pulmonary blood flow is reduced. Hyperpnea can also reflect metabolic acidosis or elevated intracranial pressure.

Differentiating cardiac from pulmonary etiologies is critical. In many, though not all, cases of cardiac disease the breath sounds will be normal and the pattern of chest excursions symmetric, while wheezes, rhonchi, and chest wall abnormalities usually accompany a pulmonary process. In either case there is reduced oxygen saturation, but the patient with cyanotic cardiac disease has little response to increased ambient oxygen, whereas with pulmonary disease the saturation increase may be dramatic (hyperoxia test). An ABG may also be useful, since an elevated pCO_2 indicating impaired ventilatory status is usually not seen with cyanotic congenital heart disease unless there is associated pulmonary congestion. The chest X-ray may reveal cardiomegaly, an abnormal pulmonary circulatory pattern, or overt pulmonary parenchymal abnormalities such as atelectasis or pneumothorax.

The absence of a heart murmur does not rule out cyanotic cardiac disease; in most conditions with right-to-left shunting there is no murmur. Also, in some conditions, such as tetralogy of Fallot, the murmur may lessen as the cyanosis becomes more intense secondary to decreased pulmonary blood flow.

ED management

See p. 62 for the treatment of an acute hypoxemic attack ("spell"). For chronic cyanotic congenital heart conditions, supportive treatment is all that can be done until a surgical or catheter-directed intervention can be accomplished. Give supplemental oxygen, even though dramatic changes in saturation will not occur with oxygen alone. Secure IV access and give fluid to maintain an adequate circulating volume. Treat systemic acidosis once adequate ventilation is ensured. Most of all, immediately consult with a cardiologist to arrange for more definitive treatment and to prevent unnecessary interventions.

Indication for admission

• Central cyanosis

Bibliography

Shrivastava S: Blue babies: when to intervene. *Indian J Pediatr* 2005;72:599–602.

Silberbach M, Hannon D: Presentation of congenital heart disease in the neonate and young infant. *Pediatr Rev* 2007; 28:123–31.

Cyanotic (Tet) spells

Acute hypoxemic attacks represent a true emergency and initial treatment is crucial to long-term outcome. Usually, the underlying diagnosis is tetralogy of Fallot, or a variant, and hence the pseudonym for these attacks is Tet spells.

In a Tet spell, an acute increase in obstruction to pulmonary blood flow has occurred, either at the level of the right ventricular outflow tract within the heart or at the level of the pulmonary circulation, with a consequent increase in right-to-left shunting through an intracardiac septal defect. Alternatively, if systemic perfusion is reduced, as with hypovolemia or the development of a tachyarrhythmia, right-to-left shunting will also increase and a cyanotic spell develop.

Clinical presentation and diagnosis

Spells are particularly common in the early morning, shortly after the patient awakens, when there is a rapid shift in circulatory dynamics from the recumbent sleeping state. Prolonged agitation and crying are also cited as precipitants, but it is sometimes unclear whether the developing hypoxemia itself has caused the agitated state which is then first noticed by the parent. Also, noxious stimuli, such as phlebotomy or a bee sting, or any circumstance which leads to enhanced catecholamine output can precipitate a spell in a susceptible child.

When caring for an acutely hypoxemic infant or child, inquire about a history of congenital heart disease, which raises the possibility that a spell has occurred. Rapid diagnosis of the presence of any form of tetralogy of Fallot is a priority. Obtain a chest X-ray, which may reveal poor pulmonary blood flow and the typical "coeur en sabot" (boot-shaped heart), while the pulmonary parenchyma will be normal. Obtain an ECG to document right ventricular hypertrophy and a rightward axis and to rule out an underlying tachyarrhythmia. In such cases, the absence of a heart murmur is a worrisome indicator that pulmonary blood flow is severely compromised.

ED management

Management is directed at manipulating the relative resistances of the systemic and pulmonary vascular beds, as well as maintenance of appropriate circulating volume and heart rate. Flex the child's knees to the chest to help raise systemic tone. Some older patients will instinctively squat to achieve the same result. Give 100% oxygen, which also increases systemic resistance and may help enhance oxygen delivery. Treat any underlying arrhythmia and correct hypovolemia.

If oxygen and position changes do not break the spell, establish IV access and give morphine sulfate (0.1 mg/kg IV or subcutaneously). Although the precise mechanism of action is unclear, morphine may cause pulmonary vasodilatation and also provide a beneficial sedative effect, with consequent reduction of catecholamine secretion.

If the patient fails to demonstrate improved oxygen saturation promptly or is obtunded, give an IV fluid bolus of 20 mL/kg normal saline and obtain an ABG. Treat metabolic acidosis with sodium bicarbonate, 1–2 mEq/kg slowly IV, only if ventilation is adequate (low or normal pCO_2). If cyanosis persists, give phenylephrine (10 mcg/kg by slow IV push) to pharmacologically increase the systemic vascular resistance. Intubation and mechanical ventilation may also be necessary in severe, protracted spells.

Follow-up

• Tet spell not requiring admission: 24–48 hours

Indication for admission

• Any hypoxemic attack requiring medical attention (not responding to simple position maneuvers)

Bibliography

Shrivastava S: Blue babies: when to intervene. *Indian J Pediatr* 2005;72:599–602.

Silberbach M, Hannon D: Presentation of congenital heart disease in the neonate and young infant. *Pediatr Rev* 2007; 28:123–31.

Heart murmurs

Although congenital heart disease is present in only about 0.8% of the general population, the prevalence of heart murmurs in children approaches 50–60%, or more. Most murmurs, therefore, are "innocent" or "functional," and not pathologic.

Clinical presentation and diagnosis

Innocent (functional) murmur

Most innocent murmurs are mid-systolic, short in duration (end well before the second heart sound), and mid-frequency or "vibratory" in quality. The intensity is ≤ grade III/VI and changes with position or Valsalva maneuver. They may be heard at the apex or the base and are not associated with other findings suggestive of cardiovascular disease (wide, fixed, or paradoxical splitting of S_2; ejection click). Innocent murmurs may be increased in intensity with conditions associated with increase stroke volume, such as fever, anemia, and hyperthyroidism. Types of innocent murmurs include the following.

Still's murmur

Still's murmur occurs in over 50% of children between 4 and 10 years of age. It is vibratory, musical, or twanging, heard best in the midprecordium between the lower left sternal border and the apex; and generally grade II–III/VI in intensity. There is a normal S_2, no ejection click, and no thrill.

Pulmonic ejection murmur

A pulmonic ejection murmur is noted most often in older children and young adolescents. It is early to midsystolic, diamond-shaped, grade I–III/VI in intensity, and vibratory in quality. It is best detected in the second left intercostal space. There is a normal S_2, and no thrill, click, or diastolic murmur.

Venous hum

A venous hum can be appreciated in over 60% of children 3–6 years of age. It is heard best in the infraclavicular area, especially on the right. It is continuous in timing with diastolic accentuation, vibratory and generally grade I–II/VI in intensity. The loudness changes with rotation of the head and generally disappears with lying down or with compression of the jugular vein. Release of pressure may cause accentuation of the murmur for a few seconds. There is no thrill, systolic accentuation, or increased peripheral pulsation.

Organic murmurs

In contrast to the conditions described above, organic murmurs are the result of turbulent blood flow through abnormal cardiac structures or communications. Murmurs which are diastolic (other than a venous hum); right-sided; holosystolic; harsh in quality; associated with a thrill, ejection click, or fixed S_2 splitting; or accompanied by physical findings consistent with heart disease (cyanosis, clubbing, absent lower extremity pulses, signs of congestive heart failure) suggest that a murmur is organic.

ED management

A murmur itself does not require acute management. Rather, intervention may be necessary for the underlying disease causing the murmur (such as endocarditis). Refer all patients with murmurs that do not meet the strict criteria of an innocent or functional murmur to a pediatric cardiologist.

Per the revised American Heart Association guidelines, very few patients with organic murmurs require SBE prophylaxis prior to procedures. Patients with murmurs secondary to rheumatic heart disease do require rheumatic fever prophylaxis.

Indications for admission
- Signs of congestive heart failure or acute rheumatic fever
- Suspected or proven infective endocarditis

Bibliography
Biancaniello T: Innocent murmurs. *Circulation* 2005;111(3):e20–2.

Menashe V: Heart murmurs. *Pediatr Rev* 2007; 28:e19–22.

Poddar B, Basu S: Approach to a child with a heart murmur. *Indian J Pediatr* 2004;71:63–6.

Infective endocarditis

Infective endocarditis (IE) is an infection of the endothelium of the heart valves or great vessels. It is most commonly subacute, developing in patients with preexisting congenital heart disease, particularly valvular anomalies (aortic stenosis, prosthetic valve) and conditions associated with increased turbulence of blood flow (ventricular septal defect, aortic regurgitation). In this regard, conditions such as isolated secundum atrial septal defect are not likely to be related to IE.

A substantial percentage of IE cases occur in patients with no preexisting cardiac anomaly. These children have developed acute bacterial endocarditis and may suddenly become extremely ill.

For IE to occur, the endocardium must be exposed to potentially pathogenic bacteria. Dental treatments can result in bacteremia even without periodontal disease. Similarly, certain surgical procedures (tonsillectomy, urologic surgery) or the presence of a chronic indwelling parenteral catheter also place the patient at risk.

Clinical presentation and diagnosis

Diligence is required to suspect and treat IE and to refrain from other incorrect therapy. Inquire about any factors establishing a milieu for IE, particularly recent dental and surgical procedures, the presence of a venous catheter, and IV drug use.

Although fever in any patient with congenital heart disease raises the possibility of IE, certain situations are particularly worrisome. These are a protracted febrile illness, particularly without any obvious focus, even if thought to be of "viral" etiology; a documented change in the clinical picture, such as the development of a new heart murmur or congestive heart failure; the onset of hematuria; signs of either cutaneous emboli or embolic events to other organs; a new neurologic finding; or a focal infection such as pneumonia or meningitis.

Frequently, early signs and symptoms may be subtle. Classic findings such as change in a murmur, evidence of emboli, and splenomegaly may not be easily discernible. Nonetheless, carefully examine the conjunctivae, nail beds, palms, soles of the feet, and other skin surfaces to search for evidence of emboli, including tender nodules in the finger or toe pads (Osler nodes), small hemorrhages on the palms or soles (Janeway lesions), and linear subungual lesions (splinter hemorrhages). Perform a careful fundoscopic exam and serial auscultations, as murmurs may be transient and change may be rapid. Conversely, in fulminant acute IE, only the signs of severely compromised circulatory status may be present, without any heart murmur.

Obtain blood for a CBC, ESR, CRP, multiple blood cultures, as well as a urinalysis. The diagnosis is ultimately confirmed by obtaining positive blood cultures and/or positive findings on an echocardiogram. There may be a leukocytosis with a leftward shift, anemia, and elevation of the ESR and CRP. The urinalysis may reveal pyuria, hematuria, and proteinuria, as infective endocarditis is a cause of immune complex nephritis. Scrape any cutaneous emboli and examine after Gram's staining. If IE is being considered, consult a cardiologist to arrange for a two-dimensional echocardiogram. If a vegetation is identified, the study can indicate the diagnosis, even before the blood results have become available.

ED management

While it may sometimes be crucial to initiate treatment rapidly, it is always imperative that an alternative diagnosis not be obscured. The treatment of IE involves protracted use of appropriate antibiotics, depending on culture and sensitivity results. Attempt to obtain at least two sets of blood cultures from any febrile child at risk for IE (congenital heart disease, normal heart but chronic indwelling catheter) before antibiotics are administered. Once the cultures have been obtained give broad-spectrum IV antibiotics such as penicillin (200 000 units/kg per day div q 4 h, 18 million units/day maximum) or ceftriaxone (100 mg/kg per day, 4 g/day maximum) combined with gentamicin (3 mg/kg per day div q 8 h, 240 mg/day maximum). If there is particular suspicion for a Gram-negative organism, such as in an immunocompromised patient, use ampicillin (300 mg/kg per day div q 6 h, 12 g/day maximum) or ceftriaxone combined with gentamicin.

These recommendations may not be adequate for patients with prosthetic heart valves or other special considerations. Consult with an infectious disease expert before initiation of therapy.

Endocarditis prophylaxis

Children with congenital and acquired heart disease may require an urgent invasive procedure. In 2007, the American Heart Association, and others, published new guidelines for the consideration of appropriate antibiotics for infectious endocarditis prophylaxis. This statement dramatically changed the recommendations, so that prophylactic antibiotics are no longer indicated solely to prevent endocarditis for any genitourinary or gastrointestinal procedure. For respiratory tract procedures, if incision and/or biopsy of the respiratory mucosa is involved, give oral amoxicillin (50 mg/kg, 2 g maximum), parenteral ampicillin (50 mg/kg, 2 g maximum) or parenteral ceftriaxone (50 mg/kg, 1 g maximum). Recommendations for prophylaxis extend only to patients with prosthetic valves or conduits, previous IE, unrepaired cyanotic heart disease (even with a shunt in place), repaired congenital heart disease within the first 6 months of surgery or with a residual defect, and cardiac transplant recipients with a valvulopathy in the new heart.

Indication for admission

- Suspected or proven infective endocarditis

Bibliography

Hoyer A, Silberbach M: Infective endocarditis. *Pediatr Rev* 2005;26:394–400.

Ishiwada N, Niwa K, Tateno S, et al: Causative organism influences clinical profile and outcome of infective endocarditis in pediatric patients and adults with congenital heart disease. *Circ J* 2005;69:1266–70.

Wilson W, Taubert KA, Gewitz MH, et al: Prevention of infective endocarditis: guidelines from the American Heart Association. *Circulation* 2007;116:1736–54.

Pericardial disease

Three distinct disease processes can involve the pericardium: pericarditis, pericardial effusion, and pericardial tamponade. Infections are the most common etiology of pericardial diseases, but there are a variety of other causes in childhood (Table 3-4).

Pericarditis

Pericarditis is inflammation of the pericardium (infectious or noninfectious).

Pericardial effusion

A pericardial effusion is the accumulation of fluid in the pericardial space.

Pericardial tamponade

Pericardial tamponade is impaired cardiac output secondary to reduced ventricular filling. This is caused either by fluid accumulation in the pericardial space or by constriction of the heart from an abnormally thickened pericardium. The rapid accumulation of a small amount of fluid can produce tamponade, while chronic slow accumulation is more readily tolerated.

Clinical presentation and diagnosis

Pericarditis

Chest pain is the initial symptom in acute pericarditis. It is a constant, sharp sensation across the anterior precordium and is frequently associated with shoulder discomfort. The pain varies with position, being worse when supine and relieved when upright. Respiratory symptoms, particularly tachypnea, typically accompany the pain. There is often a history of a preceding URI. Fever is usually present and the patient may also complain of abdominal pain. There may be a history of open heart surgery in the past 10–14 days (post pericardiotomy syndrome).

Pericardial effusion

When a substantial pericardial effusion is present, the symptoms may mimic CHF. There may be tachypnea with chest retractions and nasal flaring. With impaired cardiac output, tachycardia and vasoconstriction occur, with pallor, low blood pressure, and cool extremities. Other findings secondary to systemic congestion are hepatosplenomegaly and neck vein distension.

Pericardial tamponade

Cardiac tamponade is a true medical emergency. Classic findings include hypotension, distended neck veins, muffled heart sounds, and the presence of pulsus paradoxus, a >10 mmHg fall in systolic blood pressure associated with inspiration. A fall in the blood

Table 3-4. Etiologies of pericarditis

Infections	Traumatic
Bacterial	Postpericardiotomy syndrome
H. influenzae	Chest wall injury
Staphylococcus	
Streptococcus	Oncologic
Pneumococcus	Leukemia
Viral	Lymphoma
Other (tuberculosis, fungal)	
Inflammatory	Other
Rheumatic	Drug induced (minoxidil)
Collagen	Blood dyscrasias

pressure of >20 mmHg is serious. Pulsus paradoxus may also be found in respiratory disorders such as asthma and in congestive heart failure.

On auscultation, findings depend on the amount of fluid accumulation. When inflammation is present without fluid, as in acute pericarditis, there is often a loud friction rub audible. This is a scratchy, harsh sound heard throughout the cardiac cycle. The pericardial rub diminishes in proportion to the volume of fluid collection. The heart sounds in general decrease in intensity in direct proportion to pericardial fluid volume. Particularly ominous is the agitated child with signs of reduced cardiac output and a "quiet" auscultatory examination.

Obtain an ECG and chest X-ray. With pericarditis the ECG reveals elevated ST segments and, often, generalized T-wave inversions. Diminished precordial voltage usually indicates pericardial fluid accumulation. On X-ray, the heart size is increased with pericardial effusion but may be small with pericardial constriction without fluid (constrictive pericarditis). Other laboratory tests are nonspecific. With purulent pericarditis, there is leukocytosis and an elevated ESR and CRP. However, viral diseases will often be associated with normal values of both parameters, and the highest acute-phase reactants can be seen with rheumatologic pericarditis.

ED management
The approach to the child with pericardial disease varies depending on whether there is an effusion.

Pericarditis
For pericarditis without fluid accumulation, invasive treatment is not warranted. Admit the patient, give analgesics (aspirin, ibuprofen, or indomethacin) and observe for the development of complications (effusion, tamponade, myocarditis). Steroids are usually not indicated for initial management.

Pericardial effusion
Closely follow the vital signs and degree of pulsus paradoxus, as pericardial fluid accumulation is usually a dynamic process. Rapidly changing circumstances may precipitate an

acute crisis. Consult a cardiologist and admit the patient. Diagnostic pericardiocentesis may be required, especially if purulent pericarditis is suspected.

If purulent pericarditis is suspected, provide supplemental oxygen, establish IV access, and arrange for pericardiocentesis. Obtain blood and pericardial fluid specimens and begin broad-spectrum antibiotics (nafcillin 150 mg/kg per day div q 6 h and cefotaxime 150–200 mg/kg per day div q 6 h). Substitute vancomycin (40 mg/kg per day div q 6 h) for nafcillin if MRSA is a possibility.

Pericardial tamponade

When a substantial volume of pericardial fluid has accumulated, tamponade can develop rapidly. Arrange for immediate therapeutic drainage.

Indications for admission

- Pericardial effusion (unless chronic)
- Pericarditis
- Pericardial tamponade

Bibliography

Demmler GJ: Infectious pericarditis in children. *Pediatr Infect Dis J* 2006;25:165–6.

Rheuban KS: Pericardial diseases. In Allen HD, Driscoll DJ, Shaddy RE, Feltes TF (eds), *Moss and Adams' Heart Disease in Infants, Children, and Adolescents: Including the Fetus and Young Adult*, 7th ed. Philadelphia: Lippincott Williams & Wilkins, 2008, pp. 1290–98.

Syncope

Syncope is a transient loss of consciousness, accompanied by loss of postural tone, resulting from decreased cerebral perfusion.

Clinical presentation

The unconscious period may be preceded by a history of an inciting factor, such as a noxious stimulus, an excessively warm environment, emotional upset, or exercise. The patient may report a prodrome of dizziness, diaphoresis, headache, chest pain, palpitations, visual or auditory phenomena, respiratory distress, or a history of recurrent episodes. Findings on physical examination may include diaphoresis, hypotension (sometimes postural), tachycardia or bradycardia, lethargy, or dilated pupils. Mechanisms of syncope can be classified into three groups: neurocardiovascular, cardiac, or non-neurocardiovascular.

Neurocardiovascular

Vasovagal

Vasodilatation, with pooling of blood in capacitance vessels, causes decreased blood pressure with a resultant decrease in cerebral perfusion. Usually, an associated increase in vagal tone results in bradycardia and diaphoresis. Vasodepressor syncope is often precipitated by noxious stimuli, strong emotions, or fatigue, and is common in adolescents.

Orthostatic hypotensive syncope

This occurs on assuming an erect posture. It is rare in young children, but not uncommon in normal adolescents. It may also occur if the patient is dehydrated, chronically fatigued or malnourished, has suffered an acute blood loss, or is taking vasodilator drugs. These patients can have tachycardia associated with the syncope, the so-called postural orthostatic tachycardia syndrome.

Cardioinhibitory

Parasympathetic impulses cause a severe bradycardic response.

Cardiac

Although uncommon, cardiac causes of syncope can be life threatening. The mechanism may involve hypoxemia due to cyanotic heart disease or decreased cardiac output secondary to myocardial dysfunction, arrhythmias, or obstructive lesions.

Structural lesions

Syncope can occur in patients with obstructive lesions (severe valvar or subvalvar aortic stenosis, pulmonary hypertension) secondary to low cardiac output, cyanotic heart disease (tetralogy of Fallot) secondary to hypoxia, or mitral valve prolapse. Most of these episodes occur during physical exertion; this history suggests a cardiac etiology. Generally, there are auscultatory abnormalities, such as a murmur or abnormal second heart sound, or evidence of ventricular hypertrophy on electrocardiogram.

Arrhythmias

Arrhythmias such as atrioventricular block (second or third degree) may cause syncope. Sick sinus syndrome is usually seen in the setting of repaired congenital heart disease. These patients may develop syncope secondary to severe bradycardia or sinus arrest. Syncope can also be associated with paroxysmal supraventricular tachycardia, atrial flutter, and atrial fibrillation, especially in patients with Wolff-Parkinson-White syndrome. Ventricular tachycardia or ventricular fibrillation may present with syncope in patients with repaired congenital heart disease, arrhythmogenic right ventricular dysplasia, or primary electrical disease.

Syncope is also associated with long QT syndrome (LQTS), either congenital (the Romano-Ward syndrome, deafness-associated Jervell-Lange-Neilsen syndrome) or acquired, secondary to drugs (antibiotics [clarithromycin, erythromycin], anti-arrhythmics [sotalol, ibutilide, flecainide, quinidine], tricyclic antidepressants, antipsychotics), electrolyte imbalance, or starvation diets. LQTS can lead to a specific dysrhythmia, a polymorphic ventricular tachycardia called torsade de pointes. Consider LQTS in children with a history of syncope and a corrected QT interval >0.45 seconds.

Non-neurocardiovascular syncope

Cerebral hypoxemia

Hypoxia and anemia (rare) can cause syncope secondary to decreased cerebral oxygen delivery despite normal cardiac output. Respiratory causes include breath-holding spells in infants and toddlers and hyperventilation in adolescents. The infant or child with a breath-holding spell becomes pallid or cyanotic before losing consciousness, while hyperventilating adolescents may have paresthesias or carpopedal spasm. In both, there is usually a history of emotional upset.

Hysterical fainting

Hysterical fainting occurs primarily in patients with a histrionic (theatrical) personality style. These episodes can last for up to 1 hour and usually occur in front of others. The pulse and blood pressure are normal, and there is never any associated injury.

Fasting hypoglycemia

Fasting hypoglycemia is the most common metabolic cause of syncope. Inquire about a history of diabetes or insulin use. Weakness, diaphoresis, confusion, and palpitations may occur prior to the actual syncopal episode, which is gradual in onset. Also, aspirin and ethanol ingestion can be associated with hypoglycemia.

Other causes

Consider seizures in the differential diagnosis, although true syncope lacks convulsive movements, an aura, or a postictal state. Frequent episodes of loss of consciousness suggest epilepsy. Migraine headaches involving the vertebral-basilar system can cause syncope, preceded by an aura and followed by the headache.

Diagnosis

A careful history usually suggests the diagnosis. Especially important is a description of the events leading up to the episode, particularly whether the syncope was abrupt and without warning, or preceded by lightheadedness, dizziness, sweating, palpitations, chest pain, or respiratory distress. Cardiac syncope can be sudden, without any warning. Inquire about the frequency of the attacks, any sequelae after the episode, possible drug ingestion, and family history of arrhythmia, syncope, sudden death, or deafness (which may be associated with the LQTS).

On physical examination check for orthostatic vital sign changes, odors on the breath (ethanol, ketones), and murmurs. Most cardiac etiologies can be ruled out by auscultation and a 12-lead ECG with a long rhythm strip. Causative arrhythmias such as supraventricular tachycardia, ventricular tachycardia, sick sinus syndrome, or heart block are usually not present on admission, but underlying predisposing conditions such as WPW and prolonged LQTS may be identified. If these are not found, 24-hour ambulatory monitoring is indicated when the history does not suggest another etiology for the syncope.

ED management

Unless it is clear that the patient suffered a vasovagal episode, obtain an ECG with rhythm strip and blood for hematocrit, Dextrostix, and serum glucose. The diagnosis and management of hypoglycemia (pp. 182–186) and anemia (pp. 332–336) are discussed elsewhere.

Instruct patients with orthostatic syncope to get up slowly after lying or sitting and discontinue any implicated medications. Suggest increased fluid intake, and if the blood pressure is normal, recommend additional salt intake. The autonomic dysfunction can be documented by tilt table testing. Reassurance and primary care follow-up are all that are usually needed for hyperventilation or breath-holding. Consult with a pediatric cardiologist for LQTS, WPW, or other causes of cardiac syncope.

Follow-up
- Vasovagal, hyperventilation, or breathholding episode: primary care follow-up in one week

Indications for admission
- Recurrent syncope
- Cardiac syncope likely
- Significant injury caused by the syncopal episode

Bibliography

Dovgalyuka J, Holstege C, Mattu A, Brady WJ: The electrocardiogram in the patient with syncope. Am J Emerg Med 2008; 26:221–8.

Friedman MJ, Mull CC, Sharieff GQ, Tsarouhas N: Prolonged QT syndrome in children: an uncommon but potentially fatal entity. J Emerg Med 2003;24:173–9.

McLeod KA: Syncope in childhood. Arch Dis Child 2003;88:350–3.

Dental emergencies

Nancy Dougherty

Children frequently present to the emergency department (ED) complaining of oral problems, primarily due to oral trauma or related to dental caries. Many of these problems can be diagnosed and treated by the ED physician, with subsequent referral to a dentist for consultation and/or definitive treatment.

Dental anatomy

A basic knowledge of dental anatomy is necessary for evaluating and treating dental emergencies. The tooth itself is composed of four primary layers. The dental enamel, a mineralized, crystalline material, covers the coronal portion of the tooth. It is the hardest material found in the human body. A somewhat softer material, cementum, forms the outer surface of the root. Underneath the enamel and/or cementum is a less mineralized layer called dentin. The innermost portion of the tooth is the pulp chamber, which contains nerve tissue, as well as the vascular supply for nourishing the tooth structure. Periodontal ligament fibers attach the roots of the tooth to the surrounding alveolar bone. These structures are shown in Figure 4-1.

Dental eruption

Eruption pattern of primary and permanent dentition

Awareness of normal eruption patterns for primary and permanent teeth will assist the physician in making appropriate diagnostic and treatment decisions (Table 4-1). Although the sequence of tooth eruption is fairly constant from child to child, the exact age at which a tooth erupts can vary considerably. Reassure parents that variations of up to 6 months from the average eruption date are within the normal range.

Complaints associated with dental eruption

Teething

Teething can be associated with irritable behavior (due to minor discomfort) and increased drooling. Teething infants often present to the ED with fever and diarrhea, although there is no conclusive evidence that tooth eruption is truly the cause. Therefore, evaluate the patient appropriately, and consider teething a diagnosis of exclusion.

Treat teething pain with a frozen teething toy, but advise the parents to avoid using toys with multiple parts. For more significant pain, recommend acetaminophen (15 mg/kg q 4 h), ibuprofen (10 mg/kg q 6 h), and over-the-counter teething gels containing 10–20% benzocaine.

Eruption cyst or hematoma

An eruption cyst is a fluctuant, fluid-filled sac overlying an erupting primary or permanent tooth. An eruption hematoma will have a reddish appearance due to blood filling the sac.

Table 4-1. Chronology of dental eruption

Tooth	Primary teeth (months)		Permanent teeth (years)	
	Maxillary	Mandibular	Maxillary	Mandibular
Central incisor	7½	6	7–8	6–7
Lateral incisor	9	7	8–9	7–8
Cuspid	18	16	11–12	9–10
First bicuspid	–	–	10–11	10–12
Second bicuspid	–	–	10–12	11–12
First molar	14	12	6–7	6–7
Second molar	24	20	12–13	11–13
Third molar	–	–	17–20	17–21

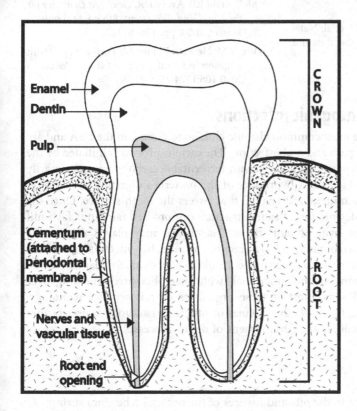

Figure 4-1. Tooth anatomy.

Eruption cysts and hematomas are benign findings and will resolve spontaneously, either through biting pressure or upon eruption of the tooth.

Eruption gingivitis

Localized inflammation of gingival tissue can sometimes be associated with tooth eruption. It is usually self-limited and can be treated with over-the-counter teething gels. However, in adolescents with erupting or impacted wisdom teeth, entrapped debris and micro-organisms may lead to infection (pericoronitis). This can cause localized tenderness and swelling or, in severe cases, fever, facial swelling, trismus, and dysphagia. See Dental abscess (p. 76) for treatment.

Natal and neonatal teeth

Natal teeth are primary teeth that are present at birth. Neonatal teeth refer to teeth that erupt in the first 30 days of life. Both usually erupt in the mandibular incisor area and, in most cases, are part of the normal primary dentition and not supernumerary. Natal and neonatal teeth pose a theoretical aspiration risk, as they often have only rudimentary roots and can be quite mobile. However, no cases of aspiration have been reported in the literature.

Traumatic injury to the infant's tongue may be caused by the sharp incisal edges of these teeth, while trauma to a nursing mother's breast may interfere with feeding. Both of these conditions are indications for extraction and require referral to a dentist.

Bibliography

Cunha RF, Boer FA, Torriani DD, et al: Natal and neonatal teeth: review of the literature. *Ped Dent* 2001;**23**:158–62.

McDonald RE, Avery DR, Dean JA: *Dentistry for the Child and Adolescent*, 8th ed. St. Louis: Mosby, 2004, pp. 176–9, 182.

Wake M, Hesketh K, Lucas J: Teething and tooth eruption in infants: a cohort study. *Pediatrics* 2000;**106**:1374–9.

Dental caries and odontogenic infections

Dental caries (cavities) are the most common chronic childhood disease in the USA and are frequently the cause of dental pain and oral infection. The carious process is initiated by the interaction of the bacteria *Streptococcus mutans* with fermentable carbohydrates, primarily sucrose. The acid that is produced as a byproduct of the bacteria's digestion of carbohy-drates can dissolve the highly mineralized enamel that covers the tooth surface. Once the enamel is destroyed, further destruction of tooth structure can proceed fairly quickly until bacteria infect the innermost layer of pulp tissue. *Lactobacilli* may play a role in the progression of the lesions. Once organisms have reached the pulp, the infection can spread through the root into the adjacent periapical tissue, resulting in a dentoalveolar infection.

Most odontogenic infections are polymicrobial, with anaerobes predominating over aerobes. Under healthy conditions, most of these organisms do not produce pathology. However, local (caries, trauma, foreign body, vascular insufficiency) and/or systemic factors (immune deficiencies) can facilitate the development of dental abscesses.

Clinical presentation
Cavities

Dental caries commonly occur in the pits and fissures of the occlusal (chewing) surfaces of posterior teeth, interproximal surfaces of molars, and smooth tooth surfaces close to the gingiva. They initially appear as dull, opaque, white discolorations which then cavitate and appear as brown holes. Although these lesions may be visible upon oral examination, they often remain asymptomatic until the infection spreads into the pulp tissue, and then present as pain upon eating sweet or cold foods. As the infection spreads, patients frequently report spontaneous pain, often interfering with sleep and eating.

Early childhood caries (ECC)

Previously termed nursing bottle caries, this is a form of rampant caries found in some young children. Recent evidence suggests that ECC is not explained totally by diet or feeding patterns. Typically, the labial and palatal surfaces of the primary maxillary incisors are the first teeth affected. If not treated, the caries can spread to the primary molars. The mandibular incisors are typically spared, except in the most severe cases. Children will often present with gross destruction of the maxillary incisors.

Dental abscess

This is a localized, purulent infection caused by dental pulp necrosis, secondary to either dental caries or trauma to a noncarious tooth. Abscesses can be chronic or acute. Chronic abscess are often asymptomatic, but can become acute, symptomatic lesions. Some painful acute abscesses are not clinically evident and require a radiograph for diagnosis. Others may present with gingival erythema, tooth mobility, tenderness to tooth percussion, soft tissue swelling, and lymphadenopathy. Sometimes, a fistulous tract develops and opens onto the gingival mucosa, forming a parulis (gum boil). This is more common in younger children, whose alveolar bone is relatively less dense.

Pericoronitis

Pericoronitis refers to inflammation or infection of the soft tissues adjacent to a partially erupted tooth. The teeth most commonly associated are the mandibular third molars (wisdom teeth). The condition is caused by food and bacteria becoming trapped under gingival tissue that partially covers the tooth. Symptoms can include localized swelling, pain, and a bad taste in the mouth due to suppuration. Frequently, there is localized lymphadenopathy and cellulitis and trismus can also develop.

Cellulitis

Localized infection from a decayed or traumatized tooth can spread through soft tissues causing cellulitis. This may be accompanied by fever, pain, trismus, and regional lymphadenopathy. Include a thorough oral examination for any patient presenting with a head or neck cellulitis, as the infection may be of odontogenic origin.

Deep fascial space infections

Oral infections can also spread to the deep fascial spaces of the head and neck. Depending on the tooth and drainage area involved, varying degrees of pain, swelling, and trismus occur. In severe cases, involvement of the sublingual, pharyngeal, retropharyngeal, or pretracheal areas can occur, leading to respiratory compromise and/or dysphagia. Ludwig's angina is a condition in which a mandibular dental abscess expands rapidly, crosses the midline, and causes airway compromise. This is usually associated with the permanent molars and is therefore uncommon in young children who have only primary teeth.

Diagnosis

A thorough intraoral evaluation is necessary for any patient with oral pain or head and neck swelling. In the absence of obvious dental caries, inquire about a history of dental trauma or past dental treatment. Inspect the oral cavity for obvious caries, gingival swelling and erythema (possible infected tooth), or a gum boil. Palpate the gums and molar occlusal surfaces for swelling and tenderness, tap each tooth with a tongue blade to identify percussion sensitivity, and check for tooth mobility. Radiographs are indicated if there is no obvious etiology for a swelling, or when numerous carious teeth are present.

ED management

Caries

Refer asymptomatic children with dental caries and no evidence of acute infection to a dentist for comprehensive care. If the patient has dental-related pain, but no soft tissue inflammation or swelling, give analgesics and refer to a dentist as soon as possible (preferably the next day). Do not prescribe antibiotics for such patients.

Localized dental abscess

Consult with a dentist to provide incision and drainage of any fluctuant area. Prescribe pain medication (ibuprofen 10 mg/kg q 6 h), or if severe, acetaminophen with codeine (0.5 mg/kg of codeine q 6 h) and oral antibiotics (penicillin (50 mg/kg per day div qid or clindamycin 20 mg/kg per day div qid), and referral to a dentist as soon as possible (either the same or next day). Pain relief is often achieved by the drainage. Treat localized pericoronitis in the same way as other localized dental abscesses. Additionally, irrigation with saline under the gingival flap that covers the affected tooth may help to alleviate discomfort.

Facial cellulitis or deep fascial space infections

Admit the patient, consult an oral surgeon, and start IV antibiotics. Use either penicillin (100,000 units/kg per day div q 6 h) or clindamycin (40 mg/kg per day div q 6 h). Carefully assess the airway; any suggestion of compromise is an indication for intubation. After initiation of antibiotic therapy, if there is a concern about the extent of a deep fascial space infection, obtain either a CT scan or an MRI.

Indications for admission

- Facial cellulitis involving periorbital region
- Evidence of deep space infection, with potential for airway compromise (sublingual, submandibular, parapharyngeal spaces)
- Systemic involvement, including fever and/or dehydration due to inability or unwillingness to eat and drink
- Patients with immune compromise (HIV, diabetes, steroid therapy, cancer chemotherapy)
- Concern about outpatient adherence to the medical and/or follow-up recommendations

Bibliography

Dahlen G: Microbiology and treatment of dental abscesses and periodontal-endodontic lesions. *Periodontology 2000* 2002;28:206–39.

Douglass AB, Douglass JM. Common dental emergencies. *Am Fam Physician* 2003;67:511–16.

McDonald RE, Avery DR, Dean JA: *Dentistry for the Child and Adolescent*, 8th ed. St. Louis: Mosby, 2004, pp. 205–10.

Oral trauma

Oral trauma is quite common in childhood; up to one-third of 5-year-olds have sustained injury to primary teeth, and one-quarter of 12-year-olds have experienced traumatic injury to permanent teeth. Causes include falls, seizures, sports injuries, motor vehicle accidents, and fights and inflicted injury. Lacerations, contusions, and abrasion of facial soft tissues, gingiva, and intra-oral mucosa are often associated with dental injuries. Fractures to facial bones and the bones that support the dentition can also occur. While dental injuries may be overlooked secondary to distracting injuries in a multiple-trauma victim, injured teeth can suffer permanent damage if not treated expeditiously.

Dental fractures

Treatment of dental fractures in the emergency department is rarely definitive, and any patient presenting with acute dental trauma requires referral to a dentist or oral surgeon within 24 hours. However, appropriate intervention provided in a timely manner in the ED is vital to prevent subsequent tooth loss and infection. See Table 4-2 for the Ellis classification of dental fractures, along with appropriate management. Recommendations for treatment of fractured primary teeth do not differ markedly from those for permanent teeth. However, depending on the age of the child at the time of trauma, and the expected longevity of the primary tooth, many dental practitioners will choose to be less aggressive in attempts to maintain a primary tooth.

Tooth displacement injuries

Oral trauma frequently results in displacement of a tooth from its normal location, rather than fracture. As with fractures, the nature of the displacement and age of the patient will influence treatment decisions. Table 4-3 lists various displacement injuries and appropriate ED treatment.

Oral soft tissue injuries

Lacerations

Lacerations of the lips, tongue, and oral mucosa are common in children of all ages. Lip lacerations which cross the vermilion border may present a cosmetic problem, since precise opposition of the wound margins is necessary for proper repair. Often, a child will present with lacerations of both the inner and outer surface of the lip. It is essential to identify whether these are two separate lesions or are, in fact, a communicating through-and-through laceration. Tongue lacerations occur frequently when children fall and accidentally bite a protruding tongue.

Punctures

Falling while running with an object in the mouth can cause soft tissue punctures. A puncture wound to the palate may represent a significant injury, especially if the soft palate is involved. Of particular concern are deep or dirty wounds, foreign-body contamination, and ongoing bleeding.

Bony fractures

Alveolar bone fractures

The alveoli are the bony processes (in both the maxilla and mandible) into which the teeth are embedded. The most common site for alveolar fractures is in the area of the maxillary

Table 4-2. Ellis classification of dental fractures

Fracture class and type	Presentation	ED management
I: Enamel, only	Piece of tooth edge missing	No acute treatment Elective dental referral
II: Enamel and dentin	Dentin appears yellow	Immediate dental consult
III: Enamel, dentin, and pulp	Pulp appears pink or red	Immediate dental consult
IV: Complete crown (enamel dentin, and pulp)		Immediate dental consult
V: Involves the root		Immediate dental consult if coronal portion of tooth is loose or displaced

Table 4-3. Dental displacement injuries

Injury	Presentation	ED management
Concussion	Tooth is tender to percussion	Soft diet for several days
	Not displaced or mobile	Dental follow-up within a few days
Subluxation	Tooth is tender to percussion	Soft diet for several days
	Not displaced, but is mobile	If tooth is very mobile, consult a dentist for possible splinting in ED
		Dental follow-up within a few days
Intrusion	Tooth is pushed into alveolar bone; ↑ risk of pulp necrosis and root resorption	Do not reposition in ED
		Refer to dentist within 24 hours
Extrusion/ lateral luxation	Tooth is displaced, but not completely avulsed; ↑ risk of pulp necrosis	Minor displacement not interfering with bite: refer to dentist within 24 hours
		Severe displacement and/or mobility:
		Primary tooth: extract
		Permanent tooth: reposition and splint
Avulsion	Tooth is displaced completely from dental arch and/or mouth; ↑ risk of pulp necrosis and root resorption	Primary tooth: do *not* reimplant Permanent tooth:
		Prognosis depends on time tooth is out of the mouth
		Place tooth in Hanks Balanced Salt Solution (HBSS) while awaiting immediate dental consultation

incisors. Clinical findings may include displacement and/or mobility of multiple teeth, along with mobility of the adjacent bone. Gingival bleeding is also commonly seen.

Mandibular fractures

The mandible is a strong cortical bone with several weak areas that are susceptible to fracture. The necks of the condyles (below the temperomandibular joints) and the body of the mandible where the mental foramen are located are common sites for fracture. Frequently, the mandible will sustain multiple fractures resulting from one traumatic event. Clinical findings in mandibular fractures include painful jaw movement, malocclusion of the teeth, inability to close the mouth, and deviation of the mandible to one side during opening. Gingival bleeding, ecchymoses, intraoral edema, and paresthesias may also be present.

Diagnosis

Evaluation of airway, vital signs, mental status, and cranial nerves is essential as part of the initial assessment. Obtain the history of the traumatic event, as well as the past medical history, including tetanus status and allergies. Treatment of life-threatening injuries obviously takes precedence. Once the patient is stabilized, a systematic approach to physical evaluation of the face is necessary so that subtle injuries are not missed.

Extraoral examination

- Inspect the face for asymmetry.
- Evaluate any abrasions, swelling, ecchymoses, and lacerations and check for the presence of foreign bodies.
- Palpate the facial bones for tenderness or discontinuities that may represent a fracture.
- Assess the integrity of the facial skeleton: place one hand on the anterior maxillary teeth and the other on the nasal bridge. Movement of the maxillary incisors and hard palate alone indicate a LeFort I fracture. Movement of the nasal bridge indicates a LeFort II fracture. Movement of the entire face indicates a LeFort III fracture.
- Ask a cooperative patient to bite down hard on a tongue blade. Inability to do so or pain when doing so may indicate a mandibular fracture.
- Note any deviations in mandibular opening and closing, and ask the patient if their bite feels normal.

Intraoral examination

- Evaluate soft tissues for bleeding, swelling, lacerations, and abrasions.
- Thoroughly examine wounds for foreign bodies (including tooth fragments).
- Assess each tooth for mobility and fracture. Suspect an alveolar fracture if several adjacent teeth move as one unit.

Radiologic studies

Depending on the location and severity of the injuries, obtain the following radiologic studies:

- Upper face: axial and coronal CT scan. A skull series and Waters view radiographs are an alternative.
- Middle face: axial and coronal CT scan. As an alternative, obtain a Waters view, posteroanterior, submental vertex, and occlusal radiographs.

- Lower face: panoramic radiograph. Posteroanterior, submental vertex, and occlusal are an alternative.
- If a condylar fracture is suspected, but radiographic findings are negative, obtain a CT scan of the condyle.

ED management

Tables 4-2 and 4-3 outline treatment recommendations for dental fractures and displacement injuries.

If a dentist is not immediately available and a primary tooth is so loose as to be an aspiration hazard, extract it. Grab the tooth firmly with gauze and twist it out. Immediately consult with an oral surgeon if there is a suspicion of alveolar, mandibular, or facial bone fracture.

Suturing of lacerations is not always indicated. Small intraoral wounds that do not pose an aesthetic problem heal quickly on their own, while tongue and lip lacerations that are small and have well-approximated margins also do not require suturing. Suture lacerations that are deep or continue to bleed, lip lacerations that cross the vermilion border, and through-and-through lip and tongue lacerations. Prior to suturing, irrigate the wound thoroughly and inspect it carefully to rule out the presence of foreign bodies, including fragments of any teeth that may have fractured during trauma. Do not inject local anesthetic directly into the wound area, as this could cause tissue swelling and hinder appropriate closure of the wound. Refer lacerations that require cosmetic repair to a plastic or oral surgeon.

Puncture wounds to the palate may be complicated by vascular injury or foreign bodies. Carefully evaluate penetrating injuries for possible involvement of the carotid, palatine, and jugular blood vessels and perform a complete neurologic examination. A CT scan is indicated only if neurovascular involvement is suspected. However, consult either an oral surgeon or otolaryngologist to determine the proper management for all puncture wounds to the palate. Sedation may be necessary when a wound requires extensive debridement and/or exploration to facilitate removal of foreign bodies.

Indications for admission

- Mandibular or facial bone fractures
- Soft tissue swelling that may compromise the airway

Bibliography

Andreasen J, Andreasen F, Bakland L, Flores MT: *Traumatic Dental Injuries: A Manual*, 2nd ed. Munksgard: Blackwell, 2003.

Ceallaigh PO, Ekanaykaee K, Beirne CJ, Patton DW: Diagnosis and management of common maxillofacial injuries in the emergency department. Part 5: Dentoalveolar injuries. *Emerg Med J* 2007;24:429–30.

McTigue DJ: Diagnosis and management of dental injuries in children. *Pediatr Clin North Am* 2000;47:1067–84.

Tooth discoloration

Tooth discoloration can be broadly classified as either extrinsic or intrinsic (see Table 4-4). Extrinsic discoloration refers to staining that is caused by pigmented substances that have adhered to the outer surfaces of the teeth. Children with poor oral hygiene, xerostomia, or enamel defects are at higher risk for developing significant extrinsic discoloration. Commonly, the stain is seen in the gingival third of the tooth, adjacent to the gingiva. Extrinsic

Table 4-4. Differential diagnosis of tooth discoloration

Color	Etiologies
Extrinsic	
Brown/black	Dental plaque, iron supplementation, beverages (coffee, tea, colas), iodine, smoking, chromogenic bacteria
Green	Iron supplementation, tea, chromogenic bacteria
Orange	Chromogenic bacteria
Intrinsic: localized to one or two teeth	
White (opaque)	Trauma during enamel formation, incipient dental caries
Yellow	Trauma during enamel formation, stained resin restoration, active dental caries
Brown	Trauma during enamel formation, pulpal trauma with hemorrhage, active dental caries
Intrinsic: generalized	
White (opaque)	Mild fluorosis, amelogenesis imperfecta
Yellow	Moderate fluorosis, diseases causing hyperbilirubinemia, epidermolysis bullosa, nutritional deficiency during enamel formation
Brown	Severe fluorosis, porphyria, tetracycline
Blue/gray/black	Tetracycline, minocycline
Green	Diseases causing hyperbilirubinemia

stain may be tenacious, but can be removed by a professional dental cleaning. Intrinsic discoloration is usually caused by substances that become incorporated into the structure of the tooth during its development. This type of discoloration is present at the time of tooth eruption. Additionally, intrinsic stain can develop in a previously erupted tooth that has suffered trauma. This type of stain is secondary to hematologic products leaking from the injured pulp into the surrounding dentin and enamel. Early carious lesions may also present as an area of intrinsic stain. Intrinsic discoloration cannot be removed through tooth cleaning.

Clinical presentation and diagnosis
See Table 4-4.

ED management
Tooth discoloration is not an urgent problem and no acute management is indicated. A careful history can often suggest the diagnosis. Referral to a pediatric dentist for definitive treatment is recommended.

Bibliography

Billings RJ, Berkowitz RJ, Watson G: Teeth. *Pediatrics* 2004;113(4 Suppl):1120–7.

McDonald RE, Avery DR, Dean JA: *Dentistry for the Child and Adolescent*, 8th ed. St. Louis: Mosby, 2004, pp. 447–8.

Warren JJ, Levy SM, Kanellis MJ. Prevalence of dental fluorosis in the primary dentition. *J Public Health Dent* 2001; 61:87–91.

Oral soft tissue lesions

Oral soft tissue lesions can result from a wide range of etiologies, including infection, inflammation, trauma, and developmental anomalies. Rarely are these of an emergency nature.

Clinical presentation and diagnosis
Infections
Herpes simplex

Primary herpetic gingivostomatitis (HSV I) is a common cause of gingivostomatitis in 1–3-year-olds. After a 1–2 day prodrome of fever, malaise, and vomiting, small vesicles appear anywhere on the oral mucosa, lips, tongue, perioral skin, or cheeks. These rapidly rupture, forming 2–10-mm lesions covered by a yellowish membrane. The membrane then sloughs, leaving a shallow ulcer on an erythematous base. Fever up to 40.5°C (105°F), excessive salivation, diminished oral intake leading to dehydration, and marked local lymphadenopathy can also occur. Healing begins within 4–5 days and is usually completed within 1–2 weeks.

Recurrent herpes

Recurrent herpes ("cold sores," herpes labialis) is thought to be secondary to stress (fever, menses, sunlight exposure). It presents with small vesicles, usually limited to the outer aspects of the lips and adjacent skin, although the hard palate and gingiva can also be involved. These rupture, coalesce, and become crusted. Healing takes 1–2 weeks.

Herpangina

Herpangina is a summertime infection caused by a number of enteroviruses, particularly type A Coxsackie viruses. The lesions are found only in the posterior oral cavity, which distinguishes them from herpes or aphthous ulcers. The soft palate, uvula, tonsils, and anterior tonsillar pillars are the sites of multiple, superficial, painful ulcers. Infants may be markedly irritable with fever and drooling, and severe dysphagia can lead to dehydration. The lesions heal spontaneously over 1–2 weeks.

Hand-foot-mouth disease

Hand-foot-mouth disease is caused primarily by type A16 Coxsackie viruses. Vesicles and ulcers occurring anywhere in the oral cavity are accompanied by fever, malaise, and abdominal pain. About 75% of patients also have a characteristic exanthem consisting of vesicles on an erythematous base located in one or more of the following sites: the palms and soles, dorsum of the hands and feet, dorsal aspects of the fingers and toes, buttocks, and genitalia. The lesions usually resolve within 2 weeks.

Acute necrotizing ulcerative gingivostomatitis

Acute necrotizing ulcerative gingivostomatitis (ANUG, Vincent's stomatitis, trench mouth) is an uncommon infectious disease of adolescents and young adults, probably caused by *Fusobacterium* and spirochetes. It is associated with stress and smoking, although in rare cases there is underlying malnutrition or immune deficiency. Characteristic findings are painful gingiva that bleed easily, ulcerated interdental papillae covered by a grayish membrane, and foul-smelling breath, in addition to lymphadenopathy, malaise, and fever.

ANUG is differentiated from acute primary herpes by the punched-out appearance of the interdental papillae, the lack of vesicles, and the older age of patients with ANUG.

Candidal thrush

Thrush is most common in the first year of life. The complaint is diminished oral intake or white spots in the oral cavity. On inspection, the oral mucosa is beefy red with a curdlike white exudate on the tongue, gingiva, hard palate, or buccal mucosa. This can resemble milk, but it is not easily removed by scraping with a tongue depressor. On occasion, cracking or fissuring at the angle of the mouth, or cheilitis, is seen. Many infants simultaneously have a typical *Candida* diaper rash.

Thrush beyond the first year of life occurs in patients who have received broad-spectrum antibiotics, and those with autoimmune diseases and nutritional deficiencies. Persistent or recurrent thrush suggests possible HIV infection.

Papilloma

Papilloma (verruca vulgaris, condyloma acuminatum) can occur at any age. They present as single or multiple pedunculated or sessile nodules at any oral site. There may also be similar lesions on the skin.

Noninfectious ulcers

Aphthous ulcers

Aphthous ulcers, or canker sores, are solitary or multiple (five or fewer) very painful lesions on the non-keratinized mucosa (buccal, inner labial, ventral surface of tongue). They begin as erythematous papules that become well-circumscribed ulcers with a gray fibrinous exudate on an erythematous base. The etiology is unknown, although they are more common in families with allergies and their appearance is thought to be related to stress (infections, drugs, trauma, emotional upset). Fever is less common than with herpes. The ulcers usually last 7–14 days and recurrent episodes are the rule.

Traumatic ulcer

Usually these are single ulcers, although the size, shape, and location all vary. Inquire as to recent ingestion of hot foods (pizza often causes burns to the anterior palate), dental treatment (children often bite the lip or tongue while it is numb, or the dental drill may have scratched the tongue or cheek), and oral habits (fingernail scratches of the gingival, chewing on inside of cheek). In the absence of repeated trauma, the lesion usually heals uneventfully within 2 weeks.

Mucocele

A mucocele is a fluid-filled nodule with a translucent red or blue surface which may fluctuate in size. It occurs most commonly on the inner lower lip, secondary to the traumatic laceration of a minor salivary gland duct that permits accumulation and blockage of mucous.

Ranula

A ranula is a mucous retention cyst of a minor salivary gland. It presents as a large, soft swelling on the floor of the mouth. It may fluctuate in size and elevate the tongue.

Angular cheilitis

Angular cheilitis presents with fissures at the corners of the mouth. These may bleed, ulcerate, and develop a crusted surface. Drooling, licking of the lips, and contact allergies may play a role and some patients may have frequent recurrences. The lesions can become infected with *Candida* and/or staphylococci.

Irritation fibroma

An irritation fibroma is a reactive hyperplastic lesion, usually secondary to chronic trauma. It can be located anywhere in the oral cavity, but the most common site is on the marginal gingiva. It appears as a painless, pedunculated or sessile nodule with a smooth pink surface.

Pyogenic granuloma

A pyogenic granuloma is a reactive (irritation, trauma, poor oral hygiene) hyperplastic lesion that presents as a pedunculated or sessile nodule with a red surface. They frequently become ulcerated and bleed easily. They are more common in females and can be associated with pregnancy.

Fordyce granules

Fordyce granules are oral sebaceous glands which often become evident at puberty. They appear as yellowish, multiple small papules, commonly on the vermilion border of the lip. These are asymptomatic and benign, but sometimes can be confused with candidiasis.

Gingival and lingual lesions

Geographic tongue

Geographic tongue, or benign migratory glossitis, is a self-limited condition of unknown etiology. It presents as oval or irregular red patches in areas of desquamated papillae. While it is usually asymptomatic, some patients may complain of a burning sensation.

Coated tongue

Coated tongue, or hairy tongue, represents elongation of the filiform papillae secondary to poor oral hygiene, dehydration, and medications (antibiotics, chlorhexidine). The presentation can range from whitish coating to brown/black "hairy" appearance.

Drug-induced gingival overgrowth

Phenytoin, cyclosporin A, and calcium channel blockers can induce gingival hyperplasia. It presents with fibrous enlargement, primarily involving the interdental papillae in the anterior section of the mouth. In extreme cases, it may cover the crowns of teeth and interfere with eruption of teeth. Pain and difficulty with mastication can occur if the gingiva overgrow the occlusal surfaces of the teeth. In contrast, gingivitis presents with edematous and hemorrhagic gums.

Aggressive periodontitis

Aggressive periodontitis presents with gingival inflammation and bleeding. In severe cases, teeth may become mobile. The etiology is unknown, although it is associated with diabetes, neutropenia, and hypophosphatasia.

ED management

Ulcerative lesions

For all oral ulcers, the major therapeutic goals are pain relief and maintenance of oral hygiene, so that adequate oral intake can continue. In patients who are not immunocompromised, these conditions are self-limiting, and palliative treatment is all that is needed.

A number of options exist for pain management, but none is universally successful. Viscous lidocaine (2%) swabbed onto the lesions offers temporary relief, but caution the parents to not allow the child to rinse and spit the lidocaine (absorption of excessive amount). In addition, it is contraindicated for pharyngeal lesions (depression of the gag reflex). An alternative is a 1:1 solution of Maalox/diphenhydramine or Kaopectate/diphenhydramine swabbed onto the lesions, but avoid using large quantities. Over-the-counter analgesic sprays offer only short-term relief, but they are safe and well-tolerated. Systemic analgesics such as acetaminophen (15 mg/kg per 4 h) and ibuprofen (10 mg/kg per 6 h) can be helpful in the management of both pain and fever.

Emphasize the importance of encouraging oral intake. Ice cream, gelatin, milk shakes, and pudding are often tolerated by children experiencing oral pain.

Acute necrotizing ulcerative gingivitis

Although ANUG is an ulcerative disorder, its bacterial etiology requires specific treatment in addition to the palliative measures discussed previously. Give a 7-day course of penicillin VK (50 mg/kg per day div qid), metronidazole (15 mg/kg per day div tid), or clindamycin (20 mg/kg per day div qid). In addition, refer the patient to a dentist for treatment within 24–48 hours for debridement of necrotic gingival tissue.

Candidiasis

Treat with nystatin oral suspension (100,000 units/ml). Advise older patients to rinse with 4 mL for 2 minutes qid. If the patient is not old enough to rinse and spit, instruct the parent to place 1–2 mL along both sides of the buccal mucosa qid. In addition, keep the patient NPO for at least 30 minutes following administration of the nystatin. For patients who are immunocompromised, consult with the child's primary care physician or an infectious disease specialist, as more aggressive treatment may be needed.

Papillomas

Refer the patient to an oral surgeon for elective excisional biopsy and possible laser ablation of the lesions.

Mucocoele, ranula

Refer the patient to an oral surgeon for excisional biopsy and removal.

Angular cheilitis

Although the etiology of angular cheilitis is multifactorial, the lesions can often become infected with *Candida albicans* and/or staphylococci. Treat with topical miconazole ointment, which has both antifungal and antibacterial properties, applied to the corners of the mouth qid. Refer the patient to a primary care provider to address any underlying conditions, such as drooling, frequent lip licking, and lip incompetence.

Irritation fibroma, pyogenic granuloma

Refer the patient to an oral surgeon for excisional biopsy.

Fordyce granules

These papules require no treatment other than reassuring the family that the finding is benign.

Geographic tongue

No treatment is indicated if the condition is asymptomatic. If the patient complains of burning sensation, treat with a 1:1 mixture of diphenhydramine and Maalox, either used as a rinse or swabbed directly onto the painful area. Also advise the patient to avoid hot, spicy foods.

Coated tongue, hairy tongue

No emergency treatment required, but treat any underlying systemic illnesses that can cause fever and dehydration. Encourage adequate hydration and recommend brushing of the tongue.

Gingival hyperplasia (drug induced)

Refer the patient to a dentist for evaluation of hygiene and possible need for surgical resection of the tissue.

Periodontal disease, gingival bleeding

Take a careful medical history, noting the duration and severity of the current complaint. Since local factors are the most common causes for gingival bleeding, look for poor oral hygiene, tooth eruption, foreign-body entrapment, and self-injurious behaviors. If no local etiology can be identified, consider hormonal changes (puberty), thrombocytopenia, leukemia, clotting defects, and diabetes.

Follow-up

- Ulcerative lesions due to viral infection: immediately for severely diminished oral intake, otherwise 2–3 days
- ANUG: dentist in 24–48 hours
- Candidiasis: 1–2 weeks
- Papillomas, mucocoeles, ranulas, fibromas, pyogenic granulomas: oral surgeon within several days
- Gingival hyperplasia: dentist within several days
- Periodontitis, gingival bleeding with known local etiology: dentist within several days

Indication for admission

- Dehydration or inability to tolerate oral intake secondary to pain

Bibliography

Pinkham JR, Fields HW Jr, McTigue DJ, Casamassino PS, Nowak A: *Pediatric Dentistry: Infancy Through Adolescence*, 4th ed. St. Louis: Elsevier Saunders, 2005, pp. 9–60.

Sciubba JJ: Oral mucosal diseases in the office setting – part I: aphthous stomatitis and herpes simplex infections. *Gen Dent* 2007;55:347–54.

Scully C, Welbury R, Flaitz C, de Almeida OP: *A Color Atlas of Orofacial Health & Disease in Children and Adolescents*, 2nd ed. London: Martin Dunitz, 2002.

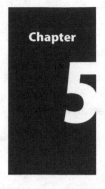

Chapter

5

Dermatologic emergencies

Alexandra D. McCollum and Sheila F. Friedlander

Dermatology is a visual specialty, and an accurate description of a "rash" makes it more likely that the practitioner will be able to classify a particular eruption and rapidly arrive at the right diagnosis. This chapter begins with definitions of dermatologic terms, which when used in conjunction with Table 5-1 can serve as a guide to the most common diagnoses.

Definition of terms

Primary lesions

Macule

A flat, non-palpable, superficial skin color change that is <1 cm in diameter. A macule can be red, brown, yellow, or white.

Patch

A macule that is >1 cm in diameter.

Papule

A firm, palpable, elevated lesion that is <1 cm in diameter. A papule may be flat-topped, dome-shaped, or pointed.

Plaque

A papule that is >1 cm in lateral diameter. It is a broad, elevated, flat-topped solid lesion often formed by a confluence of several papules. In contrast to a nodule, it does not possess increased depth, and is a "plateau," rather than a "glacier."

Nodule

A papule that is enlarged in all three dimensions: length, width, and depth. It may be dome-shaped or slope-shouldered, but the discriminating characteristic is increased depth compared to a papule or plaque.

Tumor

A large nodule.

Wheal

An evanescent, edematous, smooth, raised, pink to red lesion. The classic description is "hive-like."

Table 5-1. Dermatological diagnosis by type of eruption

Erythematous papules, nodules, and plaques

Papules

Insect bite (papular urticaria)	Erythema toxicum neonatorum
Drug reaction	Miliaria rubra
Viral exanthema	Candidiasis
Scarlet fever	Kawasaki disease
Papular acrodermatitis (Gianotti-Crosti)	

Nodules

Erythema nodosum	Furuncle/carbuncle
Pyogenic granuloma	Granuloma annulare[a]

Plaques

Cellulitis	Granuloma annulare
Tinea corporis	Contact dermatitis[b]
Psoriasis	Lupus erythematosus
Pityriasis rosea	Erythema chronicum migrans
Fixed drug eruption	Erythema marginatum

Eczematous lesions

Atopic dermatitis	Langerhans cell histiocytosis
Scabies	Diaper dermatitis
Seborrheic dermatitis	Acrodermatitis enteropathica
Contact dermatitis	

Papulosquamous diseases

Psoriasis	Secondary syphilis
Pityriasis rosea	Tinea
Id reaction	Lichen planus
Scabies	Lupus erythematosus

Pustular eruptions

Acne	Miliaria pustulosa
Candidiasis	Infantile acropustulosis
Folliculitis	Transient neonatal pustular melanosis
Bacteremia	Erythema toxicum neonatorum
Gonococcemia	Impetigo

Skin-colored papules and nodules

Granuloma annulare[a]	Verruca

Table 5-1. (cont.)

Molluscum contagiosum[c]	Dermoid cyst
Keloid	
Reddish brown papules and nodules	
Dermatofibroma	Pilomatricoma
Neurofibroma	Mastocytoma
Vascular lesions	
Nevus simplex	Port wine stain
Cutis marmorata	Pyogenic granuloma
Hemangioma of infancy	
Reactive erythematous eruptions	
Drug eruptions	Erythema multiforme
Erythema marginatum	Urticaria
Erythema migrans	Viral exanthema
Photodermatitis	Contact dermatitis
Palpable purpura	
Idiopathic thrombocytopenic purpura	Coagulopathy
Rocky Mountain spotted fever	Sepsis/DIC
Henoch-Schönlein purpura	Subacute bacterial endocarditis
Meningococcemia	TORCH infections
Vesicobullous	
Vesicular	
Dyshydrotic eczema	Miliaria crystallina
Scabies	Hand-foot-mouth disease
Herpes simplex	Varicella zoster
Eczema herpeticum	
Bullous	
Bullous impetigo	Staphylococcal scalded skin syndrome
Erythema multiforme major	Toxic epidermal necrolysis
Epidermolysis bullosa	Pemphigus
Contact dermatitis – poison ivy	Photodermatitis
White lesions	
Patches and plaques	
Pityriasis alba	Tinea versicolor
Post-inflammatory	Verrucae

Table 5-1. (cont.)

Ash leaf macules	Vitiligo
Papules	
Keratosis pilaris	Molluscum contagiosum[c]
Milia	

Notes: [a]Granuloma annulare can be either erythematous or skin-colored and presents as a papule which later develops into a nodule or plaque.
[b]Contact dermatitis can present as erythematous papules, vesicles, plaques or mixed morphology in a well demarcated distribution.
[c]Molluscum contagiosum can be skin-colored or have a white opalescent center often with umbilication.

Vesicle

A sharply circumscribed, elevated, clear fluid-filled lesion that is <1 cm in diameter. A vesicle is often thin-walled and fragile, so it ruptures easily. Therefore, patients may present instead with small erosions (de-roofed vesicles).

Bulla

A vesicle that is >1 cm in diameter. A bulla may arise as a single large blister or through the coalescence of several vesicles.

Pustule

An elevated lesion containing purulent exudate that is white, yellow, or green, rather than clear. This lesion is usually filled with polymorphonuclear leukocytes.

Secondary lesions

These changes in the skin usually occur over time as the primary lesions evolve, sometimes as a result of manipulation of the skin through scratching or rubbing.

Scale

An accumulation of excessive layers of stratum corneum, resulting from abnormal differentiation and shedding of cornified keratinocytes. A scale may be greasy and yellowish, silvery and mica-like, fine and barely visible, or large, adherent, and lamellar.

Crust

A crust (scab) results from dried serum (yellow), blood or bloody exudate (dark red or brown), or purulent exudate (green or yellowish green) overlying areas of lost or damaged epidermis. A crust can be thick, tough, and black secondary to hemorrhage and necrosis.

Erosion

A moist, slightly depressed lesion in which part or all of the epidermis has been visibly lost or denuded. Erosions do not extend into the underlying dermis or subcutaneous tissue, so they heal without scarring.

Ulcer

An ulcer results from loss of both the epidermis and dermis, resulting in a punched out lesion which may be filled with crust or necrotic skin. Alternatively, the base may be visible as a moist red surface. Ulcers heal with a scar.

Excoriation

A linear traumatic abrasion caused by scratching, rubbing, or scrubbing. Excoriations occur in pruritic disorders.

Lichenification

Thickening of the skin with an accentuation of the normal skin markings, often accompanied by scale, resulting in skin that feels tough and leather-like. It is a result of habitual scratching and rubbing and is a classic feature of atopic dermatitis.

Atrophy

A change demonstrated by thinning of the epidermis and the loss of skin markings. The skin wrinkles when subjected to pressure. When the dermis is involved the area may be slightly depressed.

Scar

A permanent fibrotic skin change following damage to the dermis. Initially a scar is pink or violaceous, becoming white, sclerotic, and shiny over time.

Acne

Acne vulgaris is a disorder of the pilosebaceous follicles. It is the most common skin disease of the second and third decades, with onset at puberty and an incidence approaching 100% between the ages of 14 and 17 in females and 16 and 19 in males. Acne can be caused or exacerbated by medications, including phenytoin, isoniazid, iodides and bromides, and lithium. It can be associated with polycystic ovarian syndrome secondary to increased levels of circulating androgens. In the neonatal period acne is secondary to maternal hormonal stimulation of sebaceous glands which have not yet involuted to a prepubertal immature state. Infantile acne, presenting in the post-neonatal period, may sometimes require therapy and rarely leads to scarring. Steroid acne is a folliculitis most commonly caused by the prolonged use of topical or systemic corticosteroids or adrenocorticotropic hormones.

Clinical presentation

Acne vulgaris primarily involves sites where pilosebaceous glands are most numerous (face, chest, upper back). The initial lesions are the pathognomonic open (blackheads) and closed (whiteheads) comedones. As the disease progresses, inflammatory lesions are seen, including papules, pustules, nodules, and cysts. The resolution phase is characterized by post-inflammatory hyperpigmentation and scarring. Neonatal acne presents with erythematous papules and pustules, rather than comedones, on the nose and cheeks. The typical lesions of steroid acne are small erythematous papules and pustules, without comedones, primarily located on the back and chest.

Diagnosis

The diagnosis of acne vulgaris is usually straightforward, although a number of conditions may have a similar appearance. Adenoma sebaceum appears as pink papules on the face of prepubertal patients with tuberous sclerosis. Other cutaneous manifestations (ash-leaf spots, Shagreen patch, periungual fibromas) are generally present. Verruca (warts) and molluscum contagiosum cause flesh-colored papules without comedones or an inflammatory response. In an infant, seborrhea is often misdiagnosed as neonatal acne. Associated cradle cap and retroauricular scaling distinguish seborrhea.

Although comedones can be found in children as young as 6–7 years of age, consider androgen excess (gonadal or adrenal tumors; congenital adrenal hyperplasia) if there is inflammatory acne in a prepubertal child.

ED management

Acne vulgaris is a chronic disease. To help prevent permanent scarring, initiate treatment in the ED, but refer the patient to a primary care setting for ongoing care. The therapeutic measures appropriate for ED use are summarized below.

Topical treatment

Benzoyl peroxide (BPO; 2.5–10%)

Benzoyl peroxide (BPO) is an effective keratolytic and antibacterial agent that is useful for comedones and mild inflammatory lesions. Common side effects are redness, drying, and scaling of the skin.

Retinoic acid (tretinoin)

Retinoic acid is derived from vitamin A and is extremely useful for treating comedonal acne. Severe skin irritation, peeling, and photosensitization can result. Therefore, start treatment on an every-other-day basis and instruct the patient to apply only at night. To minimize these side effects, instruct the patient to limit face washing and to be sure the face is dry prior to applying retinoic acid. Do not use in females who may be pregnant. Similar products include topical adapalene and tazarotene.

Topical antibiotics

Topical antibiotics are a useful adjunct in mild to moderate inflammatory acne. Clindamycin (1%) and erythromycin (2%) are effective without the same risk of side effects seen with oral administration.

There are many combination products on the market (BPO with an antibiotic or retinoic acid with an antibiotic) which may be easier for the patient but may be more costly.

Systemic treatment

Oral antibiotics

Reserve these for unresponsive acne or patients who have sensitivity to topical products. A minimum 4-week course is usually required before any improvement occurs. Use tetracycline, minocycline, or doxycycline for patients older than 8 years of age and not pregnant. Side effects include gastrointestinal upset, photosensitization, candida vaginitis, vertigo, and rarely, pseudotumor cerebri. Use erythromycin for younger patients (<9 years) or when sun exposure is a concern. The high degree of resistance to this drug makes it a poor choice for the older population.

Other systemic treatments

Defer the initiation of medications such as isotretinoin and oral contraceptives to the primary care provider.

Treat mild comedonal acne with a BPO cleanser (2.5–10%) daily or bid, depending on the degree of dryness. Add retinoic acid 0.025% cream every other night, and gradually increase to every night use. This combination is particularly effective, as the tretinoin facilitates absorption of the BPO, but irritation may preclude use of both products. Alternatively, use topical antibiotics (1% clindamycin gel or solution; 2% erythromycin gel or solution) as the second drug, every morning. Do not use topical antibiotics as monotherapy, since resistance is more likely to occur.

Treat steroid acne with topical BPO, a topical antibiotic (as described above), and discontinuation of the steroids, if possible. The management of an adolescent with acne associated with polycystic ovaries includes either a combination oral contraceptive or progestin with topical therapies (described above). Multi-disciplinary follow-up is recommended. No therapy, other than reassurance, is required for neonatal acne.

Follow-up
* Primary care follow-up in 2–6 weeks

Bibliography
Gollnick H, Cunliffe W, Berson D, et al: Management of acne: a report from a global alliance to improve outcomes in acne. *J Am Acad Derm* 2003;49(1 Suppl):S1–38.

Krakowski AC, Stendardo S, Eichenfield LF: Practical considerations in acne treatment

and the clinical impact of topical combination therapy. *Ped Derm* 2008;25 Suppl 1:1–14.

Tom WL, Fallon Friedlander S: Acne through the ages: case-based observations through childhood and adolescence. *Clin Pediatr (Phila)* 2008;47:639–51.

Alopecia

Alopecia is relatively common and, usually, a benign disorder in children. It is categorized as either localized or diffuse, and then further subcategorized as either scarring or non-scarring. The most common causes of localized alopecia include tinea capitis (pp. 129–132) and alopecia areata (presumed autoimmune disorder). Other causes of localized alopecias result from trauma or traction secondary to hair care techniques (braiding, straightening, blow drying) or trichotillomania, the purposeful removal of hair by the patient. These disorders are usually non-scarring and transient, but severe inflammatory forms of tinea capitis (kerion) can lead to permanent scarring. Classically scarring forms of alopecia include discoid lupus and lichen planopilaris.

The most common cause of diffuse alopecia in children is telogen effluvium. In most instances, the patient has recently suffered a significant stress (high fever, crash diet, parturition, convulsion, psychosocial event). Other etiologies include: chemotherapeutic agents (cyclophosphamide, vincristine), drugs (propranolol, warfarin), radiation, toxins (lead, boric acid), endocrinopathies (hyper- and hypothyroidism, hypoparathyroidism), nutritional deficiencies (zinc, vitamin A), secondary syphilis, and systemic lupus erythematous.

Clinical presentation

Localized alopecia

Alopecia areata

Alopecia areata is characterized by the sudden (possibly overnight) appearance of sharply demarcated round or oval patches of hair loss without associated scalp inflammation or scarring. Regrowth may occur in some areas while the disease progresses elsewhere. In 5–10% of cases, the lesions may expand to involve the entire scalp (alopecia totalis) or all the body hair (alopecia universalis). At the margin of active lesions, there are loose, easily plucked, "exclamation point" hairs with shortened bulbs and small stumps. The course is variable, but up to 95% of children have complete regrowth within 1 year.

Tinea capitis

Tinea capitis causes patchy alopecia with scaling and erythema similar to seborrheic dermatitis. Within the patch, "black dots" (infected hairs which are broken off at the scalp level) may be seen. A minority of cases fluoresce under Wood's lamp exposure. An allergic vesicular and pustular reaction (kerion) can develop acutely. The kerion appears as a sharply demarcated, indurated, boggy lesion that can be associated with fever, leukocytosis, and lymphadenopathy.

Traumatic and traction alopecia

Traumatic and traction alopecia occur where the hair is being pulled, as from braiding, or on the occiput of a young infant who remains supine all day. Characteristically, hair loss is incomplete; short (1–2 cm) hairs are found at the margins or within the affected area. These hairs are firmly rooted in normal-appearing scalp.

Trichotillomania

Trichotillomania primarily occurs in school-age girls. The patches of alopecia are not well demarcated, and there are well-rooted residual hairs of varying length. In some cases the eyebrows and eyelashes are also affected.

Male-pattern baldness

Male-pattern baldness is a genetically determined bilateral frontoparietal recession with thinning over the vertex. It can also occur in females taking oral contraceptives.

Diffuse alopecia

With diffuse disorders of any etiology the scalp generally has a normal appearance, and hairs are easily plucked from the periphery of areas of alopecia.

Diagnosis

For localized conditions, a careful examination of the scalp facilitates making the correct diagnosis. A careful history may suggest the stressful incident which caused a diffuse alopecia. If a previously undiagnosed systemic disorder such as syphilis, thyroid disease, lupus, or hypoparathyroidism is suspected, obtain the appropriate blood tests (VDRL, thyroid function tests, FANA, or calcium). See Table 5-2 for the differential diagnosis of alopecia.

Table 5-2. Differential diagnosis of alopecia

Diagnosis	Differentiating features
Alopecia areata	Sudden onset; no scalp inflammation
	Sharply demarcated patches with total hair loss
	Exclamation point hairs at margins
Tinea capitis	Patchy/poorly demarcated with scalp inflammation and scaling
	Black dots within the patch
	KOH-positive: chains of spores
Traction/trauma	Poorly demarcated areas of incomplete hair loss
	Occurs in scalp areas subjected to friction or pulling
	No scalp inflammation
Trichotillomania	Poorly demarcated, irregular-shaped areas of incomplete hair loss
	Eyelashes and eyebrows may also be involved
	History suggests psychopathology
Androgenetic	Bilateral frontoparietal recession and thinning over the vertex
	Begins in teenaged years
	No scalp inflammation
Telogen effluvium	History of emotional or physical stressors
	Diffuse thinning without scalp inflammation
	Positive hair pull test: >2–3 hairs removed at a time

ED management

Refer the patient to a dermatologist when the diagnosis is in doubt or when there is presence of a kerion, a history of treatment failure, or a chronic or scarring alopecia.

Localized alopecia

Most cases of alopecia areata require no treatment other than reassurance. If the lesions persist or become particularly widespread, refer the patient to a dermatologist. A change of hair care techniques or reassuring an infant's parents is usually all that is necessary for traction or traumatic alopecia. Refer the patient with trichotillomania to a primary care setting for further psychosocial evaluation. See pp. 129–131 for the treatment of tinea capitis.

Diffuse alopecia

The management of most cases primarily involves avoiding the offending agent, drug, or toxin (if possible), or treating the primary condition (lupus, thyroid disease, etc.). Stress-related hair loss is usually self-limited, with complete regrowth without any specific treatment. Refer the patient to a primary care provider.

Bibliography

Nield LS, Keri JE, Kamat D: Alopecia in the general pediatric clinic: who to treat, who to refer. *Clin Pediatr (Phila)* 2006; 45:605–12.

Paller AS, Mancini AJ: Alopecia. In *Hurwitz's Textbook of Clinical Pediatric Dermatology*, 3rd ed. Philadelphia: WB Saunders, 2006, pp. 26–30.

Price VH: Androgenetic alopecia in adolescents. *Cutis* 2003;71:115–21.

Atopic dermatitis

Atopic dermatitis is a disease that predisposes the skin to excessive dryness and pruritus. The majority of patients have a family history of allergy, asthma, hay fever, or eczema, and about half of affected children will develop one of these other diseases. It is now generally believed that childhood eczema is a disorder involving both skin barrier defects and immunologic dysregulation.

Clinical presentation

Atopic dermatitis can be categorized into three different age-dependent phases that may or may not follow one another. Pruritus and dry skin are the hallmarks at all ages. The infantile stage occurs between birth and three years and is characterized by erythema, papules, and vesicles on the face, neck, chest, and extensor surfaces of the extremities. In older children subacute and chronic papular and scaly lichenified lesions occur on the flexor aspects of the neck, arms, and legs. The antecubital and popliteal fossae are particularly involved. The adolescent and adult forms blend into the childhood phase with marked lichenification and flexural, hand, and foot involvement.

Other manifestations in children and adolescents may include nummular eczema (well-demarcated papular coin lesions) and pityriasis alba (discrete hypopigmented macules).

At any age the severe pruritus causes scratching which can lead to secondary bacterial infection. The superimposed pyoderma can confuse the clinical picture. Secondary herpes-virus infection (eczema herpeticum, pp. 116–118) can also occur and become generalized in atopic patients.

Atopic individuals can have a number of associated findings, including accentuated palmar creases, white dermatographism (blanching of the skin when stroked), and Dennie-Morgan folds or pleats (an extra groove of the lower eyelid). Keratosis pilaris (follicular hyperkeratosis) presents with scaly perifollicular papules with central hairs resulting in a "chicken skin" or "goose bump" appearance.

Diagnosis

The diagnosis of atopic dermatitis is suggested by a family history of atopy, a personal history of allergies or asthma, dry and pruritic skin, and the typical location of the lesions that blend into the surrounding normal skin. In infants, seborrheic dermatitis causes a salmon-colored, greasy eruption of the face, scalp and intertriginous area that is not pruritic. The eruption of a contact dermatitis (pp. 102–103) has a sharp border with the uninvolved skin and the history may suggest the offending agent. The lesions of tinea corporis (pp. 129–131) usually have central clearing and a raised scaly border. Bacterial infections (pp. 98–99) are not preceded by pruritus and are generally more localized than atopic rashes. Psoriatic lesions are usually well demarcated with a silvery scale. The lesions of scabies (pp. 122–123) do not follow the usual sites of predilection that eczema does, and the family or personal history of atopy may be negative. However, a secondary autoeczematization process may occur with scabies that makes differentiation between eczema and scabies difficult.

ED management

Atopic dermatitis is a chronic condition that is best managed in the primary care setting, but therapy can be initiated in the ED. The goals of therapy are to hydrate the skin, prevent itching, and treat the inflammation. Instruct the patient to use oatmeal baths, oils and soap substitutes (Cetaphil, Aveeno), avoid excessive bathing, and use emollients on slightly damp skin after bathing (Vaseline, Eucerin, Aquaphor, Lubriderm). Hydroxyzine (2 mg/kg per day div qid) is an effective anti-pruritic agent.

Prescribe a moderate-potency topical corticosteroid ointment (0.1% triamcinolone, 0.05% fluticasone, 0.1% mometasone) for the body and extremities. However, use only a low-potency ointment (1% hydrocortisone, 0.05% aclomethasone, desonide 0.05%) on the face, and limit it to a 2-week course. Do not use oral steroids without consulting a dermatologist. Tacrolimus 0.03% and pimecrolimus are nonsteroidal immunomodulators that can be used on both the face and body, but inform the patient and family of the Black Box warning now present on these products, as well as the need for photoprotection while using them.

More extensive and recalcitrant disease may benefit from wet-wrap dressings or oatmeal baths. As an alternative, instruct the family to apply a mild- to moderate-potency topical steroid, cover with wet kerlex or wet pajamas, and then place dry dressings or clothing over the treated sites.

Treat acute, oozing lesions with Burrow's solution or tap water on open dressings for 20 minutes qid. If there is a secondary bacterial infection, use topical mupirocin tid on localized areas of involvement, but treat more extensive infections with 40 mg/kg per day of cefadroxil or cephalexin (both div bid). If MRSA is a concern, either use clindamycin (20 mg/kg per day div q 6 h) or add trimethoprim-sulfamethoxazole (8 mg/kg per day of TMP div bid) to the cephalosporin. Because of the recent increase in methicillin-resistant staphylococcal infections, obtain cultures before treatment and arrange careful follow-up to document adequate response to treatment.

Follow-up

- Primary care follow-up in 1–2 weeks

Indications for admission

- Severe involvement in a patient who cannot be treated adequately at home or shows signs of secondary infection that would be best treated with intravenous antibiotics
- Evidence of eczema herpeticum

Bibliography

Fleischer AB Jr: Diagnosis and management of common dermatoses in children: atopic, seborrheic, and contact dermatitis. *Clin Pediatr (Phila)* 2008; 47:332–46.

Krakowski AC, Eichenfield LF, Dohil MA: Management of atopic dermatitis in the pediatric population. *Pediatrics* 2008;122:812–24.

Ong PY, Boguniewicz M: Atopic dermatitis. *Prim Care* 2008;35:105–17.

Bacterial skin infections

Bacterial skin infections, or pyodermas, are most commonly caused by group A *Streptococcus* and *Staphylococcus aureus*. Impetigo, folliculitis, furunculosis, and cellulitis are the usual forms of infection.

Staphylococcal scalded skin syndrome (SSSS) is not a true cutaneous infection, but may be a manifestation of one. It is an acute exfoliative dermatosis caused by an epidermolytic toxin produced by phage group II strains of staphylococci, types 3A, 3B, 3C, 55, and 71. SSSS must be distinguished from toxic epidermal necrolysis of TEN (pp. 107–108).

Clinical presentation and diagnosis

Impetigo

The most common type of bacterial skin infection is impetigo contagiosum caused by group A *Streptococcus* or *Staphylococcus aureus*. The eruption usually appears on the face and extremities. Small erythematous macules develop into vesicles that rupture, leaving a typical honey-colored crust that is easily removed, but recurs. Fever and regional lymphadenopathy may also occur. Some cases of impetigo are caused by nephritogenic strains of *Streptococcus* and subsequent acute glomerulonephritis occasionally occurs. Impetigo is extremely contagious, spreading by autoinoculation (satellite lesions), close contact, and fomites (towels). It is more common in the warm, humid summer months.

Bullous impetigo is usually caused by phage group II staphylococci. Yellowish vesicles on the face, extremities, and trunk rupture, leaving well-demarcated, erythematous, circular macules with a "collarette of scale." Fever and lymphadenopathy may occur.

Folliculitis

Folliculitis is a pyoderma involving the hair follicles, particularly in areas subjected to sweating, friction, scratching, and shaving. Coagulase-positive *Staphylococcus* is the most frequent etiologic agent. Folliculitis presents as pruritic, round-topped pustules most commonly seen on the scalp, face, thighs, and buttocks. If the diagnosis is uncertain, examine the pustule under magnification (otoscope). The hallmark of a folliculitis is the presence of a hair shaft in most lesions.

Furunculosis

Furunculosis is a deep follicular infection, usually arising from a preceding folliculitis. Furuncles (boils) are tender, erythematous 1–5 cm nodules that become fluctuant, then suppurate. They are seen in hair-bearing areas that are subject to perspiration and friction, including the face, thighs, buttocks, and scalp. In contrast, an abscess is usually a solitary lesion that is not associated with hair follicles. Risk factors for recurrent furunculosis include chronic nasal colonization with staphylococcus, diabetes mellitus, obesity, corticosteroid treatment, immunoglobulin deficiency, neutropenia of any etiology, and defective neutrophils (chronic granulomatous disease, Chediak-Higashi syndrome). Other family members may be the source of the recurrent infections. Also, recurrent folliculitis is a risk factor for infection with community-acquired methicillin-resistant *S. aureus*.

Cellulitis

Cellulitis, an infection involving the subcutaneous tissues, causes poorly demarcated, tender, erythematous swelling. It is often associated with fever, local lymphadenopathy, and proximal lymphangitic streaking. Sites of infection are often areas subjected to superficial trauma, such as the face and extremities. Common pathogens include coagulase-positive *Staphylococcus* and group A *Streptococcus;* infections with *S. pneumoniae* are rare.

Erysipelas

Erysipelas is an uncommon superficial cellulitis caused by group A *Streptococcus,* It begins as a small area of redness that progresses to a tense, erythematous, tender, well-demarcated plaque.

Staphylococcal scalded skin syndrome (SSSS)

SSSS usually occurs in children <6 years of age. It begins abruptly, with a generalized macular erythema after a period of fever and irritability. There may be a pharyngitis, conjunctivitis, rhinorrhea, or discrete staphylococcal infection. The eruption becomes scarlatiniform (sandpaperlike) and tender, with wrinkling, bullae, sheetlike exfoliation, and a positive Nikolsky's sign (a peeling of normal-appearing skin with light pressure). Crusting around the mouth and sometimes nose and eyes is typical, but mucous membrane involvement is rare. Despite the marked skin tenderness and irritability, these patients do not appear toxic. If hydration is maintained, recovery occurs in 1–2 weeks.

Early in the course, SSSS may resemble scarlet fever (pp. 391–392; nontender skin, pharyngitis, and strawberry tongue, negative Nikolsky), Kawasaki disease (pp. 395–396; erythema of the conjunctiva, lips, and oral mucosa, strawberry tongue, negative Nikolsky), and Stevens-Johnson syndrome or TEN (target lesions, mucous membrane involvement, positive Nikolsky). The diagnosis of SSSS is confirmed by isolation of staphylococci from an orifice or rarely the blood; it cannot be recovered from bullae or areas of exfoliation.

ED management

Consider the local prevalence of methicillin-resistant *S. aureus* when deciding which oral antibiotic to prescribe. If there is a significant concern, use clindamycin or trimethoprim-sulfamethoxazole.

Impetigo

Treat with mupirocin ointment (2%) tid and good local hygiene. For more extensive disease, or if mupirocin is unavailable or ineffective, treat for 7–10 days with cefadroxil (40 mg/kg per day div bid), cephalexin (40 mg/kg per day div bid), or amoxicillin-clavulanate (875/125 formulation, 45 mg/kg per day of amoxicillin div bid). If MRSA is a concern, either use clindamycin (20 mg/kg per day div q 6 h) or add trimethoprim-sulfamethoxazole (8 mg/kg per day of TMP div bid) to the above regimen. Treat weeping lesions with tap water or 5% Burrow's solution on open dressings for 10 minutes tid.

Folliculitis

Folliculitis occasionally responds to 7–14 days of treatment with a topical antibiotic (mupirocin 2%, clindamycin 1%). If the response is inadequate, treat with the same oral antibiotics as for impetigo, for 7–10 days.

Furunculosis and cellulitis

Treat with the same oral antibiotics as for impetigo. Warm soaks q 2 h are a helpful adjunct to antibiotic therapy. Delineate the margins of the infection with a pen so that the response to therapy can be objectively assessed. Incision and drainage are indicated if the area is fluctuant; obtain a culture of the pus. However, if there is fever, proximal lymphadenopathy, and/or lymphangitic streaking, admit the patient and treat with IV nafcillin (100 mg/kg per day div q 6 h), cefazolin (50 mg/kg per day div q 8 h), or clindamycin (40 mg/kg per day div q 6 h). Treat a patient with an immune deficiency with IV nafcillin (150 mg/kg per day div q 6 h).

Erysipelas

Treat with penicillin (250 mg qid) for 10 days. Admit for IV antibiotics (as for furunculosis and cellulitis) if there is an inadequate response.

Staphylococcal scalded skin syndrome

If SSSS is suspected, obtain a CBC, electrolytes, blood culture, and polymerase chain reaction (PCR) for the toxin (if available). Obtain cultures and Gram's stains from the nose, throat, conjunctiva, and other potential foci of infection (the exfoliation is toxin-mediated so exfoliated sites will be sterile). Consult a dermatologist, who may perform a skin biopsy to confirm the diagnosis. Admit the patient and treat with IV antistaphylococcal antibiotics, either nafcillin 150 mg/kg per day div q 6 h, or vancomycin 40 mg/kg per day div q 6 h if MRSA is a possibility.

Follow-up

- Impetigo: 2–3 days, if no improvement
- Folliculitis: primary care follow-up in 1–2 weeks
- Furunculosis, cellulitis, and erysipelas: 2–3 days

Indications for admission

- Furunculosis or cellulitis in a patient with an immune deficiency
- Fever, proximal lymphadenopathy, and lymphangitic streaking in association with cellulitis or other deep skin infection
- Inadequate response to outpatient management
- Suspected staphylococcal scalded skin syndrome

Bibliography

Abrahamian FM, Talan DA, Moran GJ: Management of skin and soft-tissue infections in the emergency department. *Infect Dis Clin North Am* 2008;22:89–116.

Gorwitz RJ: A review of community-associated methicillin-resistant Staphylococcus aureus skin and soft tissue infections. *Pediatr Infect Dis J* 2008;27:1–7.

Khangura S, Wallace J, Kissoon N, Kodeeswaran T: Management of cellulitis in a pediatric emergency department. *Pediatr Emerg Care* 2007;23: 805–11.

Candida

Candidiasis is caused by the fungus *Candida albicans*, which inhabits the gastrointestinal tract of young infants and the vaginal vault of mature females. Factors that predispose to candidiasis include local heat or moisture, systemic antibiotics, diabetes mellitus, and corticosteroids.

Clinical presentation

Cutaneous candidiasis

Cutaneous candidiasis is most frequently found in the intertriginous and diaper areas. It is characterized by moist, beefy red, well-demarcated macules with raised, scaly edges. Satellite vesicles and pustules may be seen near the borders. Primary infection in the diaper region causes a perianal rash, and secondary infection of a diaper rash of any other etiology is very common.

Oral candidiasis

Oral candidiasis (thrush) presents in the first weeks of life with loosely adherent, cheesy white plaques on the tongue, soft and hard palates, and buccal mucosa. The mucosal surfaces are beefy red, and the lesions bleed when scraped lightly with a tongue blade. These lesions are often painful, and a marked decrease in oral intake can occur in young infants. Thrush in older patients is usually associated with some underlying condition (immunosuppression, broad-spectrum antibiotics), but it can occur in otherwise healthy infants. Recurrent thrush can be seen in HIV-infected children; esophageal candidiasis occurs in up to 20% of these patients.

Perlèche

Perlèche (angular cheilitis) presents as erythema and fissuring at the corners of the mouth. It may be associated with overbite, braccs, poor mouth closure, or lip smacking.

Diagnosis

The typical intense erythema, scaly border, and satellite lesions suggest the diagnosis of cutaneous candidiasis. Contact diaper rashes usually do not involve the intertriginous areas, while seborrheic diaper eruptions are often associated with cradle cap and postauricular scaling. When the diagnosis is in doubt, scrape the border of the eruption and examine the scale under a microscope after mixing with 10–20% KOH. Budding yeasts and pseudohyphae are seen with *Candida*.

Thrush is often confused with milk, but the latter can easily be scraped from the oral mucosa without causing any bleeding.

Angular cheilitis can resemble impetigo, but the characteristic honey-colored crust is not present. The perioral eruption of herpes simplex presents with grouped vesicles, which are not usually located at the corners of the mouth.

ED management

Many topical agents are available, including nystatin, miconazole, clotrimazole, and econazole. Apply one of these creams tid or qid to cutaneous eruptions and perlèche. The "-azoles" are preferred in the inguinal region or when it is difficult to distinguish tinea from monilia. Avoid combination products containing neomycin, which can be sensitizing. Do not prescribe steroid-containing combination preparations, as over-use in very young children can lead to striae and thinning of the skin, particularly in the diaper area. If the eruption is markedly inflamed, use a low-potency topical corticosteroid such as hydrocortisone 1–2.5% bid for 48–72 hours in addition to a topical antifungal. Instruct parents to change the child's diapers frequently and to avoid irritating, possibly sensitizing, cleansing agents. The additional use of a barrier product containing zinc oxide is often helpful.

For thrush, instill 1 mL of a nystatin oral suspension in each side of the mouth qid, after feedings, until 5 days after the lesions have resolved. Advise the parent to rub persistent lesions with a gauze pad soaked with nystatin suspension and to discard any old pacifiers. Suspect an underlying immunodeficiency in children with persistent or recurrent thrush in the absence of antibiotic use. For these patients, use clotrimazole troches or ketoconazole (see HIV-related emergencies, pp. 374–384). Systemic fluconazole therapy may be necessary in severe, persistent, or unresponsive cases.

Follow-up

- Primary care follow-up in 1–2 weeks

Bibliography

Humphrey S, Bergman JN, Au S: Practical management strategies for diaper dermatitis. *Skin Therapy Lett* 2006;11:1–6.

Nield LS, Kamat D: Prevention, diagnosis, and management of diaper dermatitis. *Clin Pediatr (Phila)* 2007;46:480–6.

Pankhurst CL: Candidiasis (oropharyngeal). *Clin Evid* 2006;15:1849–63.

Contact dermatitis

Irritant contact dermatitis is the most common form of contact dermatitis and is a nonallergic, as well as nonspecific, reaction of the skin to an irritant. The most common irritants are water (prolonged or repeated exposure), soaps, detergents, acids, alkalis, saliva, urine, and feces.

Allergic contact dermatitis is less common and affects up to 20% of the pediatric population. It is secondary to a delayed type IV hypersensitivity response that depends on a genetic predisposition, site, and duration of the contact, as well as previous exposure and sensitization. Common causes include *Rhus* genus plants (poison ivy, oak, and sumac), nickel, latex, rubber, shoes, cosmetics, adhesives, neomycin, bacitracin, and thimerosol.

Phytophotodermatitis is a non-immunologic, acute phototoxic reaction, which can occur after contact with plants containing psoralens and subsequent exposure to UV light. Plants commonly associated with this response include lemon, lime, bergamot, celery, carrot, parsley, parsnip, fennel, dill, fig, mustard, and buttercup.

Clinical presentation

Irritant contact dermatitis presents within minutes to hours of the contact as an acute eczematous reaction, with erythema, scaling, swelling, vesicles, and erosions of varying severity at the site of the contact (perioral, dorsum of hands). Lesions may be linear and have a sharp demarcation between the involved and uninvolved skin.

Allergic contact dermatitis presents within hours or days with erythema, edema, and vesicles, most commonly on the hands and face, but also seen on the feet, eyelids, ears, neck, axillae, and periumbilical area. Once again, the lesions may be linear and have a sharp demarcation between the involved and uninvolved skin.

Phytophotodermatitis reactions may be eczematous and erythematous, with prominent vesicles and bullae, located in areas of psoralen contact. The cutaneous reaction may assume bizarre digitate, linear, or drip patterns. The rash often resolves with subsequent hyperpigmentation.

Diagnosis

Inquire about exposure to possible offending agents (new soap, detergent, shoes, or foods, or playing in the woods) and whether there have been previous similar episodes or known sensitivity to a substance. On examination, the presence of an eczematoid eruption either in nontypical locations or in a linear pattern is highly suggestive of contact dermatitis, as are the sharp borders of the rash (atopic eczema blends into neighboring normal skin). Phototoxic reactions can easily be confused with child abuse, burns, or herpes simplex.

ED management

Meticulous allergen avoidance is the key to management and, in minor cases, is sufficient treatment. Otherwise, treat an acute dermatitis with open wet dressings (tap water, normal saline, 5% Burrow's solution) PRN, soothing baths (Aveeno, oatmeal) qd, and antihistamines (hydroxyzine 2 mg/kg per day div tid or diphenhydramine 5 mg/kg per day div qid). For intense inflammation or pruritus, prescribe a low- to medium-potency topical corticosteroid (see Table 5-3) bid for 2 weeks.

Use a systemic corticosteroid for a dermatitis that is widespread or involves the mucous membranes or eyelids. Start with 0.5–1.5 mg/kg per day (40 mg/day maximum) of prednisone or prednisolone, then taper over 10–14 days to prevent a rebound in the eruption.

For a chronic dermatitis the above modalities may be effective, but refer the patient to dermatology for definitive diagnosis and treatment.

Follow-up

- As needed based on severity; if on systemic steroids follow up in 2 weeks

Indication for admission

- Severe disease with extensive involvement involving mucous membranes or threatening the eyes or upper respiratory tract

Bibliography

Carlsen K, Weismann K: Phytophotodermatitis in 19 children admitted to hospital and their differential diagnoses: child abuse and herpes simplex virus infection. J Am Acad Derm 2007;57(5 Suppl): S88–91.

Militello G, Jacob SE, Crawford GH: Allergic contact dermatitis in children. Curr Opin Pediatr 2006;18:385–90.

Slodownik D, Lee A, Nixon R: Irritant contact dermatitis: a review. Australas J Dermatol 2008;49:1–9.

Diaper dermatitis

Diaper rashes can begin as early as the first month of life and may persist or wax and wane over the next 2 or 3 years. Diaper rash can be caused by irritant contact dermatitis, infection (bacterial, fungal), nutritional deficiencies (zinc, biotin, fatty acid, protein), dermatologic disorders (seborrhea, psoriasis, Langerhans cell histiocytosis), metabolic

Table 5-3. Potency of topical corticosteroids

Class: potency	Generic name	Brand name	Strength/form
VII: lowest	Hydrocortisone acetate	Cortifoam	0.1% lotion/ointment/foam
	Hydrocortisone	Hytone, Cortaid	0.25–2.5% lotion/ointment/ solution
VI: low	Desonide	Desowen	0.05% cream
	Flucinolone acetonide	Synalar	0.01% cream/solution
	Aclometasone	Aclovate	0.05% cream/ointment
V: low/medium	Hydrocortisone butyrate	Locomid	0.1% ointment/solution
	Prednicarbate	Dermatop	0.1% cream
IV to III: medium/high medium	Mometasone	Elocon	0.1% cream
	Fluticasone proprionate	Cutivate	0.05% cream; 0.005% ointment
	Betamethasone valerate	Luxiq	0.1% cream/ointment/lotion/ foam
	Clocortolone pivalate	Cloderm	0.1% cream
II to I: high	Flucinonide	Lidex	0.05% cream/ointment/gel/ foam

Note: The duration of topical corticosteroid use varies by disease severity and location. Most patients will respond to 1–2 weeks of application q day or bid. Longer courses require close follow-up. Do not use high-potency topical corticosteroids in the facial and intertriginous areas because it can lead to atrophy, striae, and telangiectasias. Extensive use of any potency topical steroids over large body surface areas for prolonged periods may lead to adrenal axis suppression, particularly in infants.

disorders (cystic fibrosis, maple syrup urine disease, methylmalonic acidemia, organic aciduria), or abuse/neglect. *Candida* superinfection commonly occurs with a diaper rash of any other etiology.

Clinical presentation

Irritant and allergic contact dermatitis

Irritant and allergic contact dermatitis are usually located on the convex surfaces of the buttocks, genitalia, and lower abdomen, sparing the intertriginous folds. The eruption is shiny, erythematous, and scaly. Secondary candidal infection is common.

Candida

Candida infections may be primary, with perianal erythema, or secondary. Beefy red erythema with well-demarcated, raised scaly borders and satellite papules, pustules, and vesicles are seen. Involvement of the intertriginous creases and associated oral thrush are common, and the eruption can spread up the abdomen and down the thighs. The scrotum is often involved in males. Consider secondary candidiasis if a diaper rash does not respond to the usual therapeutic measures. Persistent or frequently recurring diaper candidiasis can occur in HIV-infected children.

Seborrheic dermatitis

Seborrheic dermatitis presents as nonpruritic, salmon-colored, greasy scales on a well-demarcated erythematous base. Characteristically, a similar eruption is simultaneously seen on the face, along with scaling of the scalp and retroauricular areas. Involvement of the intertriginous creases is common, and secondary candidiasis can occur.

Atopic dermatitis

Atopic dermatitis causes a moist, erythematous diaper rash in association with a similar eruption on the face, trunk, and extensor surfaces of the extremities. These infants are extremely unhappy because of the intense pruritus. The onset is between 2 and 6 months of age, and usually the family history is positive for allergies, eczema, hay fever, or asthma.

Congenital syphilis

Congenital syphilis usually presents between 2 and 6 months of age with erythematous papulosquamous plaques, and hemorrhagic bullae of the anogenital region, back, buttocks, thighs, and palms and soles.

Langerhans cell histiocytosis (histiocytosis X)

Histiocytosis may cause a diaper eruption that resembles seborrhea, but is more discretely papular. These papules may feel firm or slightly infiltrated or indurated and can appear hemorrhagic or purpuric. Furthermore, ulceration may occur, which is rare in seborrhea or psoriasis.

Acrodermatitis enteropathica

Acrodermatitis enteropathica in the diaper area can resemble candidiasis or psoriasis. However, there may be a vesiculobullous eruption of the face, hands, and feet, as well as paronychial changes. The patient may also have diarrhea, cachexia, and alopecia.

Psoriasis

Psoriasis can occasionally occur in the first few years of life. It is characterized by the presence of well-demarcated red plaques which are often covered with copious amounts of white or silver (micaceous) scales. New lesions are often small, 1–3 mm papules which subsequently enlarge and coalesce with adjacent lesions to form large plaques. Common sites for psoriatic lesions are the elbows, scalp, knees, and lumbosacral region.

Perianal streptococcal disease

Perianal group A streptococcal infection is characterized by a persistent, bright red, usually tender eruption which is sharply demarcated from the adjacent normal skin. There can be perianal tenderness and itching, and occasionally rectal pain, painful defecation, anal fissures, and secondary stool withholding.

Diagnosis

In general, the clinical presentations are sufficiently different, making the diagnosis apparent. When the picture is not typical, a secondary *Candida* infection of an irritant, contact, or seborrheic dermatitis has most likely occurred. This can be confirmed, if necessary, by microscopic examination of some scales which have been mixed with 10–20% KOH and heated gently. Budding yeasts and pseudohyphae are seen in *Candida* infections. A dermatophyte infection can also be confirmed (branching hyphae and spores).

Pruritus is the key to diagnosing atopic dermatitis. Consider congenital syphilis if there are lesions on the palms and soles or histiocytosis X if the eruption is papular. If the infant appears malnourished, with chronic diarrhea and alopecia, consider acrodermatitis. Psoriasis is suggested by the typical distribution and morphology of the lesions. Perianal streptococcal infection can be confirmed by obtaining a bacterial culture.

ED management

In general, meticulous diaper care is the cornerstone of management for all types of diaper rashes. Recommend frequent diaper changes, gentle cleansing (Cetaphil and Aveeno), and liberal use of barrier products (zinc oxide, petrolatum, A&D ointment) with every diaper change. Air drying and loose-fitting diapers are also key steps in treating and preventing a diaper rash. If the rash is inflammatory, discontinue all harsh soaps, powders, and perfumed products (including baby wipes). Also, since *Candida* super-infection is common with diaper rash of other etiologies, add antifungal therapy (see below) in refractory cases.

Treat inflammation secondary to irritants, contact dermatitis, seborrhea, or atopic dermatitis with a mild topical steroid (see Table 5-3) after diaper changing.

Many topical agents are available for the treatment of *Candida*, including nystatin, miconazole, and clotrimazole. Apply one of these creams tid or qid with a diaper change. The "-azoles" are preferred in the diaper region or when it is difficult to distinguish tinea from monilia. Nystatin (mycostatin) is only effective against *Candida* and other yeast fungi; it is not effective against dermatophyte infections. Add oral Nystatin (1 mL each side of the mouth tid after feeding) if there is oral thrush or a recurrent candidal diaper rash.

Treat perianal streptococcal infection with penicillin VK (50 mg/kg per day div qid) or 40 mg/kg per day div qid of either cephalexin or erythromycin.

A persistent diaper eruption may be the presenting sign of an underlying systemic disorder (immunodeficiency, histiocytosis X, acrodermatitis enteropathica, psoriasis). Refer the patient to a dermatologist if the rash does not respond to these routine measures or the infant is not thriving or has recurrent infections.

Follow-up

- Perianal streptococcal infection: 2–3 days
- Other diaper rashes: primary care follow-up

Bibliography

Gupta AK, Skinner AR: Management of diaper dermatitis. *Int J Dermatol* 2004;43:830–4.

Humphrey S, Bergman JN, Au S: Practical management strategies for diaper dermatitis. *Skin Therapy Lett* 2006;11:1–6.

Scheinfeld N: Diaper dermatitis: a review and brief survey of eruptions of the diaper area. *Am J Clin Dermatol* 2005; 6:273–81.

Drug eruptions and severe drug reactions

Any drug can cause adverse reactions and these frequently involve the skin. The most common offending agents are the penicillins, sulfonamides, and anticonvulsants. In general, suspect the reaction is drug-related when a drug has just been prescribed within the past 6 weeks or has been used inconsistently in the recent past. Unfortunately there are no tests that can confirm that an eruption is due to a particular agent. The priority in the ED is expeditious diagnosis and treatment of serious drug reactions and anaphylaxis.

There are four common drug-related cutaneous eruption patterns: exanthematous, urticarial, fixed drug eruption, and phototoxic/allergic drug eruptions. Of particular concern are the more serious drug reactions with cutaneous manifestations. These include serum sickness-like reactions (SSLR), drug reaction with eosinophilia and systemic symptoms (DRESS), Stevens–Johnson syndrome (SJS) and toxic epidermal necrolysis (TEN).

Clinical presentation and diagnosis

Exanthematous cutaneous eruption

This is the most common drug eruption. It is most frequently caused by amoxicillin and ampicillin ("amoxicillin rash"), developing in about 5–10% of patients taking either medication. The rash is an erythematous, nonpruritic, macular eruption primarily on the trunk, face, and extremities. The typical onset is between days 4 and 8, although the rash can occur after the first or last dose. This is not a true allergy and does not necessitate discontinuing the drug or avoiding penicillins in the future.

Erythema multiforme

Erythema multiforme (EM) is most often a postinfectious rather than drug-related disorder (see pp. 111–112). EM manifests over a period of 12–24 hours, preceded by a mild and short-lived prodromal phase consisting of URI symptoms. The typical target-shaped fixed lesions, with or without blisters, occur in a symmetric, primarily acral distribution, with or without oral mucosal involvement.

Stevens–Johnson syndrome and toxic epidermal necrolysis

Stevens-Johnson syndrome (SJS) and toxic epidermal necrolysis (TEN) are severe conditions involving blistering of two or more mucosal surfaces, widespread lesions, and systemic involvement with fever and generalized malaise. One-third of children with SJS will have episcleritis and purulent conjunctivitis. The associated fever and pharyngitis is frequently misdiagnosed as an infection.

Serum sickness

Serum sickness typically follows the administration of a drug, and is characterized by fever, lymphadenopathy, rash, arthritis, and/or arthralgias. Antigen-antibody complexes are deposited throughout the vascular system and lead to an intense inflammatory response and the associated symptomatology.

See Table 5-4 for the diagnosis and management of the common types of drug eruptions. See Table 5-5 for the diagnosis of other types of drug eruptions. See Table 5-6 for the diagnosis and management of severe drug eruptions.

Table 5-4. Drug eruptions

Eruption type	Associated drugs	Presentation	Management
Exanthematous	Amoxicillin, ampicillin	Morbilliform or scarlatiniform	Continue medication
	Antiepileptics	Generalized, symmetric	Antihistamines
	NSAIDs	Centripetally progressive	Avoid sunlight
	Anti-Tb drugs		
Urticarial	Penicillins, cephalosporins	Evanescent, pruritic	Discontinue medication
	Sulfonamides	Edematous wheals, papules, plaques	Antihistamines
	NSAIDs, opiates	Angioedema may develop	Cool emollients
	Anti-Tb drugs	Dermatographism may be present	
Fixed drug	Sulfonamides, tetracyclines	Solitary or multiple	Discontinue medication
	Acetaminophen, NSAIDs	Erythematous or violaceous	
	Ciprofloxacin, metronidazole	Distinct patches or plaques	
	Penicillins, anti-Tb drugs	Face, trunk, genitalia	
Photosensitivity			
Phototoxic	Tetracyclines, griseofulvin	Sunburn	Discontinue medication
	Fluoroquinalones	May be edematous	Avoid sunlight
	NSAIDs, diuretics	Dose-dependent	Antihistamines
	Antipsychotics		Systemic steroids (if severe)
Photoallergic	Sunscreen, fragrance, latex	Eczematous and pruritic	Same as for phototoxic
	NSAIDs, thiazides		
	Sulfonamides		

ED management

Patients with DRESS, SJS, and TEN can deteriorate quickly from dehydration and internal organ involvement. Therefore, prompt recognition and intervention may be life-saving as these processes all carry significant mortality.

For most other drug eruptions the only treatment required is discontinuing the offending agent. However, there is a wide spectrum of severity and treatment will vary accordingly.

Table 5-5. Other types of drug eruptions

Type of eruption	Most common causes
Acneiform	Corticosteroids, diphenylhydantoin, isoniazid, lithium, oral contraceptives
Erythema multiforme	Sulfonamides, penicillins, barbiturates, phenytoin, carbamazepine
Erythema nodosum	Sulfonamides, phenytoin, oral contraceptives
Lupus-like	Procainamide, hydralazine
Purpura	Penicillins, sulfonamides, oral contraceptives

Table 5-6. Serious drug reactions

Diagnosis	Drugs	Onset	Symptoms	Cutaneous findings	Treatment
SSLR	Cefaclor	1–3 wks	Fever	Erythema and urticaria	Discontinue medication
	Beta-lactams		Arthralgia	Pruritus	Antihistamines
	Sulfonamides		Lymphadenopathy		Topical steroids
	Macrolides				Systemic steroids (severe)
DRESS	Antiepileptics	1–6 wks	Fever	Initially macular and erythematous	Discontinue medication
	Sulfonamides		Lymphadenopathy	Becomes papulovesicular, then exfoliative	Systemic steroids (severe)
				Facial edema	
				Mucous membrane involvement	
SJS	Antiepileptics	1–8 wks	1–14 day prodrome:	Abrupt eruption of target lesions	Supportive care
	Sulfonamides		Fever, conjunctivitis, pharyngitis, rhinitis,	1–3 days after mucous membrane involvement	Meticulous wound care
	Beta-lactams Barbiturates		Arthralgia, myalgia,		Severe cases: burns unit
	Macrolides		vomiting, diarrhea		

Table 5-6. (cont.)

Diagnosis	Drugs	Onset	Symptoms	Cutaneous findings	Treatment
	NSAIDs		→ ↑↑ mucous membrane erosion		
TEN	Antiepileptics	1–8 wks	Same as for SJS, but ↓ mucous membrane involvement	Abrupt onset with caudal spread	PICU or burn unit
	Sulfonamides			Painful erythroderma	Meticulous wound/eye care
	Beta-lactams			Targetoid violaceous lesions →	Maintain airway, hydration
	Barbiturates		↑ systemic symptoms	flaccid blisters (face, trunk) →	30% mortality
	Macrolides		↑ skin involvement	few hours: widespread sheet-like epidermal loss	
	NSAIDs				
				+ Nikolsky's sign	

In general, treat pruritus with hydroxyzine (2 mg/kg per day div tid) or diphenhydramine (5 mg/kg per day div qid) and a low-potency topical corticosteroid (see Table 5-6).

The treatment of anaphylaxis (pp. 30–34), acne (pp. 91–93), erythema multiforme (pp. 111–112), erythema nodosum (pp. 112–113), and urticaria (pp. 36–38) is discussed elsewhere.

Indications for admission
- DRESS
- TEN
- SJS
- Anaphylactic reaction

Bibliography

Knowles SR, Shear NH: Recognition and management of severe cutaneous drug reactions. *Dermatol Clin* 2007; 25:245–53.

Segal AR, Doherty KM, Leggott J, Zlotoff B: Cutaneous reactions to drugs in children. *Pediatrics* 2007;**120**:e1082–94.

Wolf R, Orion E, Marcos B, Matz H: Life-threatening acute adverse cutaneous drug reactions. *Clin Derm* 2005;**23**:171–81.

Erythema annulare

Erythema annulare manifests as an erythematous annular lesion with a raised, non-indurated border and a clear center. The lesion enlarges centrifugally and there may be a fine collarette of scale left behind as the lesions progress. There can be single or multiple lesions on the trunk, buttocks, and thighs, but the hands and feet are usually spared. The etiology is unknown, but is thought to be a hypersensitivity reaction to an underlying condition such as dermatophyte, bacterial or viral infection, malignancy, or immunologic disorder. The lesions may be slightly pruritic but are often asymptomatic. The process is self-limiting but can last weeks to months with successive crops of lesions developing. Symptomatic treatment with antihistamines and a low-potency corticosteroid is variably effective.

Erythema marginatum

Erythema marginatum presents with distinctive, annular, expanding, polycyclic macules limited to the trunk and proximal extremities. These evanescent, pink lesions develop clear centers and serpiginous borders. The rash occurs in up to 10% of patients with active rheumatic fever and follows the onset of migratory arthritis by a few days (pp. 668–671).

Erythema multiforme

Erythema multiforme (EM) (see also p. 107) is a hypersensitivity reaction, most often to an infectious agent. In children, 50% of cases are associated with HSV Type 1, but other viral infections (EBV, hepatitis, adenovirus), bacterial infections (tuberculosis, *Staphylococcus*, group A *Streptococcus*, *Gonococcus*, *Mycoplasma*), and fungi (coccidiomycosis, histoplasmosis) are also implicated. EM is rarely associated with medications (penicillins, sulfonamides, tetracycline, phenytoin), collagen vascular diseases (lupus, rheumatoid arthritis), pregnancy, poison ivy, and neoplasms (leukemia, lymphoma).

Clinical presentation

EM occurs in all age groups, although it is uncommon in children <3 years of age. A short prodromal phase, with symptoms of cough, coryza, sore throat, and myalgias, can precede the eruption by 1–10 days. The classic lesions are dusky red, flat, round macules and target-shaped wheals, with a vesicle or bullae in the center, and occasionally with petechiae within the margins. The eruption can occur anywhere but typically involves the palms and soles, dorsal surfaces of the hands and feet, and extensor surfaces of the arms and legs. The eruption involves the oral mucous membranes in 25–50% of children. The eruption is fixed for 1 week, then resolves over 2–3 weeks, but recurrences may occur. In contrast to urticaria, the rash is symmetric and fixed. Superficial ulceration and hemorrhagic crusting of the mucous membranes also occur. There may be severe eye involvement, with conjunctivitis and keratitis. Lesions appear in successive crops over 10–15 days, after which slow resolution occurs.

Diagnosis

When the characteristic target lesions are present, there is little difficulty in making the diagnosis. However, erythema multiforme is most often confused with urticaria (pp. 36–38), in which the plaques are pruritic and individual lesions last less than 24 hours.

Lupus erythematosus can present with red to purple, annular, polycyclic, urticarial plaques. As with EM, the eruption is on the extensor surfaces of the arms and legs and dorsal aspects of the hands and feet, as well as the mucous membranes and palms and soles. In neonatal lupus erythematous, papules and persistent annular plaques are most concentrated on sun-exposed areas

ED management

If an etiology is not apparent (drug history, herpes, hepatitis, pharyngitis, pregnancy, poison ivy eruption), but the patient appears well, a viral infection is the probable cause and work-up can be deferred. If the patient appears ill, obtain a heterophile antibody, cold agglutinins, and hepatitis surface antigen (HBsAg), and place a PPD. Also obtain a throat culture if there is a pharyngitis, and a chest X-ray if there are lower respiratory tract symptoms.

Appropriately treat any underlying illness (erythromycin for mycoplasma, etc.). In mild cases, all that is needed is acetaminophen (15 mg/kg q 4 h) and wet compresses (normal saline or 5% Burrow's solution) tid for localized bullae. Diphenhydramine/Maalox/viscous lidocaine (1:1:1) rinses may ease the debilitating oral pain of the mucous membrane involvement. Consult an ophthalmologist for any ocular involvement. In rapidly progressing and severe cases admit the patient and consult a dermatologist.

Follow-up

- Ill-appearing patient with erythema multiforme: 2–3 days to check PPD and laboratory results

Indications for admission

- Inability to take liquids adequately
- Suspected Stevens-Johnson syndrome

Bibliography

Khalili B, Bahna SL: Pathogenesis and recent therapeutic trends in Stevens-Johnson syndrome and toxic epidermal necrolysis. *Ann Allergy Asthma Immunol* 2006; 97:272–80.

Leaute-Labreze C, Lamireau T, Chawki D, et al: Diagnosis, classification, and management of erythema multiforme and Stevens-Johnson syndrome. *Arch Dis Child* 2000;83: 347–52.

Letko E, Papaliodis DN, Papaliodis GN, et al: Stevens-Johnson syndrome and toxic epidermal necrolysis: a review of the literature. *Ann Allergy Asthma Immunol* 2005;94:419–36.

Erythema nodosum

Erythema nodosum (EN) is a hypersensitivity reaction that occurs most commonly in patients with respiratory infections, particularly group A streptococcal pharyngitis and primary tuberculosis. Other associations include fungal infections (coccidioidomycosis, histoplasmosis, dermatophytosis), Lyme disease, infectious mononucleosis, cat scratch disease, *Mycoplasma pneumoniae*, pregnancy, inflammatory bowel disease, sarcoidosis, lymphoma, leukemia, and drug reactions (bromides, sulfonamides, oral contraceptives). Erythema nodosum is more common in females, patients >10 years of age, and in the spring and fall.

Clinical presentation

Erythema nodosum presents with multiple, 1–5 cm, oval, red, progressing to purple-colored, slightly elevated nodules symmetrically distributed over the pretibial area. Less commonly, lesions occur on the extensor surfaces of the arms, thighs, face, and neck. Nodules can be warm and extremely tender and frequently are accompanied by arthralgias. Strep-induced erythema nodosum typically appears within 3 weeks of the infection. The eruption then usually disappears without scarring within 6 weeks. There may be recurrences over a period of weeks to months, but rarely thereafter.

Diagnosis

Usually the nodules are so characteristic that there is little difficulty in making the diagnosis. Insect bites are pruritic and not symmetrically distributed; bruises are usually not elevated and resolve over several days; and a cellulitis is hot, usually unilateral, not well demarcated, and often associated with lymphangitic streaking or local lymphadenopathy.

Inquire about a history of upper respiratory infection, tick bites, trauma, recent travel, possible tuberculosis exposure, and medication use. Obtain a rapid strep test or a throat culture and place a 5TU PPD. If tuberculosis, sarcoid, or a systemic fungal infection is suspected, also obtain a chest X-ray.

ED management

The priority is treatment of the underlying disease or eliminating the offending drug. Bed rest, leg elevation, and ibuprofen (10 mg/kg q 6 h) are helpful. Refer atypical, persistent, or recurrent cases to a dermatologist.

Follow-up

- As per the underlying illness

Bibliography

Mert A, Ozaras R, Tabak F, et al: Erythema nodosum: an experience of 10 years. *Scand J Infect Dis* 2004;36:424–7.

Requena L, Sánchez Yus E: Erythema nodosum. *Semin Cutan Med Surg* 2007;26:114–25.

Schwartz RA, Nervi SJ: Erythema nodosum: a sign of systemic disease. *Am Fam Physician* 2007;75:695–700.

Granuloma annulare

Granuloma annulare (GA) is a relatively common cutaneous disorder of unknown etiology. Although GA may occur at any age, 40% of the cases appear in children <15 years of age.

Clinical presentation

The classic lesion of GA is a nonscaling erythematous to flesh-colored annular plaque. Dome-shaped or slightly flattened papules, 3–6 mm in diameter, may also be seen. These papules may be skin-colored, pink, or violaceous and are typically arranged in the form of a ring. Ring size may vary from 1 to 10 cm in diameter and multiple rings are present in

Table 5-7. Differential diagnosis of annular lesions

Diagnosis	Morphology	Size	Location	Duration	Associated findings
Erythema migrans	Rapidly enlarging	>5 cm	Trunk	4–8 weeks	Fever, malaise, headache
	Round or oval plaques		Peripheral		Arthralgia
	Annular or targetoid		extremities		History of tick bite
Erythema multiforme	Erythematous to violaceous	1–5 cm	Symmetrical	>7 days	Nonspecific viral URI
	Targetoid plaques		Acral		Streptococcal pharyngitis
			Palms and soles		Herpes infection
					Infectious mononucleosis
Granuloma annulare	Pink to violaceous	1–5 cm	Distal extremities	Months–years	Asymptomatic
	Smooth papules and plaques				
Nummular eczema	Scaly plaques	1–5 cm	Extremities	Weeks to months	Pruritus
	Excoriations				Follicular prominence
Tinea corporis	Scaly plaques	Varies	Anywhere	Weeks to months	Cat or dog exposure
	Central clearing				
Urticaria	Erythematous and edematous papules and plaques	Varies	Generalized	Usually <24 hours	Pruritus Angioneurotic edema

Source: Adapted with permission from Nopper A, Markus R, Esterly N: When its' not ringworm: annular lesions of childhood. *Pediatr Ann* 1998;27:136–48.

about 50% of patients. GA may occur on any part of the body, but it usually begins on the lateral or dorsal surfaces of the feet, hands, and fingers.

Diagnosis

Granuloma annulare must be distinguished from other annular eruptions, particularly tinea corporis, which is a scaling disease (GA has no scale). Erythema migrans (Lyme disease) can present as a single annular plaque with central clearing. To differentiate these, use low-power magnification (otoscope) to inspect the lesion. With GA there classically are individual papules that form the ring. In addition, on palpation the individual papules of GA can be appreciated, as opposed to the continuous ring of erythema migrans. See Table 5-7 for the differential diagnosis of annular lesions.

ED management

The lesions of GA usually disappear spontaneously, often within several months to several years, with no residual scarring. If GA is severe or generalized, consult a dermatologist, who may obtain a biopsy and/or treat with topical or intralesional corticosteroids.

Follow-up

- 1–2 weeks

Bibliography

Cyr PR: Diagnosis and management of granuloma annulare. *Am Fam Physician* 2006;74:1729–34.

Dahl MV. Granuloma annulare. In Freedberg IW, Eisen AZ, Wolff K, Austen KF,

Goldsmith LA, Katz SI (eds), *Dermatology in General Medicine*, 6th ed. New York: McGraw Hill, 2003, pp. 980–985.

Hsu S, Le EH, Khoshevis MR: Differential diagnosis of annular lesions. *Am Fam Physician* 2001;64:289–96.

Herpes simplex

Herpes simplex infections are caused by two major antigenic types, although the clinical diseases are indistinguishable. Herpes simplex 1 was traditionally responsible for nongenital infections, while type 2 was the agent in sexually transmitted disease. However, this distinction is no longer valid.

After primary spread by person-to-person contact, the virus remains latent in sensory ganglia, with reactivation at a later time. Reactivating stimuli include fever, local trauma, stress, menstruation, and ultraviolet light.

Clinical presentation

The hallmark of herpes infection is a cluster of vesicles on an erythematous base. In general, recurrent disease is associated with fewer constitutional symptoms, smaller vesicles, closer grouping of lesions, and a shorter clinical course than the primary infection.

Gingivostomatitis and labialis

Gingivostomatitis and labialis are common in infants and young children. With primary infection, fever, malaise, sore throat, salivation, and cervical adenopathy occur in association with vesicles in the oral cavity. These vesicles then ulcerate, while the gingiva are erythematous, swollen, and tend to bleed easily. Decreased oral intake may lead to dehydration in infants. Resolution takes 10–14 days.

Recurrent infection is often preceded by burning or tingling in the affected areas for hours to several days. The lesions occur on the cheeks, chin, and vermilion borders of the lips, but generally not in the mouth. The grouped vesicles dry quickly and form a crust. Healing occurs in 5–14 days, but secondary impetiginization can occur.

Genitalis

In females, primary vulvovaginitis is characterized by malaise, fever, vaginal burning, and severe dysuria. The vesicles and erosions may be superficial or deep, involve the vagina, labia, and perineum, and coalesce into large ulcers. In males, the disease affects the penile shaft, glans, urethra, and scrotum. The lesions are painful single or multiple vesicles that rapidly erode and form a crust. Bilateral tender adenopathy is usually present in both genders. Recurrent disease occurs with a prodrome of pain or tingling, followed by the clustered vesicles, which rupture and form ulcers. The course is 10–14 days, with pain, dysuria, and lymphadenopathy.

Neonatal herpes

Neonatal disease occurs either as an ascending infection after premature rupture of the membranes or by direct spread to the neonate during passage through an infected birth canal. Neonatal infection can be asymptomatic or present as a local infection or disseminated life-threatening disease. Generally, the infant becomes ill during the first 1–2 weeks of life when oral or cutaneous vesicles are noted, most commonly on the face or scalp. Fever, lethargy, and hepatosplenomegaly can occur, and with dissemination there may be ocular (keratoconjunctivitis), CNS (encephalitis), and pulmonary (pneumonia) involvement. Dissemination can also occur in the absence of cutaneous lesions. A similar spectrum of disease can occur in immunocompromised patients of any age.

Keratoconjunctivitis

Primary ocular disease presents as a purulent conjunctivitis with edema, vesicles, and corneal ulcers. In contrast to other etiologies of conjunctivitis, pain and photophobia are common because the cornea is involved. With recurrent disease, keratitis or corneal ulcers occur in association with a vesicular eruption of the conjunctiva, eyelids, periorbital skin, and tip of the nose.

Whitlow

Herpetic whitlow results from inoculation of the virus into the fingers, causing a painful, localized vesiculobullous eruption with swelling and erythema. It is usually found distally on the finger that the child habitually sucks. The course is 10–21 days.

Eczema herpeticum (Kaposi's varicelliform eruption)

This occurs in a patient with underlying atopic dermatitis. There are monomorphous (identical) ovoid, eroded, or vesicular lesions that may be associated with fever and toxicity. The lesions may be confused with a secondary bacterial infection.

Diagnosis

Always suspect herpes when there are grouped vesicles on an erythematous base. The presumptive diagnosis of a herpetic infection can be confirmed by performing a Tzanck smear: open the vesicle, blot up the fluid, scrape the bottom and roof of the lesion onto a glass slide, and stain with Wright's or Giemsa stain. Multinucleated giant cells are seen in herpes. If available, direct fluorescent antibody evaluation of a smear is often more practical in the acute care setting. The diagnosis can be confirmed by culturing the virus from vesicle fluid; this requires at least 24–48 hours.

Gingivostomatitis and labialis

The differential diagnosis of mouth sores is discussed on pp. 75–76. Vincent's angina is an acute gingivitis, occurring in adolescents and young adults, that resembles herpes without buccal involvement. Stevens-Johnson syndrome may be associated with cutaneous lesions, and hand-foot-mouth disease is often associated with vesicular lesions on the hands and feet. Recurrent herpes labialis is most often confused with impetigo, although the crust in impetigo has a typical honey color.

Genitalis

Herpes is the major cause of vesicles and ulcers of the genitalia, but confusion with syphilis is common. The diagnosis of sexually transmitted diseases is summarized on pp. 314–325.

Neonatal herpes

Neonatal herpes can resemble any of the transplacental TORCH infections or bacterial sepsis, especially when there are no cutaneous lesions. A complete sepsis work-up (including lumbar puncture) and TORCH titers are indicated for infants presenting in this manner. Do not dismiss the possibility of neonatal herpes even if the mother reports no active lesions at the time of the delivery or there is no known history of the disease.

Keratoconjunctivitis

See pp. 151–153 for other etiologies for a "red eye." The symptoms of ocular pain and photophobia along with the intense conjunctival involvement do not occur with a routine viral or bacterial conjunctivitis. In recurrent infection, be suspicious of ocular involvement if a vesicular eruption is noted on the tip of the nose, since the innervation is the same.

Whitlow

A whitlow can resemble a paronychia (swelling along the lateral side of the nail) or bullous impetigo (flaccid bulla with yellowish pus inside). The diagnosis is made clinically, but if it is uncertain, obtain a Tzanck prep and Gram's stain of the fluid, DFA (if available), and bacterial and viral cultures.

ED management

The mainstays of therapy for children with herpetic gingivostomatitis, labialis, and whitlow are analgesia (acetaminophen, ibuprofen), soaks (sitz baths, 5% Burrow's solution), and patience. Prescribe oral acyclovir (80 mg/kg per day div q 8 h to a maximum of 1200 mg/24 hours) only when symptoms are severe; IV acyclovir (15 mg/kg per day div q 8 h) may be necessary in children who cannot take PO. On occasion, an infant with severe oral disease can become dehydrated and require intravenous fluids. For patients with significant gingivostomatitis that interferes with adequate intake, swab the lesions with viscous lidocaine (2%). However, use it judiciously, as viscous lidocaine can cause seizures and has known cardiotoxic effects if large quantities are absorbed (when used as a rinse or for lesions in the posterior pharynx).

Genitalis

The management is summarized on pp. xx–yy. In general, treating primary or recurrent disease results in faster resolution of the pain and pruritus as well as decreased new lesion formation. Also, suppressive therapy can reduce the frequency of recurrences.

Eczema herpeticum (Kaposi's varicelliform eruption)

Treat with PO or IV acyclovir, depending on the severity of the eruption and toxicity of the patient.

Keratoconjunctivitis

Refer any patient with suspected herpetic keratoconjunctivitis to an ophthalmologist for further evaluation and treatment (acyclovir ophthalmic ointment). Never prescribe ocular corticosteroids, which may facilitate spread of the infection.

Neonates and immunocompromised patients

Admit the patient and treat with IV acyclovir (60 mg/kg per day div q 8 h) for 21 days. Attempt to culture the virus from mucocutaneous lesions, urine, saliva, and cerebrospinal fluid.

Whitlow

Confirm the diagnosis with a Tzanck smear DFA, or culture, if necessary. Treat symptomatically but consider acyclovir and avoid surgical incision.

Follow-up

- Gingivostomatitis and labialis: 1–2 days if no improvement
- Keratoconjunctivitis: as per the ophthalmologist
- Whitlow: primary care follow-up in 1–2 weeks

Indications for admission

- Herpetic infection in a neonate or immunocompromised patient
- Poor oral intake and dehydration in an infant with gingivostomatitis
- Eczema herpeticum (Kaposi's varicelliform eruption)

Bibliography

Kimberlin DW: Herpes simplex virus infections in neonates and early childhood. *Semin Pediatr Infect Dis* 2005;16:271–81.

Kolokotronis A, Doumas S: Herpes simplex virus infection, with particular reference to the progression and complications of primary herpetic gingivostomatitis. *Clin Microbiol Infect* 2006;12:202–11.

Hypopigmented lesions

White or light patches of skin (depigmented or hypopigmented) are caused by either a decrease in number of melanocytes or a decrease in the amount of melanin within the keratocytes. Table 5-8 describes the various presentations of disorders of hypopigmentation.

ED management

Pityriasis alba

There is no effective treatment, although most children outgrow the disease by early to mid-adolescence. Occasionally, therapy with a very mild topical steroid (1% hydrocortisone

Table 5-8. Differential diagnosis of hypopigmented lesions

Diagnosis	Morphology	Distribution	Differentiating features
Pityriasis alba	Small, sharply demarcated	Cheeks	Preadolescents
	Minimal scale	Upper trunk	Worse in summer
	Accentuated in dark skin	Upper extremities	History of atopy
			Wood's lamp and KOH (−)
Tinea versicolor (pityriasis versicolor)	Well-demarcated	Upper trunk	Worse in summer
	Oval macules and patches	Back, neck	Wood's lamp (+): yellow-green
	Powdery scale	Upper arms	KOH (+): "spaghetti and meatballs"
Postinflammatory hypopigmentation	Irregularly shaped patches	Sites of previous inflammation (i.e. eczema, psoriasis)	History of previous inflammatory disorder
			Wood's lamp and KOH (−)
Tuberous Sclerosis	"Ash leaf" spots	Trunk	Other stigmata:
	Well-demarcated patches		Adenoma sebaceum Shagreen patches Periungual fibromas
			Wood's lamp and KOH (−)
Vitiligo	Oval or irregular	Anywhere	Positive family history
	Macules or patches	Axillae	Other autoimmune disorders
	Coalesce →larger patches	Genitalia	Wood's lamp and KOH (−)
		Periorbital	Ivory white, hyperpigmented border
		Acral	Can be segmental

cream, bid) and moisturizers may diminish the demarcation between normal and whiter skin. Stress to the family that sun protection is imperative because the affected areas cannot tan normally and may be more susceptible to burning, while tanning of the surrounding skin accentuates the difference between the normal and hypopigmented skin.

Tinea versicolor

The treatment is discussed on pp. 130–131.

Postinflammatory hypopigmentation

Since the defect is primarily epidermal, postinflammatory hypopigmentation generally improves over time without any therapy.

Tuberous sclerosis

There is no treatment. Rather, refer the patient to a primary care provider to investigate for other stigmata of the disease.

Vitiligo

The single most important piece of advice is for the patient to use appropriate sun protection, as areas of vitiligo are unable to tan normally and therefore are not protected from the sun.

Follow-up

• Primary care follow-up in 2–4 weeks

Bibliography

Huggins RH, Schwartz RA, Janniger CK: Childhood vitiligo. *Cutis* 2007;79:277–80.

Lio PA: Little white spots: an approach to hypopigmented macules. *Arch Dis Child Educ Pract Ed* 2008;93:98–102.

Mollet I, Ongenae K, Naeyaert JM: Origin, clinical presentation, and diagnosis of hypomelanotic skin disorders. *Dermatol Clin* 2007;25:363–71.

Infestations: lice

Three varieties of lice, the head louse, the body louse, and the pubic louse, parasitize humans. The head louse is transmitted by direct personal contact, by contact with infected upholstery, and by sharing hats, combs, brushes, and towels. Body and pubic lice are acquired via bedding, clothing, and person-to-person (sexual) contact. The body louse can carry rickettsial disease (typhus and trench fever) and spirochetal disease (relapsing fever).

Clinical presentation

Pediculosis capitis (head lice)

The patient usually presents with pruritus of the scalp, ears, and back of the neck at the hairline. They may also exhibit an eczematous eruption on the scalp and neck. Nits (eggs) are oval and yellow-white, measuring 0.3–0.8 mm in size. They are found close to the scalp, firmly cemented to the hair around the ears and the occiput. They project from the side of the hair shaft and do not surround it. Nits more than 1.25 cm (0.5 in) from the scalp are probably no longer viable. Adult lice are usually not seen. Secondary impetigo, folliculitis, or furunculosis is common and may mask the primary disease.

Pediculosis corporis (body lice)

These lice live in the lining and seams of clothing and occasionally emerge to bite the host. Erythematous macules become intensely pruritic papules and urticarial wheals, with secondary eczematization and impetiginization.

Pediculosis pubis (pubic lice; "crabs")

Itching is frequently the initial symptom, but secondary infection is common. Pubic and axillary hair and the eyelashes can be affected. The organisms can be identified as brownish crawling "flecks" and nits may be seen attached to the hair shafts. Lice bites can cause nonblanching gray-blue macules (maculae cerulae) on the lower abdomen and thighs.

Diagnosis

The diagnosis of lice infestation is based on the history of possible contact, itching, and visualization of the lice or nits. Nits fluoresce under Wood's lamp examination, and microscopic identification of a nit confirms the diagnosis. Body and pubic lice infestation may resemble eczema or folliculitis. Body lice can also simulate scabies.

ED management

Treat pruritus associated with any infestation with hydroxyzine (2 mg/kg per day div qid) or diphenhydramine (5 mg/kg per day div qid).

Pediculosis capitis

Treat with either a permethrin or pyrethrin-based shampoo. Instruct the parents to apply a single 10-minute application of a permethrin (Nix), after first shampooing and towel-drying the scalp. An equally effective alternative is two 10-minute applications of a pyrethrin-based product (A200, Rid), 1 week apart. Treat all contacts at the same time. Recommend that the parents use a fine-toothed comb to remove nits. Instruct the family to wash the clothing and bedding in very hot water (>52°C, 125°F) for 10 minutes followed by high-heat drying, and to place all hats, combs, and headgear in a plastic bag until after the second shampoo.

As a result of increasing resistance in many urban areas, a variety of other topical agents are now being used. Malathion is the most effective of these, but it is flammable and malodorous. Other options include the use of Cetaphil cleanser applied to the entire scalp with subsequent blow-drying of the hair. High-heat blow-drying of the scalp has also been found effective. Elimite (5% permethrin) applied overnight is also effective.

Pubic lice

Apply a pyrethrin-based product for 10 minutes, then repeat in 1 week. Advise the patient to have all sexual contacts treated.

Body lice

Frequent bathing and laundering (>52°C [125°F] for at least 10 minutes) of clothing and bedding followed by high-heat drying are all that is usually necessary. If lice are noted, treat with a pyrethrin: apply to the entire body from the jawline down, leave on overnight, then wash off in the morning.

Eyelash lice

Treat with petrolatum, applied bid for 8 days. Mechanically remove any nits.

Follow-up

- Primary care follow-up in 1–2 weeks

Infestations: scabies

Scabies is caused by *S. scabiei* and is a common infestation, with the highest prevalence in children <2 years old. It is acquired by close personal contact, although spread via fomites (clothing, linen, and towels) is possible, as the mite can survive for 2–5 days away from humans. The average person is infested with only about 10–15 organisms, so pruritus is presumed to be secondary to an acquired sensitivity to the mite and its feces and eggs. Pruritus begins about 3 weeks after the primary infestation, or sooner if the individual has been previously sensitized.

Clinical presentation

The usual complaint is generalized pruritus, especially interfering with sleep at night. The most common sites of involvement are the interdigital webs, flexor aspects of the wrists, extensor surfaces of the elbows, and nipples, axillae, perineum, and abdomen. The head, neck, palms, and soles can be infected in infants and young children. The eruption varies, based on the duration of infection and degree of sensitization of the patient. Papules, pustules, vesicles, and burrows (elevated, white serpiginous tracts), excoriations, and eczematization may be seen. Other family members may complain of itching and there may be a history of contact with an infected person.

Diagnosis

Scabies is a "great imitator" of other pruritic eruptions. The diagnosis is suggested by a history of contact with an infected person, the intense pruritus, and the variable nature of the lesions. Atopic dermatitis most commonly occurs on the flexor surfaces; involvement of the interdigital webs is uncommon. The lesions of pityriasis rosea are well circumscribed and not on the distal extremities. With folliculitis, a hair shaft can be seen in each papule. Since the lesions of scabies can become impetiginized, differentiation can be very difficult, although pruritus is not as intense in impetigo.

To confirm the diagnosis, place a drop of mineral oil on a burrow, then gently scrape the top off with a no. 15 scalpel blade. Place the scrapings on a microscope slide, cover with a coverslip, and examine at 10× magnification. The diagnosis is confirmed by finding eggs, mites, or oval brown feces.

ED management

Start treatment if the diagnosis of scabies is confirmed or the clinical suspicion is high. Permethrin 5% (Elimite cream) is still the drug of choice for scabies in patients >2 months of age. Massage the cream into the skin from head to toe, and leave it on for 8–14 hours (preferably at night before bed). Treat the scalp of infants. Treat all close contacts, including babysitters, simultaneously. Launder bedclothes and linens (hot-water wash and high-heat dry), or store them away for at least 1 week. Repeat the treatment 7–10 days later. Treat the pruritus with hydroxyzine (2 mg/kg per day div tid) or diphenhydramine (5 mg/kg per day div qid).

Bibliography

Burkhart CG, Burkhart CN: Head lice therapies
revisited. *Dermatol Online J* 2006;12:3.

Karthikeyan K: Scabies in children. *Arch Dis
Child Educ Pract Ed* 2007;92:ep65–9.

Lebwohl M, Clark L, Levitt J: Therapy for head
lice based on life cycle, resistance, and
safety considerations. *Pediatrics* 2007;
119:965–74.

Neonatal rashes

Compared to a child or adult, the skin of a newborn is thinner, sweats less, and has less hair
and fewer melanocytes. As a result, newborn skin appears dry and scaly, and is more likely
to develop blisters or erosions in response to minor traumas. In addition, infants have an
increased body surface area, which places them at increased risk for the absorption of, and
potential toxicities from, any topically applied agent. Fortunately, most neonatal eruptions
are transient and harmless.

Clinical presentation and diagnosis

Cutis marmorata

Cutis marmorata is a reticulated, bluish-red mottling or vascular network that is seen when
the infant is exposed to cold or in distress, and improves when warm. No treatment is
indicated and this benign, physiologic condition resolves by early childhood. Extreme,
persistent forms may be associated with Down syndrome, Cornelia de Lange syndrome
and Trisomy 18. In the uncommon condition cutis marmorata telangectatica congenita the
changes are persistent, with a deeply violaceous color and atrophy.

Erythema toxicum neonatorum

Erythema toxicum is a self-limited papulovesicular eruption that is very common in full-
term newborns in the first week of life. It appears in the first 24 hours of life and lasts as late
as 2 weeks of age. It is characterized by a combination of small (<3 mm) papules
surrounded by an erythematous rim and yellowish pustules on an erythematous macular
base. The lesions can be anywhere on the body, although the palms and soles are usually
spared. Despite the appearance, the infant is well, with no other signs of illness. If
confirmation is necessary, unroof a pustule and obtain a Gram's or Wright stain of the
contents. Eosinophils are characteristic of erythema toxicum, in contrast to the neutrophils
seen with a bacterial infection. In addition, the contents are sterile.

Milia

Milia are tiny (<2 mm), white cysts that are commonly seen on the cheeks, nose, chin, and
forehead of about 50% of newborns. They typically disappear, without treatment, within the
first few months of life.

Miliaria

Miliaria (heat rash) is a group of disorders caused by keratinous obstruction of the eccrine
sweat ducts. Miliaria can occur in any season, often secondary to overdressing an infant.
There are two main types of heat rash. Miliaria rubra (prickly heat) is the more common
type and occurs on covered skin, especially where there is friction from clothing. It is
characterized by pruritic, erythematous 1–2 mm papules and vesicles that are grouped in
clusters with surrounding erythema. Miliaria crystallina (sudamina) is a more superficial

form of miliaria and is characterized by 1–2 mm, clear, thin-walled vesicles on otherwise normal skin. The rash is asymptomatic and occurs primarily in the intertriginous areas. Sunburn can cause this type of miliaria.

Mongolian spots (dermal melanocytosis of infancy)

Mongolian spots are poorly circumscribed, dark brown to blue/black patches that are usually found over the lumbosacral area and buttocks. They are very common in newborns, occurring in more than 90% of African-Americans and native Americans, 80% of Asians, and 70% of Hispanics. Mongolian spots are present at birth and most fade over the first few years of life, while others persist into adulthood. They may be single or multiple, and can vary in size from a few mm to >10 cm in diameter. Although they can be confused with ecchymoses, Mongolian spots do not undergo the color changes seen with bruising or a coagulopathy. Extensive, persistent Mongolian spots have been reported in association with lysosomal storage diseases, such as GM1 gangliosidosis and Hurler syndrome.

Neonatal acne

Neonatal acne is thought to be secondary to maternal and infantile androgens stimulating sebaceous glands that have not yet involuted to a prepubertal immature state. It presents at birth or in the first few weeks of life with erythematous papules and pustules and comedones exclusively on the face. A variant of neonatal acne is thought to be related to the presence of pityrosporum in the pilosebaceous unit. The course is usually self-limited over the first 3 months of life and washing with mild soap and water is all that is required. In severe cases, use a mild topical treatment, such as benzoyl peroxide 2.5–5%. A more extensive evaluation is necessary if there are other signs of hyperandrogenism (pubic or axillary hair).

Neonatal herpes

Herpes occurs by either an ascending infection after premature rupture of the membranes or direct spread to the neonate during passage through an infected birth canal. Neonatal infection can be asymptomatic or present as a local infection or disseminated life-threatening disease. Generally, the infant becomes ill during the first week of life when oral or cutaneous vesicles are noted, most commonly on the face or scalp. Fever, lethargy, and hepatosplenomegaly can occur, and with dissemination there may be ocular (keratoconjunctivitis), CNS (encephalitis), and pulmonary (pneumonia) involvement. Dissemination can also occur in the absence of cutaneous lesions.

Seborrhea

Seborrheic dermatitis is characterized by erythematous skin and yellowish scaling on the scalp, face, ears, neck, intertriginous areas, and diaper region. The disease usually presents between 2 and 8 weeks of age. The eruption may progress to involve the forehead and face, with the development of characteristic salmon-colored greasy scales on a well-demarcated erythematous base known as cradle cap. In the diaper area, the eruption has a similar appearance with involvement of intertriginous areas. Secondary candidal infection can occur.

Transient neonatal pustular melanosis

Transient pustular melanosis is a self-limited neonatal eruption of unknown etiology. In contrast to erythema toxicum, it is present at birth, occurring in 5% of Black and less than 1% of White newborns. It is characterized by clusters of vesicles and pustules, found primarily on the chin, forehead, nape, trunk, and lower legs. The lesions easily rupture within 24–48 hours, leaving a collarette of scale with resultant hyperpigmentation which fades over subsequent months. As with erythema toxicum, the contents are sterile, but neutrophils are seen on Gram's or Wright stain.

ED management

Reassurance is all that is needed for erythema toxicum, milia, Mongolian spots, neonatal acne, and transient neonatal pustular melanosis.

Miliaria

Management consists of cool baths and avoidance of overheating. Parents may overdress an infant, mistakenly attempting to keep the baby's hands and feet warm. Advise them that the proper amount of clothing can be ascertained by feeling the infant's neck or upper back, which should be comfortably warm and not hot and sweaty. Cornstarch will keep inter-triginous areas dry.

Seborrhea

Usually treating the infant's scalp also clears the remainder of the eruption. Adherent scale can be removed by gently massaging mineral oil, white petrolatum, or ketoconazole 2% cream into the scalp and leaving it on for 15 minutes. Afterward, brush the scalp gently or comb with a fine-toothed comb, then shampoo. For more severe cases, an antiseborrheic shampoo containing zinc pyrithione or selenium sulfide is effective when used twice weekly. Treat severe facial eruptions with a short course (3–5 days) of 1% hydrocortisone cream bid. Intertriginous areas may require a topical antifungal cream as well to prevent secondary yeast infection.

Neonatal herpes

Since neonatal herpes can resemble any of the transplacental TORCH infections or bacterial sepsis, especially when there are no cutaneous lesions, perform a complete sepsis work-up (including lumbar puncture) and obtain TORCH titers for infants presenting in this manner. Do not dismiss the possibility of neonatal herpes if the mother denies ever having herpes or having active disease at the time of delivery. The treatment of neonatal herpes is detailed on pp. 116–125.

Follow-up

- Primary care follow-up in 1–2 weeks

Indication for admission

- Neonatal herpes

Bibliography

Caviness AC, Demmler GJ, Selwyn BJ: Clinical and laboratory features of neonatal herpes simplex virus infection: a case-control study. *Pediatr Infect Dis J* 2008;27:425–30.

Lucky A: Transient benign cutaneous lesions in the newborn. In Eichenfield LF, Frieden IJ,

Esterly NB (eds), *Textbook of Neonatal Dermatology*. Philadelphia: W.B. Saunders, 2008, pp. 184–5.

O'Connor NR, McLaughlin MR, Ham P: Newborn skin: Part I. Common rashes. *Am Fam Physician* 2008;77:47–52.

Palpable purpura

Vascular reactions are categorized as blanching (nonpurpuric) and nonblanching (purpuric). Most vascular reactions involve only dilatation of the blood vessels, with no extravasation of blood, so that the eruption blanches and fades completely when direct pressure is applied. In a purpuric eruption, there is extravasation of blood and the lesions do not blanch completely. Palpable purpura are nonblanching, slightly elevated lesions.

The distinction between palpable and nonpalpable purpura is of critical importance, as nonpalpable purpura often represent bruises or ecchymoses, caused by trauma or a clotting abnormality. However, severe fulminant infectious disorders, such as meningococcemia, can present with purpuric lesions that may not be palpable. In contrast, palpable purpura almost always signifies some type of vasculitis, secondary to a serious disease. Possible etiologies include meningococcemia with coagulopathy, SBE, SLE, Rocky Mountain spotted fever, HSP, and drug reactions.

Clinical presentation

Palpable purpura presents as elevated, nonblanching, erythematous to violaceous plaques and nodules. Dependent areas, such as the legs and feet, are the most common sites.

Henoch-Schönlein purpura (HSP) is the most common vasculitis of childhood and classically presents with nonthrombocytopenic purpura, along with some combination of abdominal pain, arthritis, and glomerulonephritis. Purpuric lesions are most concentrated on the buttocks and extensor surfaces of the lower extremities. The majority of cases of HSP are preceded by a URI and there are reports of familial HSP.

Diagnosis

Rapidly obtain a complete history, including medication use, previous illnesses, travel, tick bite, and whether there has been fever, other rashes, headache, or arthralgias. Maintain a high suspicion for sepsis (high fever, lethargy, or toxicity in association with petechiae and palpable purpura), especially meningococcemia.

In general, the purpura is not palpable in cases of physical abuse. Also, the history, distribution of the lesions (face, back, arms), and different types of injuries (burns, linear marks, fractures) suggest the diagnosis.

See the appropriate sections for the evaluation of patients with possible SLE (pp. 679–681), SBE (pp. 64–65), and Rocky Mountain spotted fever (pp. 418–420).

ED management

The priority in evaluating a nonblanching vascular process is to expeditiously rule out or treat sepsis or other serious vasculitic disorders. Any patient who exhibits purpuric lesions in an extensive distribution or of a long-standing nature merits evaluation for possible underlying infectious, autoimmune or hematologic disorders, or child abuse.

If the patient is febrile or appears toxic, treat palpable purpura as bacterial sepsis until proven otherwise. Immediately obtain a CBC, blood and urine cultures, and begin treatment with broad-spectrum antibiotics. If meningitis cannot be ruled out clinically, perform a lumbar puncture.

If HSP is suspected, assess renal function by measuring the blood pressure and obtaining a basic serum chemistry and urinalysis. Treat a drug eruption (pp. 107–110) by discontinuing the offending agent. If there is any suspicion for child abuse, contact the child protection team and social services and document diligently.

Indications for admission

- Possible sepsis
- Acute abdomen or renal compromise

Bibliography

Ballinger S: Henoch-Schönlein purpura. *Curr Opin Rheumatol* 2003;15: 591–4.

Katsambas A, Stefanaki C: Life-threatening purpura and vasculitis. *Clin Dermatol* 2005;23:227–37.

Ting TV, Hashkes PJ: Update on childhood vasculitides. *Curr Opin Rheumatol* 2004;16:560–5.

Pityriasis rosea

Pityriasis rosea is a benign self-limited eruption of unknown etiology, but presumed to be viral in origin because of the frequent prodromal symptoms, seasonal clustering, and lifelong immunity that develops in 98% of patients. However, person-to-person transmission has not been confirmed.

Clinical presentation

Pityriasis rosea occurs predominantly in adolescents and young adults, and less commonly in children <5 years of age. After a variable prodrome of malaise, about 75% of cases present with an initial lesion called a herald patch. This is a 2–5 cm scaling erythematous plaque with a "collarette of scale" (the scaling forms a circle within the borders of the plaque), seen anywhere on the body. The generalized eruption that follows 2–21 days later characteristically consists of small, ovoid papules also with a collarette of scale. The long axes of these lesions follow the cleavage lines on the back and trunk in a so-called Christmas tree pattern. This can be more easily appreciated by having the patient twist his or her spine at the waist and by examining the axillae. In older patients the rash spares the distal extremities, face, and scalp. In younger children, the head and neck may be affected and papules, vesicles, or pustules may be seen. Lesions continue to occur for upto 2 weeks, with clearing in 6–10 weeks. Postinflammatory hypo- or hyperpigmentation can result.

Diagnosis

The history of the herald patch and the characteristic nature of the lesions of the generalized eruption usually suffice to confirm the diagnosis of pityriasis rosea. However, the herald patch may resemble a tinea corporis infection, although these grow slowly and are not followed by a generalized eruption. The lesions of erythema migrans are not scaly, expand more rapidly, and grow to larger dimensions than a herald patch. See Table 5-7 for the differential diagnosis of annular lesions.

Several other diseases are characterized by diffuse erythema and scaling, including guttate psoriasis, nummular eczema, drug reactions, and seborrheic dermatitis, but the face and distal extremities are often involved and there is no Christmas tree pattern. The eruption of secondary syphilis can look very similar, but may involve the palms and soles. Obtain a VDRL if the patient is sexually active.

ED management

For most patients no treatment is necessary. Topical antipruritics or oral antihistamines (hydroxyzine 2 mg/kg per day div tid; diphenhydramine 5 mg/kg per day div qid) alleviate the pruritus. Topical corticosteroids may be useful in very inflammatory cases, but do not shorten the course of the disease. Ultraviolet light or sunlight exposure may hasten the resolution of the rash. Refer patients with lesions persisting for more than 12 weeks to a dermatologist.

Follow-up

• Primary care follow-up in 2–4 weeks

Bibliography

Chuh A, Lee A, Zawar V, Sciallis G, Kempf W: Pityriasis rosea–an update. *Indian J Dermatol Venereol Leprol* 2005;71:311–5.

Stulberg DL, Wolfrey J: Pityriasis rosea. *Am Fam Physician* 2004;69:87–91.

Wyndham M: Pityriasis rosea. *Community Pract* 2008;81:16.

Psoriasis

Psoriasis is an inherited disorder of unknown etiology that was previously thought to be uncommon in childhood. However, 27% of patients develop the disease before age 15, 10% before age 10, and 6.5% before age 5. Patients with active lesions present at birth (congenital psoriasis) have also been reported.

Clinical presentation

Psoriasis is characterized by well-demarcated red plaques which are often covered with copious amounts of white or silver (micaceous) scales. New lesions present as small, 1–3 mm papules that subsequently enlarge and coalesce with adjacent lesions to form large plaques. Partial coalescence can result in gyrate or serpiginous plaques. Linear psoriatic plaques induced by local cutaneous trauma may also occur, reflecting the Koebner phenomenon. The most common sites for psoriasis are the elbows, scalp, knees, genitalia, lumbosacral region, and extensor surfaces of the arms and legs. In infants, psoriasis may also present in the diaper area. Nail changes are also often present, including nail plate pitting, onycholysis, and yellowish discoloration of the nail plate ("oil drop").

Guttate psoriasis presents with a sudden outbreak of hundreds of small, red, drop-like (guttate), nonconfluent papules. The lesions are generally symmetrical and are distributed on the trunk and proximal aspects of the extremities. Guttate psoriasis is often triggered by group A streptococcal infection.

Diagnosis

Classic lesions of psoriasis are not difficult to diagnose, especially when there is a positive family history. The only other similar common disease that exhibits the Koebner phenomenon is lichen planus, in which the papules are usually pruritic and limited to a few areas of the body, including the flexor surfaces and oral mucosa. Pityriasis rosea can be differentiated on the basis of the herald patch and the "Christmas tree" distribution on the torso. A positive KOH preparation confirms the diagnosis of tinea corporis. If the diagnosis remains in doubt, consult a dermatologist who can perform a skin biopsy.

ED management
If the psoriasis is mild and limited to only a few sites, therapy may be initiated in the ED. Recommend mild soaps or cleansers (Dove or Cetaphil), moisturizers, and mild- to moderate-potency topical steroids. Treat scalp psoriasis with thick adherent plaques with P&S liquid or Derma-Smoothe oil, applied overnight, followed 6–8 hours later by an antiseborrheic tar or steroid shampoo. It is important to explain to patients that psoriasis is a chronic condition that is treated but not cured and that there are often alternating periods of exacerbation and remission. Refer patients with psoriasis to a dermatologist.

Follow-up
• Dermatology follow-up in 2–4 weeks

Bibliography
Belazarian L. New insights and therapies for teenage psoriasis. *Curr Opin Pediatr* 2008;20:419–24.

Benoit S, Hamm H: Childhood psoriasis. *Clin Dermatol* 2007;25:555–62.

Tinea
Superficial dermatophytoses are called tinea. The name of any particular tinea infection is based on the clinical location and the species of infecting organism (e.g. *Trichophyton tonsurans* tinea capitis).

Clinical presentation
Tinea capitis
Tinea capitis is caused by infection of the hair shaft. Patchy alopecia with scaling, erythema, and infected hairs that are broken off at scalp level (black dots) are seen. Lymphadenopathy of the cervical and suboccipital regions is often present. Patients may also present with a nonspecific, "seborrheic dermatitis-like" picture, with minimal diffuse hair loss and scale. An acute hypersensitivity reaction with a boggy, inflammatory mass (kerion) can develop.

Tinea corporis
Tinea corporis, or ringworm, is an infection of the glabrous (nonhairy) skin. Infection occurs via contact with an infected individual, infected animal (kitten or puppy), and fomites. The lesions are well-circumscribed annular patches or plaques, with central clearing, and a raised, scaly, papular, or vesicular border.

Tinea cruris
Tinea cruris, or "jock itch," is an infection of the groin and upper thighs that is rare before puberty. More frequent in hot, humid environments and in obese or very athletic individuals, tinea cruris is exacerbated by tight-fitting and chafing clothing. Sharply demarcated, bilaterally symmetric, scaly, erythematous plaques that spare the scrotum and labia are typical. Secondary candidal infection can occur, but is rare.

Tinea pedis

Tinea pedis, or "athlete's foot," is a pruritic eruption that is less common in prepubertal children. Findings range from mild scaling to marked erythema, maceration, fissuring, and vesiculation involving the toes and interdigital webs. The infection may spread to the soles and sides of the feet, but the dorsal aspects of the toes are usually spared. An allergic response to the fungus (id reaction) occasionally causes an erythematous vesicular eruption on the trunk, upper extremities, and palms.

Tinea unguium

Tinea unguium (onychomycosis) is a fungal infection of the nail plate that can be a primary infection or occur in association with dermatophytosis elsewhere (hands, feet). The infection usually begins at the distal/lateral edges of the nail, which become discolored, lusterless, and friable with subungal hyperkeratosis and separation of the distal nail from the nail bed (onycholysis).

Tinea versicolor

Tinea versicolor (pityriasis versicolor) is an infection of the upper trunk and back, proximal arms, and neck that is particularly common in warm climates. The causative organism is *Pityrosporum orbiculare* (previously called *Malassezia furfur*), a dimorphous yeast form that is not a dermatophyte. Hypo- or hyperpigmented, well-demarcated, scaling, oval macules with little or no erythema or pruritus are seen. It is diagnosed more commonly in the summertime, as the involved areas will not tan while the surrounding uninfected skin does.

Diagnosis

To differentiate fungal infections from other conditions, scrape the lesions and mix the scale with a 10–20% potassium hydroxide solution, heat gently and examine microscopically. Birefringent septate hyphae are seen in dermatophyte skin infections, and multiple spores surrounding a hair shaft are seen in tinea capitis. Tinea versicolor has a characteristic "spaghetti and meatballs" appearance on examination, which represents short hyphae and spores. If the diagnosis is in doubt, culture the fungus on Sabouraud's agar or dermatophyte test medium (DTM). Tinea versicolor requires oil supplementation to grow, and the lab must be notified, although this is usually a diagnostic concern only in immunocompromised patients. Finally, a minority of tinea capitis and all tinea versicolor infections will fluoresce under Wood's lamp examination.

Tinea capitis is the only common etiology of childhood alopecia that causes scalp inflammation. The eruption may fluoresce under a Wood's lamp and black dots may be seen. The scalp is normal in alopecia areata and trichotillomania, while seborrheic dermatitis causes scaling without hair loss. Bacterial infections of the scalp are uncommon; usually there is no hair loss as with a kerion. Bacterial folliculitis of the scalp will show discrete perifollicular erythema and purulence.

Tinea corporis can resemble contact dermatitis, the herald patch of pityriasis rosea, erythema migrans, and nummular eczema. The characteristic central clearing and raised, well-demarcated scaly border usually suggest the diagnosis.

Tinea cruris can be confused with contact dermatitis, intertrigo, and erythrasma, a *Corynebacterium* infection that fluoresces coral-red under Wood's lamp examination. In addition, secondary candidal infection can occur and confuse the picture, but a broad-spectrum topical antifungal such as miconazole will treat both dermatophytes and *Candida*.

Before the diagnosis of tinea pedis is made in a prepubertal patient, consider dyshydrotic eczema, atopic dermatitis, and contact dermatitis, which can involve the dorsum of the foot. The id reaction is characterized by the absence of fungus in the area of the reaction, an identifiable focus of fungal infection (usually on the feet), and spontaneous clearing when the primary fungal infection is eradicated.

Tinea unguium must be confirmed with a positive culture, as psoriasis, eczema, trauma, and congenital ectodermal syndromes all have a similar appearance.

Tinea versicolor resembles pityriasis alba, postinflammatory hypopigmentation, vitiligo, seborrheic dermatitis, and secondary syphilis. However, none of these conditions fluoresces under Wood's lamp examination, and all are KOH-negative.

ED management

Tinea capitis

Tinea capitis cannot be treated topically. Obtain a culture prior to treating the patient with oral griseofulvin (20–25 mg/kg per day microsize; 10–15 mg/kg per day ultramicrosize) for 6–8 weeks. Leukopenia, neutropenia, and hepatotoxicity are uncommon side effects. If therapy extends longer than 8 weeks, obtain a CBC and LFTs. Oral terbinafine is a treatment option. Use selenium (Selsun) or ketoconazole shampoo twice a week to decrease the period of infectivity. Counsel families that regrowth of hair may take months. Inquire about other symptomatic contacts and suggest evaluation for those individuals, as they may serve as an infectious focus in the house.

Tinea corporis, tinea cruris, tinea pedis

Treat with clotrimazole, miconazole, or terbinafine, bid or tid, for 4 weeks. In addition, soak inflammatory lesions with normal saline or 5% Burrow's solution compresses. Keep affected areas dry; this is particularly important for tinea pedis and tinea cruris, where antifungal powders are helpful. Instruct the patient to wear cotton (instead of synthetic) underwear and socks to help dissipate moisture.

Tinea unguium

The treatment is oral griseofulvin. However, in view of the long course (6–18 months) of therapy and high recurrence rate, refer the patient to a dermatologist rather than initiating treatment in the ED.

Tinea versicolor

Treat for 2 weeks with either 2.5% selenium sulfide shampoo or ketoconazole shampoo 3 days in a row, then monthly. Advise the patient to apply the shampoo to the affected skin daily, for 5 minutes, prior to rinsing. Topical antifungals are also effective but more expensive. Some patients will require monthly prophylaxis consisting of one treatment. Inform the patient that the normal skin pigment will not return until after the treated lesions are exposed to ultraviolet light.

Follow-up

- Primary care follow-up in 2 weeks
- Tinea unguium: dermatologist within 2 weeks

Bibliography

Andrews MD, Burns M: Common tinea infections in children. *Am Fam Physician* 2008;77:1415–20.

Crespo-Erchiga V, Florencio VD: Malassezia yeasts and pityriasis versicolor. *Curr Opin Infect Dis* 2006;19:139–47.

González U, Seaton T, Bergus G, Jacobson J, Martínez-Monzón C: Systemic antifungal therapy for tinea capitis in children. *Cochrane Database Syst Rev* 2007;CD004685.

Möhrenschlager M, Seidl HP, Ring J, Abeck D: Pediatric tinea capitis: recognition and management. *Am J Clin Dermatol* 2005;6:203–13.

Verrucae and molluscum

Verrucae, or warts, occur in 5–10% of children between the ages of 10 and 16 years. They are benign tumors of the epidermis caused by a DNA (papilloma) virus that spreads via autoinoculation and person-to-person contact. Local trauma seems to promote infection with the virus, so that lesions are most common on the fingers, hands, elbows, and plantar surfaces. The incubation period is 1–6 months and, while the course is extremely variable, two-thirds of all lesions spontaneously resolve within 2 years. A patient can have from one to several hundred warts.

Molluscum contagiosum is an eruption caused by a virus of the pox group, spread by direct person-to-person contact and autoinoculation. The disease occurs at any age, but is most common between 3 and 15 years.

Clinical presentation

Common warts

Common warts (verruca vulgaris) occur predominantly on the dorsal surfaces of the hands and the periungual regions. They usually begin as pinpoint, flesh-colored papules that grow larger (1–10 mm), with roughened surfaces, grayish color, and sharply demarcated borders. Often these lesions are studded with black dots (thrombosed capillaries).

Flat warts

Flat warts (verruca plana) are tan to flesh-colored, soft, flat, small (2–6 mm) papules that occur primarily on the face, neck, arms, and hands. These are particularly common in shaved areas. Contiguous lesions can become confluent and plaquelike.

Plantar warts

Plantar warts (verruca plantaris) usually occur in weightbearing areas of the sole of the foot. They are flat, with sharp margins, and black dots are seen within the lesions. Pressure forces them into the tissues of the foot and this leads to marked tenderness when walking. They often coalesce into a single large plaque called a mosaic wart.

Venereal warts

Venereal warts (condylomata acuminata) are soft, reddish pink, filiform lesions that may coalesce into larger, cauliflower-like clusters. They are located primarily on the genitalia and around the anus. Proctoscopic examination may reveal involvement of the rectal mucosa as well. Condylomata acuminata are usually sexually transmitted, although they can spread from a caretaker diapering or by autoinoculation from warts elsewhere on the body. Nonetheless, sexual abuse is a concern when venereal warts are found on a young child.

While the vast majority of anogenital warts found in children <2 years of age are the result of maternal perinatal transmission, the initial onset of lesions in older patients is of more concern for sexual abuse. In general, the older the prepubertal child is at first presentation of genital warts, the greater is the likelihood of sexual transmission.

Molluscum

The lesions start as small papules that typically grow to 3–6 mm in diameter, but they can be as large as 2–3 cm. They usually are flesh-colored or opalescent and dome-shaped, with a central umbilication. Papules are found on the face, trunk, extremities, and pubic region, either alone or in clusters, and number from one to several hundred. The duration of individual lesions is variable; although most resolve within 9–12 months, some may persist for 2–3 years. Chronic conjunctivitis or keratitis may occur with eyelid lesions. Particularly severe eruptions with thousands of lesions can occur in patients with atopic dermatitis or depressed cellular immunity.

Diagnosis

The diagnosis of common or flat warts can be confirmed by the absence of skin markings over the lesions and the presence of black dots (thrombosed dermal capillaries) beneath the surface. Gentle paring with a scalpel causes small bleeding points which represent intact capillaries.

Periungual warts can be confused with the periungual fibromas of tuberous sclerosis. However, other cutaneous manifestations of tuberous sclerosis usually are present (adenoma sebaceum, ash-leaf spots, Shagreen patches).

Plantar warts may resemble calluses, corns, and black heel (talon noir). Calluses do not have sharp, well-demarcated margins and no black dots are seen. Corns typically occur at the metatarsalphalangeal joints. There are no black dots, but they have sharp margins and a characteristic translucent particle at the core. Skin markings over the lesion remain intact. Black heel occurs in athletes who make frequent sudden stops, causing blackish pinpoint hemorrhages. The margin is not well demarcated, and paring does not reveal bleeding points.

Condylomata acuminata must be differentiated from the condylomata lata of secondary syphilis. The latter are 1–3 cm grayish pink nodules occurring in the same regions. Dark-field microscopy or serology (VDRL and FTA) is necessary to confirm the diagnosis.

The diagnosis of molluscum is usually easily established by the distinctive appearance of the flesh-colored papules with central umbilication. To verify the diagnosis, opening a papule will reveal a small central core, which resembles a cluster of grapes when visualized under magnification.

ED management

Since untreated lesions often spontaneously resolve within several months to years, watchful waiting is often the best approach. If there are cosmetic concerns, or if the lesions continue to spread, refer the patient to a primary care setting. However, keratolytic therapy may be instituted in the ED for a patient with a few lesions. Give salicylic acid (10–16%) with lactic acid (10–16%) in flexible collodion and instruct the patient to apply daily after bathing, then cover the wart for 24 hours with a waterproof adhesive bandage. Repeat the procedure after paring the wart with the side of a scalpel or rubbing with a washcloth, emery board, or pumice stone. Commercially available salicylic acid plaster is useful for plantar warts. Cut it to fit the lesion, tape it in place for 4–5 days, then pare the necrotic tissue and reapply the plaster, if necessary. Inform the family that multiple reapplications will probably be necessary.

Refer patients with lesions on the face, multiple hand warts, periungual and subungual warts, large plantar warts, or venereal warts to a dermatologist for other available therapies, which include liquid nitrogen, cantharidin, electrodessication and curettage, and podophyllin. See pp. 583–586 for the evaluation and management of possible sexual abuse.

Reassure patients with molluscum that the disorder is benign, and refer them to a dermatologist for treatment if desired. Cantharidin or curettage is usually effective, but defer this to the primary care setting

Follow-up

* Primary care or dermatology follow-up in 1–2 weeks

Bibliography

Brown J, Janniger CK, Schwartz RA, Silverberg NB: Childhood molluscum contagiosum. *Int J Dermatol* 2006; 45:93–9.

Herman BE, Corneli HM: A practical approach to warts in the emergency department. *Pediatr Emerg Care* 2008;24:246–51.

Lio P: Warts, molluscum and things that go bump on the skin: a practical guide. *Arch Dis Child Educ Pract Ed* 2007;92:ep119–24.

ENT emergencies

Jeffrey Keller and Stephanie R. Lichten

Acute otitis media

Acute otitis media (AOM) is a suppurative infection of the middle ear caused by bacteria and viruses. It accounts for up to one-third of pediatric acute healthcare visits. The incidence is highest during the winter months, secondary to the greater frequency of viral upper respiratory infections (URIs). Children with normal immunity may have multiple episodes in a year. Risk factors for AOM include daycare attendance, second-hand smoke exposure, use of a pacifier, bottle feeding, and a family history of ear infections. Children with Down's syndrome or craniofacial abnormalities are at an increased risk of otitis media.

The most common bacterial etiology identified is *Streptococcus pneumoniae* (30–40%), which is now decreasing in frequency secondary to vaccination, followed by nontypable *Haemophilus influenzae* (20–30%), *Moraxella catarrhalis* (10–20%), and *Streptococcus pyogenes*. The Gram-negative enteric organisms (*Escherichia coli, Klebsiella, Proteus, Pseudomonas*) and *Staphylococcus aureus* are responsible for about 15% of cases in the first few months of life, but are exceedingly rare afterward. Viruses, including parainfluenza, respiratory syncitial virus, influenza, adenovirus, and enterovirus are common pathogens (up to 50% of cases). Anaerobes, *Mycoplasma pneumoniae*, and *Chlamydia trachomatis* are not significant pathogens.

Clinical presentation

Acute otitis media is usually preceded by a URI with cough and rhinorrhea. Ear symptoms begin 2–3 days later and may include fever, pain, dizziness, buzzing in the ear, or decreased hearing. In infants, there are nonspecific symptoms, such as irritability, increased crying, decreased feeding, sleep disturbance, vomiting, or diarrhea. In many cases, the patient has only fever, a persistent URI, or behavioral changes (cranky, not feeding or sleeping well). Ear tugging is an unreliable sign of AOM. Occasionally, there is a history of severe ear pain that improved abruptly when a bloody or yellowish discharge began to drain from the external canal (tympanic membrane perforation). In summary, clinical history alone is an inaccurate predictor of AOM; therefore, examine the ears of a patient with any of the symptoms mentioned above, even if otoscopy in the previous 24–36 hours did not reveal an otitis media.

Diagnosis

The American Academy of Pediatrics and the American Academy of Family Physicians practice guidelines state that the diagnosis of AOM must meet the following three criteria: rapid onset, the presence of middle ear effusion (MEE), and signs and symptoms of middle ear inflammation.

Table 6-1. Differential diagnosis of otalgia

Diagnosis	Differentiating features
Acute myringitis	Inflammation of tympanic membrane Bullae possible
Dental abscess	Edema, erythema or tenderness of gingiva
Otitis externa	Pain on traction of pinna
Parotitis	Edema over angle of mandible
Pharyngitis	Erythema, exudate or herpangina on oropharyngeal examination
Serous otitis media	Dark, retracted tympanic membrane Air–fluid level or bubbles behind tympanic membrane Inflammation of Stensen's duct
TMJ disease	Pain with palpation of TMJ, especially with mouth opening/closing

Examine the tympanic membrane (TM) for shape (concave, retracted, bulging), color (pearly gray, injected, erythematous, yellow), the presence of landmarks (light reflex, malleus), and mobility. Redness alone is not sufficient to make the diagnosis, since crying can cause erythema of the drum. Perform pneumatic otoscopy, focusing on the light reflex. Decreased mobility of the tympanic membrane, which can be confirmed by tympanometry (flat tympanogram), is the most sensitive indicator of a middle ear effusion. A combination of erythema, bulging with or without a purulent effusion, loss of normal anatomic landmarks, and decreased mobility are characteristic of an acute otitis media. Tympanic membrane perforation with recent onset of bloody or purulent ear discharge is also diagnostic. The history of a recent URI, complaints of ear pain, and constitutional symptoms such as listlessness and fever are insufficient to make the diagnosis without the typical otoscopic findings. See Table 6-1 for the differential diagnosis of otalgia.

The optimal position for examination varies with the age of the patient. Examine infants and young children supine on the table, restrained by an adult. Place an older child on the parent's lap, seated face-to-face with the examiner. One of the parent's arms can tightly embrace the child, while the other holds the patient's head.

In some cases there may be impacted cerumen in the ear canal obstructing the view of the tympanic membrane. Remove cerumen by curetting or irrigating with warm water 20 minutes after instilling several drops of hydrogen peroxide (if no tympanic membrane perforation is suspected).

ED management

Despite the presence of an otitis media, perform a thorough physical examination to be certain that the patient does not have a more serious infection, such as meningitis. If the patient is toxic-appearing, admit for aggressive inpatient parenteral management.

The American Academy of Pediatrics practice guideline recommends a 48–72 hour period of observation, without antimicrobial treatment, for selected children ≥6 months of age in whom follow-up can be ensured if symptoms worsen (Table 6-2). Treat children <6 months with antibiotics when the diagnosis of AOM is either certain or probable (uncertain). See Table 6-3 for antibiotic choices and doses.

Table 6-2. Treatment guidelines for AOM by age

Age	Certain diagnosis	Uncertain diagnosis
<6 months	Antibiotics	Antibiotics
6 months – 2 years	Antibiotics	Antibiotics[a]
		Observation[b]
>2 years	Antibiotics[a]	Observation
	Observation[b]	

Notes: [a]Antibiotics: for temperature >102° F (38.9° C) or severe otalgia not relieved by topical or oral medication.
[b]Observation: for temperature ≤102° F (38.9° C) and mild otalgia or otalgia resolved with topical or oral medication.

Table 6-3. Antibiotic doses for otitis media and sinusitis

Antibiotic	Dose	Notes
Amoxicillin	80–90 mg/kg per day div bid	First choice if not penicillin-allergic
Amoxicillin-clavulanate ES[a]	90 mg/kg of amoxicillin div bid	Use for treatment failure after 3 days
Azithromycin	first day 10 mg/kg q day days 2–5 5 mg/kg q day	Use for type 1 penicillin hypersensitivity[b]
	or 30 mg/kg once	
	or 10 mg/kg per day × 3 days	
Cefdinir	14 mg/kg per day div q day or bid	Use for non-type 1 penicillin hypersensitivity
Cefpodoxime	10 mg/kg per day div q day or bid	Use for non-type 1 penicillin hypersensitivity
Ceftriaxone IM	Unable to take PO: 50 mg/kg × 1	
	Treatment failure: 50 mg/kg per day × 3	
Cefuroxime	30 mg/kg per day div bid	Non-type 1 penicillin hypersensitivity
Clarithromycin	15 mg/kg per day div bid	Use for type 1 penicillin hypersensitivity[b]
Clindamycin	20 mg/kg per day div qid	Use for type 1 penicillin hypersensitivity[b]
Erythromycin-sulfisoxazole	50 mg/kg per day of erythro div qid	Use for type 1 penicillin hypersensitivity[b]
Trimethoprim/sulfamethoxazole	8–10 mg/kg of TMP div bid	Use for type 1 penicillin hypersensitivity[b]

Notes: [a]Consider as first choice for otitis-conjunctivitis syndrome because of high prevalence of penicillinase resistance among non-typable H. flu (most common etiologic agent).
[b]Urticaria or anaphylaxis

Regardless of the treatment option, pain management is critical. Use topical analgesia (benzocaine otic drops, 1–2 drops qid) and/or acetaminophen (15 mg/kg q 4 h) or ibuprofen (10 mg/kg q 6 h). In the ED, instilling a single dose of one to two drops of 2% viscous lidocaine may ameliorate extreme discomfort. Do not recommend antihistamine-decongestant combinations. Instruct the parents to return in 2–3 days if the child remains symptomatic (fever, ear pain, decreased hearing) or is not improving. If AOM is confirmed on re-examination, initiate antibiotic treatment. Patients whose symptoms are worsening at any time or who have continued symptoms at the completion of treatment require re-examination.

Under 2 months of age

Treat an afebrile, well-appearing infant <2 months of age with amoxicillin. However, if there is fever (≥38.1°C; 100.6°F), toxicity, irritability, evidence of a systemic infection, a complicated neonatal course, or a previous hospitalization with antibiotic treatment, admit the patient (see Evaluation of the febrile child, pp. 370–373), perform an evaluation for sepsis, and treat with IV antibiotics.

A sterile effusion occurs in more than 40% of children following an acute otitis media. This usually resolves without intervention, although a temporary conductive hearing loss can persist until the effusion resolves.

Tympanocentesis is indicated for systemic toxicity, severe unremitting pain, inadequate response to conventional therapy, or a suppurative complication (facial nerve paralysis, mastoiditis, meningitis, brain abscess), and may be necessary in some immunocompromised patients. Obtain an otolaryngology consult.

Follow-up
- Patient not treated with antibiotics: 2–3 days
- Patient treated with antibiotics: 2–3 days if still febrile or at the completion of therapy if still symptomatic

Indications for admission
- Infant <1 month of age with temperature ≥ 38.1°C (100.6°F)
- Toxic appearance
- Immunocompromised patient with fever
- Suppurative complication (mastoiditis, meningitis, brain abscess) or seventh nerve palsy

Bibliography

American Academy of Pediatrics Subcommittee on Management of Acute Otitis Media: Diagnosis and management of acute otitis media. *Pediatrics* 2004;**113**:1451–65.

Barenkamp SJ: Implementing guidelines for the treatment of acute otitis media. *Adv Pediatr* 2006;**53**:241–54.

Coleman C, Moore M: Decongestants and antihistamines for acute otitis media in children. *Cochrane Database Syst Rev* 2008; Jul **16**(3):CD001727.

Rovers MM, Glasziou P, Appelman CL, et al: Antibiotics for acute otitis media: a meta-analysis with individual patient data. *Lancet* 2006;**368**: 1429–35.

Cervical lymphadenopathy

Palpable cervical lymph nodes >1 cm in diameter are present in approximately 80–90% of preschool and young, school-age children, especially if they have had a recent upper respiratory tract infection. Nonetheless, consider cervical lymphadenopathy in three broad etiologic categories: reactive, adenitis, or associated with systemic illness.

Clinical presentation

Reactive

Most enlarged cervical lymph nodes are reactive, found in conjunction with a viral or bacterial infection of the head or neck. These nodes are generally benign and no work-up or specific treatment is necessary.

Most often the presentation reflects the primary illness (URI, pharyngitis, etc.). Other complaints include a neck mass, stiff neck (unwillingness to move the neck side to side), or torticollis. Reactive nodes are usually multiple, discrete, firm, smaller than 1–2 cm in diameter, nontender, and mobile. The overlying skin is neither erythematous nor adherent. In general, reactive adenopathy subsides in 2–3 weeks, but it can persist.

Adenitis

An adenitis is an infection of the lymph node itself, most commonly (60–85%) caused by *Staphylococcus aureus* or group A *Streptococcus*, although viral and anaerobic infections have been implicated. Atypical *Mycobacterium* and *Mycobacterium tuberculosis* can result in a node with all the signs of acute infection. Cat scratch disease (Bartonellosis) may cause cervical, axillary, or inguinal adenitis.

With an adenitis, the node becomes enlarged, tender, and fluctuant. The overlying skin is warm, erythematous, and occasionally adherent. The hallmarks of an atypical mycobacterium infection are the presence of skin erythema overlying a nontender lymph node in an afebrile, otherwise well-appearing child. The node often suppurates. Cat scratch disease is characterized by a papule at the site of the scratch, followed in 5–60 days by regional lymphadenitis. Despite the impressive lymphadenopathy, the patient usually appears well, although 30% may have fever.

Systemic disease

Systemic diseases, especially infectious mononucleosis and mono-like syndromes (cyto-megalovirus, toxoplasmosis, leptospirosis, brucellosis, and tularemia), sarcoidosis, Kawasaki syndrome, and HIV, can cause cervical as well as generalized lymphadenopathy. Some medications, such as phenytoin and isoniazid, can cause generalized lymphadenopathy. The possibility of a malignancy (leukemia, Hodgkin's disease, non-Hodgkin's lymphoma, neuroblastoma) is always a concern.

Mononucleosis and mono-like illnesses (pp. 386–388) can present with generalized tender lymphadenopathy, sometimes in association with an exudative pharyngitis, macular rash, and hepatosplenomegaly. These nodes are firm and mobile. Kawasaki disease (pp. 395–396) and HIV (pp. 374–380) are discussed elsewhere.

A malignant node is fixed, hard, and matted. It is frequently supraclavicular in location and may be described as persistent or continuously growing. Weight loss, weakness, pallor, night sweats, fever, petechiae, and ecchymoses are other possible findings.

Diagnosis

Perform a thorough examination of the head, neck, teeth, and gums to find a source of infection draining into the affected node(s). Weakness, fever, rash, hepatosplenomegaly,

Table 6-4. Differential diagnosis of cervical lymphadenopathy

Diagnosis	Differentiating features
Branchial cleft cyst	Smooth and fluctuant along the lower anterior border of SCM muscle
Cervical ribs	Bilateral, hard, immobile masses
Cystic hygroma	Soft, compressible
	Usually transilluminates
Dermoid cyst	Midline mass with calcifications on X-ray
Hemangioma	Present at birth
	Red or bluish color
Kawasaki	Nonpurulent conjunctivitis and mucous membrane changes, Polymorphic rash
	Edema of dorsum of extremities
Malignancy	May have: weight loss, pallor, bleeding, fever, hepatosplenomegaly
	Node is fixed, hard, matted, and persistent or growing
Meningitis	Nuchal rigidity, photophobia, toxicity
Parotitis	Swelling obscures the angle of the jaw
	Intraoral exam: edema, erythema, or drainage from Stensen's duct
Thyroglossal duct cyst	Midline mass between thyroid bone and suprasternal notch
	Moves up when patient sticks out tongue

and generalized lymphadenopathy are all indicative of a systemic disease. See Table 6-4 for the differential diagnosis of cervical adenitis.

There are seven features of the affected node(s) to consider.

Single or multiple (unilateral or bilateral)

Enlargement of a single node generally occurs in an adenitis, although tuberculous adenitis causes bilateral involvement. Reactive adenopathy and systemic diseases most often result in multiple, bilateral involvement.

Location(s)

The location of a reactive node can suggest the site of the primary infection (preauricular-conjunctiva or external ear canal; occipital-scalp; submental and submandibular-intraoral). Supraclavicular adenopathy is suspicious for a malignancy, while occipital adenopathy suggests a viral illness (particularly roseola and rubella). Generalized lymphadenopathy most commonly occurs during mononucleosis or a mono-like infection, although leukemia is a possible etiology.

Size

Reactive nodes are typically small (<2 cm). Massive enlargement can occur with an atypical *Mycobacterium* infection.

Rate of growth

Nodes that slowly enlarge suggest a malignancy, while rapid enlargement occurs in an infected or reactive node.

Mobility

In general, a freely movable node is benign. A node that is fixed to adjacent structures or matted to other nodes suggests a malignancy, mycobacterial infection, or cat scratch disease.

Consistency

Soft or firm nodes are benign, while fluctuance occurs in adenitis. A rubbery consistency is noted in sarcoidosis and malignant nodes are usually rock hard.

Overlying skin

Bacterial adenitis causes erythema and warmth of the overlying skin. However, adherence occurs in cat scratch disease and atypical *Mycobacterium* infection. A reactive node does not affect the overlying skin.

ED management

Reactive

"Benign" reactive nodes found in conjunction with a head or neck infection require treatment of the primary illness, only. If the pharynx is erythematous, obtain a rapid strep test or a throat culture. Benign nodes can be followed without intervention, although persistence for more than 4–6 weeks may indicate the need for further testing. Reassure the family and arrange for primary care follow-up.

Adenitis

When bacterial adenitis is diagnosed, obtain a throat culture or rapid strep test and give an oral antibiotic with staphylococcal and streptococcal coverage such as cefadroxil (40 mg/kg per day div bid) or cephalexin (40 mg/kg per day div q 6 hr). Alternatives are cefprozil (20 mg/kg per day div bid), cefuroxime (30 mg/kg per day div bid), or azithromycin (12 mg/kg q day). If MRSA is a concern, either use clindamycin (20 mg/kg per day div q 6 hr) or add trimethoprim-sulfamethoxazole (8 mg/kg per day of TMP div bid) to one of the above regimens. However, use penicillin VK (<27 kg: 250 mg qid; >27 kg: 500 mg qid) if the adenitis is secondary to intraoral or dental disease. Warm compresses, applied for 15–30 minutes every 3–4 hours, are also necessary. Have the patient return in 2–3 days. If there is clinical improvement, or a positive strep test or culture, continue the antibiotics for a total of 10 days. If the node has not responded to antibiotics and warm compresses, change to either clindamycin (20 mg/kg per day div qid) or amoxicillin-clavulanate (875/125 formu-lation; 45 mg/kg per day of amoxicillin div bid) and follow up in two more days. If the node becomes fluctuant arrange for an incision and drainage.

Admit patients who are toxic or have nodes unresponsive to oral antibiotic therapy for parenteral treatment: nafcillin 150 mg/kg per day div q 6 h, ceftriaxone 100 mg/kg per day div q 12 h, or cefazolin 75 mg/kg per day div q 8 hr. Use clindamycin (40 mg/kg per day div q 6 h) if MRSA is a concern. Obtain a CBC with differential, heterophile antibody, and a blood culture prior to starting intravenous therapy. Indications for a node biopsy include age >10 years, persistent and unexplained weight loss or fever, skin ulceration or fixation to the node, supraclavicular location, or continuously increasing size.

If atypical mycobacterial infection is suspected, surgical curettage/excision is required as the infection is frequently resistant to antitubercular medication. Avoid incision and drainage, which can result in a chronic fistula. If tuberculosis is suspected because of possible exposure or travel, place a 5 TU PPD. If the PPD is positive, consider *Mycobacterium* as the cause of the infection. Obtain a chest X-ray and admit the patient for surgical consultation, collection of culture specimens, and institution of antituberculous therapy (pp. 423–427).

Systemic disease

When a mononucleosis syndrome is suspected, obtain a heterophile antibody or monospot test. Treatment is supportive. Note that the heterophile antibody may be negative early in the disease and in young or immunocompromised patients. If a malignancy is suspected, the initial evaluation includes a chest X-ray and CBC with differential and reticulocyte count prior to hematology consultation. See pp. xx–yy for the treatment of parotitis.

Follow-up
- Bacterial adenitis: 2–3 days

Indications for admission
- Cervical adenitis associated with toxicity or inadequate oral intake
- Cervical adenitis unresponsive to outpatient treatment
- Evaluation of a suspected malignancy
- Institution of antituberculous therapy

Bibliography

Gosche JR, Vick L: Acute, subacute, and chronic cervical lymphadenitis in children. *Semin Pediatr Surg* 2006;**15**:99–106.

Leung AK, Robson WL: Childhood cervical lymphadenopathy. *J Pediatr Health Care* 2004;**18**:3–7.

Tracy TF Jr, Muratore CS: Management of common head and neck masses. *Semin Pediatr Surg* 2007;**16**:3–13.

Epistaxis

Epistaxis usually originates from the anterior nasal septum (Kiesselbach's area). Trauma (nose picking, punch, fall), URIs, excessive use of decongestants or topical nasal steroids, an overly dry environment, and foreign bodies are predisposing factors. Rarely, structural abnormalities (hemangioma, telangiectasia, or angiofibroma), a bleeding diathesis (usually thrombocytopenia), or hypertension is involved. While children are often rushed into the ED because of "massive" blood loss, clinically significant bleeding is unusual.

Clinical presentation

Usually an anterior septal source is evident. It is rare for the bleeding to be bilateral, but blood crossing behind the nasal septum can mimic a bilateral bleed. Sometimes, if the site is posterior or if the child is sleeping, the blood may present as hematemesis.

Diagnosis

Examine the nasal cavity with the child sitting on the parent's lap, using a bright light (otoscope). If a bleeding source is found, the examination may be terminated, as multiple sites are unusual, except in the case of a fractured nasal septum. If the patient has suffered nasal trauma, look for a septal hematoma, which appears as a bluish-black mass on the anterior septum, filling the nasal cavity. Occasionally, a mucosal hemangioma or telangiectasia is seen. If no cause is found, but blood is noted trickling down the throat, assume that there is a posterior source.

Examine the skin for hemangiomata or telangiectasias, which may also be present in the nasal cavity. Pallor, tachycardia, gallop rhythm, or orthostatic vital sign changes suggest significant blood loss. Jaundice, petechiae, purpura, lymphadenopathy, and hepatosplenomegaly may reflect a bleeding diathesis.

In general, no work-up is required for a nosebleed in an otherwise well child with an anterior septal source. Obtain a hematocrit if anemia is suspected, but evaluate for a bleeding diathesis (pp. 337–339) if the patient has any of the physical findings enumerated above, a long history of recurrent nosebleeds, easy bruising, hemarthrosis, multiple subconjunctival hemorrhages, or a family history of excessive bleeding.

ED management

Most anterior bleeds respond to pressure. Pinch the nares together for a full 5 minutes with the child sitting upright (to prevent swallowing of blood). If this is unsuccessful, soak a cotton ball with 1:1000 aqueous epinephrine or 0.05% oxymetazoline solution and place it in the nasal cavity. Alternatively, pack the nose with petrolatum-impregnated gauze, merocel nasal packing, or Gelfoam. If the patient has recurrent bleeds, after hemostasis is obtained, apply topical anesthesia with 4% lidocaine or benzocaine and cauterize the site for 3 seconds with a silver nitrate stick. Treat hemangiomata or telangiectasias in the same way, but do not use cautery if a bleeding diathesis is suspected (possible tissue slough). Humidification, saline nose drops during the day, and the application of petrolatum (Vaseline) to the septum at bedtime help reduce the recurrence of nose bleeds. If a nasal septal hematoma is suspected, consult an otolaryngologist for immediate drainage, to prevent a septal abscess and subsequent nasal deformities.

If routine measures are ineffective or the source is posterior, either consult an otolaryngologist or place a posterior pack. Anesthetize the nose with a topical anesthetic (as above), insert a posterior nasal balloon pack (Epistat or Rhinostat), blow up the posterior balloon, pull anteriorly until it fits snugly in the nasopharynx, and then inflate the anterior balloon until the bleeding stops. Fill both balloons with saline solution. If nasal balloon packs are not available, pass an uninflated Foley catheter through the nose into the pharynx, inflate the balloon, then pull the catheter back until it fits snugly posteriorly in the nose. Fill the nose with petrolatum-impregnated gauze up to the balloon and place a clamp across the catheter where it exits the nose. If an anterior or posterior nasal pack is placed, give the patient broad-spectrum antibiotics to prevent an acute sinusitis (see Table 6-3). Otolaryngology consultation is indicated.

Follow-up

- Unilateral anterior pack: 48 hours for pack removal

Indications for admission

- Bilateral anterior pack
- Posterior pack
- Bleeding diathesis or significant blood loss

Bibliography

Gifford TO, Orlandi RR: Epistaxis. *Otolaryngol Clin North Am* 2008;41:525–36.

McGarry G: Nosebleeds in children. *Clin Evid* 2006;15:496–9.

Foreign bodies

Foreign bodies found in the nose or ear commonly include inanimate objects (toys, earrings, etc.), vegetable material, and insects. The nose is the most common site of foreign-body impaction in children <3 years of age, and the ear is the most frequent site in patients between 3 and 8 years of age. However, the signs and symptoms of a foreign body may be subtle, and there may be no clear history of insertion. Button batteries require immediate removal to prevent alkaline burns, necrosis, or perforation secondary to chemical leakage or electrical current.

Clinical presentation and diagnosis

Aural

A foreign body in the ear can cause pain, tinnitus, and, in the case of a live insect, extreme discomfort. Recurrent otitis externa raises the possibility of an aural foreign body. Although usually a benign condition, inexpert attempts at removal can push the object further into the canal, perforate the eardrum, and cause bleeding and swelling of the canal.

Nasal

A nasal foreign body presents with a unilateral foul-smelling discharge with unilateral obstruction. Usually the object can be seen anteriorly in the nose, but swelling of the mucosa can obscure visualization.

Esophageal

An esophageal foreign body (pp. 144–145) is an unusual but potentially serious problem. Most objects pass into the stomach. However, possible sites for lodging include the inferior margin of the cricoid cartilage, the level of the aortic arch, and the area just superior to the diaphragm. Symptoms may include pain, dysphagia, vomiting, and dyspnea (secondary to laryngeal compression), although a patient may be asymptomatic. Subsequent edema can cause esophageal obstruction (dysphagia and drooling), upper airway obstruction, and possible perforation leading to mediastinitis.

ED management

Aural

Usually, a foreign body in the external auditory canal is easily removed with suction, a wire loop, curette, or small alligator forceps, while irrigation can be used for nonvegetable objects. Prior to attempting to remove a live insect, drown it with mineral oil. Do not instill any solution if a tympanic membrane perforation is suspected (blood in the canal in association with ear pain). Arrange for otolaryngology consultation if the object cannot be removed.

Nasal

Most nasal foreign bodies become impacted between the anterior nasal septum and the inferior turbinate. Prior to attempting to remove the foreign body, anesthetize the nasal mucosa with 4% lidocaine spray and suction any nasal discharge with a frazier-tip catheter to enhance visualization. Use a nasal speculum with either a curette or an alligator forceps to remove the object. Routine use of topical decongestants is not recommended, as it may allow the object to migrate further posteriorly and result in aspiration. Antibiotics are not required after successful removal of the foreign body. As an alternative, large foreign bodies can be removed by applying positive pressure via a mouth-to-mouth forced breath by the caregiver while occluding the opposite (unobstructed) nostril. Consult with an otolaryngologist if removal is unsuccessful or if the object is in the posterior nasal cavity.

Esophageal

Most esophageal foreign bodies, whether round, irregular, or sharp, will pass without difficulty. However, drooling, dysphagia, stridor, or substernal pain or fullness suggests that the object may be lodged in the esophagus. In such cases obtain antero-posterior and lateral soft tissue neck X-rays to determine the presence and number of radio-opaque foreign bodies and whether the object(s) is in the esophagus or trachea. An esophageal foreign body typically aligns in a coronal orientation while a laryngeal or tracheal foreign body lies in the sagittal plane. If it is not clear whether the foreign body is radio-opaque, obtain a searching image X-ray by placing an identical object in a cup of water next to the patient.

A patient with minimal symptoms can be monitored for 12–24 hours to see if the object passes spontaneously. However, if the patient is symptomatic arrange for removal, under general anesthesia, through rigid esophagoscopy. If a disk battery (pp. 144–145) or sharp object is identified in the esophagus, consult an otolaryngologist to arrange expeditious removal under general anesthesia.

Follow-up

- Sharp foreign body that has passed into the stomach: obtain a follow-up abdominal X-ray in 1 week
- Blunt foreign body (including button battery) that has passed into the stomach: return at once if vomiting or abdominal pain occur

Indications for admission

- Esophageal foreign body which has been present >12–24 hours
- Symptomatic patient

Bibliography

Digoy GP: Diagnosis and management of upper aerodigestive tract foreign bodies. *Otolaryngol Clin North Am* 2008;41: 485–96.

Kadish H: Ear and nose foreign bodies: "It is all about the tools". *Clin Pediatr (Phila)* 2005;44:665–70.

Osman EZ, Swift A: Management of foreign bodies in the ears and upper aerodigestive tract. *Br J Hosp Med (Lond)* 2007;68:M189–91.

Mastoiditis

Mastoiditis is a bacterial infection of the mastoid bone and air cells usually caused by an untreated acute otitis media. Although the incidence of mastoiditis has decreased significantly with the introduction of antibiotics, it remains the most common complication of otitis media, with an incidence of about 6 cases/100 000 non-immunocompromised children <14 years of age. It most often occurs in children <2 years of age.

Streptococcus pneumoniae remains the most common cause of mastoiditis. However, universal vaccination is causing a decrease in the number of cases while increasing the cases secondary to multidrug-resistant *S. pneumoniae*. Other etiologies are *Pseudomonas aeruginosa*, *S. aureus*, *S. pyogenes*, and nontypable *Haemophilus influenzae*.

Clinical presentation

Mastoiditis often takes a few weeks to develop and typically follows an untreated or incompletely treated otitis media. The physical findings include swelling, erythema, and tenderness over the mastoid process behind the ear. The auricle is typically displaced antero-inferiorly because of mastoid swelling, and in some cases a fluctuant collection of purulent material can be palpated on the lateral surface of the mastoid process (e.g. subperiosteal abscess). The ipsilateral tympanic membrane is frequently, but not always, erythematous and bulging. Edema and sagging of the posterior external auditory canal wall may be seen upon careful examination of the external auditory canal. Fever >38.3°C (101°F) is common.

Since the advent of pneumococcal vaccination, patients are presenting with more complicated and severe disease, including subperiosteal abscesses. This usually requires surgical intervention in addition to antibiotics.

Diagnosis and ED management

If mastoiditis is suspected based on clinical findings, obtain an axial/coronal CT scan of the temporal bones to rule out possible extension of infection beyond the mastoid. Clouding of the mastoid air cells and loss of the intermastoid cell septa secondary to the osteomyelitic process are seen in coalescent mastoiditis. The radiographic findings of fluid in the middle ear and mastoid without the loss of bony septa may be the result of a recent otitis media and do not necessarily indicate acute mastoiditis, in the absence of the typical clinical findings. Plain mastoid radiographs are not necessary.

Admit all children with acute mastoiditis, consult an otolaryngologist, and treat with IV ceftriaxone (100 mg/kg per day div q 12 h) and clindamycin (40 mg/kg per day div q 6 hr). Tympanocentesis can be helpful in obtaining fluid for Gram's stain and culture. Surgical drainage is indicated if a subperiosteal or intracranial abscess is seen on CT scan or if the patient does not improve clinically with 24–48 hours of intravenous antibiotics.

Indication for admission

* Mastoiditis

Bibliography

Agrawal S, Husein M, MacRae D: Complications of otitis media: an evolving state. *J Otolaryngol* 2005;34 Suppl 1:S33–9.

Leskinen K: Complications of acute otitis media in children. *Curr Allergy Asthma Rep* 2005;5:308–12.

Roddy MG, Glazier SS, Agrawal D: Pediatric mastoiditis in the pneumococcal conjugate vaccine era: symptom duration guides empiric antimicrobial therapy *Pediatr Emerg Care* 2007;23:779–84.

Neck masses

Although the majority of neck masses in children are benign enlarged lymph nodes, the possibility of a malignancy is often a concern. In general, neck masses can be considered in four categories: lymph nodes (pp. 139–140), congenital masses, benign tumors, and malignancies.

Clinical presentation and diagnosis

Congenital masses

Branchial cleft cyst

A branchial cleft cyst is often not diagnosed until late childhood or early adulthood (average age 13 years), when it becomes infected. It presents as a discrete, erythematous, tender, fluctuant mass in the lateral neck, typically anterior to the sternocleidomastoid muscle. On occasion, there is a fistula anterior to the muscle with an orifice that drains mucus and retracts with swallowing. If the acute infection is properly treated with antibiotics, the cyst shrinks, but may reexpand during subsequent upper respiratory infections.

Thyroglossal duct cyst

A thyroglossal duct cyst usually presents as an asymptomatic midline neck mass at or below the level of the hyoid bone. The sexes are affected equally, and 50% of cases present prior to age 10 years. These frequently become infected and respond to antibiotics, only to reemerge during the next URI. In between, the mass is cystic or solid, nontender, and mobile. The pathognomonic feature is elevation of the mass when the tongue is protruded. Occasionally, it contains ectopic thyroid tissue.

Congenital muscular torticollis

Congenital muscular torticollis, or fibromatosis colli, presents at 1–2 weeks of age as a hard, nontender mass within the body of the sternocleidomastoid. Characteristically, the head is tilted to the affected side, the baby faces away from the lesion, and there can be flattening of the unaffected side of the head. The family may report that the baby looks in one direction only.

Benign tumors

Cystic hygroma

A cystic hygroma usually presents as an irregular, soft, painless, compressible lateral neck mass that transilluminates and can increase in size during straining. Fifty percent are present at birth and 90% are noted during the first 2 years of life. Massive enlargement can cause obstruction of the airway or the esophagus. Typical locations are the submental, preauricular, and submandibular areas.

Hemangioma

Hemangiomas are more frequently present at birth, and all present during the first year of life. Unlike cystic hygromas, there is a 3:1 female preponderance. Most are of the cavernous type, often located within the parotid gland in the preauricular area. Infection or hemorrhage can cause acute enlargement, and the mass becomes bluish in color when the infant is crying or straining.

Dermoid cyst

A dermoid cyst typically is an asymptomatic, cystic midline mass located in the submental region. A teratoma has a similar presentation, but calcifications or teeth are often seen on X-ray.

Malignant tumors

About one-quarter of all the malignancies of childhood occur in the neck and more than half of these are either Hodgkin's disease (p. 148) or lymphosarcoma. Hodgkin's disease usually (80%) presents in the upper neck as a painless, hard or firm, fixed, slowly enlarging unilateral node. Most patients are >5 years old. Forty percent of non-Hodgkin's lymphomas present extranodally in the neck throughout the pediatric age range, and the disease is often (40%) bilateral. A slowly growing, hard or rubbery, fixed mass is seen. Weight loss and hepatosplenomegaly are features of both diseases.

A rhabdomyosarcoma can originate in the nasopharynx or ear; symptoms are determined by the site. A nasopharyngeal mass presents as chronic adenoidal hypertrophy, with adenoidal facies, snoring, mouth breathing, serous otitis, and a serosanguinous nasal discharge. There may also be extension to the base of the skull with cranial nerve deficits. A mass in the ear causes chronic otitis, ear discharge, and mastoiditis. Weight loss can occur with a mass in either location. Other rare neck malignancies include fibrosarcoma (mandible most common site), thyroid cancer (history of neck irradiation), and both primary (causing Horner's syndrome) and metastatic (located in orbit or nasopharynx) neuroblastoma.

ED management

Congenital masses

Treat an infected branchial cleft cyst or thyroglossal duct cyst with cephalexin (40 mg/kg per day div q12 hr), cefadroxil (40 mg/kg per day div bid), or amoxicillin-clavulanate (90 mg/kg per day of amoxicillin div bid), and warm soaks every 2 hours. If MRSA is a concern, either use clindamycin (20 mg/kg per day div q 6 hr) or add trimethoprim-sulfamethoxazole (8 mg/kg per day of TMP div bid) to one of the above regimens. Since these lesions have a tendency to become reinfected, refer the patient to an otolaryngologist so that elective excision can be performed.

A neck ultrasound or thyroid scan is a prerequisite for thyroglossal duct excision, as the cyst may contain all of the patient's thyroid tissue. Instruct the parents of a child with a sternocleidomastoid tumor and torticollis to perform stretching exercises, four times a day:

straighten the head into a midline position, then rotate the head to the affected side and hold for 10 seconds.

Benign tumors

If there are no signs or symptoms of airway compromise, referral to an otolaryngologist is indicated for patients with massive enlargement of a cystic hygroma or hemangioma or extreme disfigurement. On occasion, a dermatologist or plastic surgeon should see the child so that cosmetic reconstruction can be planned. Dermoids and teratomas require elective excision.

Malignant tumors

If a malignancy is suspected (hard, nontender, slowly growing mass; systemic signs and symptoms; a clinical picture consistent with a mass in the ear or nasopharynx), obtain a CBC, reticulocyte count, and a chest X-ray to rule out mediastinal or hilar node enlargement. Admit the patient, and consult an oncologist.

Follow-up

• Infected branchial cleft cyst or thyroglossal duct cyst: 48–72 hours

Indications for admission

• Airway or esophageal obstruction
• Suspected malignancy

Bibliography

Foley DS, Fallat ME: Thyroglossal duct and other congenital midline cervical anomalies. *Semin Pediatr Surg* 2006;15:70–5.

Tracy TF Jr, Muratore CS: Management of common head and neck masses. *Semin Pediatr Surg* 2007;16:3–13.

Waldhausen JH: Branchial cleft and arch anomalies in children. *Semin Pediatr Surg* 2006;15:64–9.

Otitis externa

Acute otitis externa (AOE), also known as swimmer's ear, is an inflammation of the external auditory canal. It generally occurs in the summertime, when swimming leads to the trapping of excess moisture in the external auditory canal. Local trauma, eczema, foreign bodies, and immunocompromise are additional risk factors. This results in a mixed infection of fungi (*Aspergillus* and *Candida*) and bacteria (*Pseudomonas*, *Klebsiella*, *S. aureus*, and *Enterobacter*).

Clinical presentation and diagnosis

Generally there is a history of recent swimming or of manipulation of the external canal with a pointed object or q-tip. The patient is usually afebrile, but complaining of ear pain and itching, with a thick white, yellow, or green discharge from the external canal. Extreme discomfort when pulling the pinna or tragus distinguishes the discharge of otitis externa from that caused by a perforated tympanic membrane. Otoscopy is significant for an erythematous external canal, which can be so swollen that it prevents visualization of the tympanic membrane. In the absence of a history of swimming or ear canal manipulation, consider a foreign-body impaction.

ED management

Treat otitis externa with a topical, broad-spectrum antibiotic ear drop. Preparations that contain hydrocortisone often reduce swelling more effectively. Use acetic acid with or without hydrocortisone (3–5 drops tid × 7 days), ciprofloxacin-hydrocortisone (3 drops bid × 7 days), ofloxacin (5 drops bid <12 years, 10 drops bid ≥12 years, × 10 days), or polymyxin B-neomycin-hydrocortisone (3–5 drops tid × 7 days). If a perforated tympanic membrane cannot be ruled out, use a preparation that is less caustic to the middle ear structures, such as polymyxin B-neomycin-hydrocortisone suspension, rather than the solution. Instill the drops either directly into the canal or onto a cotton earwick, which ensures delivery of the drug throughout the external canal. In addition, keep the canal dry; further swimming is not permitted unless the child wears earplugs. Complete resolution takes 5–7 days. If the child is prone to recurrences, use two drops of a prophylactic mixture of half rubbing (isopropyl) alcohol/half water after every swim. If there is no improvement in 2 days, refer the patient to an otolaryngologist for cleaning of the ear canal and possible ear wick placement.

Severe otitis externa with associated cellulitis of the pinna requires admission for systemic antibiotics. Consult an otolaryngologist.

Follow-up

• 48 hours, if the symptoms do not begin to improve.

Bibliography

Roland PS, Belcher BP, Bettis R, et al: A single topical agent is clinically equivalent to the combination of topical and oral antibiotic treatment for otitis externa. *Am J Otolaryngol* 2008;**29**:255–61.

Thio D, Reece P, Herdman R: Necrotizing otitis externa: a painless reminder. *Eur Arch Otorhinolaryngol* 2008;**265**:907–10.

Parotitis

Sialoadenitis is an acute inflammatory process of one or more of the salivary glands, with the most frequently affected being the parotid gland. Parotitis results from salivary stasis, secondary to viruses (mumps, Coxsackie viruses), bacteria (*Staphylococcus aureus, Streptococcus viridans, Streptococcus pneumoniae*), salivary duct stone (sialolith), or dehydration in chronically ill or debilitated patients.

Recurrent parotitis of childhood (RPC) is a separate clinical entity in which periodic acute episodes of parotid swelling occur in one or both parotid glands. Although the etiology is unknown, it is thought to be secondary to poor dental hygiene.

Clinical presentation

Acute parotitis presents with swelling and pain overlying the affected parotid gland, obscuring the angle of the mandible. Infectious parotitis may cause unilateral or bilateral swelling with severe tenderness. The swelling can develop rapidly and often presents during or after a meal, when salivary flow is stimulated. Intraoral examination may reveal swelling, erythema, or a discharge from the opening of Stensen's duct, which is on the buccal mucosa opposite the second upper molar. With a bacterial parotitis, purulent material can be expressed from Stenson's duct by gently massaging the affected gland.

Diagnosis

In general, an enlarged parotid is the only mass that obscures the angle of the mandible. See Table 6-4 for the differential diagnosis of neck masses.

ED management

The treatment of parotitis is aimed at increasing salivary flow in order to flush infected material from within the salivary duct and gland. Encourage hydration and recommend the use of sialogogues, such as lemon swabs or sucking candies. In addition, provide analgesia (acetaminophen 15 mg/kg q 4 hr, ibuprofen 10 mg/kg q 6 hr) and warm compresses.

If there is evidence of duct obstruction, overlying erythema and tenderness, or purulent drainage from Stenson's duct, give anti-staphylococcal antibiotics such as cephalexin (40 mg/kg per day div q 12 hr), cefadroxil (40 mg/kg per day div bid), or amoxicillin-clavulanate (90 mg/kg per day of amoxicillin div bid). If MRSA is a concern, either use clindamycin (20 mg/kg per day div q 6 hr) or add trimethoprim-sulfamethoxazole (8 mg/kg per day of TMP div bid) to the above regimens. Obtain a CT scan of the neck if the patient has persistent or recurrent parotitis, an abscess, or if an anatomic obstruction (e.g. stone) is suspected.

Recurrent parotitis of childhood responds well to medical treatment and the episodes often disappear after puberty.

Follow-up

- Parotitis: 48–72 hours

Indications for admission

- Patient toxic or unable to manage PO hydration
- Parotid abscess

Bibliography

Dayan GH, Quinlisk MP, Parker AA, et al: Recent resurgence of mumps in the United States. *N Engl J Med* 2008; 358:1580–9.

Hviid A, Rubin S, Mühlemann K: Mumps. *Lancet* 2008;371:932–44.

Periorbital and orbital cellulitis

The orbital septum is a fibrous membrane running from the periosteum of the orbital bones to the tarsal plates. It separates the skin and subcutaneous tissues from intraorbital structures. Although the clinical pictures are similar, differentiation of periorbital (preseptal) cellulitis from orbital (postseptal) cellulitis is critical.

Clinical presentation

Both periorbital and orbital cellulitis present with warm, tender, erythematous lid swelling, usually associated with fever and regional adenopathy.

Periorbital cellulitis

Periorbital cellulitis can be divided into two types. The infection may be preceded by an obvious break in the skin (insect bite, laceration, impetigo), with the causative agents being *S. aureus* or group A *Streptococcus*. More commonly, the infection occurs as a result of local spread from an ethmoid sinusitis with a *Moraxella catarrhalis* or *pneumococcus* infection. In a sinusitis-related case, the patient may have a history of a persistent nasal discharge, and the upper eyelid may be affected first, with subsequent spread to the lower lid. With either type of periorbital cellulitis, mild to moderate conjunctival swelling and hyperemia with a mucoid to purulent discharge may be present.

Orbital cellulitis

The hallmarks of a postseptal infection are proptosis, chemosis, and decreased extraocular mobility, in association with fever and toxicity. Decreased visual acuity may also occur late in the course.

Diagnosis

Distinguishing periorbital from orbital cellulitis is critical because more aggressive medical and surgical intervention may be required with the latter. Passively open the eyelids and examine the eyes for conjunctival injection, discharge, proptosis, chemosis, and decreased extraocular mobility, and check the visual acuity. If the distinction between periorbital and orbital infection is not clear on clinical grounds, obtain a non-contrast axial/coronal CT scan of the orbit and sinuses. If orbital cellulitis is suspected or confirmed, promptly consult both an otolaryngologist and an ophthalmologist.

Lid erythema and swelling may be caused by a viral or bacterial conjunctivitis (marked palpebral conjunctival injection), an insect bite (a punctum may be identified), or infectious mononucleosis (bilateral swelling with fever and pharyngitis). An allergic reaction or nephrotic syndrome can cause lid swelling (generally bilateral) in the absence of erythema, tenderness, or fever. Proptosis can be secondary to an orbital tumor although the signs of infection are usually absent, while hyperthyroid exophthalmos can be confused with proptosis.

ED management

As mentioned above, when the distinction between a periorbital and orbital infection is not clear, radiologic studies can be helpful. Since an orbital cellulitis can be a life-threatening illness, always err on the side of overdiagnosing a postseptal infection.

Periorbital cellulitis

A child with mild preseptal cellulitis secondary to a break in the skin may be treated as an outpatient with cefadroxil (40 mg/kg per day div q 12 hr), cephalexin (40 mg/kg per day div qid), amoxicillin-clavulanate (875/125 formulation, 90 mg/kg per day of amoxicillin div bid), cefuroxime (30 mg/kg per day div bid). If MRSA is a concern, either use clindamycin (20 mg/kg per day div q 6 hr) or add trimethoprim-sulfamethoxazole (8 mg/kg per day of TMP div bid) to one of the above regimens. If the infection is sinusitis-related, give a topical nasal decongestant (oxymetazoline bid) and amoxicillin-clavulanate or cefuroxime (as above). Also recommend warm compresses qid.

Admit the patient if there is a fever >39.4°C (103.0°F), significant eyelid edema, decreased extraocular mobility, inability to tolerate oral antibiotics, or signs of systemic toxicity and treat with IV antibiotics (ampicillin-sulbactam 150 mg/kg per day div q 6 hr, cefuroxime 100 mg/kg per day div q 8 hr, or vancomycin 40 mg/kg per day div q 6 hr for possible MRSA) and a topical nasal decongestant. Obtain a CBC and blood culture.

Orbital cellulitis

The IV antibiotic treatment is the same as for a preseptal cellulitis (see above), but include vancomycin in the regimen if there is any possibility of MRSA. As mentioned above, obtain an axial/coronal CT scan of the paranasal sinuses and orbits and both otolaryngology and ophthalmology consultations early in the evaluation of the patient. Abscess drainage is indicated if there is extreme toxicity, evidence of intracranial spread (focal neurologic findings), decreased visual acuity, or no response to 24 hours of antibiotics. However, treat small subperiosteal abscesses with 24–48 hours of IV antibiotics prior to surgical intervention.

Follow-up

*   Preseptal cellulitis: 24–48 hours. Instruct the family to return immediately for IV therapy if symptoms worsen

Indications for admission

*   Preseptal cellulitis associated with fever or toxicity, or unresponsive to 24–48 hours of oral antibiotics
*   Orbital cellulitis

Bibliography

Goodyear PW, Firth AL, Strachan DR, Dudley M: Periorbital swelling: the important distinction between allergy and infection. *Emerg Med J* 2004;21:240–2.

Hennemann S, Crawford P, Nguyen L, Smith PC: Clinical inquiries. What is the best initial treatment for orbital cellulitis in children? *J Fam Pract* 2007;56:662–4.

Nageswaran S, Woods CR, Benjamin DK Jr, et al: Orbital cellulitis in children. *Pediatr Infect Dis J* 2006;25:695–9.

Peritonsillar abscess

Occasionally, a bacterial pharyngitis can evolve into a peritonsillar abscess, which is a collection of purulent material between the superior pole of the tonsil and its capsule. The infection may then spread into the surrounding soft tissues. This usually occurs in an adolescent who has not been treated with antibiotics, although adequate antimicrobial coverage does not always prevent this complication. Virtually all cases of peritonsillar abscess are caused by group A beta hemolytic streptococci, although uncommonly *S. aureus* and anaerobes are implicated.

Clinical presentation

A peritonsillar abscess causes severe sore throat and toxicity, with difficulty opening the mouth (trismus), drooling, and a "hot potato" muffled voice. The tonsil is markedly erythematous and covered with a whitish exudate, while the uvula is swollen and deviated to the contralateral side. Anterior and superior to the tonsil there is soft palate swelling which is sometimes fluctuant. The head may be tilted to the unaffected side, and tender cervical adenopathy is usually prominent on the same side as the abscess. In severe cases signs of upper airway obstruction may also be present.

Diagnosis and ED management

If a peritonsillar abscess is suspected, obtain ENT consultation to determine whether incision and drainage or needle aspiration is the most appropriate course of action. In general, imaging is not necessary.

After the drainage procedure, in a mild case, in which adequate oral intake is possible, treat with antibiotics and analgesia (ibuprofen, 10 mg/kg q 6 h; acetaminophen with codeine 1 mg/kg q 6 h, 30 mg maximum). Cultures taken from the aspirates of acute peritonsillar abscess frequently yield multiple organisms, some of which are beta-lactamase producers. Therefore, give a 10-day course of amoxicillin-clavulanate (875/125 formulation, 90 mg/kg per day of amoxicillin div q 12 hr) or, if penicillin-allergic, clindamycin (30 mg/kg per day div q 6 hr). If adequate oral intake is not possible, admit the patient and treat with intravenous penicillin G (50 000–100 000 unit/kg per day div q 6 hr) or clindamycin (40 mg/kg per day div q 6 hr) and IV hydration.

Follow-up

- Peritonsillar abscess (drained): next day

Indications for admission

- Severe dysphagia preventing oral intake
- Patient not taking adequate oral fluids, status-post incision and drainage of a peritonsillar abscess

Bibliography

Lamkin RH, Portt J: An outpatient medical treatment protocol for peritonsillar abscess. *Ear Nose Throat J* 2006;85:658–60.

Millar KR, Johnson DW, Drummond D, et al: Suspected peritonsillar abscess in children. *Pediatr Emerg Care* 2007;23:431–8.

Pharyngotonsillitis

Pharyngitis is most often caused by viral infections (adenovirus, parainfluenza, rhinovirus, coronavirus, CMV, Epstein-Barr virus, Coxsackie A virus). Approximately 20–30% of cases are caused by group A beta-hemolytic *Streptococci* ("strep throat"). Other rare etiologies include *Mycoplasma*, group C and G *Streptococcus*, toxoplasmosis, *Chlamydia*, *Neisseria gonorrhea*, tularemia, and diphtheria (very rare).

Clinical presentation and diagnosis

The older child usually complains of pain or difficulty with swallowing. The toddler may act cranky or irritable, refuse food or fluids, and have sleep disturbances. Other findings may include drooling or difficulty handling secretions, fever, otalgia, and tender anterior cervical lymphadenopathy. Infection of the pharynx causes erythema of the tonsils and tonsillar pillars with or without tonsillar enlargement. In older patients epiglottitis (pp. 622–624) may present with severe dysphagia.

Viral infections

Low-grade fever (<38.3°C; 101°F) associated with conjunctivitis, rhinitis, or cough suggests a viral etiology. Tonsillar exudate, toxicity, and severe difficulty swallowing are unusual findings in the common viral infections. However, adenovirus can cause a severe pharyngitis with exudate and ulceration. Thick, gray mucus covering the tonsils can be seen in infectious mononucleosis and mono-like syndromes (CMV, toxoplasmosis, tularemia). Generalized lymphadenopathy, hepatosplenomegaly, an erythematous maculopapular rash, fever (<38.3°C; 101°F), periorbital edema, urticaria, upper airway obstruction secondary to lymphoid hyperplasia, and severe, prolonged lethargy are other manifestations of infectious mononucleosis (pp. 386–388), especially in the adolescent. Herpangina (Coxsackie viruses) causes a vesicular eruption in the posterior pharynx.

Streptococcal infection

Streptococcal infection is suggested by whitish yellow exudate on the tonsillar surface, palatal petechiae, a red uvula, tender anterior cervical lymphadenopathy, halitosis, headache, and fever >38.3°C (101°F). On occasion, associated severe abdominal pain can mimic acute appendicitis. Marked dysphagia, with drooling and difficulty breathing, occurs less frequently. An erythematous sandpaper-like scarlatiniform rash with perioral pallor may develop. Other findings are a "strawberry" tongue, accentuation of the rash in the flexion creases (Pastia's lines), and, late in the course, periungual desquamation.

ED management

Clinical evaluation alone is an inaccurate method for diagnosing strep throat. Streptococcal infection may be diagnosed either by a throat culture on 5% sheep blood agar or by a rapid agglutination test, which is useful for early diagnosis. False-negative results, although rare, are possible with all the rapid *Streptococcus* tests, so a throat culture is indicated if the rapid test is negative.

Treat pharyngitis symptomatically, with gargles, lozenges, and acetaminophen (15 mg/kg q 4 hr) or ibuprofen (10 mg/kg q 6 hr). If a rapid strep test or throat culture is positive for beta-hemolytic streptococci, treat with antibiotics to prevent rheumatic fever as well as to shorten the course of the acute pharyngitis. Therapy consists of 10 days of oral antibiotics: penicillin VK (<27 kg: 250 mg PO bid-tid; ≥ 27 kg: 500 mg PO bid-tid), cefadroxil (20 mg/kg q day), or, for penicillin-allergic patients, erythromycin ethyl succinate (40 mg/kg per day div bid or tid) or clindamycin (25 mg/kg per day div tid or qid). If compliance is not assured, give one dose of intramuscular benzathine penicillin G mixed with procaine penicillin (600,000 unit of benzathine <27 kg [60 lb]; 1,200,000 units of benzathine >27 kg [60 lb]). At least 20% of group A beta-hemolytic *Streptococci* are resistant to tetracycline, while sulfonamides (including trimethoprim-sulfamethoxazole) do not reliably eradicate acute streptococcal infections and therefore are not appropriate therapy. Patients with severe pharyngeal discomfort may benefit from a dose of dexamethasone (0.3 mg/kg PO or IM, 10 mg maximum).

When the clinical picture is suggestive of infectious mononucleosis or the patient has been suffering an unusually prolonged or severe sore throat, an evaluation for mononucleosis (pp. 386–388) is indicated. Obtain a CBC with differential to look for atypical lymphocytosis and a monospot test or heterophile antibody.

Follow-up

- Strep throat: primary care in 1 week, or sooner if symptoms worsen
- Mononucleosis: primary care follow-up in 2 weeks, to assess for splenomegaly

Indications for admission

- Severe dysphagia preventing oral intake
- Patient not taking adequate oral fluids, status post-incision and drainage of a peritonsillar abscess

Bibliography

Altamimi S, Khalil A, Khalaiwi KA, et al: Short versus standard duration antibiotic therapy for acute streptococcal pharyngitis in children. *Cochrane Database Syst Rev* 2009; (1):CD004872.

Patel NN, Patel DN: Acute exudative tonsillitis. *Am J Med* 2009;**122**:18–20.

Tanz RR, Gerber MA, Kabat W, et al: Performance of a rapid antigen-detection test and throat culture in community pediatric offices: implications for management of pharyngitis. *Pediatrics* 2009;**123**:437–44.

Retropharyngeal abscess

A retropharyngeal abscess is a complication of streptococcal pharyngitis, trauma, or an extension of a vertebral osteomyelitis. It occurs most commonly in children between the ages of 2 and 4 years but can occur at any age. Most infections are polymicrobial with *S. aureus*, group A *Streptococcus* and anaerobes such as bacterioides and pepotostreptococcus being the most common.

Clinical presentation

The patient presents with fever, drooling, respiratory distress, and hyperextension of the neck. Torticollis or limited neck movement (side to side or up and down) may also be present. On examination, there is anterior bulging of the posterior pharyngeal wall. In severe cases upper airway obstruction with stridor or stertor (harsh crackling sounds heard over the larynx or trachea) may also be present.

Diagnosis

If a retropharyngeal abscess is suspected, obtain a soft tissue lateral neck X-ray. Findings include widening of the retropharyngeal space and loss of the normal cervical lordosis. A neck CT scan with IV contrast will confirm the diagnosis and delineate the extent and location of an abscess relative to the airway and blood vessels.

ED management

Request an ENT consultation to help confirm the diagnosis, assess for airway compromise, and determine whether surgical drainage is required. Treat with beta-lactamase-resistant antibiotics, such as IV ampicillin-sulbactam (150 mg/kg per day div q 6 hr) or IV clindamycin (40 mg/kg per day div q 6 hr) if the patient is allergic to penicillin. However, if MRSA is a concern, use vancomycin (40 mg/kg per day div q 6 hr). Respiratory distress or failure to respond to medical treatment within 24–48 hours is an indication for incision and drainage in the operating room.

Indication for admission
- Retropharyngeal abscess

Bibliography

Craig FW, Schunk JE: Retropharyngeal abscess in children: clinical presentation, utility of imaging, and current management. *Pediatrics* 2003;111:1394–8.

Page NC, Bauer EM, Lieu JE: Clinical features and treatment of retropharyngeal abscess in children. *Otolaryngol Head Neck Surg* 2008;138:300–6.

Serous otitis media

Serous otitis media (SOM), also known as otitis media with effusion (OME), is the presence of nonsuppurative fluid in the middle ear. Although no overt signs of infection are seen in SOM, bacteria have been found in 30–70% of cultures of the fluid.

Clinical presentation and diagnosis

Despite adequate treatment, serous otitis frequently follows an episode of acute otitis media. Usually, there are no complaints, although an infant may be fussy when recumbent, while an older child may note decreased hearing or mild balance disturbances.

On pneumatic otoscopy, the tympanic membrane appears darkened and retracted, with decreased mobility, but without evidence of acute infection (i.e. no erythema). There may be an air–fluid level with bubbles visible behind the drum. The limited mobility can be confirmed by impedance testing (retracted tympanic membrane with negative middle ear pressure).

ED management

The best management of SOM is watchful waiting for a 3-month period. The empirical use of antihistamine-decongestant combinations is of no value, while antibiotics and corticosteroids offer only a temporary benefit and therefore are not indicated.

Refer the patient to a primary care provider to assess the frequency of acute infections. Arrange for a hearing evaluation if fluid has been present for >3 months. Myringotomy and pressure-equalizing tubes may be indicated for unresponsive, recurrent otitis media or significant conductive hearing loss (hearing threshold >20 dB), especially in a child with speech delay.

Bibliography

American Academy of Family Physicians; American Academy of Otolaryngology-Head and Neck Surgery; American Academy of Pediatrics Subcommittee on Otitis Media With Effusion: Otitis media with effusion. *Pediatrics* 2004;113: 1412–29.

Williamson I, Little P: Otitis media with effusion: the long and winding road? *Arch Dis Child* 2008;93:268–9.

Sinusitis

Sinusitis (also known as rhinosinusitis) is defined as inflammation of one or more of the paranasal sinuses, which develop as outpouchings of the nasal chamber. They enlarge as the child grows, so that the importance of a particular sinus varies with the age of the patient.

The maxillary and ethmoid cells are present at birth while the sphenoid and frontal sinuses are not aerated until approximately 5 and 7 years of age, respectively.

The organisms responsible for most cases of acute sinusitis are similar to those implicated in acute otitis media and include S. pneumoniae, nontypable H. influenzae, M. catarrhalis, and S. aureus. In contrast, anaerobes, S. aureus, alpha Streptococcus, and nontypable H. influenzae are the predominant infectious etiologies of chronic sinusitis, which is also frequently caused by a non-infectious etiology, chronic hyperplastic eosinpohilic sinusitis.

Clinical presentation

The most common signs and symptoms of acute sinusitis are dry cough (typically occurs at night or during naps), persistent (>7–10 days) nasal discharge, and fever. Children >5 years of age may complain of a headache that is accentuated by leaning forward. Younger patients (<5 years) may have malodorous breath in the absence of a pharyngeal or dental infection. Facial pain and swelling occur, but are not as common as in adults.

Diagnosis

Acute sinusitis is a common complication of viral URIs and can usually be diagnosed on clinical grounds alone. Suspect sinusitis if a patient has nasal discharge and congestion which persist longer than expected for the typical URI (>7–10 days) or worsens after 5 days. Complaints of fever, headache, and cough are variable, and children may not exhibit the classic signs and symptoms of facial tenderness or dental pain. However, observed or reported periorbital swelling or medial infraorbital discoloration of the skin suggests ethmoid sinusitis.

Radiographs are not necessary to confirm a clinical diagnosis of sinusitis in children <6 years and are of limited value in patients >6 years. If radiographic confirmation is necessary, obtain plain sinus films (Caldwell and Waters views) to detect acute maxillary, frontal, and ethmoid sinusitis. However, plain films are not adequate for identifying sphenoid disease. Reserve axial/coronal CT scans of the paranasal sinuses for patients who have not responded to medical management and may require aspiration or surgical intervention. Transillumination and ultrasound are not helpful.

Various combinations of headache, cough, fever, and nasal discharge can occur with viral URIs, influenza, or pneumonia. Malodorous breath may be secondary to a dental abscess, pharyngitis, or nasal foreign body. Cough variant asthma may also present with a nocturnal cough.

ED management

The antibiotic treatment of acute sinusitis is summarized in Table 6-3; prescribe a 14–21 day course. Amoxicillin is the first-line choice. In addition, prescribe an oral decongestant (pseudoephedrine 1 mg/kg q 6 h) and a topical nasal vasoconstrictor (oxymetazoline bid) for 48 hours, but do not use H_1 antihistamines. Treat a patient who has recurrent sinusitis (>3–4 episodes/year) with a topical nasal steroid, such as budesonide, fluticasone, or mometasone, 1 spray each nostril daily for 4–6 weeks. Adenoidectomy may be indicated for some patients with recurrent sinusitis refractory to treatment.

Drainage, irrigation, and culture of the paranasal sinuses are indicated for patients who are immunocompromised, unresponsive to medical therapy, toxic, or suffering from one of the rare intracranial complications (brain abscess, subdural empyema, cavernous sinus thrombosis or an orbital cellulitis). Nasal cultures are of limited value, as they do not accurately predict the pathogen responsible for acute sinusitis.

Admit a patient with acute frontal sinusitis if there is an air–fluid level and moderate–severe pain, and treat with IV antibiotics because of increased risk of intracranial spread. Also admit a patient with sphenoid sinusitis.

Follow-up

• Acute sinusitis: 48–72 hours. If symptoms persist, change to an alternative medication or consult an otolaryngologist for possible parenteral antibiotics and sinus drainage

Indications for admission

• Acute frontal sinusitis with an air–fluid level and moderate–severe pain
• Sphenoid sinusitis
• Systemic toxicity
• Unremitting headache or incapacitating symptoms
• Orbital cellulitis or intracranial complication

Bibliography

Duse M, Caminiti S, Zicari AM: Rhinosinusitis: prevention strategies. *Pediatr Allergy Immunol* 2007;18 Suppl:71–4.

Novembre E, Mori F, Pucci N, et al: Systemic treatment of rhinosinusitis in children. *Pediatr Allergy Immunol* 2007; 18 Suppl:56–61.

Tan R, Spector S: Pediatric sinusitis. *Curr Allergy Asthma Rep* 2007;7:421–6.

Upper respiratory infections

Upper respiratory infections (URIs) are generally mild illnesses caused by numerous organisms. However, if a URI does not resolve within 3–4 days, consider the possibility of a more serious illness (most commonly otitis media or sinusitis).

Clinical presentation

Most often, the patient is afebrile, or has a low-grade temperature, with watery or mucoid rhinorrhea. Sneezing, coughing, and conjunctival injection are other features. Infants may have noisy breathing or decreased ability to feed.

Diagnosis

Inquire about fever, cough, appetite, vomiting, diarrhea, treatments given at home, and whether anyone else at home is ill. Perform a complete examination, looking for evidence of bacterial infection such as nasal discharge (sinusitis, allergic rhinitis), otitis media, pharyngitis, and nuchal rigidity (meningitis). Auscultate the lungs for decreased breath sounds or rales (pneumonia) or wheezing (asthma or bronchiolitis).

ED management

Although there are many over-the-counter cold remedies, there are few data proving efficacy. Antihistamine-decongestant combinations available over the counter have been shown to have little effect on the common cold. Recommend rest, fluids, and acetaminophen (15 mg/kg q 4 h) or ibuprofen (10 mg/kg q 6 h) for fever. For infants, give normal saline nose drops (2 drops in one nostril at a time), followed by gentle aspiration with a bulb syringe. A vaporizer may be helpful for all age groups.

Follow-up

- Return to primary care provider if symptoms worsen (toxicity, fever >39.4°C or 103°F, ear pain) or do not resolve within 3–4 days

Bibliography

Chang CY, Sachs HC, Lee CE: Unexpected infant deaths associated with use of cough and cold medications. *Pediatrics* 2009; 123:e358–9.

Habiba A: Cold and cough medications in children: dealing with parental expectations. *Pediatrics* 2009;123:e362.

Kuehn BM: Debate continues over the safety of cold and cough medicines for children. *JAMA* 2008;300:2354–6.

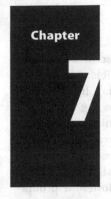

Endocrine emergencies

Joan Di Martino-Nardi

Contributing authors
Ellen F. Crain and Sandra J. Cunningham: Diabetic ketoacidosis
Morri Markowitz: Hypercalcemia and Hypocalcemia

Adrenal insufficiency

The adrenal cortex is divided into three zones: the outermost glomerulosa, which produces aldosterone, the middle fasciculata, which produces cortisol and androgens, and the innermost reticularis, which produces androgens. Cortisol production is regulated primarily by pituitary adrenocorticotropic hormone (ACTH) secretion (which in turn is regulated by the hypothalamic release of corticotrophin releasing hormone or CRH). Lesions of the hypothalamus, pituitary, or adrenal cortex may cause adrenal insufficiency (Addison's disease).

The majority of cases are of primary adrenal insufficiency (failure of the adrenal cortex), which generally leads to inadequate production of both aldosterone and cortisol. Congenital adrenal hyperplasia (CAH), an inherited defect in steroid biosynthesis, is the most common cause. Other etiologies include autoimmune adrenalitis, fulminant infections (adrenal hemorrhage in meningococcemia), trauma, HIV infection, tumor, infiltrative disease, tuberculosis, and bilateral adrenalectomy.

Secondary, or central (hypothalamic or pituitary), adrenal insufficiency results in inadequate production of cortisol. The most common etiology is exogenous steroid administration; a patient receiving supraphysiologic doses for more than 1–2 weeks is at risk for adrenal insufficiency and acute adrenal crisis. Other causes are CNS tumors, trauma, and idiopathic causes.

Acute adrenal crisis (Addisonian crisis) is a life-threatening emergency caused by relative or absolute deficiencies of cortisol and aldosterone. Crisis occurs when the adrenal gland fails to respond to stress with up to a tenfold increase in cortisol secretion. This rise in cortisol secretion is dependent on increased ACTH release. Crisis may be precipitated by bacterial or viral infections, or dental or surgical procedures. Prompt recognition of the presenting symptoms and immediate treatment is imperative.

Clinical presentation

The initial complaints are often nonspecific. The presentation may be gradual, with subtle complaints such as weakness, fatigue, malaise, anorexia, poor growth, and weight loss. With aldosterone deficiency (as occurs in primary adrenal insufficiency), salt craving may be reported and the blood pressure may be normal or low. Alternatively, there may be an acute presentation, with fever, weakness, lethargy, abdominal pain, nausea, vomiting (possibly bilious), guarding and rebound tenderness, dehydration, hypotension, and/or shock. Seizures, secondary to hypoglycemia or hyponatremia, may also occur. The presentation may also be fulminant, and sudden death can occur.

With primary adrenal insufficiency a subtle physical examination finding is skin hyperpigmentation, most often found on the lips and buccal mucosa, nipples, groin, palmar or axillary creases, and areas of old scars or friction (knees, elbows, knuckles). Skin hyper-pigmentation is a sign of increased ACTH secretion; it does not occur with secondary adrenal insufficiency (caused by pituitary or hypothalamic disease). Other possible signs include petechiae and purpura (overwhelming sepsis, usually meningococcemia), hypoglycemic seizures (glucocorticoid insufficiency), midline craniofacial malformations (e.g. septo-optic dysplasia, cleft lip/palate, holoprosencephaly), and micropenis (hypopituitarism). Central adrenal insufficiency is often associated with other hypothalamic/pituitary hormone defi-ciencies which may manifest as growth failure, delayed pubertal progression, micropenis (secondary to GH deficiency), and, in the case of CNS lesions, diabetes insipidus.

Primary adrenal insufficiency is usually associated with deficient aldosterone produc-tion with resultant significant losses of sodium and water and retention of potassium. These patients present with more severe hyponatremia, hyperkalemia, and volume depletion. As aldosterone production is primarily regulated by the renin–angiotensin enzyme system, central secondary and tertiary adrenal insufficiency are not associated with aldosterone deficiency. Autoimmune Addison's disease (primary adrenal insufficiency) may also be associated with mucocutaneous candidiasis, hypothyroidism, hypokalemia, hepatitis, viti-ligo, alopecia, and pernicious anemia.

The use of steroids for more than 2–4 weeks can cause suppression of the patient's endogenous hypothalamic/pituitary/adrenal axis. The abrupt withdrawal of steroids can then result in clinical adrenal insufficiency or acute adrenal crisis, as the patient is unable to mount an ACTH response. Acute insufficiency can also occur when there is a physiologic stress (surgery, infection, trauma) without an appropriate increase in the exogenous dose of glucocorticoids.

Congenital adrenal hyperplasia (CAH)

A female infant with CAH is usually diagnosed soon after birth because of ambiguous genitalia, ranging from mild clitoromegaly to a completely penile urethra with bilateral cryptorchidism. A male infant with CAH usually has normal external genitalia and is therefore often not diagnosed in the immediate newborn period. The patient may present at 1–3 weeks of life (or later infancy) with fatigue, poor feeding, and vomiting, resembling the clinical picture of sepsis. Alternatively, there may be a fulminant presentation with dehydration, shock, or sudden death. There may be a family history of consanguinity, CAH, or neonatal deaths. On physical examination, hyperpigmentation (as described above) may be noted, while a completely virilized girl will not have testes detected. In most states, the newborn screen includes measurement of 17OH progesterone, which will aid in the early diagnosis of the most common cause of CAH.

Diagnosis

The key to diagnosing acute adrenal crisis is to maintain a high degree of suspicion, especially in a previously well infant who has mild to moderate illness but deteriorates quickly. The prominent gastrointestinal symptoms of adrenal crisis can resemble gastroen-teritis (diarrhea is frequent), an acute abdomen (involuntary guarding and rebound tender-ness), and intestinal obstruction (bilious vomiting).

If impending or acute adrenal crisis is suspected, do not delay treatment while waiting for confirmatory laboratory tests. Initiate diagnostic testing and treatment simultaneously. Obtain blood for CBC, electrolytes, glucose, and serum cortisol, plasma renin activity, and aldosterone, while establishing IV access.

Acute primary adrenal insufficiency may cause hyponatremia, hypochloremia, and hyperkalemia with peaked T waves on ECG. Hypoglycemia and neutropenia (WBC $<5000/mm^3$) can occur, although these can also be signs of sepsis. In addition, there is increased plasma renin, increased urinary excretion of sodium if the patient is aldosterone-deficient (i.e. a salt-waster), and decreased urinary excretion of potassium.

Normally, patients in shock have an elevated serum cortisol level (> 20 mg/dL), but with adrenal insufficiency, the serum cortisol is inappropriately low. After the initial crisis, an ACTH stimulation test (Cortrosyn® 250 mcg IV with 0- and 60-minute cortisol levels), performed by an endocrinologist, may be needed to make the diagnosis of primary adrenal insufficiency. In 21-hydroxylase deficiency, an elevated 17OH progesterone confirms the diagnosis.

ED management

Once the diagnosis is suspected, therapy includes immediate, aggressive fluid management and steroid replacement. Obtain a fingerstick glucose measurement and assess possible hyperkalemia (aldosterone deficiency or resistance) by looking for peaked T waves on ECG. Infants with CAH tolerate hyperkalemia better than older children, and usually all that is needed is fluid resuscitation with normal saline. Definitive assessment of adrenal function can be performed after the acute emergency has passed.

Acute crisis

Fluid management

Clinical assessment tends to underestimate the severity of the hypovolemia. Consider the patient to be at least 10% dehydrated. Start an IV and give 20 mL/kg of normal saline over 30 minutes to 1 hour. Repeat the boluses until the patient becomes normotensive. Once the blood pressure is normal, continue with D_5 NS for patients with salt-losing adrenal insufficiency. Change non-salt losers to D_5 ½-⅔ NS, if the electrolytes are normal.

Total fluid requirements are in the range of 1.5–2 times maintenance; reassess as therapy continues. Add potassium (10–20 mEq/L) once the patient voids, as the administration of cortisol will rapidly induce kaliuresis and a fall in the serum potassium. If the patient is hypoglycemic (blood glucose <40 mg/dL), give 2–4 mL/kg of D_{10} and recheck the glucose in 15 minutes. Repeat the D_{10} if the hypoglycemia persists (blood glucose <60 mg/dL).

Corticosteroid replacement

Give a stat dose of hydrocortisone (Solu-Cortef®) IV push or IM (infant: 25 mg; small child: 50 mg; larger child or adolescent: 100 mg), followed by 25 mg/m² (or 1 mg/kg) IV or IM q 6h.

Shock

If shock persists despite the crystalloid boluses, give a plasma expander, such as plasmanate (20–40 mL/kg) or a vasopressor, such as dopamine (pp. 26–27). Vasopressors may be ineffective unless preceded by adequate cortisol replacement.

Mineralocorticoid replacement

Mineralocorticoid replacement is not necessary during the acute ED treatment because high-dose glucocorticoids with mineralocorticoid activity and normal saline are being given (steps 1 and 2). Once the patient is stable and can take oral fluids, give 9α-fluorocortisol (Florinef®) 0.1–0.3 mg PO to salt-wasters. Supplemental oral sodium may also be necessary.

Underlying pathology

Identify and treat any underlying cause of the stress. Infections are the most common precipitating factor.

Complications

ICU monitoring may be necessary, especially if the patient remains comatose or hypotensive, or the underlying pathology takes a fulminant course (sepsis). Complications of excessive fluid, salt, or steroid replacement include hypernatremia, hypokalemia, pulmonary edema, congestive heart failure, and hypervolemia.

Minor illness or stress in adrenal insufficiency

Patient taking maintenance corticosteroids (e.g. a patient with CAH or Addison's disease)

For a minor illness, such as low-grade fever ($< 38.3°$ C; $101°$ F), double the daily dose of hydrocortisone. For a moderate illness, such as fever $>102°$ F ($>38.8°$ C) and/or a bacterial infection, triple the total daily dose and divide into a q 6h dosing regimen. If the patient cannot tolerate oral medications, give the same dose IM or IV. Admission will be necessary if the patient cannot subsequently tolerate oral steroids.

Patient taking pharmacologic doses of steroids (for asthma, nephrotic syndrome, ITP, leukemia, collagen vascular diseases, etc.)

Most pharmacologic doses are greater than physiologic doses. However, if the current steroid dose is not more than twice the patient's daily maintenance of hydrocortisone ($10–15$ mg/m^2/day), double or triple the dose when the stress is trauma or surgery. If the stress is a serious infection, with an etiology that may be adversely affected by high-dose steroids (such as fungal infection in a patient with cystic fibrosis), consult with pediatric infectious disease and endocrine specialists and lower the dose to $30–50$ mg/m^2/day div q 6h. If a patient receiving a tapering dose of corticosteroids develops symptoms of adrenal insufficiency, increase the dose to the most recent dose at which he or she was asymptomatic, then initiate a more gradual taper after consulting with a pediatric endocrinologist.

Patient who has recently completed a steroid course

A history of completing a 2-week, or longer, course of corticosteroids in the previous 6 months places a patient at risk for developing Addisonian crisis. If the patient is symptomatic for an acute adrenal crisis, treat as above. If the patient is asymptomatic, obtain an early morning cortisol (normal >5 mg/dL) or arrange an ACTH stimulation test. If testing reveals adrenal insufficiency, start maintenance hydrocortisone at $10–15$ mg/m^2/day div q 8h or q 12h, although a larger dose may be needed. A re-evaluation of the patient's adrenal reserve may be indicated approximately 6 months after the last steroid course; normal results eliminate unnecessary future stress steroid doses.

It is not necessary to treat patients who received less than replacement steroid therapy for any period of time. For other patients, treatment is required only during periods of stress with a dosage equivalent of two to four times the replacement dose. If the adrenal status is uncertain, treat for presumed adrenal insufficiency, as noted above.

For all of the above scenarios, continue the oral stress dose (double or triple) of hydrocortisone for the duration of the stress, and then taper quickly, over 4–7 days, to the previous or maintenance dose. In addition, advise the family of a steroid-dependent child to obtain and wear a Medic Alert® or carry a card that indicates the presence of adrenal insufficiency, the current steroid dose (as well as the indication and the steroid doses that should be used for stress), and the prescribing physician's name and contact numbers. In addition, instruct the family members and/or caretakers to administer emergency intramuscular hydrocortisone (infant 25 mg, child 50 mg, adult 100 mg) in the event the patient has persistent vomiting or altered mental status. Remind the caretakers to check new prescriptions and expiration dates, and to have the hydrocortisone easily available in the event of an emergency.

Follow-up

- Stress doses of hydrocortisone required: daily, until the stress has resolved

Indications for admission

- Addisonian crisis
- Vomiting, inadequate oral intake, or postural vital sign changes in a patient known to be at risk for adrenal insufficiency
- Medication compliance at home is uncertain

Bibliography

New MI, Ghizzoni L, Lin-Su K: An update of congenital adrenal hyperplasia. In Lifshitz F (ed), *Pediatric Endocrinology*, New York, Informa Healthcare USA, 2007, pp. 227–45.

Riepe FG, Sippell WG: Recent advances in diagnosis, treatment, and outcome of congenital adrenal hyperplasia due to 21-hydroxylase deficiency. *Rev Endocr Metab Disord* 2007;8:349–63.

Diabetes insipidus

Diabetes insipidus (DI) is characterized by an inability to concentrate urine. The posterior pituitary secretes vasopressin in response to volume depletion, increased plasma osmolality (from hypernatremia, hyperglycemia), nausea, pain, motion sickness, vaso-vagal reactions, and a number of pharmacologic agents. Vasopressin then controls water homeostasis via reabsorption from urine.

Central diabetes insipidus is defined by a deficiency of antidiuretic hormone (ADH, vasopressin). A variety of acquired hypothalamic lesions can cause central DI, including tumors (craniopharyngioma, Langerhans cell histiocytosis, optic glioma), basilar skull fractures, neurosurgical complications, granulomatous diseases, vascular lesions, meningitis, and encephalitis. In approximately 50% of cases, however, no primary etiology can be found (idiopathic, congenital defect).

Nephrogenic DI is caused by renal unresponsiveness to ADH. The defect may be congenital, or secondary to hypercalcemia, hypokalemia, drugs (lithium, amphotericin, cisplatin, rifampin, methicillin), or chronic renal disease including ureteral obstruction, polycystic kidney disease, renal medullary cystic disease, or sickle cell disease.

Normal plasma osmolality ranges between 280 and 290 mOsm/kg. Usually, at a serum osmolality of <280 mOsm/kg, the plasma vasopressin level is ≤1 pg/mL. Above 283 mOsm/kg, the normal threshold for vasopressin release, the plasma vasopressin level rises in proportion to the plasma osmolality, up to a maximum concentration of 20 pg/mL (at a blood osmolality of 320 mOsm/kg). Peak antidiuretic effect is achieved at a vasopressin concentration of 5 pg/mL.

In contrast to the increases in vasopressin secretion with minor changes in plasma osmolality, no change in vasopressin secretion is seen until blood volume decreases by approximately 8%. Vasopressin secretion is inhibited by glucocorticoids, so that enhanced vasopressin activity occurs in primary or secondary glucocorticoid insufficiency and contributes to the hyponatremia in these conditions.

Clinical presentation

DI causes renal loss of water, which leads to excessive urine output and acute thirst. Water loss is compensated by increasing intake, so that dehydration is unusual in an awake patient. However, infants, children with altered mental status and midline brain abnormalities, and patients whose thirst centers are affected by the primary process (hydrocephalus, postconcussive syndrome) are at increased risk for hypernatremic dehydration.

An infant is usually irritable but eager to suck, often exhibiting a distinct preference for water over milk. An older child presents with the abrupt onset of polyuria and polydipsia, followed by enuresis, vomiting, and constipation. Nocturia and a preference for ice water are common. Recurrent episodes of dehydration and hypernatremia can result in poor growth and mental retardation, while polyuria and large volumes of urine can cause dilations of the urinary tract, impaired bladder function, and chronic renal failure. Unexplained fever is another possible presentation.

Abnormalities of the CNS such as irritability, altered consciousness, increased muscle tone, convulsions, and coma occur secondary to hypernatremia. These findings correlate with the degree and rapidity of the rise in serum sodium.

Diagnosis

The cardinal diagnostic features are:

- a high rate of dilute urine flow (urine output >4 mL/kg/hr)
- clinical signs of dehydration (weight loss, hypotension)
- mild to marked degree of serum hypernatremia (>150 mEq/L)
- hyperosmolality (>300 mOsm/kg)
- low urine osmolality (<300 mOsm/kg) and low specific gravity (<1.010) despite a normal or elevated serum osmolality

If the dehydration is mild, the urine osmolality is less than the serum osmolality. However, if there is severe dehydration or a low glomerular filtration rate, urine output decreases and urine osmolality increases above the serum; this may temporarily obscure the diagnosis.

Other causes of polyuria, including psychogenic water drinking (nocturia unusual), organic polydipsia (hypothalamic lesion), and osmotic diuresis (diabetes mellitus, IV contrast administration, chronic renal insufficiency), can be distinguished by the history, electrolytes, BUN, and creatinine. With a urinary tract infection there will be symptoms such as urgency, frequency, and dysuria. A large urinary volume can lead to bladder distension, which can then mimic obstructive uropathy.

ED management

If DI is suspected, obtain urine for routine analysis, as well as osmolality, sodium, potassium, and culture. Obtain blood for electrolytes, calcium, BUN, creatinine, osmolality, and ADH level. A serum osmolality >300 mOsm/kg with a urine osmolality <300 mOsm/kg establishes the diagnosis of DI. The diagnosis is also confirmed if hypernatremia and serum hyperosmolality are documented in association with large volumes of dilute urine (specific gravity $\leq$1.005, urine osmolality $\leq$ serum) that is negative for glucose. If the etiology is not clear, or the diagnosis uncertain, consult a pediatric endocrinologist and admit the patient.

In addition, perform a complete neurologic examination with visual field evaluation and arrange for an MRI of the pituitary with and without gadolinium. Normally, the posterior pituitary is seen as an area of enhanced brightness on T-1 weighted images following the administration of gadolinium. This "bright spot" is absent in both central and nephrogenic diabetes insipidus, owing to vasopressin deficiency in the former and enhanced vasopressin release in the latter. In primary polydipsia, the posterior bright spot is normal.

If the patient is dehydrated, febrile (>38.3° C; 101° F) or has a depressed level of consciousness, start treatment in the ED.

Fluid therapy

In infants and neonates, DI is best managed by providing fluid therapy alone. In infants, excessive fluid intake coupled with vasopressin therapy can result in water intoxication and hyponatremia. For all patients, pay meticulous attention to fluid management. Use a flow sheet to document fluid intake and output, replacement of urine output and insensible losses, vital signs, urine specific gravity, and serum electrolytes.

Vasopressin and vasopressin analogs (acute onset of DI)

Give antidiuretic therapy (vasopressin SQ/IM/IV or DDAVP intranasal/SQ/IV) according to the following guidelines.

Continuous vasopressin intravenous infusion

Intravenous therapy with synthetic aqueous vasopressin (Pitressin®, 20 units/mL) is indicated for central DI of acute onset or in the postoperative setting. Dilute to 0.01 units/mL (10 milliunits/mL) by adding 5 units (0.25 mL) to 500 mL NS or D_5W. Then, give 0.1–1.5 milliunits/kg/h (0.01–0.15 mL/kg/h). The effect of vasopressin is maximal within 2 hours of the start of infusion, although it has a short half life of 5–10 minutes. During the infusion, fluid intake must be limited to 1 liter/m^2/day.

Vasopressin SQ (20 units/mL)

Give 0.05–0.1 units/kg/dose q 4–6h. The onset of action is within minutes and the duration is 2–8 hours. Titrate the dose to the desired effect.

DDAVP (desmopressin 4 mcg/mL)

Dilute 1 mL DDAVP with 9 mL NS to create a 0.4 mcg/mL solution and give 0.01–0.03 mcg/kg/dose, IV or SQ, qday or bid. Intravenous DDAVP has a long half-life of 8–12 hours.

Treatment of nephrogenic diabetes insipidus

The goals of therapy are maintaining normal growth and development by providing adequate calories, decreasing urine volume, and avoiding severe dehydration. Medications used to decrease the polyuria include:

Thiazide diuretics

Thiazides promote sodium excretion by interfering with sodium reabsorption in the distal tubule of the nephron and altering inner medullary osmolality. A thiazide plus an amiloride diuretic is the most commonly used combination for the treatment of congenital X-linked nephrogenic diabetes insipidus. Give hydrochorthiazide (2mg/kg per day div bid; maximum 100 mg per day for children, 200 mg per day for adults).

Amiloride diuretics

Amiloride counteracts the thiazide-induced hypokalemia. The dose is 0.625 Mg/kg per day in patients weighing 6–20 kg; in adolescents, give 5–20 mg per day, up to a maximum of 40 mg/24 hours.

Indomethacin

Indomethacin (2 Mg/kg per day) enhances proximal tubular sodium and water reabsorption.

Indications for admission

- New onset or symptomatic DI

Bibliography

Cheetham T: Pitfalls in investigating for diabetes insipidus. *Indian Pediatr* 2008;45:452–3.

Linshaw MA: Back to basics: congenital nephrogenic diabetes insipidus. *Pediatr Rev* 2007;28:372–80.

Diabetic ketoacidosis

Diabetic ketoacidosis (DKA) may be the initial presentation of new onset Type I diabetes mellitus (DM) or a complication in a previously diagnosed patient. Diabetic ketoacidosis occurs less frequently in patients with Type II DM. Infection is the most common precipitating factor, but trauma, pregnancy, emotional stress, and noncompliance are other causes. An absolute or relative insulin deficiency is present, along with increased levels of counter-regulatory hormones (glucagon, cortisol, growth hormone, and catecholamines) leading to deranged metabolism, hyperglycemia, osmotic diuresis, hypertonic dehydration, and finally, ketoacidosis. In ketoacidosis, the acidosis is secondary to ketonemia with ß-hydroxybutyric acid and its redox partner, acetoacetate.

Clinical presentation

The patient usually presents with abdominal pain, nausea, vomiting, dehydration, fatigue, and hyperpnea. Isolated vomiting can also be a presentation of DKA. The history often reveals polydypsia, polyuria, nocturia, enuresis, and, with new-onset diabetes, recent weight-loss or lack of weight gain in a growing child. Characteristic Kussmaul breathing (deep sighing breathing) can be present, but the respirations may be depressed if the patient is severely acidotic (pH ≤6.9). Neurologic findings range from drowsiness to coma and are related to the level of hyperosmolality.

Table 7-1. Differential diagnosis of DKA

Metabolic acidosis	*Polyuria, nocturia, abdominal pain*
Severe gastroenteritis with hypovolemia	UTI
Salicylate poisoning	*Hyperglycemia*
Other ingestions	Salicylate poisoning (glucose <300 mg/dL)
Ethanol	Iron toxicity
Methanol	Hypernatremia
Ethylene glycol	Stress
Isoniazid	Sepsis
Iron	*Ketonuria (without hyperglycemia)*
Coma	Fasting states
Hypoglycemia	Gastroenteritis with vomiting
Sedative hypnotic or narcotic overdose	Anorexia of any etiology
Lactic acidosis	Salicylate poisoning
Nonketotic hyperosmolar coma	
CNS trauma, infection, bleeding	

Mild DKA

DKA is considered mild if there is ketonemia, a venous pH of 7.2–7.3, and minimal signs of dehydration. The vital signs may be normal, except for possible hyperpnea.

Moderate DKA

In moderate DKA, the venous pH is 7.1–7.2, but there are signs of moderate to severe dehydration, including dry mucous membranes and decreased skin turgor. Ketonemia is present as well.

Severe DKA

Severe DKA is defined as a venous pH <7.1, with ketonemia and severe dehydration associated with evidence of intravascular volume depletion (poor capillary refill, tachycardia, weak peripheral pulses, hypotension, orthostatic vital sign changes).

Diagnosis

In the known diabetic, consider DKA when the patient complains of abdominal pain, vomiting, or malaise. The diagnosis may be more difficult to make in a patient presenting for the first time (Table 7-1). In addition to acidosis and ketonemia, significant hyperglycemia (>500 mg/dL) is common, although DKA can occur with a glucose of 200–300 mg/dL. In fact, the glucose level is more indicative of the sugar content of what the patient has been drinking while attempting to maintain hydration than the severity of the DKA.

In DKA, sodium stores are depleted but serum sodium may be low, normal, or high, depending on the water balance. The measured sodium is lower than the true value because of the shift of water into the extracellular space (sodium decreases 1.6 mEq/L per each 100 mg/dL rise in glucose over 100 mg/dL) and the increase in serum lipid and protein levels (pseudohyponatremia). In addition, the low sodium level may reflect water retention secondary to increased secretion of antidiuretic hormone.

While there is usually a total body potassium deficit, the initial serum potassium concentration may be normal or elevated because of hemoconcentration, insulin deficiency, and the shifting of potassium into the extracellular space secondary to the hyperosmolality and metabolic acidosis. The measured potassium rises 0.6 mEq/L for every 0.1 drop in the pH, so that a low initial potassium level (<3.5 mEq/L) is an unusual and ominous finding.

Finally, in the absence of infection, the WBC count may be elevated (18,000–20,000/mm^3) in a patient with DKA, secondary to the increase in circulating catecholamines and hemoconcentration.

ED management

After a rapid evaluation of the patient's status, initiate therapy to correct fluid deficits, electrolyte imbalances, acidosis, and hyperglycemia. Avoid overly vigorous management, which can cause excessively rapid changes in glucose, osmolality, and pH, and therefore contribute to the development of complications. Treat any concomitant pathology or complications (sepsis, increased ICP, or coma).

History

Determine the duration of the current illness and any precipitating factors such as infection, trauma, or stress. If the patient is a known diabetic, document the current insulin regimen (and adherence) and the time of the last injection.

Physical examination

Focus the examination on the vital signs (including the presence of Kussmaul respirations), degree of dehydration, level of consciousness, fundoscopic examination, and possible sites of infection. If possible, weigh the patient and try to determine the premorbid weight. Document the vital signs and neurologic status at least hourly.

Initial laboratory evaluation

Obtain blood for STAT electrolytes, BUN, glucose, calcium, phosphorous, pH (venous or arterial), CBC, HgbA1c, and a bedside fingerstick glucose measurement. Also obtain a urinalysis and an ECG (check for peaked T waves). Prior to beginning insulin therapy for a patient with new-onset diabetes, send additional blood for insulin, C-peptide, and relevant autoantibodies (insulin autoantibodies [IAA], islet cell antibodies [ICA], and glutamic decarboxylase antibodies [GAD]). Also obtain blood cultures if infection is suspected.

Initial management

Place the patient on a cardiorespiratory monitor and start and maintain a flow sheet. Within the framework of the following guidelines, assess each case individually. In general, however, the goals are slow, steady rehydration over 24–48 hours, a decrease in the serum glucose of 80–100 mg/dL/h, and a stable corrected sodium while the measured sodium increases.

Fluid resuscitation

Most patients with DKA have some degree of dehydration. A premorbid weight is the best measurement of fluid loss but is often unavailable, while the traditional physical examination criteria by which the level of dehydration is assessed are unreliable. Despite significant dehydration, patients with DKA will continue to urinate until intravascular volume depletion affects the glomerular filtration rate. In general, children with moderate to severe DKA are 7–10% dehydrated.

Insert two IV catheters so that maintenance and replacement fluids and the insulin drip can be managed separately. Initially, administer a normal saline fluid bolus (20 mL/kg) over approximately 60 minutes. Reassess the patient after the initial bolus (peripheral pulses, capillary refill) and repeat, if necessary, in order to maintain adequate peripheral perfusion.

Deficit fluids

Calculate deficit fluids using recent weight loss or an estimation of percent dehydration. Replace the total deficit with normal saline, divided evenly over 24–48 hours. Use a slower rate (over 48 hours) of fluid replacement for children <2 years or, if there is severe acidosis, an elevated corrected sodium, significant hyperosmolality (>350 mOsm/kg), or a long prodromal illness. Subtract the amount of fluid given as a fluid bolus from the total deficit.

Maintenance fluids

Calculate the daily maintenance fluid requirements and administer as normal saline. Replacement of ongoing losses may be necessary, especially if there is polyuria (>5 mL/kg/h). For a polyuric patient, measure the urinary losses every 4–8 hours, and then replace half of this volume over the next 4–8 hours with ½ NS in a separate "piggy-back" line. Also replace the volume of vomitus with ½ NS in this line.

Potassium

DKA is associated with a marked depletion of total body potassium, while correction of the acidosis will exacerbate the hypokalemia. If the serum potassium is <5.0 mEq/L, add 20 mEq K acetate/L and 20 mEq K phosphate/L, *once urine output is documented*. If a serum potassium level is unavailable, obtain an ECG to look for evidence of hyperkalemia (peaked T waves, shortened QT interval) or hypokalemia (flattened T waves, widened QT interval). If the patient is hypocalcemic, use KCL instead of K phosphate. Measure the phosphorus and calcium every 4–6 hours and repeat the ECG every 2–4 hours.

Insulin and glucose

After the initial fluid resuscitation begin an insulin drip with the goal of decreasing the blood sugar by 80–100 mg/dL/h. Within the first 1–2 two hours of treatment, start the insulin drip at 0.1 units/kg/h, but do not give an insulin bolus. Add 50 units of regular insulin to 500 mL of normal saline (resultant concentration is 0.1 units/mL). Run the IV at an hourly rate equal to patient's weight in kg (i.e. 40 mL/hour for a 40 kg patient). Subtract this hourly rate from the maintenance fluids. Prior to running the drip, allow 50 mL of the mixture to flow through the IV in order to saturate insulin-binding sites in the tubing. Start the insulin drip at 0.05 units/kg/h if the patient is markedly hyperglycemic (glucose >1000 mg/dL), is <2 years of age, or has recently received a subcutaneous dose of insulin.

Add D_5 to the fluids when the glucose reaches 250–300 mg/dL, but continue the insulin infusion until the ketonemia is cleared or clearing. Adjust the rate of the drip to maintain a blood glucose of 120–180 mg/dL. Initially, lower the rate by one-half (0.5 units/kg/h), but do not decrease the insulin drip rate below 0.03 units/kg/hour. If the patient is becoming hypoglycemic at this rate, increase the dextrose in the IV solution to $D_{7.5}$–$D_{12.5}$. Calculate the glucose requirement per unit of insulin; most patients require 3–5 g of glucose/unit of insulin. Once the acidosis is resolved (pH >7.30, bicarbonate >15) and the patient can tolerate a PO diet, begin subcutaneous insulin. Stop the insulin drip one hour after the subcutaneous insulin dose.

Bicarbonate

Do not use sodium bicarbonate unless the venous pH is <7.0 or the serum bicarbonate is <6 mEq/L. The dose is 0.5–1 mEq/kg by IV infusion over 1 hour, *not as an IV push*. Mix a 50 mL ampule of sodium bicarbonate with 250 mL sterile water to create a concentration of 44 mEq/300 mL.

Example calculation

Patient with DKA who weighs 40 kg and has 10% dehydration:

Initial fluid bolus

20 mL/kg = 800 mL

Fluid deficit

10% of 40 kg = 4 kg (= 4 L or 4000 mL of fluid loss)
4000 mL (fluid deficit) – 800 mL (initial fluid bolus) = 3200 mL
3200 mL div over 24 hours = 133 mL/hour

Maintenance fluids

40 kg patient maintenance = 1900 mL/day
1900 mL div over 24 hours = 79 mL

Insulin

0.1 units/kg/h = 40 mL/h

Initial fluids

(Deficit – bolus) + (maintenance – insulin drip) = 172 mL/hour normal saline + 20 mEq K phosphate/L + 20 mEq K acetate/L

Continue normal saline until the osmolality is <310 mOsm/kg and the sodium rises to approximately 140 mEq/L as the blood sugar falls. Then, begin ½ NS. However, if the corrected sodium is >160 mEq/L, consult with a pediatric endocrinologist and use a lower sodium concentration in the IV fluid.

Laboratory assessments

Repeat the glucose and venous pH hourly. Obtain electrolytes, osmolality, BUN, and creatinine every 2 hours until the trend is normalizing, then every 4 hours until normal. Calculate the corrected sodium with each set of laboratory values:

Corrected sodium = measured sodium +1.6 X [(measured glucose – 100)/100]

Obtain calcium and phosphorus levels every 4–6 hours until the DKA is resolving. Obtain an ECG every 2–4 hours, looking for peaked T waves (hyperkalemia).

Even with meticulous care, a patient with DKA is at risk for developing cerebral edema. Risk factors include age <3 years, high BUN, low pCO_2, and failure of the serum sodium to rise as expected as the glucose falls. Signs and symptoms of increased ICP (pp. 516–17) classically occur 6–18 hours into treatment and include headache, vomiting, lethargy, disorientation, fundoscopic changes (absent venous pulsations, blurring of optic disk margins), decorticate or decerebrate posturing, and pupillary changes. Any neurologic signs at presentation, *prior* to treatment, reflect the patient's hyperosmolality.

If the patient complains of headache and becomes lethargic *during* treatment, but has a normal fundoscopic examination, obtain a stat CT scan of the head. If the patient is unresponsive, posturing, has pupillary changes, or has milder symptoms with fundoscopic abnormalities, immediately treat for increased intracranial pressure with mannitol 1 g/kg IV over 10 minutes, endotracheal intubation if airway protection is compromised because of the patient's mental status, and elevation of the head to 30°.

Also observe the patient for other problems associated with therapy for DKA, such as fluid overload with edema or CHF.

Management of mild DKA (pH >7.2)

Administer a normal saline bolus (20 mL/kg), if needed (as above). If the patient is not dehydrated, give ½NS at a maintenance rate plus deficit (based on clinical examination and recent weight loss). Give the known diabetic subcutaneous regular insulin (usually 0.1 units/kg). In the case of a new-onset diabetic not in DKA, treat with appropriate hydration and consult with a pediatric endocrinologist. Do not treat with insulin until after consultation, as such a patient is particularly sensitive to exogenous insulin. Obtain baseline measurements of serum insulin, c-peptide, HbA_{1c}, IAA, ICA, GAD antibodies, and thyroid function tests.

Hyperglycemia during stress

Hyperglycemia may occur in response to stress, such as sepsis or corticosteroid administration, although most patients with stress do not become hyperglycemic. Diabetes cannot be definitively diagnosed during another illness, but the patient requires close follow-up. Obtain IAA, ICA, and GAD antibodies to evaluate the risk of type 1 diabetes, which is greater in a child with positive antibodies, with or without known relatives with diabetes. Refer a patient with any positive antibody test to a pediatric endocrinologist, in about 6 weeks, for evaluation of glucose tolerance.

Type II diabetes

Type II Diabetes is increasing in frequency among children, though it is more commonly an incidental finding than the cause for an ED visit. It is characterized by insulin resistance and relative insulin hyposecretion. Patients can present with polydipsia, polyuria, and polyphagia, and infrequently weight loss. However, ketosis and/or acidosis are rare, unless the patient presents with a significant infection. Alternatively, glucosuria or hyperglycemia may be noted as incidental findings.

A patient with Type II diabetes is usually obese and frequently has acanthosis nigricans, most commonly on the posterior neck, but lesions may also be found on the anterior neck, the axillae, and in the groin. The blood sugar is >200 mg/dL and the fasting glucose is

>125 mg/dL. Management depends on the severity of presentation; a dehydrated patient requires IV fluid and a ketotic patient needs insulin. Also give insulin to a patient who remains hyperglycemic after a bolus of normal saline. Consult with a pediatric endocrinologist to determine whether treatment with oral agents is appropriate.

Hyperosmolar hyperglycemic state (HHS) is a serious complication of Type II DM with a mortality rate of 10–20%. It is characterized by hyperosmolarity, hyperglycemia, dehydration, and minimal ketoacidosis. The HHS can be the initial presentation of Type II DM or can occur in patients with a known history of Type II DM during an intercurrent illness. Unlike DKA, the onset is more insidious and patients may initially present with nonspecific flu-like symptoms. Plasma glucose levels (>600 mg/dL), as well as serum osmolality (>320 mOsm/kg) are significantly elevated. The bicarbonate level is generally >15 mEq/L, the venous pH >7.30, and urine and serum ketones are small or absent. Neurologic features are prominent, including stupor and coma. Volume depletion in HHS is greater than in DKA, so that patients require aggressive fluid resuscitation. Although many patients with HHS will respond to fluids alone, administer IV insulin as in DKA to facilitate correction of the hyperglycemia. Do not give insulin without adequate fluid resuscitation. Correct electrolyte imbalances as in DKA, and assess the patient for an underlying infection.

Follow-up

- Mild DKA in a known diabetic when compliance and follow-up can be assured: 1–2 days
- Stress hyperglycemia with positive antibody test: endocrinology follow-up in 6 weeks

Indications for admission

- Newly diagnosed diabetes
- Moderate or severe DKA
- Known diabetic with an intercurrent illness which limits oral rehydration or therapy (nausea and vomiting)
- HHS

Bibliography

Cooke DW, Plotnick L: Management of diabetic ketoacidosis in children and adolescents. *Pediatr Rev* 2008;29:431–6.

Koul PB: Diabetic ketoacidosis – a current appraisal of pathophysiology and management. *Clin Pediatr (Phila)* 2009;48:135–44.

Wolfsdorf J, Glaser N, Sperling MA; American Diabetes Association: Diabetic ketoacidosis in infants, children and adolescents – A consensus statement from the American Diabetes Association. *Diabetes Care* 2006;29:1150–9.

Hypercalcemia

Although serum calcium levels vary somewhat by patient age and laboratory, hypercalcemia is generally accepted to be a serum calcium >11 mg/dL or a blood ionized calcium >5.5 mg/dL. In contrast to hypocalcemia, hypercalcemia is uncommon in children.

Clinical presentation

Patients with serum calcium levels <12 mg/dL are often asymptomatic. The hallmark symptoms of hypercalcemia are pain, weakness, and cognitive impairment. The pain may be gastrointestinal in origin and be accompanied by nausea, vomiting, and constipation. In addition, there may be renal colic caused by genitourinary stone formation, with or without hematuria. Finally, the patient may have bone lesions.

Neurologic system symptoms can range from confusion or agitation to stupor and coma, with weakness eventually including the respiratory muscles. Since calcium acts as an antidiuretic hormone (ADH) antagonist, the patient may have polyuria, polydypsia, and dehydration. Long-standing hypercalcemia may lead to band keratopathy. An uncommon sign of hypercalcemia in children is hypertension.

In the Williams Syndrome, hypercalcemia may be associated with elfin facies (upturned nose, long philtrum, hypotelorism, receding chin), full lips, stellate pattern of the iris with blue eyes, strabismus, medial flare of the eyebrows, supravalvular aortic stenosis, and mental retardation. In these patients the hypercalcemia usually resolves a year or two after birth.

Diagnosis

The diagnosis of hypercalcemia is confirmed by documenting either a high ionized calcium concentration or an elevated serum calcium level in the absence of a high serum protein level. Associated serum laboratory abnormalities may include any of the following: decreased phosphorus or bicarbonate; increased BUN, alkaline phosphatase, PTH, 25-hydroxyvitamin D, 1,25-dihydroxyvitamin D, PTHrP, thyroid hormones, or vitamin A level. Urine findings may include an elevated pH ($\geq$7.0), calciuria, phosphaturia, and aminoaciduria. Radiographs may reveal generalized bone demineralization, bone tumors, resorption of subperiosteal bone in distal phalanges, nephrocalcinosis, or renal stones.

ED management

If the serum calcium is >12.0 mg/dL or the patient is symptomatic with a calcium between 11–12 mg/dL, consult a pediatric endocrinologist and begin treatment after obtaining the blood tests mentioned above. Many hypercalcemic patients are dehydrated at presentation, so that calcium levels may decline solely with rehydration. If the patient remains hypercalcemic, increase calciuresis by giving IV normal saline at 2–3 times maintenance rates, along with furosemide (1 mg/kg IV q 6h). Ensure adequate hydration before the furosemide is given, otherwise the hypercalcemia can worsen. Check the serum electrolytes at least every 6 hours during this aggressive stage of therapy. Dialysis is indicated for renal failure. There are three medication types that can be used for more long-term control, depending on the likely cause of the hypercalcemia.

Corticosteroids

Steroids reduce intestinal calcium absorption and may be particularly efficacious in malignancies. However, they may not be effective for 4-5 days and a rebound hypercalcemia can occur if treatment is discontinued abruptly. Give either prednisone 2 Mg/kg per day div bid (60 mg/day maximum) or hydrocortisone 10 Mg/kg per day div qid (300 mg/day maximum).

Calcitonin

Calcitonin is most effective in cases of immobilization or other causes of bone resorption. It may also be effective for bone pain. Typically, the calcium level will decline by 2 mg/dL after

24–48 hours, although the effects may be transient, lasting only a week or less. Give 4 units/kg SQ every 12 hours, and increase to q 6h if the hypercalcemia persists.

Bisphosphonates

These are the most effective agents at reducing bone resorption and calcium levels. Limited experience in children suggests that pamidronate 1–1.5 mg/kg (90 mg maximum) infused IV over 2–4 hours is effective. Note that the first dose may be accompanied by fever and aches, which can be treated with ibuprofen, and transient hypocalcemia can occur several days after infusion.

Indications for admission

- Treatment required for hypercalcemia

Bibliography

Benjamin RW, Moats-Staats BM, Calikoglu A, Savendahl L, Chrysis D: Hypercalcemia in children. *Pediatr Endocrinol Rev* 2008;5:778–84.

Carroll MF, Schade DS: A practical approach to hypercalcemia. *Am Fam Physician* 2003; 67:1959–66.

Hyperkalemia

Hyperkalemia is defined as a serum potassium $\geq$5.5 mEq/L. In general, elevated potassium levels are secondary to increased exogenous intake, transcellular shifts, or decreased excretion. Diagnosis and management of hyperkalemia is critical given the potential for lethal cardiac arrhythmias.

The most common causes of increased serum potassium are metabolic acidosis (DKA) and acute kidney injury (acute glomerulonephritis, acute tubular necrosis). Other etiologies include adrenal insufficiency, hypoaldosteronism, chronic renal failure, hypovolemia, ingestions (beta-blocker, digoxin), cytotoxic chemotherapy, tumor lysis syndrome, medication side-effects (succinylcholine, ace-inhibitors), trauma, rhabdomyolysis, and familial periodic paralysis. However, most often the elevated potassium reflects a pseudohyperkalemia caused by hemolysis or in association with thrombocytosis or leukocytosis.

Clinical presentation

A serum potassium <6 mEq/L is usually asymptomatic. At higher levels there may be muscle weakness, paresthesias, and flaccid paralysis, associated with asymptomatic ECG changes (see below). With further increases in serum potassium (K^+ >7.0), there is a possibility of ventricular arrhythmias. This risk is increased by hyponatremia, hypocalcemia, and acidosis.

Diagnosis

If the potassium is $\geq$6.0mEq/L, immediately obtain an ECG to identify cardiac conduction abnormalities such as peaked T waves (T wave > one-half the R or S wave) and a shortened QT interval. Later changes (K^+ >6.5–7.0) may include flattening of the P wave, lengthening of the PR interval, and widening of the QRS complex.

ED management

The treatment of hyperkalemia primarily entails enhancing potassium excretion or increasing the movement of potassium into cells as a temporary measure, as well as minimizing cardiac effects. Aggressive IV therapy is necessary for patients who are symptomatic (muscle weakness, cramps, etc.) or have ECG changes.

To shift potassium intracellularly, give 0.5–1 g/kg of glucose (2–4 mL/kg of a 25% dextrose solution) over 30 minutes concurrently with regular insulin (1 unit per 5 g of glucose given). The potassium-lowering effect occurs in 10–20 minutes, but carefully monitor the serum glucose for both hyper- and hypoglycemia. Nebulized β agonists, such as albuterol, are also effective at shifting potassium into the cells, but are less predictable than other therapies. The peak effect is 40–80 minutes after administration. Give 10–20 mg in 4 mL normal saline (4–8 times the dose used for the treatment of asthma).

If there are associated peaked T waves, QRS widening, PR lengthening, or severe hyperkalemia (K^+ >7.0) give calcium chloride (20 mg/kg IV over 3–5 min) to stabilize the cardiac membrane potential. Protecting the myocardium early in the treatment course is crucial, as the potassium-lowering effects of the other therapies may not be effective for 30–60 minutes.

To promote potassium excretion in the absence of peaked T waves, treat with polystyrene sulfonate (Kayexalate®), 1 g/kg dissolved in 4 mL of water, with sorbitol (PO or PR). This dose lowers the serum potassium by 0.5–1 mEq/L by enhancing GI excretion, but the onset is slow and duration is variable. For a patient who is not anuric, also give furosemide (1–2 mg/kg). The onset of action is within one hour, and the dose may be repeated every 6 hours. These interventions are second-line therapy which decreases total body potassium. Use them after life-threatening hyperkalemia has been managed.

In patients with acute kidney injury, life-threatening hyperkalemia (serum potassium >7 mEq/L) is an indication for dialysis.

Indications for admission
- Hyperkalemia with clinical symptoms and/or ECG changes
- Severe hyperkalemia (K^+ >7.0)

Bibliography
Evans KJ, Greenberg A: Hyperkalemia – a review. *J Intensive Care Med* 2005;20:272–90.

Schaefer TJ, Wolford RW: Disorders of potassium. *Emerg Med Clin North Am* 2005;23:723–47.

Hypernatremia

Hypernatremia is defined as a serum sodium level ≥150 mEq/L. Hypernatremia occurs when there is a relative excess of sodium compared to water. Normally, hypertonicity stimulates both the secretion of ADH and an extremely powerful compensatory thirst, which can keep up with as much as 15–20 L of pure water loss.

Patients with adipsic hypernatremia do not feel the urge to drink fluids even in the presence of hyperosmolar dehydration owing to a disruption in the regulation of thirst by the osmosensor. The hypernatremia in these patients is accelerated by events such as gastroenteritis, fever, or excessive sweating. A disordered thirst mechanism can occur in approximately 10% of patients with central diabetes insipidus. Adipsic hypernatremia can occur with malformations of the brain (holoprosencephaly, hypoplasia of the corpus callosum), vascular lesions, neoplasms, AIDS, cytomegalovirus encephalitis, pseudotumor cerebri, and empty sella turcica.

Regardless of the etiology, acute hypernatremia has a mortality of 10–70%. Morbidity of the CNS has been reported in up to two-thirds of patients, although it is unclear whether this is a result of the primary disease or the treatment. There are three categories of hypernatremia:

Low total body (TBNa); lower total body water (TBW)

Most often, this occurs in the setting of hypernatremic dehydration in infants, usually secondary to gastrointestinal losses (particularly during rotavirus infection). Osmotic diuretics (mannitol, glucose, urea) can also cause water loss in excess of salt loss.

Normal TBNa; low TBW

Central and nephrogenic diabetes insipidus cause excessive renal water loss. In central DI caused by trauma, hydrocephalus, or neoplasia there may be a concomitant derangement in the thirst mechanism further predisposing to hypernatremia. Increased insensible losses (hypermetabolic states with fever) and tachypnea can also result in hypernatremia, while restricted access to water (infants, developmentally impaired children, bedridden patients) may put a patient at increased risk.

Increased TBNa (uncommon)

Primary hyperaldosteronism, Cushing's syndrome, and salt poisoning (inappropriately mixed infant formula, salt tablet ingestion, iatrogenic sodium bicarbonate administration) result in excess body sodium. Except in the case of salt poisoning, very high serum sodium levels are unusual.

Clinical presentation

The clinical signs and symptoms result from the physiologic response to serum hypertonicity. Most conscious patients will exhibit a voracious thirst and, if given the opportunity, will drink water. If ADH and oral intake do not compensate, serum hypertonicity occurs and the brain cells shrink, leading to CNS signs and symptoms. Lethargy, alternating with irritability, and a high-pitched cry (infants) occur early and are followed by tremors and ataxia, then muscle twitching, tonic spasms, seizures (both focal and generalized), and ultimately coma.

Physical signs may include altered mental status, hypertonia, hyper-reflexia, and nuchal rigidity (secondary to hypertonia). Since intracellular fluid shifts extracellularly, the intravascular volume is maintained, so that signs of intravascular volume depletion are late findings. Chvostek's sign may be elicited occasionally, and a smooth, velvety, or doughy feel to the skin may be noted. Localizing neurologic findings suggest the possibility of CNS hemorrhage as a sequela of brain shrinkage. Also, hypocalcemia and hyperglycemia may be seen.

In a patient with DI (p. 166), signs of intravascular depletion and dehydration may be absent if the thirst mechanism and access to water are preserved. Salt poisoning may cause pulmonary edema (tachypnea, hepatomegaly, rales) and acute CNS pathology without signs of intravascular depletion. An infant exposed to extreme heat and humidity is at risk for hypernatremic dehydration; consider child abuse or neglect in such cases.

Diagnosis

Hypernatremia is usually discovered incidentally when electrolytes are obtained because of gastroenteritis, fever, altered mental status, seizures, polyuria, or polydipsia. In general,

Table 7-2. Diagnosis of hypernatremia

TBNa*	TBW†	Urine osmolality	Urine sodium
Low	Lower		
	GI losses (>800 mOsm/kg)	Hypertonic	<10 mEq/L (low)
	Osmotic diuresis	Hypertonic	>20 mEq/L (high)
Normal	Low		
	Diabetes insipidus	Isotonic/hypotonic	Variable
	Insensible losses	Hypertonic	Variable
Increased	Low/high		
	Salt poisoning	Isotonic/hypertonic	>20 mEq/L (high)

*TBNa: Total body sodium
†TBW: Total body water

since the presentation of hypernatremia is nonspecific, early diagnosis requires a high index of suspicion. Consider hypernatremia if the skin has a velvety, doughy feel, or if the clinical history fits the common etiologies.

If increased total body sodium from improper feeding technique is suspected, obtain some of the infant formula from the home and send it to the company and/or laboratory for evaluation. Also, watch how the caregiver prepares powdered formula and/or dilutes concentrated formula.

Once hypernatremia is documented, use the urine osmolality and urine sodium to categorize the patient (Table 7-2).

ED management

Be judicious in the fluid management of any patient with an electrolyte abnormality, as rapid correction carries its own risks, such as cerebral edema. If there are signs of intravascular depletion (resting tachycardia, orthostatic vital sign changes, weak peripheral pulses, poor capillary refill), give repeated boluses of 20 mL/kg of isotonic crystalloid (normal saline, Ringer's lactate) until perfusion is normalized. Hypernatremia is not a contraindication to using isotonic fluids, as these are hypotonic relative to the patient's serum; the hypernatremia will not be exacerbated.

Hyperglycemia and hypocalcemia often accompany hypernatremia. Once the intravascular volume has been restored, obtain a CBC, electrolytes, Dextrostix®, calcium, creatinine, urinalysis, urine sodium and osmolality, and any other laboratory tests pertinent to the patient's presentation.

TBNa and TBW depletion

In hypernatremic dehydration, the key to therapy is restoration of isotonicity without causing rapid fluid shifts into the brain cells. Otherwise, cerebral edema can ensue. First, give normal saline boluses until perfusion is normalized (as above). Estimate the free water deficit using the formula:

free H_2O deficit (L) = [(serum sodium level – 140)/140] × weight (kg) × 0.6

Replace the deficit over 48 hours, using $D_5\frac{1}{2}$ NS with one ampule of 10% calcium gluconate added per 500 mL of replacement fluid. Also add 40 mEq/L of potassium acetate after adequate urinary output is established. Replace ongoing losses simultaneously while closely monitoring the clinical status and serum electrolytes. The goal is a slow fall in the serum sodium of 0.5–1.0 mEq/h. Measure the sodium and glucose hourly to document the rate of sodium correction, and follow the calcium and potassium every 2–4 hours until normal levels are documented or the replacement is nearly complete. If hyperglycemia occurs, do not use insulin unless there are signs of glucose intolerance (glycosuria), as the glucose will generally correct with hydration alone. Increase the calcium infusion if hypocalcemia occurs (pp. 181–182).

TBNa normal; TBW depleted

Give maintenance fluids along with one-half of the excess urine output as D_5W. Treat central DI with vasopressin (pp. 167).

Increased TBNa/salt poisoning

Treat with peritoneal dialysis for serum sodium >200 mEq/L or if the patient has seizures or is comatose. Otherwise, give normal saline at a maintenance rate with furosemide (1 mg/kg) to achieve a net loss of sodium in excess of water.

Manage a patient with adipsic hypernatremia by limiting the daily fluid intake along with closely monitoring the body weight, urine output, clinical symptoms, and serum sodium level.

Hypertension may be the presenting sign of a patient with hyperaldosteronism, although malignant hypertension is rare. Consult a pediatric endocrinologist.

Indications for admission

- Symptomatic hypernatremia
- New-onset DI

Bibliography

Ghirardello S, Garrè ML, Rossi A, Maghnie M: The diagnosis of children with central diabetes insipidus. *J Pediatr Endocrinol Metab* 2007;**20**:359–75.

Modi N: Avoiding hypernatremia dehydration in healthy term infants. *Arch Dis Child* 2007;**92**:474–5.

Hypocalcemia

Hypocalcemia is generally accepted to be a blood ionized calcium <4.0 mg/dL, or a total serum calcium <8.5 mg/dL in the absence of hypoalbuminemia or acidosis. In the neonate these numbers are shifted down 0.5 and 1.0 mg/dL respectively. Alkalosis, which causes increased calcium binding to protein, can decrease the ionized calcium fraction without a significant change in the serum total calcium level. Severely ill children are at risk for concomitant hypocalcemia, while chronic hypocalcemia is associated with hypoparathyroid conditions and vitamin D disorders.

Clinical presentation

Clinical manifestations of hypocalcemia primarily involve the neuromuscular system. Muscle cramps and paresthesias are the hallmark symptoms. These can be sustained, producing tetany, or intermittent, as in a seizure. Contractions of the larynx can produce stridor or complete airway occlusion. Newborns may present with nonspecific symptoms of poor feeding, vomiting, and lethargy.

Characteristic signs include the Chvostek (facial muscle twitching elicited by tapping the facial nerve just anterior to the ear) and Trousseau (carpal spasm elicited by maintaining a blood pressure cuff at just above systolic pressure for <5 minutes).

Typically, the hyperventilating adolescent presents with hypocalcemic symptoms in addition to anxiety, tachypnea, and labored breathing. There may be a history of recent emotional upset or past psychiatric disorders.

Findings in patients with long-standing hypocalcemia may include cataracts and basal ganglia calcifications, along with radiographic evidence of rickets.

Diagnosis
Hyperventilation
Suspect hyperventilation-induced hypocalcemia in an older child or adolescent who presents with tachypnea, anxiety, and carpopedal spasm. If the presentation is not typical for anxiety-related hyperventilation obtain an ABG. An increased pH, decreased pCO_2, and normal pO_2 confirm the diagnosis and rule out other causes of hyperventilation, such as hypoxia or a metabolic acidosis. See Table 7-3 for the differential diagnosis of hypocalcemia.

Other etiologies
Immediately obtain an ECG to determine the corrected QT (QTc) interval, which is prolonged with hypocalcemia. In addition, obtain blood for total and/or ionized calcium, electrolytes, BUN, creatinine, phosphorus, magnesium, and liver function tests, including albumin and alkaline phosphatase.

ED management
Hyperventilation
Instruct the patient to breathe slowly in and out of a paper bag or a face mask with a reservoir attached and the side ports taped shut. This causes rebreathing of CO_2, leading to a decreased plasma pH and, thus, an increased ionized calcium. Occasionally sedation is required. Use either hydroxyzine (1 mg/kg, 20 mg maximum), diphenhydramine (1–2 mg/kg, 50 mg maximum), or a more rapid-acting anxiolytic, such as IV lorazepam (0.03 mg/kg, 1 mg maximum) or diazepam (0.05–0.2 mg/kg, 5 mg maximum). Once the hyperventilation has stopped, try to discover the precipitating cause and reassure the patient and the family as to the benign nature of the episode.

Other etiologies
Give symptomatic patients (seizures, laryngospasm, tetany) 0.2 mL/kg of 10% calcium chloride (10 mL maximum) *slowly* IV over 10–15 minutes, while continuously monitoring the ECG. The bolus may be repeated once. If symptoms persist consider other diagnostic possibilities, such as hypokalemia, hypomagnesemia, or a seizure disorder. After the bolus (es) are completed, give a continuous calcium IV infusion, starting with 200 Mg/kg per day

Table 7-3. Differential diagnosis of hypocalcemia

Diagnosis	Differentiating features
Hypoparathyroidism	↑ phosphate; normal alkaline phosphatase; ↓ PTH
Pseudohypoparathyroidism	↑ phosphorous and PTH
	Mental retardation
	Short 4th and 5th metacarpals/metatarsals
Vitamin D disorders	↓serum phosphate; ↑ alkaline phosphatase, PTH
Inadequate vitamin D intake, absorption or production	↓serum 25-hydroxy vitamin D
Inadequate hepatic 25-hydroxylation	↑ serum LFTs
Lack of renal 1-hydroxylation	Normal renal function and 25-hydroxyvitamin D
	↓ serum calcitriol
End-organ vitamin D resistance	↑ serum calcitriol
Hypernatremic dehydration	↑ serum sodium
Pancreatitis	↑ serum amylase and lipase
	Abdominal pain and vomiting
Phosphate overload (renal failure, tumor lysis, enemas)	Positive history
Severe acute illnesses	Positive history
Overwhelming sepsis	Pre-morbid finding
Rhabdomyolysis	Acute phase
Cardiac bypass surgery	Positive history

of calcium gluconate, which is equivalent to about 20 Mg/kg per day of elemental calcium. Increase the dose to 500 Mg/kg per day for neonates.

Oral calcium administration will be ineffective in hypoparathyroidism and vitamin D disorders unless calcitriol (or other appropriate forms of vitamin D) is also given. Consult a pediatric endocrinologist.

Follow-up

- Hyperventilation that seems to be a manifestation of anxiety: primary care follow-up within 1 week for evaluation and possible psychiatric referral

Indications for admission

- Hypocalcemia requiring IV treatment

Bibliography

Dawrant J, Pacaud D: Pediatric hypocalcemia - making the diagnosis. *CMAJ* 2007;177: 1494-7.

Holick MF: Resurrection of vitamin D deficiency and rickets. *J Clin Invest* 2006;116:2062-72.

Jain A, Agarwal R, Sankar MJ, Deorari AK, Paul VK: Hypocalcemia in the newborn. *Indian J Pediatr* 2008;75:165-9.

Hypoglycemia

Hypoglycemia occurs when there is failure to maintain glucose homeostasis secondary to defects in substrate, enzymes, or hormones. The definition of hypoglycemia depends upon the method by which the specimen was obtained: consider hypoglycemia to be a whole blood glucose <50 mg/dL in a full-term newborn infant, child, or adult. Recurrent hypoglycemia during the period of rapid brain growth and differentiation in infancy can result in long-term neurological sequelae, psychomotor retardation, and seizures. Therefore, prevention, rapid diagnosis, and aggressive therapy are essential to prevent these severe consequences of hypoglycemia.

Although there are many etiologies of hypoglycemia, it is most commonly seen in diabetics having an "insulin reaction" secondary to insulin overdose, skipped or late meals, or exercise without an adjustment in food intake or insulin dosage. In a nondiabetic < 8 years of age, ketotic hypoglycemia is the most frequent cause. Inadequate intake (prolonged fasting, malnutrition), gastroenteritis, ingestions (alcohol, oral hypoglycemic agents, propanolol, salicylates), hyperinsulinemia, hormone deficiencies (panhypopituitarism, growth hormone, ACTH, cortisol), liver disease or a ketogenic diet may lead to hypoglycemia.

Hypoglycemia in the newborn period may be transient or persistent. Transient neonatal hypoglycemia can be seen in an infant who was born prematurely, is small for gestational age, has erythroblastosis fetalis, has sustained birth trauma, or is the infant of a diabetic mother.

Clinical presentation

The presentation is nonspecific. Autonomic symptoms arise from both sympathetic and parasympathetic divisions and include sweating, hunger, paresthesias, tremors, pallor, anxiety, nausea, and palpitations. Glucose deprivation of the CNS causes warmth, fatigue, weakness, dizziness, headache, inability to concentrate, drowsiness, blurred vision, difficulty speaking, confusion, bizarre behavior, loss of coordination, difficulty walking, coma, and seizures.

A neonate presents with jitteriness, irritability, poor feeding, apnea, perioral cyanosis, irregular respirations or tachypnea, hypothermia, hypotonia, seizures, and an abnormal cry. An infant or older child can have gastrointestinal symptoms (hunger, nausea, abdominal pain) or neurologic complaints (headache, speech and vision disturbances, weakness, anxiety, behavior changes, short attention span, ataxia, seizures, coma). These symptoms may occur with or without the signs of catecholamine excess (sweating, pallor, tachycardia).

A patient with hypoglycemia secondary to hormone deficiencies, such as growth hormone deficiency or panhypopituitarism, may have a microphallus or undescended testes. An infant or child with a metabolic defect may present with metabolic acidosis, hepatosplenomegaly, increased uric acid and lactic acid levels, and positive urine or serum ketones.

Ketotic hypoglycemia

Ketotic hypoglycemia presents most commonly between 18 months and 5 years of age and remits spontaneously by 8–9 years. Hypoglycemia typically occurs in a lean child with decreased muscle mass when food intake is limited by anorexia or vomiting caused by an intercurrent illness. It usually presents in the morning, before breakfast or when breakfast is skipped, and in many cases the child has either skipped the evening meal or eaten poorly. Hypoglycemia occurs after 2–24 hours of fasting, and, at the time of hypoglycemia, insulin and plasma alanine levels are low, serum ketones are elevated with ketonuria, blood lactate and pyruvate levels are normal, and the concentrations of counter-regulatory hormones (growth hormone and cortisol) are increased.

Hyperinsulinism

Hyperinsulinism caused by generalized β-cell dysfunction is the most common cause of persistent hypoglycemia in infants and young children. Several distinct genetic forms of congenital hyperinsulinism have now been described. It generally presents in infants <1 year of age and there may be a history of constant hunger and frequent night-time feeds. Hypoglycemia occurs soon (usually 30 min–2 h) after feeding and is associated with negative or small urinary ketones (insulin prevents ketosis) with inappropriately low plasma ketone (β-OH-butyrate and acetoacetate) concentrations. In milder, autosomal dominant forms of hyperinsulinism, patients may not present with hypoglycemia until later in childhood or in adulthood.

Hereditary fructose intolerance

Typically, a nursing infant is asymptomatic until fruits and juices are added to the diet. It can also present following the consumption of a commercial formula containing sucrose (soy-based formulas). Fructose causes vomiting, diarrhea, and hypoglycemia acutely. Chronic exposure to fructose results in hepatomegaly, jaundice, failure to thrive, and renal tubular dysfunction.

Diagnosis

If hypoglycemia is suspected or the patient has an altered mental status or seizures, obtain a fingerstick glucose determination. Confirm any reading <60 mg/dL with a laboratory measurement of the serum glucose. If the patient is not a known diabetic, at the time of hypoglycemia, also send a urine for ketones, reducing substances, and save an aliquot for analysis of amino acids, organic acids, and acylglycines. Also obtain a "critical blood sample" for whole blood glucose, electrolytes, liver function tests, uric acid, insulin, growth hormone, cortisol, plasma ammonia, lactate, pyruvate, alanine, and C-peptide (if exogenous hyperinsulinism is suspected).

In general, vomiting associated with hypoglycemia suggests acidosis, gastroenteritis, food poisoning, or acute liver disease. Hepatomegaly, ketosis, and metabolic acidosis occur in an inborn error of metabolism, which may present in the neonatal period or later in infancy. The hypoglycemia typically occurs when feeding is interrupted, as can occur when the overnight feeding is withheld or an infection interrupts the normal feeding pattern.

The absence of ketones or their presence in only trace or small amounts is characteristic of hyperinsulinism and disorders of carnitine metabolism and fatty acid oxidation and/or ketogenesis. An elevated lactate suggests an inborn error of metabolism, while positive urine-reducing substances occur in disorders of galactose, fructose, and tyrosine metabolism. If the symptoms followed a meal, determine whether fructose or galactose was the sole sugar consumed.

Short stature, microphallus, and midline defects (cleft palate, single maxillary central incisor) suggest hypopituitarism. Increased skin pigmentation may indicate compensatory ACTH release (primary adrenal insufficiency). Hepatomegaly occurs in glycogen storage diseases, galactosemia, liver disease, and disorders of gluconeogenesis, fatty acid oxidation, and carnitine metabolism, but not in ketotic hypoglycemia.

ED management

Regardless of the etiology, the treatment of hypoglycemia is glucose. The goal of therapy is to prevent hypoglycemia in order to protect the brain from damage. Maintain the plasma glucose concentration at > 60 mg/dL.

Encourage an alert child to drink a carbohydrate-containing solution (orange juice, apple juice, soft drink with sugar). If the patient is unconscious, vomiting, or unable to take fluids orally, give a bolus of 0.5–1 g/kg of glucose IV. Give an older child 1–2 mL/kg of D_{50}, and a young child 2–4 mL/kg of D_{25}. Treat a neonate with a smaller bolus (0.25–0.5 g/kg) of D_{25} (1–2 mL/kg). Follow bolus therapy with a continuous infusion of 10% glucose, with maintenance electrolytes, at a maintenance rate. Adjust the infusion rate and concentration to maintain a glucose level of about 80 mg/dL.

Hyperinsulinism

If the hypoglycemia persists (hyperinsulinemia), consult an endocrinologist and give glucagon (<20 kg 0.5 mg, >20 kg 1 mg, IV, IM, or SQ), then 1 hour later add IV hydrocortisone (Solu-Cortef® 100 mg/m^2 for infants; 3 mg/kg for children). However, since a glycemic response to these hormones requires adequate amounts of substrates, continue the glucose infusion. Patients without hyperinsulinism typically require glucose infusion rates of 6–8 mg/kg/minute to maintain euglycemia, while children with hyperinsulinism may require glucose infusion rates that are 2–4 times greater because of their increased glucose utilization.

For hyperinsulinism meeting the above criteria, give a trial of diazoxide to suppress insulin secretion (10 Mg/kg per day, gradually increasing to 25 Mg/kg per day maximum). Other possible treatments include a long-acting somatostatin analog (Octreotide® given IV, SC or as a continuous IV infusion) and nifedipine. Glucagon can be used to stabilize the hypoglycemia in patients prior to surgery.

Ketotic hypoglycemia

Instruct the family of a child with ketotic hypoglycemia that the child must avoid prolonged periods of fasting. Recommend a bedtime snack consisting of both carbohydrate and protein to prevent further episodes of hypoglycemia. During intercurrent illness, instruct the parents to provide carbohydrate-rich drinks at frequent intervals during both day and night. Also, have the family test the urine for ketones during an intercurrent illness, as ketonuria may precede the onset of hypoglycemia by several hours. An ED visit for IV glucose may be necessary if carbohydrate-containing drinks are not tolerated. Discharge the patient when the glucose normalizes, oral intake is adequate, and close follow-up is arranged.

Follow-up

*   Ketotic hypoglycemia: primary care follow-up in 1 week

Indications for admission

*   Hypoglycemic episode in a nondiabetic, unless patient is known to have ketotic hypoglycemia and the glucose normalizes
*   Hypoglycemia in a diabetic if the cause is unclear, or self-destructive behavior is likely

Bibliography

Hussain K: Diagnosis and management of hyperinsulinaemic hypoglycaemia of infancy. *Horm Res* 2008;69:2–13.

Valayannopoulos V, Romano S, Mention K, *et al*: What's new in metabolic and genetic

hypoglycaemias – diagnosis and management. *Eur J Pediatr* 2008;167:257–65.

Wolfsdorf JI, Weinstein DA: Hypoglycemia in children, in Lifshitz F (ed). *Pediatric Endocrinology*, Marcel Dekker, New York, 2003, pp. 575–610.

Hyponatremia

Hyponatremia is defined as a serum sodium concentration ≤ 130 mEq/L. Hyponatremia may be associated with hypovolemic, euvolemic, or hypervolemic states.

Hypovolemia

Hypovolemic hyponatremia is caused by loss of sodium in excess of water. Most often this is secondary to extrarenal losses, especially gastrointestinal, but sweating (cystic fibrosis), and "third spacing" from burns, trauma, peritonitis, effusions, ascites, and pancreatitis are other etiologies. Renal salt-wasting is seen in diuretic abuse, osmotic diuresis, salt-wasting nephropathy, renal tubular acidosis (types 2 and 4), and adrenal insufficiency.

Euvolemia

The most common cause of euvolemic hyponatremia is the inappropriate secretion of ADH (SIADH) with a primary elevation in vasopressin secretion, secondary to CNS pathology (meningitis, trauma) or pulmonary disease (pneumonia, tuberculosis). Drugs, such as nicotine, morphine, barbiturates, isoproterenol, antineoplastic agents, carbamazepine, and acetaminophen have all been implicated as "antidiuretic" agents. Other etiologies are hypothyroidism and water intoxication. Glucocorticoid deficiency can cause euvolemic or hypovolemic hyponatremia.

Hypervolemia

Hypervolemic hyponatremia is characterized by edema, as in congestive heart failure, cirrhosis, nephrotic syndrome, and renal failure.

Clinical presentation

The clinical presentation of hyponatremia is determined by the intravascular volume and the absolute concentration and rate of fall of the serum sodium.

Hypovolemia

With depletion of the intravascular space, signs of hypovolemia predominate. There may be tachycardia, orthostatic vital sign changes, poor capillary refill, weight loss, and decreased skin turgor. Laboratory abnormalities include elevations of the BUN, renin, aldosterone, and uric acid, while the urinary sodium excretion is low (<10 mEq/L).

Euvolemia

The clinical findings are related to the serum sodium level. A rapid decrease to the 120–125 mEq/L range may cause gastrointestinal symptoms such as anorexia, nausea, and vomiting with agitation, headache, muscle cramps, seizures, and coma. Other neurologic signs (decreased deep tendon reflexes, pathologic reflexes, Cheyne–Stokes respiration, and pseudobulbar palsy) can be present, especially when the level is ≤120 mEq/L. The patient may be asymptomatic with a sodium <120 mEq/L if the fall in the serum sodium occurred slowly, over days to weeks.

Hypervolemia

In hypervolemia, there may be signs of fluid excess, including edema, tachycardia, hypertension, headache, pulmonary rales, and hepatomegaly.

Diagnosis

Hyponatremia is usually discovered incidentally, when electrolytes are obtained because of vomiting, dehydration, altered mental status, or seizures. Once hyponatremia is reported, rule out pseudohyponatremia as a result of increased serum proteins or lipids; usually the plasma has a milky appearance. Next, consider dilutional hyponatremia secondary to the presence of excess solutes, such as glucose or mannitol, which cause intracellular fluid to shift to the extracellular space. In a diabetic, for every 100 mg/dL increase in glucose over 100 mg/dL, the serum sodium is lowered by 1.6 mEq/L. If true hyponatremia is suspected, the next step is to assess the patient's hydration status and obtain blood for a CBC, electrolytes, and glucose, as well as a urinary sodium. If a euvolemic or hypervolemic state is likely, also obtain a vasopressin, renin, aldosterone, uric acid, cortisol, thyroid function tests, and a lipid panel, as well as urinary osmolality and creatinine.

The urinary sodium level can help distinguish among the various etiologies of hyponatremia. With dehydration and volume depletion, the proximal tubular reabsorption of sodium and water will be high, leading to a urinary sodium of less than <10 mEq/L. It will also be low in most hypervolemic states; a urine sodium >20 mEq/L suggests renal salt-wasting, SIADH, and other euvolemic conditions. With renal failure the urine sodium may be >40 mEq/L, except in acute glomerulonephritis (when it is typically low).

Patients with decreased effective intravascular volume caused by CHF, cirrhosis, nephrotic syndrome, or lung disease will present with signs of their underlying disease, which often includes peripheral edema. Patients with primary salt loss will also appear volume depleted. If the salt loss is from the kidney (e.g., diuretic therapy or polycystic kidney disease), urinary sodium will be elevated, as may be the urine volume. Salt loss from other regions (e.g., the gut in gastroenteritis or the skin in cystic fibrosis) will cause urine sodium to be low, as in other forms of systemic dehydration. Cerebral salt wasting is encountered with central nervous system insults, and results in high serum atrial natriuretic peptide concentrations, leading to high urine sodium and urine excretion.

The syndrome of inappropriate antidiuretic hormone (vasopressin) secretion (SIADH) exists when a primary elevation in vasopressin secretion is the cause of hyponatremia. It is characterized by hyponatremia, an inappropriately increased urine osmolality (>100 mOsm/kg), normal or slightly elevated plasma volume, and a normal to high urine sodium level (because of volume-induced suppression of aldosterone and elevation of atrial natriuretic peptide). Serum uric acid is low in patients with SIADH, whereas it is high in those with hyponatremia owing to systemic dehydration from other causes of decreased intravascular volume.

Consider drug-induced hyponatremia in patients taking potentially contributory medications. A careful search for a tumor (thymoma, glioma, bronchial carcinoid) causing SIADH is necessary if there is not an obvious cause. Patients will present with nonspecific symptoms of hyponatremia, such as anorexia, lethargy, weakness, and in severe cases, obtundity and convulsions. Signs of diminished intravascular volume, edema, hypothyroidism, adrenal insufficiency, and renal disease are absent by definition.

ED management

Immediately treat symptomatic hypovolemia (poor peripheral pulses, delayed capillary refill, orthostatic changes) without waiting for the laboratory confirmation of hyponatremia. Give 20 mL/kg boluses of isotonic crystalloid (normal saline, Ringer's lactate) until adequate perfusion is established. Obtain blood for serum electrolytes, BUN, and creatinine and urine for urinalysis, sodium, creatinine, and osmolality. Begin definitive therapy once the initial serum and urine studies confirm the diagnosis.

If the hyponatremia is acute and there are severe neurological symptoms secondary to a serum sodium level <125 mEq/L (lethargy, psychosis, coma, or generalized seizures, especially in younger children), give hypertonic saline (3% [513 mEq/L] or 5% [855 mEq/L]) to raise the sodium above 125 mEq/L. Replace this deficit over 4 hours, using the following formula:

Sodium needed (mEq) = (125 - patient's sodium) x (0.6) x (body weight in kg)

As a general guide, 12 mL/kg of 3% sodium chloride will result in a rise in serum sodium of approximately 10 mEq/L. Raise the serum sodium to 135 mEq/L over the subsequent 24 hours. Do not exceed a rate of correction of >0.5 mEq/L/hr or 12 mEq/day. Measure the serum sodium every 2 hours until it is >135 mEq/L and all symptoms have resolved. Subsequent treatment then depends on the initial assessment of the intravascular volume status.

If the hyponatremia is chronic, give hypertonic saline treatment cautiously, as it may result in both cell shrinkage and central pontine myelinolysis characterized by somnolence, disorientation, and aphasia, which may progress over a few weeks to quadriplegia. This becomes evident 24–48 hours after allowing too rapid a correction of hyponatremia. It has a characteristic appearance on CT and MRI, and often causes irreversible brain damage.

Hypovolemia

Replace volume with NS or D_5 NS. In adrenal insufficiency, sodium deficits are difficult to replace without corticosteroid replacement (pp. 163–4).

Euvolemia

Limiting the water intake to two-thirds maintenance, including all fluids (e.g., IV medications), may be all that is required. Immediately begin treatment of the cause of SIADH.

Hypervolemia

If the patient is edematous, restrict fluids to two-thirds maintenance and give furosemide (1 mg/kg IV) if there is pulmonary edema and respiratory compromise.

Acute treatment of hyponatremia caused by SIADH is indicated only if there is cerebral dysfunction. Because patients with SIADH have volume expansion, salt administration is not very effective in raising the serum sodium level. It is rapidly excreted in the urine owing to suppressed aldosterone levels and elevated atrial natriuretic peptide concentration.

Indications for admission

- Symptomatic hyponatremia
- Hyponatremia of undetermined etiology
- Factitious hyponatremia

Bibliography

Lin M, Liu SJ, Lim IT: Disorders of water imbalance. *Emerg Med Clin North Am* 2005;23:749–70.

Srivatsa A, Majzoub JA: Disorders of water homeostasis, in Lifshitz F: *Pediatric Endocrinology*, New York, Informa Healthcare USA, 2007, pp. 651–92.

Thyroid disorders

Hyperthyroidism primarily affects children > 6 years of age. The most common cause is diffuse toxic goiter (Graves' disease). Other etiologies include thyroiditis with hyperthyroidism, thyroid adenoma, and exogenous overdosage.

Thyrotoxicosis is the clinical manifestation of hyperthyroidism without the severe cardiovascular, thermoregulatory, gastrointestinal, and neurobehavioral symptoms associated with thyroid storm or crisis, a life-threatening complication rarely seen in children. In 50% of episodes of thyroid storm there is an identifiable precipitating factor (stress, infection, surgery, childbirth).

Euthyroid hyperthyroxinemia is the term used to describe the various conditions in which the serum T4 level, either total or free, is elevated in the absence of thyrotoxicosis. This may be caused by increased T4-binding by serum proteins, increased concentration of thyroid binding globulin (TBG), and a generalized (pituitary and peripheral tissues) resistance to thyroid hormone.

A newborn can develop neonatal Grave's disease, which occurs when the thyroid stimulating immunoglobulins of maternal Graves' disease cross the placenta and can cause transient or permanent thyroid disease in the infant. Maternal therapy with radioactive iodine or surgery does not eliminate the presence of thyroid antibodies. In contrast, neonatal hypothyroidism is a very rare emergency, but time is critical, as a delay in therapy is associated with decreased IQ. Thyroid screening, either TSH or T4, is part of the newborn screen in every US state. Patients with the highest percentile of TSH or the lowest percentile of T4 from a certain day are recalled. Therefore, false positives occur, but this is necessary to ensure that all truly hypothyroid newborns are identified. Hypothyroidism beyond the newborn period is most commonly caused by chronic autoimmune thyroiditis (Hashimoto's thyroiditis).

Clinical presentation

The onset of hyperthyroidism is gradual, with complaints of palpitations, sweating, heat intolerance, weight loss despite increased appetite, tremor, nervousness, increased frequency of bowel movements, and emotional lability. Short attention span, inability to concentrate, deteriorating school performance, attacks of dyspnea, and easy fatigability may occur. Insomnia, restless sleep, and nocturia are common and are often associated with fatigue and lethargy during the day. Children who develop Graves' disease before the age of 3 years can experience transitory speech and language delays, mental retardation, and craniosynostosis. Oligomenorrhea and irregular menses may result in the postmenarchal female. Newborns may exhibit irritability, inability to feed (breast or bottle), and inadequate weight gain. There is usually a history of maternal thyroid disease, thyroid surgery, or radioactive iodine treatment.

On examination, almost all hyperthyroid patients (except in the case of exogenous overdose) have a goiter, and a characteristic bruit may be heard over the thyroid. The skin is warm and moist, and tachycardia (particularly increased resting pulse rate), increased systolic blood pressure, and widened pulse pressure are common. Eye findings, when present, include lid retraction, staring, lid lag, and exophthalmos (see below). There may be proximal muscle weakness, brisk deep tendon reflexes, and fine tremors of the eyelids, fingers, or tongue. Although pretibial myxedema is observed in 1–2% of adults with Graves' disease, it rarely, if ever, occurs in children. Other diseases have been observed in association with Graves' disease and include Hashimoto's thyroiditis, vitiligo, systemic lupus erythematosus, rheumatoid arthritis, Addison's disease, insulin-dependent diabetes mellitus, myasthenia gravis, and pernicious anemia.

Graves' ophthalmopathy

In most children and adolescents with Graves' disease, the signs and symptoms are relatively mild and include lid lag, lid retraction, stare, proptosis, conjunctival injection, chemosis, and periorbital and eyelid edema. Less commonly, patients may complain of eye discomfort, pain, or diplopia. Severe ophthalmopathy, associated with marked chemosis, severe proptosis, periorbital ecchymosis, corneal ulceration, eye muscle paralysis, and optic atrophy, is extremely rare during childhood and adolescence. Ophthalmoplegia may be secondary to severe exophthalmos, nerve entrapment, or myasthenia gravis, which is a rare coexisting disease.

Thyroid storm

Thyroid storm is a life-threatening manifestation of thyrotoxicosis which is very rare in childhood. It often starts abruptly, with the sudden onset of severe thyrotoxic symptoms and fever (usually >38.5° C [101.3° F], often up to 41.1° C [106° F]), cardiovascular symptoms (tachycardia out of proportion to the fever, high-output cardiac failure, arrhythmias, shock), gastrointestinal dysfunction (vomiting, diarrhea, hepatomegaly, jaundice), and neurological changes (agitation, tremor, psychosis, stupor, coma). The syndrome complex may occur either in a previously undiagnosed patient or someone with poorly controlled hyperthyroidism. If left untreated, mortality rates of up to 90% have been reported. Storm can be precipitated by infection, trauma, surgery, concomitant ingestion of sympathomimetic agents (e.g., pseudoephedrine), withdrawal of antithyroid medication, and radioactive iodine therapy.

Hypothyroidism

Acquired hypothyroidism is most commonly caused by chronic autoimmune thyroiditis (Hashimoto's). It presents with a combination of poor appetite, slowing growth velocity, cold intolerance, constipation, hypotonia, poor school performance, delayed puberty, and delayed dentition. On physical examination there may be bradycardia, delayed deep tendon reflexes, and a goiter may be appreciated.

Diagnosis

The differential diagnosis of hyperthyroidism includes anxiety attack, sepsis, pheochromocytoma, gastroenteritis, and congestive heart failure. Other possible midline neck masses include thyroglossal duct cyst, dermoid cyst, cystic hygroma, and neuroblastoma (with Horner's syndrome). Exophthalmos or ophthalmoplegia can be confused with a neuroblastoma, intraorbital tumor, and orbital cellulitis. The typical gradual onset of hyperthyroidism makes the early diagnosis difficult. However, the presence of a goiter or bruit, along with other symptoms of hyperthyroidism, usually suggests the diagnosis.

If hyperthyroidism is suspected, obtain a CBC, electrolytes, and liver function tests, in addition to thyroid function tests, including T3, T4, TSH, thyroid antibodies (anti-thyroglobulin, thyroid peroxidase), and thyroid stimulating immunoglobulin (TSI). Typical findings are elevated free T4, total T4 or T3, and FT4I, with a suppressed (low) TSH. Some thyrotoxic children may present with an elevated T3 level with a normal T4 level early in the course of their thyrotoxicosis or with a thyroid nodule.

If hypothyroidism is suspected, obtain TFTs. The free T4 and total T4 will be low while the TSH is elevated.

ED management

Propylthiouracil (PTU) or methimazole are the drugs of choice for the management of hyperthyroidism. They both inhibit the synthesis and the release of thyroid hormone from the gland. Propylthiouracil has the added advantage of inhibiting the peripheral conversion of T4 to T3. Methimazole has a longer half-life (12–16 hours vs. 4–6 hours) and is about 10-fold more potent than PTU. These drugs may take 6–8 weeks to exert their antithyroid effect and they have multiple side effects.

Hyperthyroidism

To control hyperthyroidism, initially give oral PTU (5–10 Mg/kg per day div q 6–8h) *or* methimazole (0.5–1.0 Mg/kg per day div q 8–12h); after 3–4 weeks the dosing can be changed to once daily or bid). Lower doses may be effective in patients with mild disease. Side effects, both idiosyncratic and dose-related, occur in up to 20–30% of patients. The majority are mild and include elevated liver enzymes levels, mild leucopenia, rashes, and mild gastrointestinal symptoms (nausea). Although very rare, the most serious complication is agranulocytosis. Obtain a CBC if a patient complains of a sore throat or fever, or mouth ulcers occur and stop the medication if the diagnosis is confirmed.

In addition to the antithyroid medication, give oral atenolol (1–2 Mg/kg per day div q 6–8h) to treat the adrenergic symptoms.

Thyroid storm

Thyroid storm requires *immediate treatment*. After obtaining blood for T3, T4, TSH, cortisol, CBC, electrolytes, and LFTs, the goals are to decrease the thyroid hormone levels acutely and block their peripheral effects. Therapeutic intervention includes emergency and supportive care to maintain adequate respiratory and cardiovascular functions, control body temperature, treat any precipitating factors, and limit the amount of thyroid hormones available to the peripheral body tissues. Call for an immediate pediatric endocrinology consultation and initiate therapy using the following modalities:

Propranolol

Treat the symptoms of hyperthyroidism with propranolol, although it has no effect on the cause. Give a child 0.5–2.0 Mg/kg per day div q 6h (60 mg/day maximum) and an older adolescent 20–40 mg q 6h. If gastrointestinal symptoms preclude oral treatment, give 0.025 mg/kg IV over 10 minutes. The dose may be repeated three to four times, but consult a pediatric cardiologist. Possible side effects include hypotension, hypoglycemia, bronchospasm, and heart block.

PTU

Give 5–10 Mg/kg per day div q 6–8h. Propylthiouracil can be administered orally, rectally, or via nasogastric tube in dosages ranging from 100–200 mg every 4–6 hours, maximum 1200 mg/day. Alternatively, use methimazole 0.5–1.0 Mg/kg per day div q 8h. Once initial control of thyrotoxicosis has been achieved, reduce the PO PTU dosage to 5–10 Mg/kg per day div q 6–8h.

Oral iodide (Lugol's solution)

Lugol's solution is 5% iodine and 10% potassium iodide; it contains 126 mg iodine/mL, or 8 mg iodine/drop. Give children and adolescents 5–10 drops (40–80 mg iodine) PO tid at least one hour after the thionamides. Alternatively, use potassium iodide (1 gm/mL), 150–200 mg PO tid for infants <1 year of age; 300–500 mg PO tid for children and adolescents. However, propranolol is so effective in blocking the ß-adrenergic effects that iodides are often unnecessary.

Dexamethasone

Give dexamethasone (1–2 mg q 6h) or hydrocortisone (2 mg/kg as an IV bolus, then 30–45 mg/m²/day div q 6h) in extreme cases, such as a patient with heart failure, arrhythmias, severe adrenergic symptoms, or shock.

Temperature regulation

Use antipyretics (acetaminophen 15 mg/kg; ibuprofen 10 mg/kg), cooling blankets, and muscle relaxants, as needed. However, do not give aspirin, which may elevate the T4 level.

Ophthalmopathy

Because it is usually relatively mild and self-limited in the vast majority of affected children and adolescents, specific treatment is often not necessary. In general, eye findings improve in association with control of the hyperthyroidism. Occasionally, local measures may be used to treat symptoms. For example, eye drops or ointment preparations containing methylcellulose may be necessary to prevent corneal drying. Sleeping with the head elevated may help to reduce chemosis and periorbital edema. If there are severe symptoms, consult an ophthalmologist.

Hypothyroidism

If a newborn is brought to the ED with documentation of a failed thyroid screen, consult a pediatric endocrinologist and obtain blood for TSH, free and total T4, and TBG. Start treatment with thyroxine at 8–15 mcg/kg/day. The goal is to maintain the T4 in the high range of normal for newborns (10–13 mg/dL) and TSH 1–2 milliunits/mL.

Outside of the newborn period, defer treatment and promptly refer the patient to a pediatric endocrinologist.

Follow-up

- Hyperthyroidism without thyroid storm: 2–3 days
- Neonatal hypothyroidism: pediatric endocrinology follow-up 1–3 days
- Acquired hypothyroidism: pediatric endocrinology follow-up within 1 week

Indications for admission

- Thyroid storm or thyrotoxic periodic paralysis
- Hyperthyroidism with heart failure, arrhythmias, shock, or psychosis

Bibliography

Hung W, Sarlis NJ: Autoimmune and non-autoimmune hyperthyroidism in pediatric patients: a review and personal commentary on management. *Pediatr Endocrinol Rev* 2004;2:21–38.

McKeown NJ, Tews MC, Gossain VV, Shah SM: Hyperthyroidism. *Emerg Med Clin North Am* 2005;23:669–85.

Chapter 8

Environmental emergencies

Anthony J. Ciorciari

Contributing author
Katherine J. Chou: Hyperbaric oxygen therapy

Burns

Each year 450,000 children are evaluated for burn injuries. Approximately 50% of major burns occur in patients <20 years of age, and nearly one-third occur in children <10 years old. In the United States, burns are the third most frequent cause of pediatric injury-related mortality.

Common types of burn injuries are thermal (scald and flame), chemical (acids and alkalis), electrical, and radiation (sunburn). Scald burns are the most frequent type in children <5 years of age, while flame burns are most common between 5 and 13 years of age. In teenagers, burn injury most often results from accidents involving flammable liquids.

Approximately 10% of child abuse cases involve burns, accounting for 15–20% of all childhood burns. The most common mechanism is scalding. Other causes include burns from appliances, matches, and tobacco products.

Clinical presentation

The presentation and severity of a thermal injury is determined by the type and temperature of the agent causing the burn and the duration of exposure to the agent.

Determining the surface area and depth of tissue involved are priorities in evaluating the extent of a burn injury. The "rule of nines" used in older children and adolescents requires modification for infants and young children, because the percent of the total body surface area (BSA) represented by the various body parts changes with age. To estimate the BSA involved, use the patient's own hand, which, including the fingers, is approximately 0.8–1% of the BSA. Depth can be difficult to estimate, since the injury is usually not uniform in all affected areas, and the depth may progress over time. Scald burns, other than those caused by immersion, tend to be superficial, while chemical burns are typically deeper. Electrical burns (pp. 200–203) can cause tissue damage that is much deeper than suspected during the initial examination.

First-degree burns

Sunburn is the most common example of a first-degree burn. First-degree burns involve only the superficial epidermal layers. The area appears pink or light red and blanches with pressure. The burn is dry, without blister formation and is hypersensitive. Healing generally takes place within 7 days, without scarring.

Second-degree burns

Second-degree burns are also known as partial thickness burns. They are subdivided into superficial and deep partial thickness burns. Superficial partial thickness burns involve the papillary layer of the dermis. They present with blisters and bullae and are typically bright red or mottled in color. They have a moist surface, and the superficial skin can be wiped away. These burns are extremely painful. With proper care, they heal within 14–21 days with a small risk of hypertrophic scarring.

Deep partial thickness burns involve the reticular layer of the dermis. The skin may appear yellow-white or dark red (nonblanching), with a dry or mildly moist surface. There is sensation to pressure only. These injuries may be difficult to distinguish from third-degree burns and may require >21 days (up to 2 months) for healing with residual scar formation.

Third-degree burns

Third-degree, or full thickness, burns are usually caused by flame, hot grease or oil, chemicals, or prolonged immersion. All skin elements are lost, with coagulation of blood vessels. The skin is dry or leathery, grayish-white, and waxy. Thrombosed superficial veins may be visible. The patient has sensation to deep pressure only. Wound closure requires resurfacing and grafting, because the burned surface will not support the migration of normal epithelium from the unburned periphery.

Fourth-degree burns

Fourth-degree burns have the same etiologies as third-degree burns. They involve the subcutaneous layer, fascia, tendon, muscle, and/or bone. The extensive amount of necrotic tissue can produce systemic toxicity from tissue breakdown products and deep infection.

Diagnosis

The evaluation of any burn injury includes determination of the cause, location, and depth of the burn. Look for evidence of inhalation injury or other associated injuries, and note any preexisting illness. Always consider child abuse when the patient presents with burns to the buttocks or burns with a sharp delineation from immersion or the application of a hot object to the skin.

Burns can be classified as minor, moderate, or major, based on the severity of the burn and the involved BSA. See Table 8-1.

ED management
First-degree burns

Treat pain with aspirin (15 mg/kg q 4 h) or ibuprofen (10 mg/kg q 6 h). Hydrocortisone cream (1%) may help reduce the pain and swelling of severe sunburn, especially if the eyelids and face are involved, but do not apply steroids to higher-degree burns. Cool showers and baths are also helpful. Severe itching can occur after a few days and persist for more than 1 week; treat with hydroxyzine (2 mg/kg per day div tid, 50 mg/dose maximum) or diphenhydramine (5 mg/kg per day div qid, 50 mg/dose maximum).

Second-degree burns

Immediately remove any clothing that is hot or soaked with chemical. Mineral oil mixed with cool water can remove substances such as tar. To decrease the burning process, apply sterile gauze pads soaked with slightly cooled (12° C; 53.6° F) or room-temperature saline. To be effective in preventing microvascular changes, the cooling must occur within 30 minutes after the burn occurred.

Table 8-1. Burn classification

Burn type	Minor	Moderate	Major
Criteria	<5 percent TBSA	5 to 10 percent TBSA	>10 percent TBSA
	<2 percent full-thickness burn	2 to 5 percent full-thickness burn	>5 percent full-thickness burn
		Suspected inhalation injury	Any significant burn to face, eyes, ears, genitalia, hands, feet or joints
		Circumferential burn	High-voltage burn
			Known inhalation injury
			Significant associated injuries (fracture or other major trauma)

TBSA: total body surface area.
Calculate burn percentage using second- and third-degree burns only.

Before the burn is cleaned, parenteral analgesia, such as IM or IV morphine sulfate (0.10 to 0.15 mg/kg q 15–60 min, as needed), may be required. Do not attempt IV access in a burned area. Gently clean the burned surface with chlorhexidine solution (Hibiclens) and rinse thoroughly. Debride devitalized tissues using aseptic technique.

To promote restoration of mobility, open and debride blisters over joints. Also open and debride large blisters over immobile areas, but leave small blisters on immobile areas intact. If there is a concern about follow-up, debride all blisters as intact or spontaneously collapsed blisters can serve as a focus for wound infection.

Silver sulfadiazine (SSD, Silvadene) has both Gram-positive and Gram-negative activity and provides good prophylactic antibiotic coverage. It also facilitates debridement. However, do not use silver sulfadiazine on the face, for children with hypersensitivity to sulfonamides, or for infants <2 months of age (bacitracin ointment is an acceptable alternative). Use a sterile tongue depressor to apply a 2 mm layer, and cover with either a nonadherent or petrolatum-impregnated dressing, then wrap with gauze.

If the hand and fingers are involved, dress each finger individually and place the hand in a "position of function" (wrist flexed 20–30°, metacarpals flexed 60–90°, interphalangeal joints as close to 0° as possible). Use a sling to elevate the extremity above the level of the heart.

Clean and dress the burn daily. At each dressing change, remove the silver sulfadiazine completely, as it loses its antibacterial activity.

Biobrane (Woodruff Laboratories, Santa Ana, CA), a biosynthetic dressing coated with collagen peptides, is indicated for superficial second-degree burns (those with no chance of becoming third-degree burns). Apply it directly to a cleaned burn area, then cover with an absorbent dressing that should be changed every 24 hours. The Biobrane will separate on its own in 1–2 weeks. Apply it to flat surfaces, only.

Third-degree burns

If the burn encompasses <2% total BSA, with no involvement of the face, hands, feet, or perineum, the care is the same as for second-degree burns. If >2% total BSA is involved, admit the patient to a burn unit.

General approach to the burned child

1. Stop the burning process by removing burned clothing and copiously lavaging all chemical burns. Apply cool or room-temperature soaks to reverse the thermal gradient and relieve pain (second-degree burns), but avoid hypothermia.

2. Assess and maintain ventilation. Check for signs of inhalation injury (pp. 212–214); if any are present, measure the oxygen saturation and immediately perform fiberoptic laryngoscopy to rule out involvement of the upper airway. Obtain a carboxyhemoglobin level if the patient was in a closed-space fire. If there is a marked metabolic acidosis or hyperlactatemia, treat the patient for possible cyanide toxicity (see pp. 212–214).

3. Initiate IV fluid therapy for patients with >20% partial or full thickness burns. Immediately place a large-bore IV catheter in either a central or peripheral vein found in an unburned area. Treat signs of hypovolemia with a 20 mL/kg bolus of normal saline or lactated Ringer's solution. Use dopamine (5–20 mcg/kg per min) if poor perfusion persists. For patients not in shock, administer 2–4 mL/kg per %BSA burned of normal saline or lactated Ringer's solution over the first 24 hours. Give one-half of the calculated total over the first 8 hours (starting from the time of the burn incident) and the remainder over the next 16 hours. For children <30 kg add the estimated daily maintenance fluid requirement. Patients >30 kg do not need the maintenance fluids added as part of the fluid replacement. The goal is a urine output from 1 mL/kg per h in a young child to 0.5 mL/kg per h in an adolescent.

   Insert an indwelling urinary catheter using aseptic technique in any burn victim needing IV fluids. Discard any urine obtained when the catheter is inserted, as this may have been in the bladder before the burn injury. Check the urine (with a dipstick) for hemoglobin or myoglobin; if positive, obtain a microscopic urinalysis to differentiate hematuria from rhabdomyolysis. If myoglobin is present, increase the fluid rate to maintain a brisk urine output (2 mL/kg per h).

4. Take a careful history. Inquire about the cause of the burn, preexisting illnesses, chronic medications, and allergies. Suspect child abuse (pp. 580–583) if the accident occurred when the child was reportedly alone, the injury is attributed to a sibling, the history varies from one interview to another, there is a previous history of accidental trauma, the history is incompatible with the observed injury, or there is delay in seeking medical attention.

5. Ascertain the tetanus immunization status; give 0.5 mL of tetanus toxoid booster if the last immunization was >5 years ago. If the patient has received <3 tetanus toxoid boosters, give 0.5 mL of tetanus immune globulin as well as 0.5 mL of tetanus toxoid booster.

6. Perform a careful physical examination. Check for corneal injury with fluorescein staining if the lids are burned, the eyelashes have been singed, or eye damage is suspected. Evaluate the patient for associated injuries, especially fractures and head trauma, and signs of child abuse. Nonaccidental burn injuries include pattern burns, sharply demarcated burns of the hands, feet, buttocks, and perineum, and stocking-glove burn injuries.

7. Insert a nasogastric tube and attach it to suction if the burn exceeds 20% of total BSA or if there is nausea, vomiting, or abdominal distention. An ileus is common as a result of splanchnic vasoconstriction.

8. Give pain medication as needed (IV morphine sulfate, 0.1–0.15 mg/kg q 15–60 min).

9. Perform the initial burn wound care as described above.

10. Examine the patient for circumferential injuries. Remove all rings, bracelets, and restrictive clothing. Look carefully for signs of impaired circulation including cyanosis, impaired capillary refill, changes in sensation, deep tissue pain, or paresthesias. If circulatory impairment is a possibility, call a burn surgeon or a plastic surgeon as an escharotomy may be necessary.

Follow-up

- First-degree burns: return at once if blisters form
- Second- and third-degree burns: Return at once if there are any signs or symptoms of impaired circulation (numbness, tingling, or color change distal to the bandage) or infection (fever, vomiting, poor feeding, or change in mental status). Otherwise, follow-up with a primary care provider in 3–4 days

Indications for admission

- First-degree burns: total body involvement or if the patient is at risk for dehydration
- Second-degree burns: >5% total BSA in infants, >10% total BSA in children, or >15% total BSA in adolescents; or when the burns involve critical areas such as the face, hands, feet, or perineum
- Third-degree burns: >2% of the total BSA or involvement of the face, hands, feet, or perineum
- Circumferential burns
- Comorbidity (diabetes, immunodeficiency, sickle cell disease), multiple trauma
- Electrical burns from a current ≥220 volts
- Patients with a burn of any size whose family seems unable to cope with recommendations for care and follow-up
- Transfer the patient to a special burn treatment facility if the total burn is >20% total BSA, or if there are third-degree burns covering >10% of the total BSA

Guidelines for transferring the burn victim

In addition to the usual considerations when transferring any patient to another institution, there are several special concerns when transferring a burn victim.

1. The patient's airway must be securely protected. An accidental extubation in a burn victim with a swollen airway can prove fatal. A physician who is able to perform an emergency intubation and/or emergency cricothyroidotomy must accompany the patient.
2. Just prior to transport, remove all saline-soaked dressing and replace them with sterile dry gauze dressings to prevent hypothermia.
3. Treat the patient with adequate sedation and analgesia to minimize pain and agitation.

Bibliography

Diver AJ: The evolution of burn fluid resuscitation. *Int J Surg* 2008;6:345–50.

Holland AJ: Pediatric burns: the forgotten trauma of childhood. *Can J Surg* 2006;49:272–7.

Sakallioglu AE, Haberal M: Current approach to burn critical care. *Minerva Med* 2007;98:569–73.

Drowning

Drowning is a process resulting in primary respiratory impairment from submersion in a liquid medium, secondary to a liquid–air interface in the child's airway. Therefore, do not use the terms wet drowning, dry drowning, and near drowning. Approximately one-third of deaths from unintentional drowning occur in patients <19 years of age; drowning is the second most common cause of injury and death in children aged 1 month to 14 years of age. Among toddlers, most incidents occur in bathtubs and swimming pools.

Death may be caused directly by laryngospasm, or by cerebral hypoxia, carbon dioxide narcosis, or cardiac arrest.

Aspiration of either salt water or fresh water results in hypoxemia. As little as 1–3 mL/kg of water can cause pulmonary vasoconstriction and impaired gas exchange. In salt water drownings, ventilation perfusion mismatch follows intrapulmonary shunting and decreased compliance. In both fresh water and salt water drownings, surfactant is either destroyed or washed out. Compliance is reduced, and ventilation/perfusion mismatch develops.

Hypothermia is the double-edged sword of drowning. Cold water (<20°C; 68° F) decreases metabolic demands and shunting blood from nonvital to vital organs, but adverse effects such as dysrhythmias (sinus bradycardia, atrial and ventricular fibrillation, asystole) and exhaustion often occur.

Clinical presentation and diagnosis

Inquire about the site and duration of submersion, water temperature, possibility of trauma or physical abuse, drug or alcohol use, and past medical history.

A drowning victim's mental status may range from fully alert to comatose. The patient may have no signs of respiratory distress or may present with tachypnea, nasal flaring, and/or retractions. Auscultation of the lungs may reveal adventitious sounds, and any type of dysrhythmia may be seen on ECG. Among adolescents, inquire about drinking or drug use prior to the event.

Trauma is often involved in near-drowning. Pay particular attention to the possibility of head or cervical spine injuries. Consider internal injuries to the chest or abdomen, especially if the patient does not respond appropriately to resuscitation interventions. Electrolyte imbalance, hypoglycemia, and renal impairment can also occur with drowning.

ED management

Handle the patient carefully because of the possibility of cervical spine injury (pp. 702–704. Place a rectal temperature probe to confirm the core temperature, rapidly assess the airway and breathing, and provide 100% oxygen. Consult with a pediatric pulmonologist about the possibility of BiPAP for patients who are alert and able to maintain their own airway but remain hypoxic. Indications for assisted ventilation via bag-mask apparatus and endotracheal intubation are apnea, an oxygen saturation <85% while inspiring 100% oxygen, or signs of neurologic deterioration. The patient may require positive end expiratory pressure (PEEP) if there is an inadequate response to the initial ventilator settings. Treat bronchospasm with nebulized albuterol (0.03 mL/kg in 3 mL of normal saline) and repeat as needed. There is no evidence that steroids are beneficial in aspiration-induced bronchospasm.

Assess the cardiac status and continuously monitor the ECG. If the patient is pulseless, start basic life support, then advanced life support as warranted by the ECG rhythm and the clinical status. However, most resuscitation drugs are not effective in a severely hypothermic patient and are therefore contraindicated during rewarming (see Hypothermia). One exception is glucose; give 0.5–1 g/kg (1–2 mL/kg D_{50}; 0.25–0.5 mL/kg D_{25}) to any patient with altered mental status. Also give naloxone (2.0 mg IV or 4.0 mg ET) to adolescents if the history suggests a narcotic overdose.

Start at least one large-bore IV with normal saline or lactated Ringer's solution. However, give fluids cautiously since these patients are at risk for pulmonary and cerebral edema, and warm the fluids if the patient is hypothermic. Initial laboratory studies include CBC, electrolytes, BUN, creatinine, glucose, CPK, ABG, serum pregnancy test (for female patients of childbearing age), serum osmolality, and type and cross (if there is any suspicion of trauma). If the history or physical exam is suggestive, obtain a blood alcohol level and urine for toxicology. Also obtain an ECG and a chest radiograph. Other tests, such as additional X-rays or CT scans, are determined by the history of the event and serial assessments.

An initially well-appearing child may rapidly develop both pulmonary and neurologic complications any time within the first 24 hours. However, most asymptomatic children may be discharged after 8 hours observation if the physical examination, the initial chest X-ray, and all tests are normal; the physician is assured that the family is reliable; and adequate follow-up is arranged. Poor prognostic signs include a submersion duration of >9 minutes, prolonged apnea, or coma.

Follow-up
- At once if pulmonary (cough, tachypnea, dyspnea) or neurologic (altered mental status) symptoms develop, otherwise primary care follow-up in 2–3 days

Indications for admission
- History of prolonged submersion
- Respiratory or neurologic symptoms
- A patient with an abnormal chest X-ray, for at least 24 hours

Bibliography
Burford AE, Ryan LM, Stone BJ, Hirshon JM, Klein BL: Drowning and near-drowning in children and adolescents: a succinct review for emergency physicians and nurses. *Pediatr Emerg Care* 2005;21:610–6.

Meyer RJ, Theodorou AA, Berg RA: Childhood drowning. *Pediatr Rev* 2006;27:163–8.

Olshaker JS: Submersion. *Emerg Med Clin North Am* 2004;22:357–67.

Electrical injuries
Small children, especially toddlers, frequently sustain low-voltage electrical injuries when they insert objects (pins or keys) into household sockets or chew on electrical cords. Older children are more likely to sustain high-voltage electrical injuries by contacting live third rails or power lines when climbing.

Most of the harmful effects from electrical injuries are due to the heat generated, which is directly related to current, tissue resistance, and duration of contact. Serious electrical injuries are uncommon, but carry a mortality risk of approximately 40%.

Electrical injuries are usually categorized in terms of high (>1000 V) or low (<500–1000 V) voltage injuries. Household current is low-voltage (110 volts). Because voltage is directly related to current, high-voltage injuries are usually more serious than low-voltage, although a low-voltage contact applied to areas of low resistance can also cause serious injury. Exposure to an electrical socket with a wet hand can result in a current of 100 mA, which is enough to cause ventricular fibrillation. Low-voltage injuries account for about one-half to three-quarters of all deaths from electrical injuries.

Clinical presentation and diagnosis

A child who has had contact with electric current can present with first-, second-, or third-degree burns of the skin, as well as entrance and exit burns (which are usually third-degree burns). There may also be burns at flexor creases and at the oral commissure, which may be associated with delayed labial artery bleeding 2–21 days after the burn.

If the electrical current takes a vertical path, or if there is extensive skin damage, cardiac involvement is more likely. Cardiac complications include all forms of dysrhythmias, ranging from occasional ectopic atrial and/or ventricular beats, supraventricular tachycardia, first-, second-, and third-degree AV blocks, ventricular tachycardia, and ventricular fibrillation. ECG abnormalities are usually evident upon initial ED evaluation and commonly include accelerated sinus rhythm and nonspecific ST-T wave changes, although damage to the myocardium is uncommon. Pulmonary involvement can include pulmonary contusion, hemothorax, pneumothorax, and/or ventilatory arrest.

Central nervous system involvement may be due to the electrical injury itself or the subsequent fall after the event. The patient can present with any type of mental status change. Other neurologic symptoms such as paralysis can occur immediately or can be delayed for up to several days. Electric current can cause tetany of skeletal muscle and both upper and lower motor neuron findings may be noted. This can lead to all types of musculoskeletal injury, including strains, fractures and/or dislocations.

Vascular injuries directly from the electric current can include hemorrhage, either immediate or delayed, in addition to thrombosis. Renal complications can include renal failure, which may be due to either third-spacing of fluid or rhabdomyolysis.

Gastrointestinal injuries can occur in up to 25% of high-voltage injuries. The most common complication is adynamic ileus. Other conditions that may be seen include hepatic, gallbladder, and pancreatic necrosis as well as stress ulcers.

High-voltage injuries

The patient may present with a variety of complications involving a number of organ systems. Asystole, respiratory arrest, and hypoxia-induced ventricular fibrillation are the most common causes of immediate death. These injuries are associated with hemolysis, rhabdomyolysis, direct burns of the lung or viscera, cardiac dysrhythmias, neurologic injuries, renal failure, and fractures or ruptured viscera secondary to falls.

Burns are usually characteristic of high-voltage injuries. The types of burns that may be seen include the following.

Flash burns

Flash burns look like thermal burns and are treated as such.

Arc burns

These burns have a dry center (1–30 mm) with a surrounding area of congestion. These burns suggest internal injury.

Contact burns

A burn from the contacted item. These may look like flash burns early in the course of care. These burns also suggest internal injury.

Low-voltage injuries

Most low-voltage injuries initially present with a small, localized, painless, white parchment-like patch of skin. However, if a child has bitten on an electrical cord, within a few hours there can be considerable edema of the lips, tongue, and gums. Rarely, severe intraoral edema may result in airway obstruction. If the child conducts electricity, muscle paralysis and ventricular dysrhythmias may occur. Fortunately, conduction with low voltage is rare, so these are usually limited injuries.

ED management

High-voltage injuries

Rapidly assess the adequacy of the airway. Use the chin-lift maneuver without hyperextension to maintain patency if there is the possibility of a cervical spine injury, either directly from the electrical injury or from resulting trauma (e.g. fall from a tree or ladder). If the patient is not breathing, ventilate with a bag-mask resuscitator and prepare for intubation. If respirations are adequate, administer 100% oxygen via a nonrebreather mask.

Assess the cardiovascular status, obtain an ECG, and secure a large-bore IV. If the patient is pulseless and the ECG monitor reveals ventricular fibrillation or pulseless ventricular tachycardia, defibrillate with an energy level of 2 J/kg (monophasic or biphasic; see Ventricular fibrillation, pp. 22–23).

If the patient presents with signs of inadequate tissue perfusion, give a fluid bolus of 20 mL/kg of NS and repeat as needed. If the patient remains hemodynamically unstable, continue rapid intravenous hydration and start a dopamine drip at 5–20 mcg/kg per min (see Shock). However, inadequate tissue perfusion may be due to an associated thoracic, abdominal, or long-bone injury sustained after the electrical insult. Always consider major trauma in patients presenting in shock after an electrical injury.

If the patient has a normal pulse rate and blood pressure, give IV hydration with $D_5\frac{1}{2}NS$ at a rate of 1½–2 times maintenance. Aim for a urine output of at least 2–3 mL/kg per h, but do not add potassium for the first 24 hours (unless the patient has documented hypokalemia). The presence of rhabdomyolysis (hemoglobin or myoglobin on urine dipstick and/or an elevated CPK) indicates significant deep tissue injury and predicts renal failure unless a brisk urine output is quickly established.

Initial laboratory tests include blood for an ABG, CBC, electrolytes, glucose, BUN, creatinine, PT and PTT, serum osmolality, pregnancy test (for adolescent females of childbearing age), a urinalysis, and a 12-lead ECG. Do not use CPK-MB as a single criterion for myocardial infarction as it is not specific for myocardial damage in electrical injury. The role of troponin in electrical injuries has not been studied extensively.

Perform a secondary survey to check for surface thermal burns, orthopedic injuries, or evidence of compartment syndrome. If the patient presents with an altered mental status, evidence or suspicion of an intoxicant, or a distracting injury, clear the cervical spine radiographically. However, a head CT is also indicated for continued altered mental status after electrical injury.

Categorize and treat surface thermal burns in the usual fashion (see Burns, pp. 194–198).

Low-voltage injuries

Quickly assess the patency of the airway, especially if there are burns of the mouth. Perform a careful physical examination, looking for evidence of both an entrance and an exit wound. For the common electrical burn of the mouth, local wound management includes oral hygiene and direct wound care with topical bacitracin. If localized tissue charring is present and there is any suggestion of injury to underlying structures, immediate surgical consultation is necessary. When significant portions of the lips are involved (especially the oral commissure), consult a plastic surgeon or oral surgeon. Warn the parents that between 2 and 21 days after the injury, as the burned tissue begins to separate, bleeding from the labial artery may occur. This bleeding can be controlled by local pressure but occasionally requires suture ligation in the ED.

Burns that are sustained by placing a metal object into a wall socket can usually be managed with routine local burn care, only. Since cardiovascular and neurologic complications are rare, if the vital signs (particularly the pulse) and mental status are normal, in the absence of a history of loss of consciousness, tetany, wet skin, or evidence of current flow across the heart, an ECG and cardiac monitoring are not necessary.

Follow-up

- Immediate, for any signs or symptoms of impaired circulation (numbness, tingling, color change distal to the bandage) or infection (fever, vomiting, poor feeding, change in mental status), otherwise, primary care follow-up in 3–4 days

Indications for admission

- The presence of both an entrance and an exit wound
- Any neurologic or cardiovascular instability
- Patient with mouth burns unwilling or unable to take adequate fluids by mouth
- All high-voltage electrical burns

Bibliography

Celik A, Ergün O, Ozok G: Pediatric electrical injuries: a review of 38 consecutive patients. *J Pediatr Surg* 2004;39:1233–7.

Dokov W: Assessment of risk factors for death in electrical injury. *Burns* 2009;35:114–7.

Gomez R, Caucio LC: Management of burn wounds in the emergency department. *Emerg Med Clin N Am* 2007;25:135–46.

Maghsoudi H, Adyani Y, Ahmadian N: Electrical and lightning injuries. *J Burn Care Res* 2007;28:255–61.

Frostbite

Frostbite occurs when ice crystals form within the soft tissues as a consequence of prolonged exposure to cold. For this to occur, the soft tissues have to be cooled to -4 to $-2.2°C$ (24.8–28°F). Low ambient temperatures and high wind velocity quicken the freezing process. The tissue temperature is influenced by the circulation in the extremity and the cold stress, which in turn depends on the environmental temperature, wind chill, moisture, and protective insulation. Circulation in the extremity, which influences the tissue's internal heat flow, is affected by constrictive garments, the position of the extremity, local pressure, and vasospasm. The most severe damage occurs to tissues that freeze, thaw, and then refreeze. Factors that predispose to cold injury include inadequate nutrition, smoking, alcohol and drug use, fatigue, and tight clothing.

Superficial frost involves the skin only. Deep frostbite involves the underlying tissues, such as muscles and tendons.

Clinical presentation and diagnosis

Frostbite most commonly involves distal, relatively poorly perfused regions of the body, such as fingertips, toes, earlobes, and the nose. In children, areas that have poor heat-generating ability and insulation, including the cheeks and chin, are also at high risk for frostbite. However, any area of skin that is exposed to prolonged cold can be affected.

Initially, frostbite presents with a painful cold feeling and skin blanching. This is followed by numbness, while the involved area becomes waxy, white, and firm. Deeply frostbitten skin feels hard and appears white with a yellow to blue tint. Superficial frostbitten skin also feels firm, but will indent when pressure is applied. All patients experience a sensory deficit (touch, pain, temperature) in the involved region that may extend just proximal to the line of demarcation of the frostbite.

Upon thawing an area of superficial frostbite, there is a throbbing pain followed by a tingling sensation. Deeper injuries become mottled-blue, swollen, and extremely painful upon warming. Edema occurs within 3 hours after thawing; vesicles and bullae form in more severe cases after 6–48 hours. Immediately following thawing, findings such as sensation to pinprick, good color, warm tissue, and large, clear nonhemorrhagic blebs which, if the digits are involved extend completely to the tips, suggest a relatively favorable prognosis for tissue viability. Poor prognostic signs include the late occurrence of small, dark hemorrhagic blebs that do not extend to the tips of the extremities, cyanosis, and the absence of edema.

ED management

The goal of therapy, prevention of further soft tissue destruction, is accomplished via rapid rewarming. Thaw the frozen part by immersion in water heated to 37.8–42°C (100–108°F); do not use warmer water, which may cause burns. If possible, have the child move the frostbitten body part during rewarming. A whirlpool is ideal for an extremity, as thawing time is decreased when water is circulated. Carefully monitor the temperature; as the bath cools, add hotter water to maintain the desired temperature range. Avoid rubbing or massaging the frostbitten area.

The warming usually takes 15–30 minutes; remove the extremity after thawing has occurred. The endpoint is when the affected area becomes soft, develops a purple-red color, and sensation starts to return. While in the last stages of rewarming, the patient may experience severe pain and require analgesia (morphine sulfate 0.10–0.15 mg/kg IV).

After thawing, inspect the wound. Debride any ruptured blebs, apply an antibiotic ointment such as bacitracin, and apply bulky sterile dressings. Place cotton between affected fingers or toes. Again, the use of a potent analgesic such as morphine may be necessary, but prophylactic antibiotics are not indicated. Obtain plastic surgery consultation early in the course of treatment. An escharotomy is indicated if the digits are not freely mobile. Give tetanus toxoid (0.5 mL) if the last immunization was >5 years ago.

Follow-up

- Daily follow-up, until injured areas are healing well

Indication for admission

- Frostbite of hands and feet

Bibliography

Golant A, Nord RM, Paksima N, Posner MA:
Cold exposure injuries to the extremities.
J Am Acad Orthop Surg 2008;16:
704–15.

Patel NN, Patel DN: Frostbite. *Am J Med*
2008;121:765–6.

Roche-Nagle G, Murphy D, Collins A,
Sheehan S: Frostbite: management options.
Eur J Emerg Med 2008;15:173–5.

Heat-excess syndromes

Most cases of heat illnesses occur during the summer months. Environmental conditions that increase the risk include the lack of air conditioning and enclosure in a small, unventilated space such as an automobile. Extreme physical activity, underlying illness, alcohol abuse, inadequate fluid intake, and drugs such as cocaine, salicylates, amphetamines, phenothiazines, antihistamines, or anticholinergics, coupled with any of the predisposing environmental factors, increase the risk for developing hyperthermic injury.

Children are less efficient thermoregulators compared to adults. They exhibit a slower speed of acclimatization, have a lower sweating rate, and produce more metabolic heat per kilogram of body weight, placing a greater strain on thermoregulatory mechanisms. Children also have a higher set point (the change in core temperature when sweating starts) than adults.

Clinical presentation and diagnosis

Heat cramps

Heat cramps are painful muscle cramps that are probably caused by electrolyte depletion in association with insufficient blood supply to an exercising muscle. Large muscle groups, such as the hamstrings and the gastrocnemius, are most likely to be involved. Clinically, the affected muscles are contracted. However, the onset may be delayed, occurring when the patient is showering after exercise or resting. The patient has a normal mental status and normal vital signs, but the core temperature may be slightly elevated. There may or may not be sweating.

Heat exhaustion

Heat exhaustion is caused by excessive sweating associated with inadequate intake of water and salt in a hot environment. Symptoms include headache, dizziness, fatigue, syncope, visual disturbances, nausea, vomiting, malaise, myalgias, and muscle cramps. The patient is usually tachycardic and tachypneic, and may have orthostatic vital sign changes. At the time of presentation, however, sweating may not be present. The rectal temperature is typically 38–40°C (100.4–104.0°F).

Heat stroke

Heat stroke is a life-threatening emergency that occurs when the core body temperature exceeds 40.0°C (104.0°F). The estimated mortality is >50%. It is associated with acute neurologic changes, including irritability, aggression, or emotional instability, along with any of the symptoms of heat exhaustion. Heat stroke has been classified as either classic or exertional. Classic heat stroke occurs in a child secondary to poor water intake. It has a relatively slow onset, with the insidious development of anorexia, nausea, vomiting, headaches, dry skin, and progressive deterioration of mental function. Sweating is usually absent and rhabdomyolysis and hypoglycemia are uncommon. Exertional heat stroke usually occurs in a child who engages in prolonged physical activity. It presents with the rapid onset of severe prostration, headache, syncope, tachycardia, tachypnea, and hypotension. Lactic acidosis is common and rhabdomyolysis, hypoglycemia, and hypocalcemia are often present. These patients may have dry or wet skin. The most important prognostic sign is the duration, not the degree, of the hyperthermic state.

ED management

Heat cramps

Treat heat cramps by placing the patient at rest in a cool environment. In mild cases, replace salt with a salt-containing oral rehydration solution. For severe cases, start an IV and give the patient 20 mL/kg of normal saline. Obtain blood for CBC and electrolytes (including calcium and magnesium). The patient may be discharged after clinical improvement (well-hydrated, no cramps).

Heat exhaustion

Immediately place the patient in a cool environment, remove any excess clothing, and sponge with lukewarm tap water. Then increase the heat dissipation by placing fans directed to blow air across the patient. Assess the airway and breathing and administer 100% oxygen. Start a large-bore IV, give 20 mL/kg of normal saline, then reassess the patient's hydration status and response to fluids. Obtain a CBC, electrolytes, and urinalysis. Discharge the patient after cooling and volume replacement, if vital signs are normal and symptoms have resolved.

Heat stroke

Rapidly assess airway and breathing and intubate a patient who is comatose, seizing, or has an oxygen saturation <85% while breathing 100% oxygen. Obtain vital signs including a rectal temperature (use a rectal probe), and monitor the cardiac rhythm. Undress the patient completely and start the cooling process by spraying with lukewarm tap water, then positioning fans to blow air across the body. It is estimated that the evaporation of 1 g of water transfers seven times as much heat as melting 1 g of ice. However, use ice packs to the axillae, neck, and groin as supplemental treatment. Continue this aggressive cooling, at a rate of approximately 0.2°C (0.4°F) per minute until the core temperature reaches 39°C (102.2°F). Prevent shivering, which generates body heat, with IV lorazepam (0.1 mg/kg IV). Alcohol baths are contraindicated, due to the potential of alcohol intoxication. Acetaminophen and ibuprofen have no role in the treatment of heat stroke.

Start two large-bore IVs, immediately give 0.5–1 g/kg dextrose (1–2 mL/kg D_{50}; 2–4 mL/kg D_{25}), give two 20 mL/kg boluses of normal saline, then reassess the circulatory status. If the patient remains in shock after the second bolus of crystalloid, consider severe vasodilatation. Use central venous pressure (CVP) monitoring to guide further fluid therapy, since continued boluses may cause pulmonary edema. If the CVP is low, give repeated fluid boluses. If the CVP is normal, and the patient is still hypotensive, start dopamine at a rate of 2–5 mcg/kg per min. Insert a Foley catheter, and carefully monitor intake and output.

Initial laboratory studies include CBC, PT/PTT, electrolytes, BUN, creatinine, glucose, CPK, LFTs, serum osmolality, salicylate level, pregnancy test (for females of childbearing age), fibrinogen, lactate, urinalysis, and an ECG. Reassess the patient frequently to identify complications such as brain cell injury, liver and pulmonary injury, rhabdomyolysis, and disseminated intravascular coagulation.

Follow-up

- Heat cramps: primary care follow-up in 1–2 weeks
- Heat exhaustion: next day

Indication for admission

- Heat stroke

Bibliography

Glazer JL: Management of heatstroke and heat exhaustion. *Am Fam Physician* 2005;71:2133–40.

Jardine DS: Heat illness and heat stroke. *Pediatr Rev* 2007;28:249–58.

McDermott BP, Casa DJ, Ganio MS, et al: Acute whole-body cooling for exercise-induced hyperthermia: a systematic review. *J Athl Train* 2009;44:84–93.

Hyperbaric oxygen therapy

Hyperbaric oxygen therapy (HBOT) involves the administration of oxygen under increased ambient pressure. While the indications for HBOT are controversial, the most common emergency conditions which appear to benefit from HBOT are decompression sickness, air embolism, and carbon monoxide (CO) poisoning. Other indications for HBOT are listed in Table 8-2.

Decompression sickness and air emboli

Decompression sickness occurs when nitrogen in the blood comes quickly out of solution, resulting in bubble formation in the circulation and tissues. Type I decompression sickness can present with a dull deep pain (usually in a joint or tendon area), pruritus, or a rash that that may be mottling, or papular. The upper extremities are usually affected more than the lower extremities. Type II decompression sickness presents with pulmonary symptoms (cough, respiratory distress, chest discomfort), neurologic symptoms (headaches, visual disturbances, vertigo, nystagmus, paresis, paralysis, and mental status changes), and circulatory symptoms (shock or thrombus formation)

Arterial gas emboli result from leakage of air bubbles into the circulation and may cause circulatory obstruction. They may be iatrogenic (cardiovascular procedures, central line placement, lung biopsies, hemodialysis) or may be a complication of uncontrolled ascents in scuba diving.

Table 8-2. Indications for HBOT

Traditional indications	Newer indications
Carbon monoxide poisoning	Acute air embolism
Decompression sickness	Acute traumatic ischemia
Gas gangrene	Compromised skin grafts and flaps
Wound healing	Necrotizing soft tissue infections
	Osteoradionecrosis
	Soft tissue radionecrosis
	Thermal burns

Source: Adapted with permission from Weiss LD, Van Meter KW: The applications of hyperbaric oxygen therapy in emergency medicine. *Am J Emerg Med* 1992;10:558–567.

When treating both these disorders, HBOT relies upon two basic laws of physics: Boyle's law (the pressure of a gas is inversely proportional to its volume), and Henry's law (the amount of gas dissolved in solution is directly proportional to its partial pressure). HBOT causes a reduction in the size of the trapped bubbles and forces them back into solution from the circulatory system and tissues.

Carbon monoxide poisoning

Carbon monoxide competes with oxygen for hemoglobin and cytochrome binding sites. Toxicity results from direct hypoxic damage to tissues, inhibition of cellular respiration by disruption of the cytochrome system, and lipid peroxidation in the central nervous system. Signs and symptoms of carbon monoxide poisoning include fatigue, nausea, vomiting, and neurologic abnormalities ranging from headache to personality deficit to frank coma.

HBOT increases the oxygenation of the tissues, decreases the half-life of carboxyhemoglobin (COHb) from approximately 240–320 minutes (range of 128–409 minutes) at sea level (1 atmosphere absolute [ATA]) in 21% oxygen to approximately 15–30 minutes at 2.5–3.0 ATA in 100% oxygen.

Since the serum (either venous or arterial) COHb level may not reflect COHb tissue levels and often does not correlate with the degree of toxicity, the signs and symptoms of toxicity are equally important in determining the need for therapy for CO poisoning. HBOT is recommended for a patient with a history of unconsciousness after exposure to CO regardless of COHb level, a history of continued mental status change or other neurologic deficit, cardiac dysfunction or ischemia, a COHb level >25% regardless of symptoms, or for any pregnant woman with a history of CO exposure (regardless of COHb level). The only absolute contraindication to HBOT is an untreated pneumothorax.

Patients to be treated cautiously include those with significant upper respiratory infections, fever, seizure disorder, diabetes, or a history of chest surgery or pneumothorax. Also, unstable patients who have had a cardiac arrest and/or require pressors for support may experience little improvement in clinical symptoms after HBOT because of other ongoing medical problems, and they are difficult to resuscitate inside the hyperbaric chamber.

A patient who has suffered a cardiac arrest has a very poor prognosis and may not experience enough benefit from HBOT to warrant the risks.

Initial ED management and preparation for HBOT

Initial priorities include addressing the ABCs, providing 100% oxygen via a tight-fitting nonrebreather mask or endotracheal tube, and obtaining a COHb level from venous or arterial blood using a heparinized 1 mL syringe. If the patient is in respiratory distress or requires ventilatory support, secure an IV and obtain an ABG, ECG, and chest X-ray. Other tests may be indicated, including serum electrolytes, liver function tests, and creatinine. In addition, assess the patient for other traumatic injuries, smoke inhalation, or cyanide poisoning. These conditions must be fully addressed before the patient is taken into the hyperbaric chamber.

Once it is determined that HBOT is indicated, prepare the patient for the chamber. If the patient is intubated with a cuffed endotracheal tube, replace the air in the cuff with saline or water, since fluids do not compress under pressure. Change glass IV bottles, which may implode under pressure, to flexible plastic IV bags. Adjust IV drip rates manually with pressure bags. Open the nasogastric tube (if inserted) to gravity to allow for equalization of pressure between the stomach and the atmosphere. Make sure that the patient's clothing is made of cotton or flame-retardant material, and remove any fire hazards, including matches, lighters, jewelry, watches, alcohol, cosmetics, lubricants, hairsprays, cell phones, and newspapers from the patient and keep out of the chamber.

Sedate and paralyze (pp. 16–17) intubated patients to minimize the risk of extubation, and consider restraints for patients with altered mental status who may improve and awaken during treatment and injure themselves or chamber personnel. Optional considerations include prophylactic administration of a decongestant (pseudoephedrine 1 mg/kg) to an awake patient to help prevent middle ear and sinus barotrauma.

One current treatment protocol for CO poisoning involves administering 100% O_2, via a tight-fitting mask or endotracheal tube, at 2.8 ATA for two 23-minute periods interrupted by a 5-minute interval on 21% oxygen.

HBOT may result in barotrauma to any air-filled cavity which cannot equilibrate with ambient pressure. The middle ear and/or sinuses are most commonly affected. Rarely, barotrauma may cause a pneumothorax or air embolus.

Oxygen toxicity to the CNS may occur with prolonged exposure to 100% oxygen. Additionally, the seizure threshold may be lowered, and autonomic regulation of respiration may be affected. However, neurotoxicity is very unusual with the low-pressure, short-duration treatments used in most clinical situations.

Pulmonary toxicity may occur with 100% inspired oxygen at increased pressure for prolonged exposures. Although pulmonary toxicity will occur after six continuous hours of exposure to 100% O_2 at 2 ATA, no HBOT protocol requires this length of treatment.

Other side effects include accelerated cataract growth, temporary worsening of myopia or improved presbyopia, claustrophobia, and fatigue. Technical complications of HBOT include a fire risk within the chamber where oxygen is being used, and the inadequacy of equipment and personnel to perform prolonged resuscitation on a patient while pressurized within the chamber.

Follow-up

- Asymptomatic patient: next day

Indication for admission

- Any patient treated with HBOT who has continued significant respiratory, cardiovascular, or neurologic compromise

Bibliography

Buckley NA, Isbister GK, Stokes B, Juurlink DN: Hyperbaric oxygen for carbon monoxide poisoning: a systematic review and critical analysis of the evidence. *Toxicol Rev* 2005;24:75–92.

Gill AL, Bell CN: Hyperbaric oxygen: its uses, mechanisms of action and outcomes. *QJM* 2004;97:385–95.

Stoller KP: Hyperbaric oxygen and carbon monoxide poisoning: a critical review. *Neurol Res* 2007;29:146–55.

Hypothermia

Hypothermia, a core temperature ≤35°C (95°F), is usually caused by accidental exposure. At <35°C (95°F) the human body loses its ability to generate sufficient heat to maintain bodily functions. Below 30°C (86°F) the body assumes the temperature of the surrounding environment.

Children are at particular risk, because of their large body surface area, lack of fat insulation, inadequate shivering, and inability to escape a cold environment. Prolonged out-of-hospital resuscitation and cold-water immersion are common causes of hypothermia. Predisposing factors include malnutrition, hypoglycemia, major trauma, hypothyroidism, Addison's disease, and drug use or abuse (alcohol, sedatives, antidepressants). Although most cases of accidental exposure are seen in winter, hypothermia may occur in the spring and fall during wet, windy weather. Hypothermia may develop acutely within minutes in a cold-water immersion victim, or insidiously over days in a neonate in a poorly heated home.

Clinical presentation

Mild hypothermia (32–35°C; 89.6°–95°F)

The child may present with tachypnea, tachycardia, ataxia, dysarthria, and shivering. There may be loss of coordination, but the patient is hemodynamically stable.

Moderate hypothermia (32–28°C; 89.6–82.4°F)

There may be a slowing of the heart rate or dysrhythmias, as well as a loss of shivering. The mental status may also be altered.

Severe hypothermia (< 28°C; 82.4°F)

There is a change in the mental status, vascular collapse, and malignant dysrhythmias.

Diagnosis

Consider a patient with cold skin, altered mental status, and bradycardia to be hypothermic until proved otherwise. In addition, any severe injury or illness can be associated with hypothermia. Since the diagnosis of hypothermia rests on measuring the core temperature, use a thermocouple probe inserted 3–5 cm into the rectum. Do not use a tympanic thermometer, which is unreliable.

A "J," or Osborne, wave may be observed on the ECG of as many as 80% of hypothermic patients. This is a secondary wave, following the S wave, seen in aVL, aVF and throughout the chest leads. Other ECG findings include prolonged PR, QRS, and/or QT intervals.

Investigate for precipitating and complicating factors such as alcohol or drug intoxication (barbiturates, phenothiazines), near-drowning, head trauma, sepsis, or hypoglycemia. Consider other causes of hypothermia, including hypothyroidism and Addison's disease, when a patient fails to respond to rewarming measures with a rise in core temperature of at least 1°C per hour.

ED management

Classify the hypothermia as mild, moderate, or severe (see above). Passive rewarming is satisfactory for mild hypothermia. Remove all wet or cold clothing, place pre-warmed layers of blankets on the patient, give warm IV fluids (normal saline at maintenance), and administer warmed (47°C; 116.6°F), humidified oxygen.

A patient with moderate hypothermia requires active external rewarming with electric warming blankets, hot water bottles, heating pads, or warming beds. However, IV access must already be obtained and fluid therapy initiated before active rewarming is started; otherwise as vasodilatation occurs during warming, the patient can become acutely hypotensive and develop a fatal cardiac arrhythmia.

Treat severe hypothermia with active core rewarming; use warmed nasogastric, peritoneal, or pleural lavage. For peritoneal dialysis infuse a commercial dialysate, normal saline, or lactated Ringer's solution heated to 40–45°C (104 F–113°F). Place two trocars (one for infusion and one for drainage) into the peritoneal cavity. Use a dose of 15 mL/kg, and leave the fluid in place for 30 minutes, then aspirate.

Because of the very low threshold for cardiac arrhythmias, handle a hypothermia victim as gently as possible. Rapidly assess the child's airway and breathing. Intubate if the patient requires a protected airway or has an oxygen saturation <85% while breathing warmed, humidified oxygen.

Continuously monitor the cardiac rhythm, and if the patient is hypotensive, give a 20 mL/kg fluid challenge of normal saline through a large-bore IV. If peripheral vasoconstriction interferes with obtaining venous access, insert a central femoral line, but avoid catheters that enter the heart since they may induce cardiac dysrhythmias. After obtaining access and before initiating IV fluids, obtain blood for CBC, electrolytes, BUN, creatinine, calcium, magnesium, amylase, osmolality, fibrinogen, CPK, and PT and PTT.

If the patient's fingerstick reveals hypoglycemia, give glucose (0.5–1.0 g/kg IV). Treat hypotension unresponsive to fluid boluses with a dopamine drip (start at 2–5 mcg/kg per min). Place a Foley catheter and send urine for dipstick and microscopic analysis.

Ventricular fibrillation and asystole (not bradycardia) are the only indications for chest compressions since external cardiac massage can induce fatal ventricular arrhythmias in profound hypothermia. Ventricular fibrillation may occur spontaneously when the core temperature is <28°C (82.4°F). If ventricular fibrillation is present, attempt defibrillation (2 J/kg first attempt; 4 J/kg second and third attempts [monophasic and biphasic]), although electrical defibrillation and standard advanced cardiac life support drug protocols are unlikely to be successful at core temperatures of 28–30°C (82.4–86°F). Medications that improve the chances of a return of spontaneous circulation include amiodarone IV (5 mg/kg bolus) and epinephrine (0.01 mg/kg of a 1:10 000 solution). Most atrial arrhythmias are benign and disappear with rewarming.

It can be especially difficult to distinguish between hypothermia and death. Therefore, continue all resuscitative measures until the patient's core temperature is >32°C (89.6°F).

Indication for admission

- Hypothermia

Bibliography

Golant A, Nord RM, Paksima N, Posner MA: Cold exposure injuries to the extremities. *J Am Acad Orthop Surg* 2008;16:704–15.

Jurkovich GJ: Environmental cold-induced injury. *Surg Clin North Am* 2007;87:247–67.

Wira CR: Anti-arrhythmic and vasopressor medications for the treatment of ventricular fibrillation in severe hypothermia: a systematic review of the literature. *Resuscitation* 2008;78:21–9.

Inhalation injury

Inhalation injuries account for up to 50% of fire-related deaths in the United States. There are four distinct clinical entities with inhalation injuries: thermal burns of the upper airway, smoke inhalation, carbon monoxide poisoning, and cyanide poisoning. The clinical presentations, treatments, and prognoses differ, and serious life-threatening complications can occur insidiously or rapidly.

Thermal injury

Thermal burns from inhalation injuries almost never involve the lungs or lower airways because of the poor heat-carrying capacity of air and the excellent heat-dissipating capacity of the upper airway. Thermal injury above the glottis is very common and probably the most immediate life-threatening problem in a patient with inhalation injury. However, lower parenchymal injury can occur with steam burns. The extent of the injury may not be seen until 24 hours after the initial insult.

Smoke inhalation

Many of the chemical components in smoke (aldehydes and organic acids), as well as soot and particulate matter, cause direct parenchymal injury when inhaled, resulting in acute pulmonary insufficiency, pulmonary edema, and bronchopneumonia.

Carbon monoxide poisoning

Carbon monoxide (pp. 207–209) poisoning is the most common cause of fire-related deaths. It is a colorless, odorless, tasteless gas produced by incomplete combustion of carbon-containing materials (wood, fuel, paper). CO binds to hemoglobin with an affinity approximately 250 times more than oxygen, resulting in displacement of oxygen from hemoglobin and causing cellular anoxia affecting all organ systems.

Cyanide

Cyanide is released through incomplete combustion of acrylics, wool, and plastics and it is absorbed rapidly. Cyanide inhibits aerobic metabolism, reversibly binds with cytochrome oxidase, and inhibits the last step of mitochondrial oxidative phosphorylation, leading to a depletion of adenosine triphosphate.

Clinical presentation and diagnosis
Thermal injury
Thermal injury of the upper airway causes laryngeal edema and laryngospasm which can occur at any time within the first 24 hours and cause total airway obstruction within minutes. Clinically, there is a history of exposure to smoke or fire in an enclosed space, in association with cough, tachypnea, hoarseness, stridor, or carbon-tinged sputum. Burns on the head, face, or neck and singed nasal hairs may also be present.

Smoke inhalation
A patient with flame burns, the smell of smoke on the clothes, or a history of being in an enclosed smoke-filled room is at high risk for developing pulmonary injury from smoke inhalation. Hoarseness, wheezing, rales, or soot-tinged sputum may be early evidence of pulmonary insufficiency. However, the absence of these signs does not rule out parenchymal damage, since a patient who appears symptom-free 1–2 hours postinhalation may subsequently develop significant respiratory problems within a matter of hours. In general, pulmonary insufficiency with bronchospasm occurs in the first 12 hours postinhalation, pulmonary edema occurs 6–72 hours postinhalation, and bronchopneumonia occurs within 5 days postinhalation. The ABGs and chest X-rays may not deteriorate until 12–24 hours postinhalation. Therefore, if there is a suspicious history, evaluate and treat the patient for smoke inhalation.

Carbon monoxide poisoning
The measured level of carboxyhemoglobin (COHb) correlates only moderately with the clinical picture and degree of CO poisoning. Mild symptoms include dizziness, headache, and GI symptoms. Moderate symptoms include syncope, chest pain, shortness of breath, and altered mental status. Severe symptoms include dysrhythmias, hypotension, noncardiogenic pulmonary edema, seizures, coma, and ventilatory/cardiac arrest. The COHb level may not accurately reflect the degree of CO poisoning at the cellular level. Therefore, rely on the history and clinical presentation when assessing and managing an inhalation victim for CO poisoning.

Cyanide
Cyanide intoxication presents with altered mental status including seizures and coma. A lactate level ≥10 mmol/L suggests the diagnosis. Pulse oximetry is of little value because cyanide inhibits oxidative phosphorylation.

ED management
Thermal injury
Mental status changes, cough, tachypnea, hoarseness, stridor, carbon-tinged sputum, singed nasal hairs, or burns on the head, face, or neck are absolute indications for immediate direct visualization of the mouth and upper airway. This can be done in the ED with either a fiberoptic bronchoscope or a laryngoscope, but ensure that the personnel and equipment to

perform an emergency intubation or tracheostomy are at the bedside. Upon visualization of the airway, the presence of erythema, edema, dried mucosa, or small blisters on the hard palate or mucosa of the upper airway are clear indications for elective early intubation. All the other signs and symptoms mentioned above are relative indications for elective intubation.

Expectant observation of a patient with a history of or any signs or symptoms of smoke exposure is appropriate only in a facility where emergency intubation and/or tracheostomy can be performed immediately. If intubation is required, sedate the patient, if necessary. Steroids are not useful. Elective tracheostomy significantly increases the morbidity and mortality of patients with smoke inhalation and is never indicated.

Smoke inhalation

Provide humidified 100% oxygen by either a tight-fitting nonrebreather face mask or through an ETT after intubation. As with thermal injury of the upper airway, fiberoptic bronchoscopy is the standard diagnostic procedure for pulmonary injury. Treat wheezing with nebulized albuterol (0.03 mL/kg), and follow the progression of the pulmonary disease with serial ABGs and chest X-rays. Prophylactic antibiotics and steroids are contraindicated in treating inhalation injury. Good pulmonary toilet, bronchodilators, and humidified oxygen are the mainstays of treatment.

Carbon monoxide poisoning

The management of CO poisoning is discussed in detail elsewhere (see Hyperbaric oxygen therapy, pp. 207–209). However, defer hyperbaric treatment if the patient has severe burns, needs PEEP for oxygenation, or requires pressors to maintain a blood pressure. In centers which do not have a hyperbaric chamber, contact the local Poison Control Center for information as to the location of the nearest available hyperbaric center. If a hyperbaric chamber is not available, provide 100% oxygen to patients with severe CO poisoning for at least 24 hours, regardless of the COHb level. Obtain serial ABGs to follow and correct any acid–base derangements.

Cyanide

If cyanide poisoning is suspected, use the Lilly Cyanide Antidote Kit that includes amyl nitrite, sodium nitrite, and sodium thiosulfate. However, if the patient has CO poisoning, only use the sodium thiosulfate, as nitrites will induce a methhemoglobinema which may exacerbate the hypoxia secondary to elevated carboxyhemoglobin. Alternatively, use hydroxocobalamin, which chelates with the cyanide molecule (1:1) to form cyanocobalamin or vitamin B12. This is excreted in the urine and does not interfere with oxygen-carrying capacity. Contact the local Poison Control Center for appropriate pediatric dosing.

Indications for admission

- Documented thermal injury of the upper airway
- Severe CO poisoning
- Smoke inhalation with upper or lower airway injury
- History of significant smoke or fire exposure in an enclosed area

Bibliography

Endorf FW, Gamelli RL: Inhalation injury, pulmonary perturbations, and fluid resuscitation. *J Burn Care Res* 2007;28:80–3.

Geller RJ, Barthold C, Saiers JA, Hall AH: Pediatric cyanide poisoning: causes,

manifestations, management and unmet needs. *Pediatrics* 2006;188;2146–58.

Lee AS, Mellins RB: Lung injury from smoke inhalation. *Paediatr Respir Rev* 2006;7:123–8.

Lead poisoning

Lead poisoning in children is usually the result of chronic ingestion. Young children are at risk of lead exposure through pica (ingestion of lead-based paint chips), lead-contaminated dust or dirt along heavily traveled roads, and water carried by outdated lead pipes. In addition, exposure to lead can occur through burning of automobile battery casings, improperly home-glazed ceramics, or certain folk medicines (e.g. Mexican folk remedies such as azarcon and greta or cosmetics such as kohl and surma). Despite widespread lead-screening programs, children who frequent inner-city EDs may have disproportionately elevated lead levels.

Clinical presentation

The majority of patients are asymptomatic, but are brought to the ED because they have been observed eating paint chips or have an elevated microsample lead level. Although acute lead poisoning is rare, consider it in the differential of vague, nonspecific signs and symptoms such as headaches, anorexia, abdominal pain, constipation, intermittent vomiting, listlessness, or irritability. With increasing levels, encephalopathy develops with persistent vomiting, drowsiness, clumsiness, and frank ataxia. Kidney damage results in a spectrum ranging from slight aminoaciduria to a full Fanconi syndrome. High lead levels are also associated with a microcytic anemia.

A mildly elevated blood lead level (< 25 mcg/dL) is associated with decreased intelligence and impaired development. A lead level of 25–60 mcg/dL may cause headache, irritability, and anemia, while a lead level of 60–80 mcg/dL is associated with gastrointestinal symptoms and subclinical renal effects. With a level >80 mcg/dL there may be overt intoxication, with encephalopathy, increased intracranial pressure, and seizures.

Diagnosis

The risk for lead exposure is primarily determined by the patient's home environment. In most cases the nonspecific presentation may be mistaken for a viral syndrome. However, consider lead poisoning in a patient who lives in an older home (up to 1960), has a history of pica or iron-deficiency anemia, uses products from other countries (including spices, health remedies, or pottery), or has a family history of lead poisoning. Clinical features suggesting chronic lead poisoning include persistent vomiting, listlessness, irritability, clumsiness, or loss of acquired developmental skills. Although rare, lead poisoning can also present as an acute encephalopathy, afebrile seizures, or signs of increased intracranial pressure. Also consider lead poisoning if there is evidence of child abuse or neglect.

Nonspecific laboratory findings include anemia (normocytic or microcytic), basophilic stippling, and the presence of radioopaque chips on abdominal X-ray.

ED management

If lead poisoning is suspected (based on symptoms), obtain a whole blood lead level, CBC, and if there is a history of pica or the child was seen with paint chips in his or her mouth, a KUB. If the KUB is positive (radioopaque particles in the intestinal tract), give a pediatric hypertonic phosphate enema, then repeat the X-ray. The management of acute encephalopathy (pp. 216, 646), seizures (pp. 521–524), and increased intracranial pressure (pp. 516–518) are discussed elsewhere.

Management of elevated screening microsamples

BLL (mcg/dL) 5–9

If the initial test was a fingerstick, confirm with a venous specimen. Ask about adequate intake of calcium, iron, and vitamin C, and check for risks for elevated lead (pica, previous residence in a country where lead exposure is common, use of products that contain lead, adult job or hobby that involves exposure to lead) and refer the patient to their primary care provider for follow-up evaluation within 3–6 months.

BLL (mcg/dL) 10–14

As above, plus report the BLL to your local Department of Health including the patient's name, birthdate, address, and phone number.

BLL (mcg/dL) 15–44

As above, plus obtain a detailed environmental and developmental history and perform a complete physical examination. Obtain a CBC to check for iron-deficiency anemia, as well as an erythrocyte protoporphyrin (EP) level. An elevated EP reflects chronic exposure. Order a KUB if there is a suspicion of PICA. If paint chips are seen, give an enema.

BLL (mcg/dL) ≥45

As above, plus arrange for chelation therapy in the hospital or at a lead-safe facility with expertise in treating lead poisoning. Confirm the BLL with a venous specimen prior to chelation, unless the child has symptoms of encephalopathy. Inform your local Department of Health of the hospitalization for treatment.

Chelation therapy

Asymptomatic and lead level 45–60 mcg/dL

Arrange for outpatient chelation, preferably with oral dimercaptosuccinic acid (succimer). Use 10 mg/kg PO q 8 h on days 1–5, then 10 mg/kg PO q 12 h on days 6–14.

Symptomatic patient

Admit the patient and treat with two drugs, oral dimercaptosuccinic acid (as above) and $CaNa_2EDTA$ (edetate), 1000–1500 mg/m^2 per day IV infusion. Obtain pretreatment electrolytes, calcium, creatinine, and a urinalysis.

Encephalopathy

Give IM British AntiLewisite (BAL) 3–5 mg/kg q 4 h for 3–5 days, followed 4 hours later by $CaNa_2EDTA$ (as above).

Follow-up

- Asymptomatic patient with a venous lead level 5–9 mcg/dL; repeat blood lead in 3–6 months
- Asymptomatic patient with a venous lead level 10–14 mcg/dL: repeat blood lead in 3 months
- Asymptomatic patient with a venous lead level 15–24: mcg/dL repeat blood lead in 1–3 months
- Asymptomatic patient with a venous lead level 25–44 mcg/dL: repeat blood lead in 2 weeks-1 month
- Asymptomatic patient with a lead level >45 mcg/dL: repeat blood lead in 48 hours

Indications for admission

- Any symptoms of lead poisoning
- Need for chelation

Bibliography

Etzel RA (ed): *Handbook of Pediatric Environmental Health*, 2nd ed. Elk Grove Village: American Academy of Pediatrics, 2003, pp. 249–66.

Levin R, Brown MJ, Kashtock ME, et al: Lead exposures in U.S. children, 2008: implications for prevention. *Environ Health Perspect* 2008;**116**:1285–93.

Piomelli S: Childhood lead poisoning. *Pediatr Clin North Am* 2002;**49**:1285–304.

Lightning injuries

Lightning is a direct current estimated to produce, for a span of several microseconds, up to 20 000–40 000 amperes and 30 million to one billion volts. There are about 1500 human lightning strikes each year, the mortality is approximately 5–20%, and nearly three-fourths of survivors have permanent sequelae. The incidence of lightning strikes is highest in the summer months, with the majority of cases occurring in the late afternoon.

Lightning causes injury by direct strike, ground strike, splash, and blunt trauma. A direct strike is considered the most serious, as the patient absorbs the entire charge. It most often occurs when the victim is in the open or in contact with metal objects. A ground strike occurs when the lightning strikes the ground near a person; the closer the patient is to the ground strike, the more likely injury will ensue. A splash injury occurs when lightning jumps from the primary site through the air to a person. Blunt injury is the result of the expansion and explosion of rapidly cooling air, and is estimated to occur in one-third of lightning strikes.

Electrical energy follows the path of least resistance, which is nerves and blood vessels, followed by muscle, skin, and tendons. Bone and fat have the highest resistance. However, skin resistance, and therefore the extent of injury, depends on whether the skin is wet (decreased skin resistance, less penetration of deep tissues) or dry (increased skin resistance, more penetration of deep tissues).

Clinical presentation

Lightning injuries frequently affect multiple organ systems. Cutaneous burns may range from minor first-degree to severe third-degree. Dermal ferning, or feathering burn, is a reddish erythema that appears within several hours of the injury and disappears in several days. It is characteristic of lightning injuries. Burns may also present in a linear or punctate fashion, but discrete entrance and exit burns are rare.

Signs of central nervous system involvement include mental status changes, amnesia, paralysis, and seizures. Many types of brain injury have been documented, such as subdural and epidural hematoma and intraventricular hemorrhage.

Dysrhythmias, including ventricular fibrillation, ventricular tachycardia, asystole, and nonspecific ST-T wave changes, may occur but usually resolve within 24 hours. Myocardial infarction is uncommon. Vascular instability may also occur, but resolves after several hours.

Possible pulmonary injuries include pulmonary contusions and hemopneumothorax. Muscle injury can result in rhabdomyolysis and myoglobinuria. Approximately one-half of lightning victims have an eye injury, including cataracts, retinal detachment or hemorrhage, or optic nerve injury. Cataracts are most frequently unilateral and may occur immediately after the lightning strike or as late as 2 years after. Otologic injuries include tympanic membrane rupture, which occurs in over 50% of victims, and middle ear hematoma. Hearing loss may be a late sequela.

Psychiatric effects are a special late consequence among children. These include anxiety, sleep disturbances, separation anxiety, and secondary enuresis.

ED management
The management of lightning strikes is basically the same as that for electrical injuries (pp. 200–203). This includes basic and advanced life support, a full trauma examination, and neurologic, renal, and dermatologic assessment. Pay special attention to the possibility of otologic and ophthalmologic injuries common to lightning strikes.

Follow-up
- Ophthalmologic and otologic follow-up in 2–3 days
- Psychiatric follow-up within 1 month

Indication for admission
- Lightning strike victim with cardiovascular, neurologic, or renal injury (by history or direct observation in the ED)

Bibliography
Mistovich JJ, Krost WS, Limmer DD: Beyond the basics: lightning-strike injuries. *EMS Mag* 2008;37:82–7.

O'Keefe Gatewood M, Zane RD: Lightning injuries. *Emerg Med Clin North Am* 2004; 22:369–403.

Ritenour AE, Morton MJ, McManus JG, Barillo DJ, Cancio LC: Lightning injury: a review. *Burns* 2008;34:585–94.

Gastrointestinal emergencies

9

Teresa McCann and Julie Lin

Contributing authors
Ellen F. Crain and Sandra J. Cunningham: Assessment and management of dehydration

Abdominal pain

Abdominal pain is a common complaint in children. The differential is extensive (Table 9-1), so that a systematic approach is required to make an accurate diagnosis.

Clinical presentation and diagnosis

Spasm or distention of an abdominal viscus typically causes poorly localized, ill-defined visceral pain due to the bilateral, unmyelinated nature of the pain fibers. These fibers enter the spinal cord at multiple levels, leading to typical midline complaints, regardless of the anatomic location of the source of the pain. Upper gastrointestinal (GI) pathology causes epigastric discomfort; distal small bowel and proximal colonic diseases are perceived as periumbilical pain; and distal colonic pain is referred to the hypogastrium. Conversely, stimulation of the parietal peritoneum causes localized pain on the same side and at the same dermatomal level as the origin of the pain. This pain is usually sharp, well defined, and aggravated by movement or cough. Referred pain is similar to parietal pain, but occurs at a site distant to, but supplied by the same dermatome as, the involved organ.

Ask about the duration, quality, intensity, location, and radiation of the pain; and the response to defecation, urination, meals, and change in position. Determine whether there is upper or lower GI bleeding, fever, vomiting, diarrhea, night or early morning awakening, weight loss, or growth failure. Inquire about respiratory, cardiovascular or urinary symptoms, menstrual cycle, testicular pain, sexual activity, and possibility of pregnancy. Ask about past illnesses, medication, travel, family and social history, and exposure to animals or sick contacts.

Although a definitive diagnosis cannot always be made immediately, a primary goal is the early recognition of surgically correctable emergencies and potentially unstable conditions. Begin the examination with the non-threatening and painless components, leaving the abdominal and rectal examinations for the end. Quickly assess the patient's hydration status and cardiovascular/respiratory stability. Try to elicit and localize abdominal tenderness, as well as rebound tenderness or masses. A pelvic exam is necessary for all sexually active or menstruating females with lower abdominal pain.

In infancy suspect an intraabdominal surgical emergency such as malrotation with midgut volvulus or intussusception whenever there is a history of bilious or projectile vomiting and/or bleeding. The signs may be preceded or accompanied by irritability, poor feeding, and lethargy. Suspect a surgical condition if the physical examination reveals abdominal distension, a scaphoid abdomen, localized abdominal tenderness or guarding, a mass, or high-pitched or absent bowel sounds, or if the patient is ill-appearing.

Once surgical conditions are ruled out by history and physical examination, consider constipation as a cause of the pain, particularly in preschool and school-age children (see pp. 236–240).

Table 9-1. Differential diagnosis of abdominal pain

Diagnosis	Differentiating features
Gastrointestinal	
Appendicitis	Pain followed by vomiting
	Associated with low-grade fever and anorexia
	Pain starts periumbilical and migrates to RLQ
Bowel obstruction	Crampy pain which is usually periumbilical
	Associated with vomiting and abdominal distention
Cholelithiasis	Colicky pain, typically RUQ
Cholecystitis	Pain RUQ, positive Murphy's sign
Constipation	Pain is non-migratory and is relieved upon defecation
	Ampulla is frequently filled with stool on digital rectal exam
Gastroenteritis	Vomiting prior to, or simultaneously with, abdominal pain
	Pain often relieved by vomiting or bowel movement
	Diarrhea may be prominent
	Fecal leukocytes or blood present if bacterial
Hepatitis	Tenderness on exam in RUQ
	May be jaundiced
Incarcerated hernia	Usually inguinal or umbilical
	Evidence of bowel obstruction
Inflammatory bowel disease	Recurrent episodes of pain
	Associated with bloody diarrhea and abdominal distension
Intussusception	Pain and vomiting alternating with periods of lethargy
	Usually afebrile and may have guaiac positive stools 80% of patients are <2 years old
Irritable bowel	Recurrent crampy lower abdominal pain
	Episodes of non-bloody diarrhea and constipation
Lactose intolerance	Intermittent, crampy pain associated with dairy intake
Meckel's diverticulum	Painless LGI bleeding
	May perforate or lead an intussusception, causing pain
Mesenteric adenitis	Diagnosis of exclusion
Pancreatitis	Pain is epigastric, may radiate to the back
Peptic ulcer/gastritis	Pain is usually epigastric, gnawing-like, worse with fasting

Table 9-1. (cont.)

Diagnosis	Differentiating features
Gynecological/genitourinary	
Endometriosis	Cyclical, usually pelvic pain, may have irregular menses
Ovarian cyst	Pain during or shortly after menses
Menstruation	Crampy pain that subsides on day 1–2 of menses
Mittelschmerz	Lower abdominal or pelvic pain
	Occurs around the time of ovulation
Pelvic inflammatory disease	Pain is usually lower in abdomen
	Vaginal discharge or bleeding
Pregnancy	Positive serum or urine pregnancy test
Torsion	Ovarian or testicular torsion may present at any age
	Check cremasteric reflex in males
Hematology/oncology	
Henoch-Schönlein purpura	Pain may precede the rash, arthritis and nephritis
Hemolytic uremic syndrome	Pain accompanies microangiopathic hemolytic anemia
	Renal insufficiency or failure
Lymphoma	Solid tumor may cause bowel obstruction or intussusception
Porphyria	Vomiting and constipation
	Mental status changes, peripheral neuropathy
	Urinary complaints and hypertension
Sickle cell disease	Vaso-occlusive crisis or splenic sequestration
	Associated anemia
Metabolic/toxic	
Adrenal insufficiency	Chronic fatigue, weight loss
	Hypotension, hyperpigmentation,
	Hyponatremia, hyperkalemia, hypercalcemia
Diabetic ketoacidosis	Polyuria, polydypsia, polyphagia
	Kussmaul respirations
Ingestion	Detailed history is key
Pulmonary/cardiovascular	
Heart failure	Typically associated with myocarditis
	Tachycardia, diffuse ST segment changes on EKG

Table 9-1. (cont.)

Diagnosis	Differentiating features
Pneumonia (RLL)	Tachypnea and pulmonary rales are usually present
Renal	
Hydronephrosis	If acute, pain more severe with associated nausea or vomiting
Nephrolithiasis	Colicky pain, typically flank and back
	Gross or microscopic hematuria
UTI	Frequency, urgency, dysuria, flank pain, suprapubic tenderness
	Associated pyuria
Miscellaneous	
Abdominal migraine	Acute intermittent non-colicky pain
	Resolves spontaneously over several hours
Functional pain	Recurrent attacks of abdominal pain in the school-aged child
	No vomiting, diarrhea, fever or weight loss
Musculoskeletal	Pain reproduced by palpating contracted abdominal wall muscles
Streptococcal pharyngitis	Pain associated with fever and exudative pharyngitis
	Cervical or submandibular lymphadenopathy
Splenomegaly	Typically associated with viral infection such as Epstein-Barr
Trauma	Duodenal hematoma, liver or spleen laceration, or renal contusion
	Consider abuse if proposed mechanism does not match injury

If the etiology of the abdominal pain is unclear and the patient has persistent, severe symptoms, obtain a CBC, ESR and/or CRP, electrolytes, liver panel, amylase, lipase, urinalysis, and stool guaiac. If the child is too young to verbalize dysuria, obtain urine for culture. Obtain a pregnancy test for any female in whom a pelvic exam is being performed. Patients with severe or focal pain require hospitalization or further ED evaluation.

Follow-up

- No suspicion of a surgical condition, patient appears well, initial laboratory tests normal: primary care follow-up within 1 week

Indications for admission

- Suspected surgical abdomen
- Dehydration or inability to take fluids
- Persistent, severe abdominal pain

Bibliography

Leung A, Sigalet D: Acute abdominal pain in children. *Am Fam Physician* 2003;67:2321–6.

McCollough M, Sharieff GQ: Abdominal pain in children. *Pediatr Clin North Am* 2006; 53:107–37.

Acute pancreatitis

Acute pancreatitis is an infrequent but serious cause of abdominal pain in children. Although there are many conditions associated with pancreatitis (Table 9-2), the common initiating event is injury to the pancreatic acinar cells by the premature activation of digestive enzymes. This damage then attracts inflammatory cells and activates platelets and the complement system. A systemic response to the initial insult ensues, leading to oxidative stress, edema and, in severe cases, necrosis of the gland.

Table 9-2. Etiologies of pancreatitis

Infectious	Mumps, EBV, Coxsackie B, influenza A, varicella, leptospirosis, mycoplasma, HIV, CMV, hepatitis (A, B, C, E)
Metabolic	Hypertriglyceridemia (>1000 mg/dL), hyperlipidemia diabetic ketoacidosis, hypercalcemia
Medication/toxin	Ethyl alcohol, valproic acid, cimetidine, carbamazepine, corticosteroids, tetracycline, erythromycin, isoniazid, pentamidine, metronidazole, furosemide, sulfonamides, metronidazole, organophosphates
Mechanical	Trauma (handlebar injury), gallstones, tumors, choledochal cyst, pancreatic divisum, annular pancreas, status post-ERCP
Other	Idiopathic, hereditary, systemic lupus erythematosus, cystic fibrosis, inflammatory bowel disease

Clinical presentation

The classic symptoms of acute pancreatitis are abdominal pain, nausea, vomiting, and anorexia. The pain is typically located in the epigastrium, right upper quadrant, or peri-umbilical area, with radiation to the back or lower chest. Both the pain and vomiting are worsened by eating.

On physical examination the patient is often tachycardic and may be hypotensive early in the disease. Fever, when present, is often low grade. There may be tenderness in the upper abdomen, and the patient may refuse to lie supine. Guarding, rebound tenderness, abdominal distension, and decreased bowel sounds can suggest an acute surgical abdomen. With severe hemorrhagic pancreatitis, serosanguinous fluid may track through fascial planes resulting in blue discoloration of the flanks (Grey-Turner sign) or the umbilicus (Cullen sign). Signs of ascites (shifting dullness, fluid wave) or pleural effusion (decreased bowel sounds, friction rub, dullness to percussion) may be present if the disease is advanced.

Diagnosis

Obtain a serum amylase and lipase; elevations of three to four times the upper limits of normal suggest pancreatitis. However, acute pancreatitis may occur with a normal amylase, and the amylase may be elevated in a large number of other conditions (Table 9-3). In contrast, lipase is more specific, because virtually all lipase originates from the pancreas. Also, the serum half-life of lipase is longer than amylase, so it is more sensitive in diagnosing pancreatitis in cases that present 3–4 days after the onset of pain.

Table 9-3. Causes of amylase elevation

Pancreatic	Intestinal
Acute or chronic pancreatitis	Appendicitis
Pancreatic tumor	Perforated peptic ulcer
Pancreatic ductal obstruction	Intestinal obstruction
Salivary	*Miscellaneous*
Parotitis	Burns
Salivary duct obstruction	Diabetic ketoacidosis
Trauma	Macroamylasemia
Biliary	Pregnancy (ruptured ectopic)
Cholecystitis	Renal insufficiency
Biliary duct obstruction	

Other laboratory abnormalities that occur with severe pancreatitis include hypocalcemia, hypomagnesemia, hyperglycemia, and hemoconcentration. If there is associated cholelithiasis, there may be elevation of direct bilirubin, gamma-glutamyl transpeptidase (GGT), and alkaline phosphatase.

Radiologic confirmation requires either abdominal ultrasound or a CT scan. Ultrasound can document the presence of a pancreatic pseudocyst, dilated ducts, cholelithiasis, abscesses, and ascites. Abdominal CT scan is helpful in suspected traumatic pancreatitis and can also detect associated injury to the liver, spleen, and duodenum.

ED management

When the diagnosis is suspected, obtain a CBC, electrolytes, glucose, calcium, magnesium, amylase, lipase, albumin, and liver function tests (ALT, AST, GGT, bilirubin, and alkaline phosphatase). If the amylase and/or lipase is elevated, order an ultrasound or abdominal CT.

The management of pancreatitis is largely supportive and begins with keeping the patient NPO in an effort to "rest" the pancreas. Start an IV and aggressively treat signs of hypovolemia with IV fluids. Insert a nasogastric tube if there is persistent vomiting or other evidence of an ileus. Give an H_2 blocker IV to help prevent stress ulceration (ranitidine 2–4 mg/kg per day div q 8 h, 50 mg/dose maximum; famotidine 0.6–0.8 mg/kg per day div q 12 h, 40 mg/dose maximum). Reserve antibiotics for clinical signs of sepsis, necrotic pancreatitis, or multiorgan system failure.

Manage pain with hydromorphone 0.015 mg/kg per dose IV q 4 h PRN (2 mg/dose maximum). Morphine (0.1 mg/kg per dose SC or IV [5 mg maximum] for the initial dose, then titrate subsequent doses to the clinical effect) is safe to use, as it has not been shown to cause spasm of the Sphincter of Oddi. Another alternative is meperidine 1 mg/kg per dose q 4 h, but with repeated doses there is the risk of the accumulation of neurotoxic metabolites, which may cause seizures. If the patient requires multiple doses of narcotic analgesia, use a fentanyl drip or hydromorphone via a patient-controlled analgesia (PCA) pump.

Admission to an ICU is indicated for severe complications such as shock, impending renal failure, hypoxia, or significant metabolic derangements. In addition, supplemental calcium (see p. 182), magnesium, and insulin (pp. 171–172) may be needed.

Indication for admission

• Acute pancreatitis

Bibliography

Kandula L, Lowe ME: Etiology and outcome of acute pancreatitis in infants and toddlers. *J Pediatr* 2008;152:106–10.

Nydegger A, Couper RT, Oliver MR: Childhood pancreatitis. *J Gastroenterol Hepatol* 2006;21:499–509.

Appendicitis

Appendicitis is the most common childhood illness requiring emergency surgery, with a peak incidence between 15 and 24 years. It begins with obstruction of the appendiceal lumen often secondary to an appendicolith or lymphoid hyperplasia. Necrosis of the wall of the appendix ensues, followed by perforation and spillage of stool into the peritoneal cavity with subsequent peritonitis. Early diagnosis is therefore of paramount importance.

Clinical presentation

In uncomplicated appendicitis (prior to rupture), there is a short history (usually <36 hours) of pain, anorexia, nausea, and vomiting in up to 90% of cases. Early in the course colicky or persistent periumbilical pain is typical. The pain then shifts to the right lower quadrant where it is constant and severe. Low-grade fever (<38.3°C; 101°F) is common, and a change in stool pattern occurs in about 15% of patients. Other symptoms may include dysuria or labial, testicular, or penile pain. However, maintain a high index of suspicion, as many patients do not have a "classic" presentation.

On physical examination tenderness is greatest over McBurney's point, one-third of the distance along a line from the anterior superior iliac spine to the umbilicus. There may be positive psoas (pain on passive hip hyperextension consistent with retrocecal appendix) and/or obturator (pain on passive internal rotation of the thigh consistent with pelvic appendix) signs. In the case of a retrocecal appendix, the maximum tenderness and rigidity may remain in the periumbilical area or in the right flank. While palpating the left lower quadrant, discomfort may be elicited in the right lower quadrant (Rovsing's sign). Rigidity of the abdominal wall or involuntary guarding (reflexive spasm of the abdominal wall secondary to peritoneal irritation) is common in cases of perforation.

Perforation of the appendix occurs in 20–40% of patients, although the incidence varies with age. Perforation occurs in 80–100% of children <4 years old; between 10–17 years of age the rate drops to 10–20%. Pain >36 hours, frequent vomiting, dyspnea secondary to elevation of the diaphragm, lethargy in the young child, and a temperature over 38.5°C (101.3°F) suggest rupture. A diffusely tender and rigid abdomen indicates peritonitis.

Diagnosis

Careful physical examination is the key to diagnosing appendicitis. Defer the abdominal and rectal examinations for last. Gently palpate the abdomen beginning away from the right lower quadrant. If the patient's responses do not seem accurate, palpate the abdomen with the membrane of the stethoscope; the child will believe that auscultation, and not palpation, is being performed. Since appendicitis is a progressive disease, increasing abdominal pain, tenderness, and rigidity on serial physical examinations are highly suggestive of the diagnosis.

Try to elicit rebound tenderness, which occurs with inflammation of the peritoneum. In younger children, shake or percuss the abdomen, tap firmly on the feet, or ask the patient to cough, jump down from the table, or hop. In the older patient, depress the abdomen for 15–30 seconds, then remove your hand suddenly. Rebound tenderness is confirmed by finding pain on release, rather than during direct pressure.

Perform a rectal examination in any child suspected of having appendicitis. Right-sided tenderness is consistent with the diagnosis. Hard stool in the vault is suggestive of constipation, which frequently mimics appendicitis.

The differential diagnosis of appendicitis is extensive as shown in Table 9-4. In a sexually active adolescent female ectopic pregnancy, ovarian pathology, and pelvic inflammatory disease may mimic appendicitis. Perform a pelvic exam and obtain urine for a pregnancy test. Perform a genital exam, including the cremasteric reflex, to rule out testicular torsion in a male.

ED management

When the diagnosis is evident from the history and physical examination make the patient NPO, start maintenance IV hydration with $D_5\frac{1}{2}NS$, obtain a CBC, electrolytes, and type and cross-match, and consult a surgeon. If there is evidence of intravascular depletion (orthostatic vital sign changes, delayed capillary refill, hypotension), give the patient a bolus of 20 mL/kg of NS or lactated Ringer's.

In general, abdominal X-rays are not necessary. However, a KUB can suggest constipation if it reveals large amounts of stool. Resolution of the pain after an enema-induced bowel movement (3 mL/kg of a Fleet's enema, patients >10 kg) can be diagnostic. Finding an appendicolith (10% of cases) is compelling evidence of appendicitis in a symptomatic patient. A soft tissue mass or focal ileus in the right lower quadrant is also suggestive.

A focused CT scan with rectal contrast can rule out appendicitis if the appendix fills, but reserve this test for children in whom the diagnosis remains uncertain after a thorough clinical evaluation. If your suspicion of appendicitis is high, also give IV contrast to better evaluate for abscess formation. CT findings in acute appendicitis include: appendicular diameter of >6 mm; appendicolith; pericecal fat stranding; thickening of adjacent bowel walls; free peritoneal fluid; lymphadenopathy; and the presence of a phlegmon.

Conversely, an ultrasound can rule in appendicitis if a fluid-filled, noncompressible, distended, tubular mass >6 mm with no evidence of peristalsis is found. Sonography is rapid, well-tolerated by children, and does not involve ionizing radiation, but it is highly operator-dependent and is much less sensitive in cases of retroperitoneal appendix or obesity. Ultrasound is extremely useful for identifying an inflamed appendix, periappendiceal abscess, or gynecological pathology.

Obtain a chest X-ray if there is tachypnea, rales, or other pulmonary signs such as an elevated WBC in a child with a negative CT scan. A WBC >15 000/mm^3 suggests rupture or another bacterial process (pneumonia, bacterial gastroenteritis). However, do not delay surgical evaluation if the WBC is normal in a patient with a clinical picture that is suggestive of appendicitis.

Table 9-4. Differential diagnosis of appendicitis

Diagnosis	Differentiating features
Viral gastroenteritis	Vomiting prior to, or simultaneously with, abdominal pain
	Abdominal pain relieved by vomiting or a bowel movement
	Diarrhea may be prominent
Bacterial enteritis	Guaiac-positive stools and fecal leukocytosis
Intussusception	Pain and vomiting alternating with periods of lethargy
	Afebrile
	80% of patients are <2 years old
Functional abdominal pain	Recurrent attacks of abdominal pain
	No vomiting, diarrhea, fever, or weight loss
Pneumonia	Tachypnea may be present
Constipation	Pain is non-migratory and is relieved upon defecation
	Stool palpated in descending colon and ampulla
UTI	Frequency, urgency, dysuria, and flank pain
	Pyuria
Bowel obstruction	Crampy, periumbilical pain
	Abdominal distention
Mesenteric adenitis	Diagnosis of exclusion
Hepatitis	RUQ tenderness and jaundice (variable)
Pancreatitis	Epigastric pain that may radiate to the back
Urolithiasis	Colicky pain with gross or microscopic hematuria
Cholelithiasis	RUQ colicky pain
Cholecytitis	RUQ pain with positive Murphy's sign
Diabetic ketoacidosis	Polyuria, polydypsia, polyphagia
	Kussmaul respirations
HSP	Pain may precede the rash
PID	Pain in lower abdomen
	Vaginal discharge or bleeding
Intrauterine pregnancy	Positive pregnancy test
Ectopic pregnancy	Positive pregnancy test, vaginal bleeding
Testicular torsion	Tender, erythematous hemiscrotum
	Abnormal cremasteric reflex
Inflammatory bowel disease	Recurrent episodes of pain
	Bloody diarrhea and abdominal distention

Serum electrolytes may be helpful in patients with abdominal pain and dehydration. A low serum sodium (<130 mEq/L) may reflect third spacing of fluids from the ileus associated with appendicitis. A urinalysis is necessary to rule out DKA (glycosuria and ketonuria) or a UTI (pyuria). Although there can be WBCs in the urine with an appendicitis, bacteriuria is typically absent. A pelvic examination and pregnancy test are necessary for post-menarchal females with abdominal pain.

Once the diagnosis of appendicitis has been made, and agreed upon by the surgical team, start antibiotic therapy. If a nonperforated appendicitis is suspected, give cefoxitin (30 mg/kg per dose q 6 h, 12 g/day maximum) or cefotetan (30 mg/kg per day div q 12 h, 6 g/day maximum) IV, while awaiting appendectomy. If a perforated appendicitis is suspected, give broader antibiotic coverage to prevent or minimize intraperitoneal abscess formation. Use monotherapy with a very broad-spectrum antibiotic such as piperacillin-tazobactam (350 mg/kg per day div q 6 h, 3 g/dose maximum; use 175 mg/kg per day for infants <6 months) IV.

The appropriate use of analgesia does not impair diagnostic accuracy. Give morphine SC or IV (0.1 mg/kg, 5 mg maximum for the initial dose; titrate subsequent doses based upon clinical effect). Do not use nonsteroidal medications such as ketorolac if there is a possibility of surgical intervention, as this class of drugs inhibits platelet function and can cause excessive bleeding.

When appendicitis cannot be excluded, obtain a surgical consultation and admit the patient for IV hydration and observation (NPO).

Follow-up
- If appendicitis seems highly unlikely, have the patient return in 6–8 hours (still symptomatic) or sooner, if the symptoms intensify. Prescribe a clear liquid diet and no analgesics

Indication for admission
- Suspected appendicitis

Bibliography

Bundy DG, Byerley JS, Liles EA, et al: Does this child have appendicitis? *JAMA* 2007;298:438–51.

Goldin AB, Sawin RS, Garrison MM, Zerr DM, Christakis DA: Aminoglycoside-based triple-antibiotic therapy versus monotherapy for children with ruptured appendicitis. *Pediatrics* 2007;119:905–11.

McCollough M, Sharieff GQ: Abdominal pain in children. *Pediatr Clin North Am* 2006;53:107–37.

Puig S, Staudenherz A, Felder-Puig R, Paya K: Imaging of appendicitis in children and adolescents: useful or useless? A comparison of imaging techniques and a critical review of the current literature. *Semin Roentgenol* 2008; 43:22–8.

Assessment and management of dehydration
The most common causes of dehydration in children are vomiting and diarrhea.

Clinical presentation and diagnosis
Dehydration is classified by the percentage of total body water lost: mild (<5%), moderate (5–10%), and severe (>10%). A variety of signs and symptoms and ancillary data help to

Table 9-5. Assessment of degree of dehydration

Signs/symptoms	Mild (< 5%)	Moderate (5–10%)	Severe (> 10%)
Tachycardia	+/−	+	+
Dry mucous membranes	+	+	+
Depressed fontanelle	−	+	+
Sunken eyeballs	−	+	+
Abnormal skin turgor	−	+/−	+
Decreased urine output	+/−	+	+
Capillary refill time >2 s	−	+/−	+
Weak peripheral pulses	−	−	+
Hypotension	−	−	+
Hyperpnea	−	−	+
Altered mental status	−	+/−	+
Urine specific gravity	normal/high	normal/high	high
Serum acidosis	−	+/−	+

distinguish the degree of dehydration (Table 9-5). A mildly dehydrated child has dry mucous membranes and decreased urinary output with a urine specific gravity under 1.020. If the child is moderately dehydrated there are additional signs and symptoms of dehydration such as tachycardia, orthostatic changes in heart rate and blood pressure, and a depressed fontanelle in an infant. Urine specific gravity is generally greater than 1.030. A severely dehydrated child appears ill and listless and has prolonged capillary refill (>2 s), tachypnea or hyperpnea, sunken eyeballs and abnormal skin turgor (tenting). The urine specific gravity is greater than 1.035 and there is a metabolic acidosis.

ED management
The management priorities are stabilization of the patient's vital signs, replenishment of the intravascular volume and correction of electrolyte abnormalities. Assess the degree of dehydration and check for orthostatic changes in a patient old enough to cooperate. Measure the pulse and blood pressure with the patient supine for 5 minutes, and again after standing or sitting upright for 2 minutes. A pulse increase > 20 bpm and/or a fall in systolic BP > 20 mmHg are positive orthostatic findings. If the patient complains of weakness or dizziness while sitting, the test is positive. Do not have the patient stand.

No dehydration
If the patient has diarrhea but is not dehydrated and appears well, give clear fluids to maintain hydration, as well as an age-appropriate diet as tolerated. Allow a breast-fed infant to continue to nurse. If the patient also is vomiting give small amounts of clear fluids (see Mild and moderate dehydration below). Make sure that all infants and children patients can tolerate oral fluids prior to discharge.

Mild and moderate dehydration

A patient with mild or moderate dehydration can be orally rehydrated, if willing and able to tolerate fluids.

Vomiting

If the patient has been vomiting, wait 1 hour after the last vomiting episode to initiate oral fluids. For infants and toddlers, use a rehydration or maintenance solution containing 45–50 mEq/L of sodium and 25–30 g/L of glucose (Pedialyte, Infalyte, etc.). Treat an older child with an oral electrolyte solution, tea, decarbonated soda, or fruit juice. Give an infant (<1 year of age) small (5–10 mL) aliquots and an older child a larger amount (10–20 mL) of fluid every 5–15 minutes, over the next hour. Then reassess the hydration status. If the patient vomits once or twice more, give one dose of odansetron. When the patient looks well and has stopped vomiting, discharge him or her with written instructions on how to advance the diet. Instruct the parent to double the volume every hour until the child is taking 60 mL every 20 minutes without vomiting. If the patient vomits at home, instruct the parents to wait an hour, and then begin again with 10–20 mL every 15 minutes and advance every hour. If vomiting persists and the child is unable to tolerate small amounts of fluids, instruct the parent to return to the ED or contact the primary care provider. When the child patient is tolerating 60 mL every 20 minutes, the liquid diet volume can be liberalized, but restrict the diet to clear liquids for 12 hours.

Once it is clear that the child can tolerate fluids, instruct the parents to give breast milk or full-strength formula to infants and to offer carbohydrate foods, if the patient eats solid food. For an infant, recommend bananas and other fruit, cereals (mixed with formula or water), and starchy vegetables. An older patient may have rice or noodles, toast with jelly, fruits, starchy vegetables, crackers, clear soup, and chicken, in addition to the above foods. If the child continues to feel well after 48 hours, milk and other foods may be added to the diet.

Diarrhea

Start oral rehydration with an electrolyte solution (Pedialyte, Infalyte, etc.). Give a total volume of 40–50 mL/kg in small aliquots (15–30 mL) over a 3–4 hour period, while doing hourly reassessments of hydration status. Failure of oral rehydration (inability to take adequate volume orally, excessive ongoing losses) is an indication for IV rehydration therapy. Once the initial rehydration is tolerated, resume giving milk (breast or formula) to an infant, whether breast or formula fed. An infant who has large, watery stools can have the milk feedings supplemented with feedings of an oral electrolyte solution. For older infants and toddlers already taking solid foods, recommend an electrolyte solution, clear soup, or decarbonated soda with a low-fat carbohydrate diet. Recommend bananas and other fruits – rice, pasta, potatoes, bread with jam, and crackers are other options. Milk can usually be successfully reintroduced by the second day. Anti-diarrheal compounds and anti-motility agents have no role in the management of acute diarrhea.

Severe dehydration

IV fluid restoration is necessary for severe dehydration, shock, altered mental status or if the patient is unable to take fluids orally or has an altered mental status.

Initial intravascular restoration

Give fluid resuscitation with a 20 mL/kg bolus of normal saline or lactated Ringer's solution over 20–30 minutes. Obtain blood for electrolytes, BUN, creatinine, and glucose. Also obtain a urinalysis, and if the urine contains large ketones or if the child is hypoglycemic add 2 mL/kg of D_{25} (0.5 g/kg of glucose) to the bolus solution. After the first bolus reevaluate the patient using parameters such as vital signs, the presence or correction of orthostatic changes, and capillary refill. If there is a poor response to the initial bolus, repeat the infusion. However, patients with renal or cardiac disease are at risk for developing congestive heart failure and patients with sickle cell disease are at risk for acute chest syndrome; be extremely careful when assessing their fluid status. If there is a poor response to two IV boluses consider other associated organ disease or the need for central venous monitoring before giving a third bolus. Following the restoration of adequate intravascular volume, assess the need for replacement of fluid and electrolyte deficits. Calculate maintenance fluids using the Holiday-Segar method:

100 mL/kg per day for the first 10 kg (1000 mL/day) or 4 mL/kg/h for the first 10 kg

50 mL/kg per day for the next 10 kg (500 mL/day) or 2 mL/kg/h for the next 10 kg

20 mL/kg per day for each additional kg or 1 mL/kg/h for each additional kg

Replacement of fluid and electrolyte deficits

Isotonic dehydration – In isotonic dehydration the serum sodium is between 130 mEq/L and 150 mEq/L. Estimate the percent of dehydration either by physical signs and symptoms or more accurately, if a recent premorbid weight is known, although the accuracy of scales varies. Multiply the percent of dehydration by the weight of the child to calculate the fluid deficit (e.g. 10% dehydration × 20 kg child = a deficit of 2 L). Administer maintenance fluid requirements plus half of the deficit over the first 8 hours and the second half over the following 16 hours. Sodium requirements are 2–4 mEq/kg per day. In general, either $D_5\frac{1}{2}NS$ (> 2 years of age) or $D_5\frac{1}{3}NS$ (<2 years of age) is an adequate solution. Potassium requirements are 2–3 mEq/kg per day. After the patient has voided, add potassium chloride (20–40 mEq/L) to the IV bag.

Hypotonic dehydration – Hypotonic dehydration occurs when salt losses exceed water losses or when water intake exceeds required salt intake. Hyponatremia is defined as serum sodium <130 mEq/L. Use the following formula to calculate the sodium deficit to be added to the replacement fluids (see Hyponatremia, pp. 186–189):

mEq sodium required for replacement = (125 − measured sodium)

× (premorbid body weight in kg) × 0.6

Give the sodium replacement over 4 hours, but do not exceed a rate of correction of more than 0.5–1 mEq/h. An excessively rapid correction of the serum sodium may be associated with central pontine myelinolysis.

Symptomatic hyponatremia (seizures) requires a more rapid correction with hypertonic 3% saline. Three percent saline contains 513 mEq/L of Na, so that every 2 mL contains 1 mEq Na. The initial goal is to raise the serum sodium by 5 mEq, which is usually sufficient to terminate the seizures; do not exceed a rate of correction of 2 mEq/h. One mL/kg of

3% NaCl will increase the plasma sodium by approximately 1 mEq/L. Calculate the amount of 3% NaCl (mL) required as follows:

3% NaCl(mEq/L) = (125 − measured Na) × premorbid weight(kg) × 0.6

Multiple the results by 2 to determine the volume in mL.

Hypertonic dehydration – Hypernatremia is defined as a serum sodium greater than > 150 mEq/L. It occurs when solute-free water losses exceed salt losses or in the context of excessive salt intake. The degree of dehydration is more difficult to determine in these patients because the extracellular fluid space is preserved. The skin may have normal turgor but feel doughy. Calculate the free water deficit as follows:

Solute-free water deficit (mL) = (measured sodium − 145)

× 4mL/kg × (premorbid weight in kg)

(Use 3 mL/kg for serum sodium >170 mEq/L.)

Because of the potential for neurologic complications correct the serum sodium and free water deficit slowly over 48 hours, with a daily sodium decrease of 10–15 mEq/L (approximately 0.5 mEq/h). In general, $D_5\frac{1}{2}NS$ is an appropriate solution. Add one ampule of 10% calcium gluconate to each 500 mL of replacement fluid. Also, add 40 mEq/L of potassium acetate after the patient voids (see Hypernatremia, pp. 177–180).

Calculation examples

10 kg (premorbid weight) child with 10% isotonic dehydration (sodium = 140 mEq/L)

Fluid deficit (L) = premorbid weight (kg) × % dehydration
Fluid deficit (L) = 10 kg ×.10 = 1 L
Maintenance fluid = 100 mL/kg per day = 1000 mL
Sodium deficit (mEq) = fluid deficit (L) × % Na from ECF × Na (mEq/L) concentration in ECF
Sodium deficit = 1L × 0.6 × 140 mEq/L = 84 mEq
Maintenance sodium requirements = 3 mEq/kg per day = 30 mEq

Give half of deficit in the first 8 hours and the remaining half in the next 16 hours. Divide the maintenance evenly over 24 hours.
First 8 hours: fluid deficit 500 mL + maintenance 333 mL = 833 mL/8 h = 104 mL/h
Sodium deficit 42 mEq + maintenance 10 mEq = 52 mEq
Sodium concentration: 52 mEq/0.833L = 62 mEq/L

10 kg (premorbid weight) child with 10% hypotonic dehydration (sodium 115 mEq/L)

Fluid deficit and maintenance (as above)
Sodium deficit and maintenance (as above)
Additional sodium deficit = (desired Na mEq/L − measured Na mEq/L) × % Na from ECF (L/kg) × weight (kg)
Additional sodium deficit = (135 − 115) × 0.6 × 10 = 120 mEq

Give half of deficit in the first 8 hours and the remaining half in over the next 16 hours; divide the maintenance evenly over 24 hours.

First 8 hours:

Fluid deficit and maintenance = 833 mL/8 h = 104 mL/h (as above)

Sodium (deficit + maintenance) = 52 mEq (as above)

Additional sodium deficit = 60 mEq

Sodium concentration: (52 mEq + 60 mEq)/0.833 L = 134 mEq/L

10 kg (premorbid weight) child with 10% hypertonic dehydration (sodium 160 mEq/L)

Fluid deficit and maintenance (as above)

Sodium maintenance (as above)

Solute-free water deficit = 4 mL/kg × weight (kg) × (measured sodium – desired sodium)

Solute-free water deficit = 4 mL/kg × 10 kg × (160–145) = 600 mL

Solute fluid deficit = total fluid deficit – free water deficit

Solute fluid deficit = 1000 mL – 600 mL = 400 mL (0.4L)

Solute sodium deficit = solute fluid deficit (L) × (% sodium from ECF) × (desired sodium mEq/L)

Solute sodium deficit = 0.4L × 0.6 × 145 mEq/L = 35 mEq

Give half of the free water deficit + the total solute fluid deficit + solute sodium deficit + maintenance sodium and fluid divided over the first 24 hours.

Fluids: 300 mL + 400 mL + 1000 mL = 1700 mL/day = 71 mL/h

Sodium maintenance + solute sodium deficit = 65 mEq

Sodium concentration: (65 mEq/1.7 L = 38 mEq/L

Follow-up

- Mild or moderate dehydration: Primary care follow-up the next day or return to the ED if unable to tolerate oral fluids

Indications for admission

- Significant ongoing fluid losses and/or inability to tolerate oral fluids
- Severe dehydration
- Hypotonic or hypertonic dehydration

Bibliography

Atherly-John YC, Cunningham SJ, Crain EF: A randomized trial of oral vs. intravenous rehydration in a pediatric emergency department. *Arch Pediatr Adolesc Med* 2002;156:1240–3.

Custer JW, Rau RE: *Johns Hopkins: Harriet Lane Handbook*, 18th ed. St. Louis: Mosby-Year Book, 2009, pp. 301–325.

King CK, Glass R, Bresee JS, Dugan C, Centers for Disease Control and Prevention, et al.: Managing acute gastroenteritis among children: oral rehydration, maintenance and nutritional therapy. *MMWR Recomm Rep* 2003;52 (RR-16):1–16.

Steiner MJ, DeWalt DA, Byerley JS: Is this child dehydrated? *JAMA* 2004;291:2746–54.

Colic

Colic (paroxysmal fussing of infancy) is a well-accepted entity whose etiology and pathogenesis are poorly understood.

Clinical presentation

Typically, at 2 or 3 weeks of age, an otherwise well baby begins to become fussy with periods of prolonged crying. The behavior peaks at 2 months and typically resolves by 3 months of age, although in 30% of cases the symptoms extend into the fourth and fifth months of life.

In mild cases, the fussiness occurs only in the evening or has some other regular diurnal pattern. There may be associated rhythmic kicking, grimacing, and flatus. Vomiting, diarrhea, constipation, and failure to thrive are not features of colic, and in between episodes the infant appears comfortable and alert. The crying may not respond to the parents' attempts at comforting or may stop only to resume when the infant is put down. Notably, the physical and neurologic examinations are normal. In the ED, the parents are concerned about the baby being ill, or they are exhausted and want relief.

Diagnosis

The key to making the diagnosis of colic is the parents' statement that the infant is perfectly fine between paroxysms. Perform a complete physical examination. If the baby cries during the examination, have him or her suck on a gloved finger or nipple. If this does not stop the crying, place the infant in the prone position or over your shoulder. When distracted, the colicky baby will appear alert and will suck vigorously on a nipple or pacifier. Upon gentle palpation, the abdomen is soft and nontender.

Several conditions other than colic can present as nothing more than fussiness or excessive crying. Therefore, a thorough history and physical examination must be completed. See Table 9-6 for the differential diagnosis of colic.

ED management

The goal of the ED examination is to rule out other conditions that can present with colicky pain. Perform a complete physical examination, including a rectal exam with stool for guaiac. Once the diagnosis is made, reassure the parents that the infant is not seriously ill and that colic is a self-limited phenomenon among well infants. There is no definite cure or universally accepted therapy for colic. Instead, the lack of a recognized etiology has led to the existence of a number of controversial remedies. Dispel any of the commonly held myths about colic, including that medications are beneficial, that infants are "spoiled" by excessive holding, and that colic is caused by parental inexperience and anxiety. Reassure the parents and offer them suggestions that may mitigate a crying attack, such as increased holding and rocking of the baby, more frequent feeding, use of a pacifier, and environmental changes (stroller ride, infant swing, car ride).

If there is suspicion of cow's milk allergy, refer the family to a primary care provider, who may decide to change to an elemental formula. Do not advise a nursing mother to discontinue breast-feeding, but have her try a dairy-free diet for several days. Avoid antispasmodics, which have not proved effective and may have side effects. Encourage the parents to burp the infant frequently during and after the feeding if they are not already doing so.

Table 9-6. Differential diagnosis of colic

Diagnosis	Differentiating features
Allergic colitis	Guaiac-positive stools
Congenital glaucoma	Excessive tearing; abnormal red reflex
Congestive heart failure	Tachypnea and diaphoresis during feeding; failure to thrive
Constipation/diarrhea	Change in stooling pattern; anal fissure
Corneal abrasion	Conjunctival hyperemia, excessive tearing
Gastroesophageal reflux	Regurgitation; irritability related to feeds
Hair tourniquet syndrome	Swelling of a digit, penis, or clitoris
Incarcerated hernia	Mass in inguinal region
Infantile spasms	Attacks occur in clusters throughout the day
Infection/sepsis	Fever, vomiting, diarrhea, lethargy, or decreased feeding
SVT	Pallor, poor feeding
Trauma	Swelling over affected site; decreased movement

Follow-up

- Primary care follow-up within the week
- Arrange for psychosocial support if the family can no longer cope with the crying

Bibliography

Fireman L: Colic. *Pediatr Rev* 2006;27:357–8.

Savino F: Focus on infantile colic. *Acta Paediatr* 2007;96:1259–64.

Wade S: Extracts from "clinical evidence": Infantile colic. *BMJ* 2006;439–47.

Constipation

Constipation is either a delay or difficulty in defecation, which then persists for at least 2 weeks. Most often, constipation is a transient disturbance precipitated by a medication, brief illness, anal fissure, traumatic toileting experience, or a period of poor diet. While a very small number of patients have an organic disorder causing their constipation, it remains a common cause of abdominal pain and ED visits.

Clinical presentation

In infancy, stools tend to be pasty or "mustard-like" in consistency. More than 90% of infants in the first 3 months of life have between one and seven bowel movements per day, although the frequency in breast-fed infants ranges from a small stool with each feeding to one soft stool every 7 days. It is common for an infant to strain and grunt with defecation and the passage of soft stools; this does not represent constipation. Rather, stool consistency (hard, pellet-like or adult-like formed stools) defines constipation in infancy.

After infancy, the most common presentation of constipation is hard, infrequent, large, or painful stools. The toddler may voluntarily withhold large stools, leading to chronic incomplete evacuation and subsequent impaction and fecal incontinence (encopresis). Therefore, neither a history of soft stool consistency nor daily bowel movements rules out constipation. After the child is toilet trained, constipation is frequently not recognized unless there are other related symptoms. In a school-age child, constipation may be associated with acute or chronic abdominal pain, which may be so intense that it can mimic appendicitis or intussusception. Young girls may also present with recurrent urinary tract infections.

Diagnosis

The vast majority of patients will have functional or idiopathic constipation, with no objective evidence of a pathologic condition. In most cases, a thorough history and physical examination is sufficient to make the diagnosis.

Always ask about the onset and duration of symptoms, whether there was delay in passing meconium at birth (>24 h), and whether there were symptoms in the neonatal period. Obtain a complete dietary history, including fluid intake, toileting history, and medication use (including prior therapy for constipation). Establish whether there are associated symptoms such as abdominal distension, vomiting, poor weight gain and growth, or the recent onset of gait abnormalities, urinary incontinence or lower extremity weakness.

On physical examination, assess growth by plotting the child's weight and height on a growth chart. On the abdominal examination, determine whether there is distension or palpable retained stool in the abdomen. Perform a careful neurologic examination of the lower extremities focusing on tone, strength, reflexes, sensation, and gait. Inspect the perineal tissues and anus for local inflammation, fissures, or fecal soiling. Assess placement of the anus relative to the tip of the coccyx and the vaginal fourchette or base of the scrotum.

Before performing a rectal examination, inspect the sacrum for signs of a hair tuft or deep dimple that may indicate an underlying spinal anomaly. Then, assess anal sphincter tone, rectal size, and the size and consistency of stool in the rectum. A properly done rectal examination should not be painful or traumatic to the child. The differential diagnosis of constipation appears in Table 9-7.

It is unnecessary to obtain an abdominal X-ray when attempting to diagnose consti- pation, if the rectum is filled with large amounts of stool. However, an X-ray may be helpful in the child with a history that strongly suggests constipation, but without evidence of impaction on physical examination.

ED management

The ultimate goals of treatment are to establish dietary and behavioral patterns in the child and family that compensate for a tendency to constipation. This includes increas- ing dietary fiber and fluid intake, as well as altering toileting behavior utilizing the gastrocolic reflex. In the emergency department, rescue management includes rectal disimpaction if the patient is in severe discomfort. As an alternative, administer a Fleets enema (3 mL/kg for children >10 kg), which can be repeated once. Use an adult Fleets enema for children weighing ≥40 kg. Medical management is necessary at home to stimulate gastrointestinal motility and hydrate the stool while dietary and behavioral adjustments are made.

A summary of pharmacologic products indicated in the treatment of constipation can be found in Table 9-8. The choice of medication(s) depends upon the patient's age and whether fecal impaction is present. For infants <1 year old, dietary changes are key.

Table 9-7. Etiologies of constipation

Functional/idiopathic

Developmental	Cognitive impairment
	Attention deficit disorder
Situational	Coercive toilet training
	Toilet phobia
	School bathroom avoidance
	Excessive parental interventions
	Sexual abuse
Psychiatric	Depression
Reduced stool volume	Low fiber diet; dehydration
	Underfeeding

Organic

Gastrointestinal	Milk protein allergy
	Hirschsprung's disease
	Gluten enteropathy
Anatomic malformations	Imperforate anus, anal stenosis
	Anteriorly displaced anus
	Pelvic mass
Metabolic	Hypothyroidism; hypercalcemia
	Cystic fibrosis
	Diabetes mellitus
Neuropathic	Spinal cord abnormalities (tethered cord, trauma)
	Static encephalopathy
Abnormal musculature	Prune belly
	Gastroschisis
	Down syndrome
Drugs	Opiates, phenobarbital, sucralfate, antacids, antihypertensives; anticholinergics; antidepressants, sympathomimetics
Other	Heavy metal ingestion (lead)
	Vitamin D intoxication
	Botulism

Table 9-8. Treatment of constipation

Medication	Dose	Notes
Osmotic agents		
Lactulose	1–3 mL/kg per day in div doses (70% solution)	Flatulence, cramping
Sorbitol	1–3 mL/kg per day in div doses (70% solution)	Same as Lactulose
Barley malt extract	2–10 mL/240 mL of milk or juice	Unpleasant odor, good for bottle feeders
Magnesium hydroxide	1–3 mL/kg per day of 400 mg/5 mL	Can cause Mg poisoning in infants
	Also available as 800 mg/5 mL	
Magnesium citrate	<6 yrs 1–3 mL/kg per day div q day or bid	Same as Mg hydroxide
	6–12 yrs: 100–150 mL/day div q day or bid	
	>12 yrs: 150–300 mL/day div q day or bid	
PEG solution	Disimpact: 1–1.5 g/kg per day for 3 days	
	Maintenance: 1 g/kg per day	
PEG powder (Miralax)	<12 yrs 1 g/kg per day (maximum 17 g); >12 yrs 17 g/day	Mix in 8 oz juice or water
		Single or divided doses
Phosphate enema	6 mL/kg up to 135 mL (do not use if <2 yrs)	Risk of severe ↑phosphate with ↓calcium
Lubricants		
Mineral oil	Disimpact: 15–30 mL/yr of age (240 mL/day maximum)	Lipoid pneumonia if aspirated
	Maintenance: 1–3 mL/kg per day (do not use if <1 yr)	
Stimulants		
Senna	2–6 yrs 2.5–7.5 mL/day; 6–12 yrs 5–15 mL/day	Idiosyncratic hepatitis
	(8.8 mg sennosides/5 mL)	Melanosis coli
Bisacodyl (Dulcolax)	≥2 yrs 0.5–1 suppository	Abdominal pain; hypokalemia
Stool softeners		
Docosate sodium (Colace)	<3 yrs 10–40 mg/day; 3–6 yrs 20–60 mg/day	Very bitter, give with tasty liquid
	6–12 yrs 40–150 mg/day; >12 yrs 50–400 mg/day	Divide into 1–4 daily doses

Increase the fluid intake, especially juices containing sorbitol (prune, pear, apple) and institute a 1-week trial of a hydrolyzed formula such as Carnation Good Start. For infants <2 months of age, mix the juice with water in a 1:1 ratio, titrating intake according to stool consistency. Barley malt extract, corn syrup, or lactulose can also be used as stool softeners. Dark Karo syrup is safe and not a potential source of *Clostridium botulinum*; add 1 teaspoon to 2–4 oz of water, titrating the intake according to stool consistency. Do not use mineral oil, because of the risk of aspiration and the development of lipoid pneumonia. Prescribe polyethylene glycol electrolyte (PEG) solution (1 g/kg up to 17 g in juice daily) for children >2 years for at least 1 month or until follow-up is ensured while behavioral and dietary changes are under way.

Follow-up

• Constipation without impaction: primary care follow-up in 1–2 weeks
• Impaction: 2 days

Indications for admission

• Severe constipation with emesis and dehydration
• Serious underlying disorder (Hirschsprung's disease)

Bibliography

Montgomery DF, Navarro F: Management of constipation and encopresis in children. *J Pediatr Health Care* 2008;22:199–204.

North American Society for Pediatric Gastroenterology, Hepatology and Nutrition: Evaluation and treatment of constipation in children: summary of updated recommendations of the North American Society for Pediatric gastroenterology, Hepatology and Nutrition. *J Pediatr Gastroenterol Nutr* 2006;43: 405–7.

Diarrhea

Gastroenteritis is secondary only to respiratory illness as a cause of childhood morbidity worldwide. In the United States, acute gastroenteritis is responsible for 4% of all outpatient visits and up to 10% of hospitalizations among children under 5 years of age.

In developed countries with a temperate climate, most gastroenteritis is caused by viral infection; bacterial, parasitic, and protozoal illnesses are less frequent but not uncommon. In viral infection, diarrhea is non-inflammatory and results from an enteropathy in which the death of mature villus-tip cells (responsible for disaccharide digestion and monosaccharide absorption) causes an osmotic diarrhea due to the malabsorption of sugars. The pathophysiology of bacterial diarrhea involves a combination of impaired water absorption due to the inflammatory process and often a secretory toxin elaborated by the bacteria. Invasive bacterial disease in the colon results in frequent, small, bloody, often mucoid stools known as dysentery. Occasionally, both toxic and inflammatory processes are operative.

Clinical presentation

The symptoms and signs of gastroenteritis are vomiting, abdominal pain, and diarrhea typically with fever. See Table 9-9 for the more common causes of acute diarrhea and their differentiating features.

Table 9-9. Differential diagnosis of acute diarrhea

Diagnosis	Differentiating features
Rotavirus	Peak age <2 years; wintertime
	Fever, vomiting, watery, nonbloody diarrhea
Norovirus (Norwalk virus)	Epidemic outbreaks; school-age to adults
	Watery, nonbloody diarrhea
	Can have headache, malaise, and myalgias
Enteric adenovirus	Peak age <4 years; year-round
	Watery, nonbloody diarrhea
Salmonella (non-typhi)	Abdominal cramps; bloody diarrhea
	Bacteremia in 5–10% of infant cases
	Sources: contaminated meat/eggs/poultry; reptiles
Enterohemorrhagic *E. coli*	Peak age <5 years; summertime
	Watery, then bloody diarrhea; severe abdominal pain
	Can lead to HUS
	Sources: undercooked meat, unpasteurized milk/cider
Enterotoxigenic *E. coli*	Major cause of traveler's diarrhea
	Moderate abdominal pain; watery diarrhea
Shigella	Risk factors: daycare or crowded conditions
	Can have high fever; voluminous, bloody stools
	Seizures can occur early and precede the diarrhea
Campylobacter	Watery or bloody stools
	Most <1 week duration, but can be prolonged IBD-like
	Sources: undercooked poultry, unpasteurized milk, pets
Yersinia enterocolitica	More common in young children and in cooler climates
	Can mimic appendicitis in older children
	Sources: undercooked pork, unpasteurized milk, well water
Giardia lamblia	Epidemics: daycare, contaminated water
	Afebrile; foul-smelling stools; flatulence; distention
Other infections	Associated with UTI, otitis media, sepsis, pneumonia
Antibiotic-related	*C. difficile*: fever, toxicity, pain
	Mucoid or bloody stools
Toddler's diarrhea	Viral gastroenteritis weeks to months prior
	Large stools with food particles; exacerbated by juice
Milk protein allergy	Presents <3 months old with mucoid, bloody stools

Table 9-9. (cont.)

Diagnosis	Differentiating features
Appendicitis	Periumbilical then RLQ pain
	Vomiting predominates
Intussusception	Intermittent colicky abdominal pain
	Currant jelly stools
Onset of chronic illness	IBD; celiac disease; cystic fibrosis

Table 9-10. Stool studies

Gross examination

Blood, mucus, pus: bacterial infection

Microscopic examination

Add 1–2 drops of methylene blue to stool mucus

Cover with a coverslip

Look for WBCs under high-dry power

>5 WBC/HPF: bacterial infection

Chemical examination

Stool pH: Extract water from diaper and check with urine dipstick

pH ≤5: viral infection or carbohydrate malabsorption

Stool-reducing substances:

In a test tube, mix 2 drops of stool water with 10 drops of tap water.

Add Clinitest tablet and check for reducing substances (compare to accompanying chart in Clinitest box).

Positive reducing substances: viral infection or carbohydrate malabsorption

Diagnosis

Inquire about the onset and duration of symptoms (acute diarrhea lasts <2 weeks), the frequency and volume of diarrhea, the appearance of the stool, and associated symptoms such as fever and vomiting. Determine what and how much the child has been eating and drinking. The sorbitol in apple and grape juice may exacerbate diarrhea. Ask about the child's urine output and general activity level.

If there is a history of persistent (>2 weeks) or bloody diarrhea, test the stool for fecal leukocytes and blood (see Table 9-10); obtain a stool culture if the tests are positive or the illness otherwise suggests a bacterial etiology.

With a viral diarrhea, malabsorbed sugars are present either as reducing substances or converted to acids, and fecal leukocytes are absent. If indicated (i.e. cohorting of patients during an epidemic, diagnosis unclear, unusually sick patient), send a stool sample for rapid enzyme immunoassay for rotavirus. However, if the stools are grossly bloody, obtain a culture for bacterial pathogens (*E. coli* 0157:H7, *Salmonella*, *Shigella*, *Yersinia*, *Campylobacter*, *C. difficile* toxin).

E. coli 0157:H7 is responsible for 90% of cases of the hemolytic uremic syndrome (HUS) in the United States. HUS occurs 3–12 days after the onset of diarrhea and is characterized by a triad of microangiopathic hemolytic anemia, thrombocytopenia, and oliguria or anuria. Clinically the child is pale, irritable, and edematous. Obtain a CBC with platelet count, BUN, creatinine, and electrolytes if the patient has proven *E. coli* 0157:H7 infection or is suspected of having HUS.

With milk protein allergy, all stool cultures are negative, and typically the bleeding stops after switching to an elemental formula (Nutramigen, Alimentum) or eliminating cow's milk from the mother's diet in a breast-fed infant. In 20–40% of cases, there is cross-reaction with soy formula.

Consider inflammatory bowel disease in children who have either persistent or bloody diarrhea or diarrhea in conjunction with constitutional symptoms, fever, weight loss, oral ulcers, arthralgia, or uveitis. A neuroblastoma or ganglioneuroma may cause chronic watery diarrhea, while bulky, greasy, foul-smelling stools are associated with celiac disease, cystic fibrosis, and pancreatic insufficiency.

ED management

The goals of management include: (1) recognition, treatment, and prevention of dehydration; (2) prescription of dietary therapy that maximizes nutrient retention; (3) recognition of invasive or potentially invasive infection; and (4) management of the public health aspects of acute gastroenteritis.

Determination of hydration status is the first priority. Use the patient's premorbid weight, vital signs, and clinical characteristics (Table 9-1) to estimate the degree of dehydration. See pp. 229–234 for the management of dehydration.

Continue to feed milk (formula or breast) to an infant, or an age-appropriate diet to a child, if the patient is not dehydrated or as soon as rehydration is complete. Guidelines do not exist for the use of a soy formula in acute infantile gastroenteritis with suspected temporary lactase deficiency. However, it is reasonable to prescribe a switch to a soy formula for an infant less than 6 months of age who develops dehydration, is malnourished (less than 5th percentile weight for height), has a significant underlying medical condition, or has diarrhea that does not improve on cow's milk formula after 5 days of illness. As a general rule, do not recommend pharmacologic agents to treat acute diarrhea.

Empiric antibiotic treatment of suspected bacterial gastroenteritis is rarely necessary and may prolong *Salmonella* excretion. More importantly, antibiotic treatment has been epidemiologically linked to HUS and a worse outcome in *E. coli* 0157:H7 infection. The treatment of *E. coli* 0157:H7 is supportive, but consult a nephrologist in the event that HUS develops.

Treat proven *Shigella* with trimethoprim-sulfamethoxazole (8 mg/kg per day of TMP div bid) for 5 days and *Campylobacter* with erythromycin (40 mg/kg per day div tid or qid) for 5–7 days. Guidelines for treating *Salmonella* in infants are presented in Table 9-11. Do not treat uncomplicated, noninvasive *Salmonella* infections unless the patient is less than 3 months of age, immunocompromised, has chronic gastrointestinal disease (inflammatory bowel disease, celiac disease), or has severe colitis.

Table 9-11. Management of infants less than 1 year with diarrhea not requiring hospitalization at the initial visit

	Age	Management
I. First evaluation		
A. Colitis (dysentery fecal WBCs)	0–12 months	Stool culture
		CBC and blood culture if <3 months or if child appears ill
B. No colitis or diarrhea <5 days	0–12 months	No stool culture
		Evaluate for nonbacterial causes if indicated
C. Exposure to *Salmonella*	0–3 months	Stool and blood cultures
		CBC
II. Follow-up evaluation		
A. Diarrhea ≥5 days	0–12 months	Stool culture
B. Stool culture positive[a] and blood culture positive	0–12 months	Admit[b] and treat with antibiotics[c]
C. Stool culture positive[a] and blood culture negative		
1. Toxic, ill, immunocompromised	0–12 months	Admit[b] and treat with antibiotics[c]
2. Febrile, well-appearing	≤3 months	Admit[b] and treat with antibiotics[c]
3. Febrile, improving	3–12 months	Blood culture
		TMP-SMX[d] (blood culture pending)
4. Afebrile, improving	≤3 months	Oral antibiotics[e]
	3–12 months	Reexamine and observe at home
D. Stool culture positive[a] but blood culture not obtained at first visit		
		See category IIC
		CBC and blood culture

Notes: [a]Stool culture positive for salmonella.
[b] Includes evaluation for focal infection of meninges, bone, urinary tract, and other sites.
[c] Cefotaxime or ceftriaxone.
[d] 8 mg/kg per day of TMP div bid.
[e] Oral/TMP-SMX pending sensitivities. If <1 month of age, consult an infectious disease specialist
Source: Adapted from *Pediatr Infect Dis J* 1988;7:620, with permission.

Treat *C. difficile*-associated pseudomembranous colitis for 7–10 days with PO or IV metronidazole (30 mg/kg per day div qid, maximum 2 g/day) or, alternatively, with oral vancomycin (40 mg/kg per day div qid, maximum 500 mg/day).

Have all family members practice meticulous hand-washing during a diarrheal illness. Report enteric pathogen infection to the public health authorities. Exclude from day care children with diarrhea that overflows the diaper, those with bloody stools until treated or resolved, and patients with *Shigella* or *E. coli* 0157:H7 until stool cultures are negative.

Follow-up
- Mild or no dehydration: contact primary care provider in 2–3 days

Indications for admission
- >5% dehydration
- Failure of oral rehydration
- Inability to take fluids orally
- Febrile infant less than 3 months of age with suspected or proven *Salmonella* enteritis or any child with *Salmonella* bacteremia
- Hemolytic-uremic syndrome complicating *E. coli* 0157:H7 infection
- Severe infection with clinical toxicity caused by any enteric pathogen

Bibliography

American Academy of Pediatrics: Practice parameter: the management of acute gastroenteritis in young children. *Pediatrics* 1996;97:424–36.

Committee on Infectious Diseases, *American Academy of Pediatrics: 2006 Report of the Committee on Infectious Diseases*, 27th ed. Elk Grove, IL: American Academy of Pediatrics, 2006, pp. 858–60.

Murphy MS: Management of bloody diarrhoea in children in primary care. *BMJ* 2008;336:1010–5.

Ochoa TJ, Salazar-Lindo E, Cleary TG: Management of children with infection-associated persistent diarrhea. *Semin Pediatr Infect Dis* 2004;15:229–36.

Gallbladder and gallstone disease

Three types of gallbladder disease occur in children and adolescents: calculous cholecystitis, acalculous cholecystitis, and acute hydrops of the gallbladder. Transient obstruction of the cystic duct may lead to a brief episode of biliary colic without subsequent cholecystitis.

Calculous cholecystitis

Calculous cholecystitis occurs when a gallstone obstructs the cystic duct or, less commonly, the common duct. This results in swelling and inflammation of the gallbladder. Factors predisposing to gallstone formation are chronic hemolytic disorders (sickle cell, hereditary spherocytosis, etc.), prolonged parenteral nutrition, chronic liver disease, obesity, pregnancy, malabsorption (ileal resection, Crohn's disease, cystic fibrosis, etc.), prolonged fasting or rapid weight reduction, chemotherapy, a history of abdominal surgery, and a family history of gallstone disease. In younger children there may be no predisposing factors.

Acalculous cholecystitis

Acalculous cholecystitis refers to an acutely distended, inflamed gallbladder in the absence of an obstructing gallstone. It occurs as a postoperative complication or as a result of sepsis or systemic infection, Rocky Mountain Spotted Fever, typhoid fever, *Shigella*, or viral gastrointestinal or respiratory infections. In 50% of cases, acalculous cholecystitis is idiopathic.

Acute hydrops

Acute hydrops of the gallbladder is an acute non-inflammatory swelling of the gallbladder without gallstones. It is primarily recognized as a complication of Kawasaki disease (5–20% of patients), but it also occurs in viral hepatitis, streptococcal pharyngitis, staphylococcal infection, Henoch-Schönlein purpura, nephrotic syndrome, mesenteric adenitis, and Sjögren's syndrome. Hydrops can also occur in children receiving long-term parenteral nutrition.

Clinical presentation

Calculous cholecystitis

Biliary "colic" and acute cholecystitis both present with the sudden onset of non-crampy pain, which rapidly becomes severe. In biliary colic, the severe pain lasts for 1–3 hours and then moderates into a dull ache over 30–90 minutes. With cholecystitis, the severe pain persists for >6–12 hours. Most commonly, the pain is in the right upper quadrant or epigastrium, although it can be periumbilical or diffuse. In one-third of patients, the pain radiates to the back, scapula, shoulder, or arm. Associated symptoms include anorexia, nausea, vomiting, and low-grade fever. As the gallbladder inflammation progresses, there may be local peritoneal inflammation with associated peritoneal pain.

On physical examination, the enlarged gallbladder is appreciated in one-third of cases, and there is often guarding of the right upper quadrant. Murphy's sign (inspiratory arrest with deep palpation of the right upper quadrant) and Boas' sign (tenderness or hyperesthesia over the right scapula) may be appreciated. Only 15–20% of patients develop jaundice. Two-thirds of cases of acute cholecystitis resolve spontaneously over the course of 2–3 days, although there may be progression to gallbladder necrosis and perforation with either localized abscess formation or peritonitis.

Acalculous cholecystitis and hydrops

Acalculous cholecystitis and acute hydrops of the gallbladder have a clinical presentation that is indistinguishable from gallstone disease. In younger patients, the presentation is nonspecific, with right-sided pain, vomiting, and sometimes fever. There may be a palpable mass at the right costal margin.

Diagnosis

Obtain blood for a CBC, hepatic profile, amylase, lipase, and electrolytes. Cholecystitis is associated with increased serum alkaline phosphatase and direct bilirubin, as well as leukocytosis. An ultrasound is usually sufficient to make the diagnosis of gallbladder disease.

See Table 9-12 for the differential diagnosis of right upper quadrant pain, which is the most common symptom of gallbladder disease.

Table 9-12. Differential diagnosis of right upper quadrant abdominal pain

Diagnosis	Differentiating features
Biliary tract disease	
Gallbladder disease	Pain radiates around to back/scapula
	Ultrasound is diagnostic
Cholecystitis	Low-grade fever, variable jaundice
	Positive Murphy's and/or Boas' signs
Choledochal cyst	Palpable mass, seen on ultrasound
Hydrops	Fever is rare (except with Kawasaki)
	Palpable RUQ mass
Cholelithiasis	Pain may worsen with meals
Liver disease	
Hepatic abscess	Insidious pain, fever, leukocytosis, elevated ESR
Hepatitis	Hepatomegaly
	↑ ALT/AST (4–100 times normal)
Other diagnoses	
Appendicitis (retrocecal)	Fever, vomiting, rebound tenderness
Fitz-Hugh-Curtis	Positive gonorrheal and/or chlamydial cultures
	Signs of PID are variable
Pancreatitis	Pain radiates straight to back
	↑ amylase and lipase
Peptic ulcer disease	Pain may be relieved with meals
Pyelonephritis	Fever, CVA tenderness, pyuria
Renal stones	Colicky pain, hematuria
RLL pneumonia	Tachypnea, fever, cough

ED management

If gallbladder disease is suspected, make the patient NPO, secure an IV, obtain the blood tests mentioned above, and order an ultrasound. In questionable cases, obtain a cholescinti-graphic (HIDA) scan or oral cholecystogram. Non-filling of the gallbladder is diagnostic of cholecystitis.

If cholecystitis or hydrops is diagnosed, obtain a surgical consultation, and defer giving any pain medications until the surgeon has seen the patient. Urgent surgery is indicated for peritonitis, perforation, or progression of symptoms with worsening pain and fever while under observation. Do not use ceftriaxone in suspected gallbladder disease as it may cause sludging of the gallbladder contents. Management of acute hydrops is usually supportive and concurrent with treatment of any associated illness.

Indication for admission

- Suspected cholecystitis or hydrops of the gallbladder

Bibliography

Broderick A: Gallbladder diseases. In Kleinmnan RE, Walker WA (eds). *Walker's Pediatric Gastrointestinal Disease: Physiology Diagnosis, Management*, 5th ed. PMPH-USA, 2008, pp. 1173–84.

Parks RW: Biliary tract emergencies. *Hosp Med* 2002;**63**:226–9.

Yusoff IF, Barkun JS, Barkun AN: Diagnosis and management of cholecystitis and cholangitis. *Gastroenterol Clin North Am* 2003;**32**:1145–68.

Hepatomegaly

It is not unusual to palpate the liver below the costal margin in infants and young children. A liver edge >3.5 cm below the costal margin in infants and >2 cm in children suggests hepatomegaly. Normal liver spans determined by percussion and palpation are 4.5–5 cm at 1 week of age, 7–8 cm for 12-year-old boys, and 6–6.5 cm for 12-year-old girls.

Clinical presentation and diagnosis

Apparent liver enlargement may be caused by downward displacement secondary to intrathoracic conditions (hyperinflation secondary to asthma or bronchiolitis, pneumothorax), subdiaphragmatic or retroperitoneal masses, and thoracic deformities.

True liver enlargement results from inflammation, storage disorders, infiltrative processes, congestion, and obstruction. The most common cause of hepatomegaly is infectious mononucleosis or a mono-like syndrome (CMV, toxoplasmosis). Malaise, weakness, fever, pharyngitis, generalized lymphadenopathy, and splenomegaly are associated findings. Other common causes include viral hepatitis (vomiting, jaundice, dark urine, acholic stools), cirrhosis and chronic liver disease (jaundice, spider angiomata, splenomegaly, ascites, hemorrhoids), hemolytic anemias such as thalassemia (peculiar facies, jaundice), and congestive heart failure (tachypnea, rales, cardiomegaly, edema).

Serious, but less common, diseases include leukemia (pallor, bleeding, fever) and cystic fibrosis (failure to thrive, recurrent pulmonary illnesses). Rare etiologies include storage disorders (Pompe's disease, Tay-Sachs disease, tyrosinemia, von Gierke's disease, galactosemia), drugs (acetaminophen overdose, carbon tetrachloride, methotrexate, chlorambucil), Wilson's disease, alpha-1-antitrypsin deficiency, hepatoma, liver hemangiomatosis, malaria, and liver abscesses. In the newborn consider congenital TORCH infection, neonatal hepatitis, and obstructive conditions (biliary atresia, choledochal cyst).

ED management

If the patient does not appear seriously ill or jaundiced, a mono-like illness is most likely. Obtain a CBC with differential, heterophile antibody, liver function tests, and a hepatitis screen. If the diagnosis remains uncertain, refer the patient for further evaluation.

Jaundice, excessive vomiting, altered mentation, failure to thrive, and/or abnormal bleeding demand an immediate work-up. In addition to the laboratory tests mentioned above, obtain a PT, PTT, and glucose. Further evaluation is dictated by the clinical picture and may include a bone marrow aspiration, abdominal CT scan, liver–spleen scan, liver ultrasound, sweat chloride, alpha-1-antitrypsin assay, and/or liver biopsy.

Follow-up

- Hepatomegaly without jaundice or ill appearance: primary care follow-up in one week

Indications for admission

- Signs and symptoms of hepatic failure
- Severe vomiting that prevents adequate oral intake
- Suspicion of serious disease (leukemia, heart failure, cirrhosis, etc.) for evaluation and management

Bibliography

Clayton PT: Diagnosis of inherited disorders of liver metabolism. *J Inherit Metab Dis* 2003;26: 135–46.

Mishra A, Pant N, Chadha R, Choudhury SR: Choledochal cysts in infancy and childhood. *Indian J Pediatr* 2007;74:937–43.

Wolf AD, Lavine JE: Hepatomegaly in neonates and children. *Pediatr Rev* 2000;21:303–10.

Intussusception

Intussusception is the most frequent cause of intestinal obstruction in infants over 3 months of age. It can occur at any age, although 60% of patients are <1 year and 80% are <2 years of age. Anatomically, there is an invagination of one part of the bowel into the lumen of the distal adjoining part. Although the most common type is an ileocolic, intussusception may occur at any level of the GI tract.

In the majority of cases, no etiology for the intussusception can be identified. However, a lead point such as a polyp, lymphoma, Meckel's diverticulum, or bowel hematoma (as in Henoch-Schönlein purpura) is present in 5–10% of cases, especially in those >6 years of age. Mesenteric venous engorgement due to compression between the layers of the intussuscepted bowel causes mucous secretion and blood seepage, leading to the typical currant jelly stools. If the compression is not relieved, necrosis of the bowel with subsequent perforation and peritonitis can occur.

Clinical presentation

Intussusception usually presents with the acute onset of intermittent abdominal pain and vomiting in a previously well infant. The classic triad of colicky abdominal pain, vomiting, and bloody stool is present in only about 25% of cases. The pain lasts from 1 to 5 minutes, recurring every 5–20 minutes. During these paroxysms the baby may cry out, draw up his/her legs, and appear extremely uncomfortable. In between episodes the patient may initially appear well, but eventually becomes lethargic and apathetic. Vomiting follows the pain and, in the case of an ileoileal intussusception, may contain bile and suggest an intestinal obstruction. Classic currant jelly stools are present early in only 10%. In some cases, a currant jelly stool is found only with a rectal examination. Constipation, nonspecific diarrhea, and fever may also occur. With recurrent intussusception and spontaneous reduction, symptoms may be subacute or chronic over a period of a few days to weeks.

Initially the abdomen is soft between episodes of pain, but later it becomes distended and tender. In 85% of cases a sausage-like mass can be palpated in the right lower quadrant or upper abdomen. When the intussusception has progressed into the transverse colon, there may be absence of palpable viscera in the right lower quadrant (Dance's sign). An abdominal mass may be appreciated on rectal examination and stool for occult blood is positive in 75% of cases. Bowel sounds are initially hyperactive and then become hypoactive or absent.

Occasionally lethargy will be the most prominent presenting sign. A history of crampy abdominal pain and vomiting demands a careful physical examination for an abdominal mass and rectal bleeding. Consider the possibility of intussusception in any child with altered mental status.

Diagnosis

If the clinical suspicion of intussusception is high, prompt confirmation is necessary, as persistence of the intestinal obstruction may increase the child's risk for surgical intervention. Prone and supine plain abdominal radiographs are a useful screening tool. Normally, the transverse colon and rectosigmoid are filled with air when a patient is supine; the ascending and descending colons are air-filled when prone. The inability to fill the ascending colon is highly suggestive of intussusception, while the leading edge of the intussusceptum may be seen as a curvilinear density in the transverse colon. The diagnosis can be confirmed with an ultrasound, looking for the target sign on transverse view and the pseudokidney sign on longitudinal view. In addition, color Doppler can be used to assess blood flow to the involved segment of bowel.

Ultimately, a contrast enema, preferably with air, is both the diagnostic and therapeutic procedure of choice. In up to 90% of cases, the enema will reduce the intussusception.

ED management

If intussusception is suspected, immediately notify a pediatric surgeon and radiologist. Insert an IV and give a bolus of 10–20 mL/kg of NS, followed by maintenance fluids. Timely diagnosis and intervention are paramount. If the patient is stable, obtain an air contrast enema as soon as possible. However, if intussusception is confirmed and there are signs of perforation or peritonitis, start IV piperacillin–tozobactam (<6 months of age: 200 mg/kg per day div q 6 h; >6 months of age: 350 mg/kg per day div q 6 h, 3 g/dose maximum) and prepare for emergency laparotomy. Surgery is also indicated if the radiologist is unsuccessful in reducing the intussusception.

Admit all patients with suspected or confirmed intussusception, as the immediate recurrence risk is about 10%. The majority of recurrent cases occur in the first 24 hours following reduction.

Indication for admission

* Suspected intussusception

Bibliography

Cera SM: Intestinal intussusception. *Clin Colon Rectal Surg* 2008;21:106–13.

McCollough M, Sharieff GQ: Abdominal pain in children. *Pediatr Clin North Am* 2006; 53:107–37.

Jaundice

The goals of the ED evaluation of the icteric child include rapid diagnosis of the acutely treatable causes of jaundice (sepsis, obstruction, metabolic disease), identification of patients in acute or impending liver failure, prophylaxis of susceptible contacts when icterus is caused by viral hepatitis, and reassurance when jaundice is physiologic or related to breast feeding.

Clinical presentation

Unconjugated hyperbilirubinemia is characterized by elevation of the indirect bilirubin fraction, while the direct bilirubin is less than 15% of the total, there is no bilirubin in the urine, and the stool color is normal. In conjugated hyperbilirubinemia, the total bilirubin is elevated, the direct bilirubin is greater than 15% of the total, bilirubin is found in the urine, and the stools may be acholic. In newborns, jaundice progresses in a cephalocaudal manner with increasing concentrations of total serum bilirubin.

Neonates and infants
Unconjugated hyperbilirubinemia

Full-term, well-appearing neonates with unconjugated hyperbilirubinemia are likely to have physiologic jaundice. Bilirubin levels peak at 3 days and then start to decrease, typically resolving by 10 days of life. The total bilirubin generally does not exceed 12 mg/dL at any time and the direct bilirubin is less than 2 mg/dL.

Breast-fed infants may have prolonged unconjugated hyperbilirubinemia lasting several weeks. These infants have no evidence of blood group incompatibility, hemolytic disease, or infection.

Conjugated hyperbilirubinemia

Conjugated hyperbilirubinemia is never physiologic. Cholestasis is an indication of hepatocellular dysfunction, biliary obstruction, or a metabolic disorder. In infants, biliary atresia and neonatal hepatitis are the most common etiologies.

Children and adolescents
Unconjugated hyperbilirubinemia

The most common causes of unconjugated hyperbilirubinemia are hemolytic disorders. Gilbert's syndrome is characterized by mild, fluctuating unconjugated hyperbilirubinemia with levels between 2 and 5 mg/dL, normal liver function and transaminases, and no evidence of hemolysis.

Conjugated hyperbilirubinemia

Toxin-induced or viral hepatitis are the most common etiologies. Clinically apparent icteric hepatitis is most commonly caused by hepatitis A (HAV), hepatitis B (HBV), or hepatitis C (HCV) (see pp. 269–270). See Table 9-13 for a list of the most common hepatotoxins.

Diagnosis

Differentiate true icterus from carotenemia. Carotenemia is a nonpathologic accumulation of dietary carotene that causes yellow skin color without scleral icterus in infants and toddlers. In the jaundiced child, scleral icterus can be appreciated at a total serum bilirubin concentration of approximately 3.0 mg/dL, so that icterus is often noted before jaundice is appreciated.

In infants, unconjugated hyperbilirubinemia that does not fit the pattern of physiologic or breast milk jaundice and is not due to hemolytic disorders may be caused by dehydration, polycythemia, hypothyroidism, infection (particularly UTI), Crigler-Najjar syndrome, and pyloric stenosis in a vomiting infant.

Table 9-13. Most common hepatotoxins

Medications		
Acetaminophen	Estrogens	Ketoconazole
Amiodarone	Haloperidol	Penicillins
Anticonvulsants	Halothane	Retinoids
Antineoplastics	Immunosuppressives	Sulfonamides
Aspirin	Isoniazid	Zidovudine
Erythromycin		
Environmental		
Aflatoxins	Arsenic	Ma huang/ephedra
Amanita mushroom	Carbon tetrachloride	Vinyl chloride

See Table 9-14 for the differential diagnosis of jaundice. See pp. 270–272 for the diagnostic evaluation of suspected viral hepatitis.

ED management

If an infant is jaundiced, obtain total and direct bilirubin levels. Calculate the indirect or unconjugated bilirubin level by subtracting the direct bilirubin from the total bilirubin level. Infants with unconjugated hyperbilirubinemia may be sent home if they have physiologic jaundice. The Subcommittee on Hyperbilirubinemia of the American Academy of Pediatrics has published guidelines for the management of hyperbilirubinemia in newborn infants ≥35 weeks and recommend phototherapy in an otherwise healthy neonate ≥38 weeks for levels >15 mg/dL at 48 hours and >18 mg/dL at 72 hours. See Figure 9-1 for more specific guidelines for phototherapy using a nomogram.

If the infant has conjugated hyperbilirubinemia, obtain blood for culture, albumin, hepatic profile, PT, PTT, CBC, and hepatitis serologies and urine for culture, urinalysis, and reducing substances. Consult with a gastroenterologist, and admit the patient to facilitate the evaluation.

As discussed above, the diagnostic approach to the older child with suspected viral hepatitis is outlined elsewhere. There is no specific therapy for acute viral hepatitis. See the section on liver failure (pp. 256–257) if the patient has coagulopathy, hypoglycemia, or encephalopathy, or returns to the ED with progressive jaundice.

Follow-up

- Breast milk or physiologic jaundice: primary care follow-up the next day

Indications for admission

- Newborn requiring phototherapy
- Infant with conjugated hyperbilirubinemia
- Fulminant hepatitis, with hypoglycemia, coagulopathy, encephalopathy, or vomiting precluding adequate oral intake

Table 9-14. Differential diagnosis of jaundice

Diagnosis	Differentiating features
Unconjugated: neonates and infants	
Physiologic jaundice	Presents 1–3 days of life and resolves by 10 days
	Total bili <15 mg/dL
Breast milk jaundice	Presents after 4 days and may last for weeks
Dehydration	Often due to poor breast-feeding (breast-feeding jaundice)
ABO/Rh incompatibility	Coombs positive
Other hemolytic disorders	Coombs negative
Polycythemia	Plethora, lethargy/irritability, jitteriness
Sequestered blood	Cephalohematoma, bruising, CNS hemorrhage
Infection/sepsis	UTI can present with jaundice, which may be conjugated
Hypothyroidism	Delayed stooling after birth
	Macroglossia, large fontanelles
Crigler-Najjar syndrome	Presents 1–3 days of life
	Total bili >15 mg/dL
Unconjugated: children and adolescents	
Hemolytic disorders	Associated anemia
Gilbert syndrome	Intermittent jaundice
	Presents postpuberty when ill/stressed
Conjugated: neonates and infants	
Neonatal hepatitis	Diagnosis usually requires liver biopsy
Biliary atresia	Presents in first 2 months of life, usually full-term
Congenital infection	CMV most common
	HSV, HIV, parvovirus B19, syphilis
TPN cholestasis	Usually after 2 weeks of TPN
	Reverses when TPN stopped
Genetic/metabolic disease	Galactosemia, α1-antitrypsin deficiency, cystic fibrosis
Choledochal cyst	Usually prenatal diagnosis
Conjugated: children and adolescents	
Viral hepatitis	Prodrome of fever, vomiting
	RUQ pain then hepatomegaly
Hepatotoxins	See Table 9-13 for list of most common
Autoimmune hepatitis	(+) ANA and α-SMA, α-LKM-1, or α-SLA
Cholelithiasis	Sickle cell, pregnancy, obesity/weight loss

Table 9-14. (cont.)

Diagnosis	Differentiating features
Wilson disease	Presents at 8–14 years
	Low serum ceruloplasmin
Dubin-Johnson syndrome	Presents postpuberty
	Worse with illness, stress/OCPs

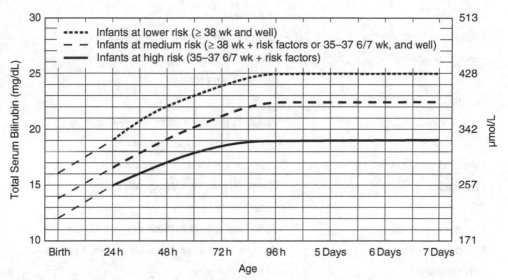

Figure 9-1. Guidelines for phototherapy in hospitalized infants > 35 weeks' gestation. Use total bilirubin. Do not subtract direct reacting or conjugated bilirubin. Risk factors: isoimmune hemolytic disease, G6PD deficiency, asphyxia, significant lethargy, temperature instability, sepsis, and acidosis. If infant is well and 35–36 6/7 weeks (median risk) can individualize TSB levels for exchange based on actual gestational age. Reproduced with permission from http://pediatrics.aappublications.org/cgi/ content/full/114/1/297.

Bibliography

Harb R: Conjugated hyperbilirubinemia: screening and treatment in older infants and children. *Pediatr Rev* 2007;**28**:83–91.

Moyer V: Guideline for the evaluation of cholestatic jaundice in infants: recommendations of the North American Society for Pediatric Gastroenterology, Hepatology and Nutrition. *J Pediatr Gastro Nutr* 2004;**39**:115–28.

Subcommittee on Hyperbilirubinemia: Management of hyperbilirubinemia in the newborn infant 35 or more weeks of gestation. *Pediatrics* 2004;**114**:297–316.

Liver failure

Acute liver failure is a devastating disease that results from the rapid destruction of hepatocytes, leading to progressive jaundice, coagulopathy, and encephalopathy over a period of weeks to months. Although it is rare in children, early recognition and treatment is critical, as mortality can reach 90% in the absence of liver transplant. Although the list of etiologies of acute liver failure in childhood (Table 9-15) is long, in most cases no definite cause is found, especially in those <3 years old.

Table 9-15. Causes of acute liver failure

Diagnosis	Differentiating features
Drugs/toxins	
Acetaminophen	↑AST/ALT to 400 × normal
	Bilirubin normal
Anticonvulsants	Phenytoin, carbamazepine, phenobarbital
Isoniazid	Affects <0.3% pts <20 years old
	Not dose-related
Idiosyncratic drug reaction	Green tea, weight loss agents, ephedra
Amanita poisoning	Recent mushroom ingestion
	Severe GI symptoms
Genetic	
Galactosemia	Failure to thrive; cataracts, *E.coli* sepsis
	(+) urine-reducing substances
Fatty acid oxidation defect	↑ammonia, nonketotic hypoglycemia
Tyrosinemia	Onset <6 months, cabbage-like odor
	Renal tubular acidosis
Iron storage disease	Autosomal recessive; presents in adulthood
Mitochondrial disorders	Acidosis, ↑ammonia, ↑pyruvate/lactate, ↓glucose
Wilson's disease	Hemolytic anemia
	Kayser-Fleischer rings, chorea, ataxia
	Immune dysregulation
Autoimmune hepatitis	Evidence of chronic disease: ascites, spider angiomata
Infectious	
Hepatitis A–D	Infrequent, unless related to chronic infection
Herpes simplex virus	Usually no skin lesions, requires histology
Epstein-Barr virus	Severe disease in immunocompromised host
Cytomegalovirus	Severe disease in immunocompromised host
Vascular	
Budd-Chiari syndrome	Abdominal pain, hepatomegaly, ascites
Ischemic hepatitis	CHF, shock, vasculitis, thrombosis
Other	
Malignancy	Metastatic disease
	Primary leukemia/lymphoma

Clinical presentation

Acute liver failure is characterized by the rapid development of severe liver damage, with associated synthetic dysfunction and encephalopathy, in a patient without prior liver disease. In adults, hepatic encephalopathy develops within 8 weeks of jaundice. In children, particularly infants, evidence of encephalopathy may not be apparent until the terminal stages of disease. While most patients initially present with jaundice, many report having preceding nausea, vomiting, abdominal pain, anorexia, and malaise. Hepatic encephalopathy can be graded based upon changes in consciousness:

- Stage 1: mild confusion, decreased attention, irritability, and reversal of sleep cycles
- Stage 2: drowsiness, personality changes, and intermittent disorientation
- Stage 3: gross disorientation, marked confusion, and slurred speech
- Stage 4: coma.

For children <4 years of age, coma is divided into three stages: early – inconsolable crying, sleep reversal and inattention to task; mid – somnolence, stupor, and combativeness; and late – coma, with or without arousal to painful stimuli.

Complications of acute liver failure include hypotension, cerebral edema, coagulopathy, acidosis, hypoglycemia, electrolyte disturbances, renal failure, and sepsis.

Diagnosis

Inquire about possible exposure to hepatitis, through blood products, travel, and sexual activity. In infants also ask about exposure to herpes and cytomegalovirus. Take a detailed medication history, which includes the use of herbal remedies, weight loss products, glue sniffing, cocaine use, and exposure to industrial chemicals. Ask about previous infections and risks for HIV, as immunodeficient patients are at risk for severe hepatitis.

On physical examination assess the patient for the presence of jaundice, scleral icterus, viral skin lesions, and purpura or petechiae. Perform a careful abdominal exam assessing both liver and spleen size and a meticulous neurologic exam looking for alteration in mental status and signs of increased intracranial pressure (increased muscle tone, hyperventilation, unequal or dilated pupils with sluggish response to light, focal seizures, papilledema, trismus, posturing, or loss of brainstem reflexes). Test for asterixis, a forward flapping of the hands when the patient's arms are extended and wrists are dorsiflexed. Smell the breath for fetor hepaticus which is a musty, sweet, or fecal odor to the breath. Some forms of liver failure occur without marked jaundice and the liver size may be increased, normal, or small.

Obtain a CBC with differential, electrolytes, BUN, creatinine, and hepatic profile (AST, ALT, CPK, LDH, alkaline phosphatase, bilirubin, total protein and albumin), PT, PTT, INR, fibrinogen, type and hold, ammonia, acetaminophen level, and a viral hepatitis panel, including CMV, HSV and EBV. If clinically indicated, send a βHCG, HIV, autoantibody serology, ceruloplasmin, lactate, and pyruvate levels.

ED management

The priorities in the ED are the prompt recognition of acute liver failure and early management of potential complications, especially cerebral edema. Frequent assessment of neurologic status is critical.

Insert an IV and infuse a 10% dextrose solution at a maintenance rate. Monitor the glucose frequently (every 1–2 hours) and maintain a serum glucose level of at least 40–60 mg/dL. If liver failure is secondary to acetaminophen ingestion, give N-acetylcysteine (NAC) 150 mg/kg in 250 ml D_5W over 1 hour (see pp. 448–449). Intravenous NAC is contraindicated in patients with a sulfa allergy.

Administer vitamin K (10 mg subcutaneously for 3 days) to patients with coagulopathy (INR>1.5 or PT>15). As prophylaxis against GI bleeding, also give either ranitidine (2–4 mg/kg per day div q 8 h, 50 mg/dose maximum) or famotidine (0.6–0.8 mg/kg per day div q 12 h, 40 mg/dose maximum). If there is active bleeding or the patient requires an invasive procedure, including central line placement, give fresh frozen plasma to maintain an INR of 1.5. In addition, give a platelet transfusion if the count is <50 000/mL and administer cryoprecipitate if the fibrinogen level is >100 mg/dL.

If the patient has grade 3 or 4 encephalopathy, avoid medication with sedative properties, elevate the head of bed to 30°, and use cooling blankets to keep core temperature at 37°C. Obtain a head CT and consider intubation for airway protection.

Admit the patient to an ICU where the multi-system complications of acute liver failure can be continually assessed and managed.

Indication for admission

* Acute hepatic failure

Bibliography

Bucuvalas J, Yazigi N, Squires RH Jr: Acute liver failure in children. *Clin Liver Dis* 2006;10: 149–68.

Dhawan A: Etiology and prognosis of acute liver failure in children. *Liver Transpl* 2008;14(S2): S80–S84.

Fontana RJ: Acute liver failure including acetaminophen overdose. *Med Clin North Am* 2008;92:761–94.

Lower gastrointestinal bleeding

Lower gastrointestinal (LGI) bleeding is a common complaint during childhood and is defined as intestinal bleeding distal to the ligament of Treitz. Most LGI bleeds are minor and not hemodynamically significant. Although severe LGI bleeding is rare, it demands a careful, coordinated approach.

Clinical presentation

Patients with a LGI bleed may present with hematochezia, melena, or occult blood loss without gross blood. Hematochezia is bright or dark red blood per rectum and is usually indicative of colonic or rectal bleeding, but can be seen with a severe, rapid upper GI bleed. Melena is tarry jet-black stool that is characteristically malodorous. Melena implies blood loss of 50–100 mL/day, usually from an upper GI source but also from the small intestine or ascending colon.

Diagnosis

Confirm that the red or black color in the stool is truly blood by obtaining stool for guaiac. Beets, gelatin, artificially colored drinks, and certain medications may turn the stools red.

Iron, Pepto-Bismol, blueberries, spinach, and licorice can cause stools to have a dark appearance. Undercooked meat and peroxidase-containing fruits and vegetables can cause false-positive stool guaiac tests.

Bright red blood or streaking of blood on the stool surface suggests a low rectal lesion, such as an anal fissure or a polyp. In contrast, blood originating from the small bowel (polyp, gastroenteritis, intussusception, HSP, Meckel's diverticulum, vascular malformation) varies from maroon to bright red depending on the volume and transit time. Flecks of blood admixed with mucus in a diarrheal stool is indicative of colonic inflammation (colitis, inflammatory bowel disease).

Once the presence of blood is confirmed, inquire about a history of fever, vomiting, diarrhea, or constipation. Ask about NSAID or steroid use (ulcer, gastritis, erosion); prior antibiotic use (pseudomembranous colitis); previous bleeding episodes (Meckel's diverticulum, polyps); weight loss or arthralgias (inflammatory bowel disease); and jaundice, liver disease or a complicated neonatal course with umbilical vein catheterization (varices).

On physical examination, look for signs of liver disease (jaundice, hepatosplenomegaly, caput medusae), purpura (Henoch-Schönlein purpura), perioral pigmentation (Peutz-Jeghers syndrome), an abdominal mass (intussusception, volvulus), and an anal fissure or sentinel tag. Perform a rectal examination on all patients to check for polyp, mass, intussusception, or constipation and to test the stool for blood.

Anal fissures, allergic colitis (cow's milk protein allergy) in infants, and infectious colitis are the most common causes of LGI bleeding in children. The infectious agent causing colitis is most likely viral or bacterial, but *Entamoeba histolytica* can also lead to LGI bleeding. Many cases of rectal bleeding in children over 1 year of age are due to polyps, from which the bleeding is usually not severe.

There are several syndromes with multiple polyps and cutaneous findings, such as Peutz-Jeghers (perioral pigmentation), Gardner's (bony and soft tissue tumors), and Cronkhite-Canada (alopecia, dystrophic nails) syndromes. Although rare, both syndromic and nonsyndromic forms of vascular malformations may cause GI bleeding, and many affected children will also have cutaneous findings. In the blue-rubber bleb nevus syndrome there are small (<1 cm), dark, cutaneous and gastrointestinal hemangiomas. In hereditary hemorrhagic telangiectasias, there are telangiectasias on the lips, tongue, ears, fingertips, or nail beds.

The differential diagnosis of LGI bleeding is summarized in Table 9-16.

ED management

Stabilization of the vital signs is the priority. Check for signs of volume depletion (orthostatic vital sign changes, skin color and temperature, capillary refill, mental status). If volume depletion is present or bleeding is ongoing in the ED, insert a large-bore IV and resuscitate with isotonic fluid followed by whole blood if bleeding persists (see Shock, p. 23). Obtain blood for CBC, PT and PTT, type and cross-match, electrolytes, glucose, and liver function tests, and consult a radiologist, gastroenterologist, and a pediatric surgeon.

If the patient has significant unexplained LGI bleeding, insert a nasogastric tube and lavage with 5 mL/kg of room temperature normal saline. Bright-red blood or coffee grounds on lavage is consistent with an upper GI source of bleeding; however, a negative lavage does not rule out a duodenal bleeding site.

Obtain an abdominal flat plate X-ray in any child whose LGI bleeding is associated with vomiting or abdominal pain to look for signs of intestinal obstruction (intussusception,

Table 9-16. Differential diagnosis of LGI bleeding

Diagnosis	Differentiating features
Anal fissure	Blood-streaked stool or blood passed following defecation
	History of constipation
	May have sentinel skin tag
Coagulopathy	Petechiae, purpura, other bleeding sites
Colitis	Frequent bloody, mucoid stools
Allergic	Formula-fed infant
	Breast-fed if mother is ingesting milk
Hirschsprung's	Fever, vomiting, abdominal pain; history of constipation
Infectious	Abdominal pain, tenesmus
Inflammatory	Fever, weight loss, poor growth
	Extraintestinal symptoms
Pseudomembranous	*Clostridium difficile* (+)
	Recent antibiotic treatment
Duplication of the bowel	May contain ectopic gastric mucosa and mimic a Meckel's
Hemolytic-uremic syndrome	Follows acute diarrheal illness
	Commonly *E. coli* 0157:H7
Hemorrhoids	Teens with constipation
	Infants with portal hypertension
Henoch-Schönlein purpura	Colicky abdominal pain; arthralgias; hematuria
	Symmetric purpuric rash on lower extremities, buttocks
Intussusception	Intermittent colicky abdominal pain; vomiting
	Sausage-shaped mass in RUQ while RLQ feels empty
	Currant jelly stools
Massive UGI bleeding	May occur with gastroesophageal varices, ulcers
Meckel's diverticulum	Painless voluminous bleeding
Polyp	Painless bright-red blood
	May have mucocutaneous lesions
Vascular malformations	Painless bleeding
	May have cutaneous lesions
Midgut volvulus	Bright-red or maroon bleeding in infant or toddler
	Possible bilious vomiting and abdominal mass

volvulus, duplication). Brisk, painless bleeding is most often due to Meckel's diverticulum, and a Meckel's scan is indicated.

If the patient is having bloody diarrhea, obtain a stool smear for neutrophils, which suggests a bacterial etiology (see Stool studies, Table 9-4). If PMNs are present, collect a stool sample for culture. Also obtain a CBC and blood culture if the patient is febrile (>38.9°C; 102°F) and less than 3 months of age.

GI bleeding due to severe colitis warrants both an investigation for infection and lower endoscopy to evaluate the possibility of inflammatory bowel disease. Note that severe colonic bleeding in the hemolytic-uremic syndrome may occur in the absence of stool leukocytes.

Treat an anal fissure in a well-appearing infant less than 1 year of age with petrolatum to the anus at each diaper change, and use dietary measures to treat coexistent constipation.

Treat suspected cow's milk protein intolerance by switching a formula-fed infant to a protein hydrolysate formula (Alimentum, Nutramigen). Advise the breast-feeding mother to discontinue cow's milk protein from her diet and to begin a calcium supplement. Arrange for follow-up within 2–3 days.

Patients with stable vital signs who definitely have a polyp (past history, polyp seen or palpated) may be discharged with referrals to a primary care provider and a pediatric gastro-enterologist. If the bleeding consists of more than streaking or anemia is suspected (history of significant blood loss, pallor, tachycardia), obtain a hematocrit. Obtain an ESR for suspected inflammatory bowel disease (weight loss in association with abdominal pain or arthralgias).

The ED management of constipation (pp. 238–240), intussusception (p. 250), volvulus (p. 258), and gastroenteritis (p. 243–244) are detailed elsewhere.

Follow-up
- Cow's milk protein intolerance: 2–3 days
- Polyp (with stable vital signs): pediatric gastroenterologist in 1 to 2 weeks

Indications for admission
- Signs of intravascular volume depletion
- UGI bleeding or significant LGI bleeding
- Infants <3 months of age with fever and colitis (PMNs in stool)
- Severe abdominal pain

Bibliography
Arvola T, Ruuska T, Keränen J, et al: Rectal bleeding in infancy: clinical, allergological, and microbiological examination. *Pediatrics* 2006;117:e760–8.

Boyle JT: Gastrointestinal bleeding in infants and children. *Pediatr Rev* 2008;29:39–52.

Upper gastrointestinal bleeding
Upper gastrointestinal (UGI) bleeding is always concerning and occasionally life threatening. By definition, the source of an UGI bleed is proximal to the ligament of Treitz.

Clinical presentation

A patient with an UGI bleed may present with one, or a combination, of the following: (1) hematemesis, which is vomiting of bright-red blood or coffee-ground material, (2) melena, which is a tarry black stool containing digested blood, and (3) hematochezia, which is bright-red blood per rectum seen in severe and rapid UGI bleeding. Clinically, the presentation may range from asymptomatic anemia to dizziness, dyspnea, or hypovolemic shock.

Diagnosis

Confirm the presence of blood. Red-colored foods or medications can easily be mistaken for hematemesis, and some foods (blueberries) and iron-supplements can cause black-colored stools. When the only evidence of bleeding is melena, confirm the diagnosis of an UGI bleed by passing a nasogastric tube and aspirating the stomach contents. A negative lavage, however, does not rule out a bleed. Test the stool, vomitus, or aspirate with stool guaiac/ Hemoccult or Gastroccult. Undercooked meat and peroxidase-containing fruits and vegetables can cause false-positive reactions.

If blood is confirmed, consider non-GI sources, which are more common than true UGI bleeds. Ask about recent epistaxis, pharyngitis, dental work, orofacial trauma, and hemoptysis. Determine whether the patient has taken any medications associated with UGI bleeding (NSAIDs, anticoagulants, corticosteroids). Establish any family history of peptic ulcer disease, *Heliocobacter pylori*, or inflammatory bowel disease. Peptic disease in young children may present atypically with generalized abdominal pain, nocturnal or early morning pain, and pain related to meals (causing exacerbation or relief). Consider alcoholic gastritis in adolescents. An antecedent history of splenomegaly or prematurity raises the possibility of esophageal varices. Ask about umbilical vein catheterization, omphalitis, or congenital anomalies and about risk factors for liver disease.

On physical examination, focus on the vital signs (including orthostatic changes) and signs of shock (skin color, temperature, and capillary refill). Check the skin for petechiae or purpura and examine the nose and oropharynx carefully for a source of bleeding.

The differential diagnosis of UGI bleeding is summarized in Table 9-17.

ED management
Unstable patient

The priority is the recognition and treatment of shock. Begin fluid resuscitation if the patient has orthostatic changes, tachycardia, prolonged capillary refill, and/or altered sensorium. Elevate the patient's legs, administer oxygen, start two large-bore IVs and give a fluid bolus with 20 mL/kg of normal saline or Ringer's lactate. Obtain a stat CBC and type and cross. If coagulopathy or liver disease is suspected, obtain a PT, PTT, albumin, and liver enzymes.

Correct any coagulation defects with vitamin K, fresh frozen plasma, or platelets. Have packed RBCs available and give a transfusion if there is brisk bleeding associated with anemia and hemodynamic compromise. Pass a nasogastric tube and lavage with 3–5 mL/kg of room-temperature normal saline. This will reduce the volume of blood loss but does not stop bleeding. Assess continued bleeding by repeated lavages. In the rare instance in which persistent UGI bleeding is brisk enough to require ongoing transfusions, consult a pediatric surgeon or gastroenterologist for vasopressin or octreotide therapy (for esophageal varices) or to arrange for emergency measures to control the bleeding.

Table 9-17. Differential diagnosis of UGI bleeding

Diagnosis	Differentiating features
Any age	
Coagulopathy	Petechiae and purpura
	Other bleeding sites
Esophagitis	Associated GERD, infection, immunosuppression
Gastritis/ulcer disease	*H. pylori*
	Stressed patient
	Medications (NSAIDs, steroids, anticoagulants)
Mallory–Weiss tear	Forceful or repeated vomiting or retching
UGI obstruction	Persistent vomiting, which can be bilious
	Abdominal distention, irritability
Neonate	
Breast-feeding	Mother with cracked nipples or mastitis
Hemorrhagic disease (HDN)	Presents on days 1–5 of life
	Breast-fed baby born at home is at risk
Milk protein allergy	Streaks of blood and mucous in stool; rash
Stress gastritis	Stressful delivery, serious infection, or anoxic event
Swallowed maternal blood	Apt test to differentiate fetal from maternal blood
Infant	
AVM/hemangioma	May have associated cutaneous lesions
Congenital factor deficiency	Bleeding disproportionate to trauma
GI duplication	Presence of heterotopic mucosa can cause ulcer/bleeding
Reflux esophagitis	Regurgitation, vomiting, irritability, poor feeding
Child and adolescent	
Caustic ingestion	Drooling, oropharyngeal burns, refusal to swallow
Crohn's disease	Weight loss, low-grade fever
	Extraintestinal manifestations
Esophageal foreign body	Antecedent choking event, drooling, refusal to swallow
Esophageal varices	Voluminous/painless bleed
	Splenomegaly, caput medusae
Swallowed blood	Dental, nasal, pharyngeal, or pulmonary bleeding source
Trauma/duodenal hematoma	Blunt trauma may be trivial causing gradual obstruction

Stable patient

If the patient is hemodynamically stable, obtain the same laboratory studies (see above), pass a nasogastric tube, and lavage to detect acute ongoing bleeding. Treat continuing bleeding with lavage and an H_2 antagonist (ranitidine 1 mg/kg IV q 8 h, 50 mg maximum per dose). Upper endoscopy is indicated for ongoing bleeding, UGI bleeding accompanied by peptic symptoms, and a significant drop in hematocrit, regardless of the presence of active bleeding. Prescribe antacid therapy and/or an H_2 blocking agent pending endoscopy.

A hemodynamically stable patient who presents with hematemesis without peptic symptoms may be discharged if not actively bleeding. Observe the patient for several hours and document that the hematocrit is normal, stool guaiac is negative, and gastric lavage is clear.

Follow-up

• Hemodynamically stable patient without peptic symptoms or active bleeding: 2–3 days

Indication for admission

• Ongoing UGI bleeding or persistent peptic symptoms

Bibliography

Boyle JT: Gastrointestinal bleeding in infants and children. *Pediatr Rev* 2008;**29**:39–52.

Chawla S, Seth D, Mahajan P, Kamat D: Upper gastrointestinal bleeding in children. *Clin Pediatr (Phila)* 2007;**46**:16–21.

Czinn SJ: *Helicobacter pylori* infection: detection, investigation, and management. *J Pediatr* 2005;**146**:S21–S26.

Meckel's diverticulum

Meckel's diverticulum is the most common intestinal malformation, occurring in approximately 2% of the population. It is caused by an incomplete obliteration of the omphalomesenteric (vitelline) duct and is usually located within the terminal 100 cm of the ileum. About one-half of cases contain ectopic mucosa, usually (90%) gastric, but ectopic pancreatic, small bowel, or colonic mucosa can also be present. Meckel's diverticulum is the most common cause of massive lower gastrointestinal bleeding in children.

Clinical presentation

Clinical symptoms occur in 4–25% of cases of Meckel's diverticulum and are due to complications, including hemorrhage, obstruction, or diverticulitis. Bleeding occurs in 40–60% of symptomatic patients, secondary to ulceration of the ileal mucosa adjacent to the ectopic gastric tissue. Many children present with massive painless rectal bleeding. Alternatively, chronic blood loss or tarry stools can occur.

Intestinal obstruction, presenting with abdominal pain and vomiting which can be bilious, occurs in 20% of symptomatic patients. This can be secondary to intussusception with the diverticulum acting as a lead point, volvulus around the fixed tip of the diverticulum, internal herniation, or incarceration in an inguinal hernia. One-half of cases of intussusception due to Meckel's diverticulum occur in infancy, with a presentation that is identical to idiopathic intussusception.

Diverticulitis and perforation occasionally occur, possibly secondary to peptic ulceration. These are clinically indistinguishable from acute appendicitis, although the area of most intense pain is closer to the midline.

Diagnosis and ED management

The ED management, as well as the differential diagnosis, is dictated by the presenting symptom. (See Abdominal pain, pp. 219–222; Lower gastrointestinal bleeding, pp. 257–260; Intussusception, pp. 249–250; and Acute appendicitis, pp. 225–228).

A history of previous episodes of lower gastrointestinal bleeding is important, as many patients with a bleeding Meckel's diverticulum will have had a similar episode in the past. Once it has been established that the bleeding is coming from the lower gastrointestinal tract, insert a large-bore IV if there is active bleeding, orthostatic vital sign changes, tachycardia, or hypotension. Give fluid resuscitation with normal saline boluses (20 mL/kg) as needed. Obtain blood for a CBC with differential, platelet count, type and cross-match, PT, and PTT.

Order a technetium-99m pertechnetate scintiscan (Meckel's scan) for a stable patient with painless LGI bleeding. It is a simple and noninvasive method for identifying a Meckel's diverticulum with ectopic gastric mucosa, with a sensitivity of 80–90% and a specificity of >95%. To increase the accuracy of the scan, give oral cimetidine (20 mg/kg per day), or for an emergency scan, subcutaneous pentagastrin (6 mcg/kg). Notify a surgeon when a patient presents with a possible Meckel's diverticulum as surgery may be required on an emergency basis, after correction of anemia or fluid and electrolyte imbalances.

Indications for admission

- Positive Meckel's scan
- Significant LGI blood loss with evidence of hypovolemia
- Intestinal obstruction or suspected surgical abdomen

Bibliography

Levy AD, Hobbs CM: From the archives of the AFIP. Meckel diverticulum: radiologic features with pathologic correlation. *Radiographics* 2004;24:565–87.

Menezes M, Tareen F, Saeed A, Khan N, Puri P: Symptomatic Meckel's diverticulum in children: a 16-year review. *Pediatr Surg Int* 2008;24:575–7.

Sagar J, Kumar V, Shah DK: Meckel's diverticulum: a systematic review. *J R Soc Med* 2006;99:501–5.

Pyloric stenosis

Consider the possibility of pyloric stenosis in an infant with nonbilious emesis, particularly in the absence of fever or diarrhea. It is five times more common in boys than girls, usually occurs in full-term infants, and in about 5–7% of cases there is a positive family history in a parent or sibling.

Clinical presentation

Infants with pyloric stenosis usually present between 2 and 8 weeks of life with nonbilious, nonbloody emesis that is initially intermittent, and is often attributed to gastroesophageal reflux, overfeeding, or cow's milk intolerance. As the muscular hypertrophy progresses, the emesis becomes projectile or forceful, occurring after each feed. Parents often note that the infant appears hungry after vomiting and demands refeeding. As the vomiting continues, the infant can become dehydrated with worsening malnutrition, weight loss, and lethargy.

Diagnosis

The diagnosis can be confirmed by appreciating a small mobile mass ("olive") slightly above and to the right of the umbilicus. Palpate for the olive-size pylorus either during a feed or immediately after vomiting, when the abdominal musculature is relaxed. Peristaltic gastric waves, traveling from the left upper quadrant to the right lower quadrant, may be seen after a feed and just before forceful emesis occurs.

Obtain an abdominal ultrasound to confirm the diagnosis and accurately measure the pylorus. A wall thickness >3 mm and a channel length >16 mm are diagnostic. If the ultrasound is negative or equivocal, but the clinical picture is suggestive of pyloric stenosis, repeat the study on subsequent days to look for progression of the muscular hypertrophy. If ultrasound is unavailable, obtain an upper gastrointestinal radiographic contrast study. A dilated stomach with outlet obstruction and/or a narrowed, elongated pyloric channel that swings upward (string sign) confirms the diagnosis.

Because the obstruction is proximal to the ampulla of Vater, recurrent vomiting causes a hypokalemic, hypochloremic metabolic alkalosis. Due to heightened physician awareness and the availability of radiographic studies, these metabolic abnormalities are not always present at the time of diagnosis. Elevated hemoglobin and hematocrit levels are secondary to hemoconcentration. Mild indirect hyperbilirubinemia is present in 20% of patients secondary to decreased hepatic glucuronyl transferase activity.

The most common alternative diagnoses are gastroesophageal reflux and improper feeding practices (large nipple hole, failure to burp the infant, etc.). The differential diagnosis is summarized in Table 9-18.

ED management

If an olive is palpated, make the patient NPO, insert a nasogastric tube if there is persistent emesis, and obtain blood for a CBC, electrolytes, and type and hold. Start an IV and give a 20 mL/kg bolus of NS if the infant appears dehydrated. Otherwise, infuse $D_5\frac{1}{4}$ to $D_5\frac{1}{2}$NS at a rate appropriate to the patient's weight and hydration status. When the patient is voiding well, add 20 mEq/L of KCl. Pyloromyotomy is not urgent. Therefore, delay surgery until any fluid and electrolyte imbalances are corrected (chloride >100 mEq/L and bicarbonate <25 mEq/L).

If an olive is not appreciated, ultrasonography may identify an enlarged pylorus. If ultrasound is not available, but the patient is well-hydrated, observe the parent feeding an oral electrolyte maintenance solution. A patient who does not vomit can be discharged, with daily follow-up. If the patient vomits the feed or appears dehydrated, obtain radiographic studies and admit the infant to the hospital for further evaluation.

Follow-up

- Infant can tolerate oral fluids and does not appear dehydrated: the next day

Indications for admission

- Suspected or confirmed pyloric stenosis
- Inability to tolerate oral feedings

Table 9-18. Differential diagnosis of pyloric stenosis

Diagnosis	Differentiating features
Adrenal insufficiency	Nonprojectile; ambiguous genitalia (female)
Antral web or atresia	Present in first week of life
Duodenal stenosis/atresia	Bilious vomiting; history of polyhydramnios
Gastroenteritis	Fever and/or diarrhea
Gastroesophageal reflux	Nonprojectile
Improper feeding practices	Nonprojectile; well-nourished
Increased ICP	Enlarging head circumference; split sutures
	VIth nerve palsy
Inborn error of metabolism	Lethargy; poor feeding; metabolic acidosis
Midgut volvulus	Bilious vomiting
	Guaiac-positive stool
Sepsis	Fever, toxicity

Bibliography

Aspelund G, Langer JC: Current management of hypertrophic pyloric stenosis. *Semin Pediatr Surg* 2007;16:27–33.

Leaphart CL, Borland K, Kane TD, Hackam DJ: Hypertrophic pyloric stenosis in newborns younger than 21 days: remodeling the path of surgical intervention. *J Pediatr Surg* 2008;43:998–1001.

McVay MR, Copeland DR, McMahon LE, et al: Surgeon-performed ultrasound for diagnosis of pyloric stenosis is accurate, reproducible, and clinically valuable. *J Pediatr Surg* 2009;44:169–71.

Rectal prolapse

Rectal prolapse is usually a benign, self-limited condition that occurs predominantly in the first 4 years of life, with the highest incidence in the first year.

Clinical presentation and diagnosis

Rectal prolapse appears as a sausage-shaped, dark red mass that protrudes from the anus. It occurs during defecation and often recedes spontaneously by the time the child reaches medical attention. An underlying or predisposing condition can usually be identified (see Table 9-19).

A protruding polyp or hemorrhoid can easily be differentiated from a prolapsed rectum by simple inspection, as they do not involve the entire anal circumference.

ED management

If the prolapsed rectum does not reduce spontaneously, lubricate the prolapsed tissue and gently reduce it manually. Treat any underlying constipation or diarrhea. Perform careful physical and neurologic examinations, paying careful attention to the anus, spine, and lower

Table 9-19. Conditions associated with rectal prolapse

Chronic constipation	Parasitic infections
Diarrheal diseases	Pertussis
Ehlers-Danlos syndrome	Rectal polyps or neoplasms
Hirschsprung's disease	Spinal cord lesions (meningomyelocele)
Malnutrition	Ulcerative colitis

extremities. Refer the patient to a primary care setting to arrange for serial stool collections for ova and parasites and, if there have been recurrent unexplained episodes of prolapse, a sweat chloride test (to rule out cystic fibrosis).

Follow-up

• Primary care follow-up within 1 week

Bibliography

Antao B, Bradley V, Roberts JP, Shawis R: Management of rectal prolapse in children. *Dis Colon Rectum* 2005;48: 1620–5.

Siafakas C, Vottler TP, Andersen JM: Rectal prolapse in pediatrics. *Clin Pediatr (Phila)* 1999;38:63–72.

Umbilical lesions

Most umbilical lesions are benign. The umbilical cord begins to dry shortly after birth and typically separates completely and falls off by the end of the second week (mean 7–10 days). Delayed separation, defined as after 3 weeks of age, is most commonly caused by vigorous use of antiseptics to clean the cord and is rarely secondary to abnormal neutrophil function.

Clinical presentation

Granuloma

The most common of all umbilical lesions is persistence of granulation tissue at the site of cord separation. This presents as a reddish mass protruding from the umbilicus. There may be a small amount of a blood-tinged discharge.

Umbilical hernia

An umbilical hernia presents as a bulging out of the umbilicus that is most prominent when the baby is crying or stooling. The hernia can be quite large and occurs more commonly in African-Americans. The hernia typically closes by 2 or 3 years of age as the abdominal musculature grows. Very rarely, a piece of mesentery can become incarcerated, causing local pain and tenderness.

Omphalitis

In newborns a small rim of erythema around the umbilicus can be normal. In contrast, omphalitis presents with a foul odor and erythematous streaking, particularly in the direction of the liver. The infant may have fever, irritability, decreased oral intake, and lethargy.

Persistent omphalomesenteric duct and urachus

After the cord separates a persistent omphalomesenteric duct may present with fecal drainage. A persistent urachus may allow the drainage of urine from the umbilicus. Either remnant may also persist as a blind sinus with a purulent or egg-white discharge.

Diagnosis

Normally, once the umbilical cord separates, there is no erythema or tenderness of the surrounding skin, although there can be a small amount of blood-tinged, non-foul-smelling discharge.

Examine the umbilicus for any masses, erythema, and odor, and note the quality of the discharge, if any. Look for signs of local pain and tenderness, which could signify an incarcerated hernia or omphalitis. If the drainage smells like feces consider a persistent omphalomesenteric duct, while a large amount of clear watery discharge suggests a persistent urachus. Purulent drainage or material resembling egg whites suggests a persistent sinus secondary to one of the two preceding conditions. A febrile and sick-appearing infant is more likely to have omphalitis.

ED management
Umbilical hernia

The treatment is education and reassurance since most umbilical hernias resolve without intervention. Surgical repair is not indicated until the child is at least 3 years old; however, instruct the parents to seek medical attention if the hernia cannot be easily reduced. If the patient presents with incarcerated mesentery, manually reduce the incarceration and arrange for surgical repair. Urgent surgical reduction is required if bowel incarcerates (very rare).

Granuloma

The treatment is cauterization with a silver nitrate stick. Moisten the stick with tap water and apply to the granuloma until the entire surface changes from a pinkish-red to a grayish color. Avoid contact with normal skin. Advise the family to not bathe the baby for several days. See the infant in 1 week and repeat the cauterization, if necessary. If the mass is particularly large when first seen, tie a ligature (3–0 nylon) around the base, and see the patient again in 1 week. At that time, sever the granuloma at its base, and then cauterize the stump.

Omphalitis

Omphalitis is potentially life-threatening. Perform a full sepsis work-up, including a culture of any discharge, admit the infant, and treat with IV nafcillin (100 mg/kg per day div q 6 h). In communities with a high prevalence of methicillin-resistant *S. aureus*, use vancomycin (40 mg/kg per day div q 6 h) instead. Consider anaerobic infection in the case of severe necrotizing omphalitis. The infant will appear toxic, with associated cellulitis or peritonitis. Add either clindamycin (40 mg/kg per day div q 6 h) or metronidazole (30 mg/kg per day div q 8 h).

Omphalomesenteric and urachal remnants

If a persistent omphalomesenteric duct or urachus is suspected, consult with a pediatric surgeon to confirm the diagnosis.

Delayed cord separation

If the presumed etiology is not excessive antiseptic use, obtain a CBC with differential. Regardless of the cause, instruct the parents to keep the cord dry and refer the infant to a primary care provider for follow-up within 1 week.

Follow-up

- Umbilical granuloma, delayed cord separation: primary care visit in 1 week

Indications for admission

- Omphalitis
- Incarcerated or strangulated umbilical hernia

Bibliography

Berseth CL, Poenaru D: Structural anomalies of the gastrointestinal tract. In Taeusch HW, Ballard RA, Gleason CA, et al. (eds). *Avery's Diseases of the Newborn*. Philadelphia: Elsevier Health Sciences, 2004, pp. 1118–9.

Fraser N: Neonatal omphalitis: a review of its serious complications. *Acta Paediatr* 2006;95:519–22.

Pomeranz A: Anomalies, abnormalities, and care of the umbilicus. *Pediatr Clin North Am* 2004;51:819–27.

Viral hepatitis

Most cases of viral hepatitis are caused by hepatitis A (HAV), hepatitis B (HBV), or hepatitis C (HCV). Universal vaccination of all infants and children has been recommended for HBV since 1992 and for HAV since 1999. This has resulted in an 81% decrease in hepatitis B infection from 1990 to 2006 and a 90% decrease in hepatitis A infection from 1995 to 2006.

HCV accounts for approximately 90% of what was formerly known as non-A non-B hepatitis. Intravenous drug use is the major risk factor for acquiring HCV. Patients who have received blood products or tattoos or are undergoing hemodialysis are also at risk, while sexual and perinatal transmission can also occur. There is no vaccine available to prevent hepatitis C infection.

Hepatitis D (delta hepatitis) only occurs in patients infected with hepatitis B. Hepatitis E is clinically similar to A but is not endemic in the United States. Although most cases occur in travelers from endemic areas, such as Asia, Africa, and Mexico, the incidence of sporadic cases in the non-traveler in industrialized countries is growing.

Other infections can cause acute hepatitis. These include Epstein-Barr virus, cytomegalovirus, varicella, toxoplasmosis, and *Leptospira*. Both icteric and nonicteric hepatitis may also complicate HIV infection.

Clinical presentation

Anicteric hepatitis is the most common form of hepatitis (up to 90% of cases) and many patients with hepatitis A or C may be completely asymptomatic. Clinically apparent icteric hepatitis caused by the any of the hepatitis viruses can resemble other infectious and non-infectious causes of acute hepatitis (Table 9-20). In general, the symptoms of HAV, HBV, and HCV are the same early in the course of the disease. During the prodromal phase, viral hepatitis may resemble a flu-like illness or gastroenteritis, with fever, lethargy, anorexia,

Table 9-20. Differential diagnosis of viral hepatitis

Diagnosis	Differentiating features
Acetaminophen toxicity	Aminotransferase elevation out of proportion to jaundice
Alpha-1 antitrypsin deficiency	Neonatal hepatitis or hepatic failure in older children
Anticonvulsants	Carbamazepine, phenobarbital, phenytoin
Autoimmune hepatitis	GGT and alkaline phosphatase usually normal
	May have evidence of chronic liver disease:
	hepatomegaly spider angiomata, palmar erythema
Cystic fibrosis	Malabsorption/poor growth
	Chronic respiratory symptoms
Inborn error of metabolism	Acidosis, hypoglycemia, ↑ammonia
	Failure to thrive
Ischemia	CHF, shock, thrombosis, vasculitis
Mitochondrial disorder	Lactic acidosis with ↑ lactate/pyruvate ratio Hypoglycemia, ↑direct bili, ↑ammonia,
Non-alcoholic steato-hepatitis/ fatty liver disease	Obese
Non-hepatitis viruses	Fever, lymphadenopathy, splenomegaly
Systemic lupus	Arthritis, nephritis, cytopenia, malar rash
	↑ESR/CRP, positive ANA
Wilson's disease	Chorea, ataxia
	Kayser-Fleischer rings
	Hemolytic anemia

nausea, vomiting, and right upper quadrant abdominal pain for about 1 week. The spleen is usually not palpable. In addition, with HBV, urticaria, purpura, papular acrodermatitis (Gianotti-Crosti syndrome), arthralgias, or arthritis may also occur. Lymphadenopathy is not a feature of HAV, HBV, or HCV. The epidemiologic and clinical characteristics are summarized in Table 9-21.

Although most young children with acute hepatitis are without jaundice, 30% of cases of HBV will present with jaundice. The icteric phase lasts 1–4 weeks, with complete recovery in the majority of patients. A prolonged cholestatic form is rare in children. In about 0.1–1% of all cases, a fulminant hepatitis results in hepatic coma and possibly death.

Although infection with HAV is not associated with long-term sequelae, both HBV and HCV can progress to chronic liver disease, cirrhosis, and hepatocellular carcinoma. Acute HCV progresses to chronic disease in up to 70% of patients and end-stage liver disease occurs in 10% of patients. There is also a carrier state for HBV that can be asymptomatic or associated with chronic liver disease.

Table 9-21. Clinical and epidemiologic characteristics of HAV, HBV and HCV

	HAV	HBV	HCV
Clinical features			
Peak pediatric incidence	1st decade	2nd decade/neonatal	2nd decade/neonatal
Route	Fecal-oral	Parenteral/sexual/perinatal	Parenteral/sexual/perinatal
Incubation	15–50 days	40–180 days	2–26 weeks
Onset	Acute	Subacute	Subacute
Fever > 38.3°C (101°F)	Common	Less common	Rare
Anorexia	Severe	Moderate	Moderate
Nausea/vomiting	Common	Less common	Less common
Rash	Rare	Common	Rare
Arthralgias/arthritis	Rare	Common	Rare
Epidemiologic features			
Common-source epidemic	Yes	No	No
Day care center contact	Yes	No	No
IV drug use	No	Yes	Yes
Blood, blood products, dialysis	No	Yes	Yes
Homosexuality	?	Yes	Yes

Infectious mononucleosis may manifest as isolated hepatitis or a syndrome that includes pharyngitis and splenomegaly. Lymphadenopathy occurs in Epstein-Barr, CMV, and HIV infections.

Diagnosis

If hepatitis is suspected, obtain a CBC, differential, albumin, hepatic profile, PT, PTT, INR, electrolytes, glucose, an acute hepatitis serology panel (hepatitis B surface antigen [HBsAg], surface antibody [anti-HBs], core antibody [anti-HBc], and IgM anti-HAV and anti-HCV), acetaminophen level, and heterophile antibody. If an autoimmune process is being considered, send an ESR or CRP, antinuclear antibodies (ANA), anti-smooth muscle antibodies (ASMA), and antibodies to liver and kidney microsomes (anti-LKM).

In general, transaminases (ALT [SGPT], AST [SGOT]) increase during the prodromal period and return to normal after the appearance of jaundice. Conjugated hyperbilirubinemia predominates during the icteric stage and bilirubin levels may be extremely high if there is associated renal disease or hemolysis. Alkaline phosphatase is elevated but albumin is normal. Leukopenia with atypical lymphocytes may be seen during the prodrome.

Suspect HAV if the patient is in day care, has just returned from travel to an endemic area, or has a history of possible exposure to contaminated food or shellfish. The presence

Table 9-22. Hepatitis B serology

Stage of disease	HBsAg	anti-HBs	anti-HBc
Incubation	+	–	–
Acute illness	+	–	+
Early convalescence (serologic gap)	–	–	+
Resolved infection (<6 months ago)	–	+	+
Post-recovery (infection >6 months ago)	–	+	+
Chronic carrier	+	–	+
Post-vaccination	–	+	–

of anti-HAV IgM confirms HAV infection within the previous 4 weeks, while anti-HAV IgG implies infection that occurred more than 4 weeks prior to testing or successful immunization.

The primary test for diagnosing HBV is the surface antigen (HBsAg), which appears in the blood 4–6 weeks after exposure, but 1 week to 2 months before any elevation of the transaminases. HBsAg usually disappears 1–13 weeks after the onset of clinical disease. Persistence beyond 6 months defines chronic carriage or chronic hepatitis. Antibody to HBV surface antigen is protective, lasts indefinitely, and implies recovery from infection and absence of infectivity. It does not appear until there is resolution of the clinical hepatitis and is usually not measurable until several weeks after the disappearance of HBsAg. As a result, there can be a serologic "gap" when both HBsAg and anti-HBs are absent from the blood. This gap is filled by core antibody which is not protective. Anti-HBs can also indicate successful immunization when present without HBcAb. HBV serology is summarized in Table 9-22.

During the prodromal phase, viral hepatitis may be confused with a flu-like illness or gastroenteritis. A tender enlarged liver, hyperbilirubinemia, and increased transaminases suggest the correct diagnosis. During the icteric stage, consider other causes of jaundice such as obstruction (right upper quadrant colicky pain and mass), toxins, and drugs. Carotenemia occurs in infants and is confirmed by the absence of scleral icterus and a normal serum bilirubin. Other causes of elevated transaminases include alpha-1-antitrypsin deficiency, Budd-Chiari syndrome, congestive heart failure, Wilson's disease, autoimmune hepatitis, and steatohepatitis. In the neonate intrauterine infections (TORCH), metabolic disease (galactosemia), biliary atresia, and a choledochal cyst are the major differential diagnoses.

ED management

The diagnostic approach to a child with suspected viral hepatitis is outlined above. There is no specific therapy for acute viral hepatitis. Intravenous hydration may be necessary for patients with severe vomiting. Treat a coagulopathy (INR >1.5 or PT >15) with vitamin K, 10 mg subcutaneously daily for 3 days. As prophylaxis against gastrointestinal bleeding give ranitidine (2–4 mg/kg per day div q 8 h, 50 mg/dose maximum) or famotidine (0.6–0.8 mg/kg per day div q 12 h, 40 mg/dose maximum). A fulminant course characterized by progressive jaundice and encephalopathy occurs in <1% of patients. See the section on liver failure (pp. 254–257) if the patient has coagulopathy, hypoglycemia, encephalopathy, or returns to the ED with progressive jaundice.

Postexposure prophylaxis

In the situation where the serologic status of the source of the exposure is unknown, promptly test the source for acute viral hepatitis serologies (HA IgM, HBsAg, IgM anti-HBcAb, heterophile) and proceed with prophylaxis for hepatitis A or B, if indicated.

Hepatitis A postexposure prophylaxis

Give immune globulin (IG) within 2 weeks of exposure to all previously unimmunized household members or sexual contacts of a person who has serologically confirmed HAV infection. The dose is 0.02 mL/kg IM, 3 mL maximum, in each buttock for an infant or small child and 5 mL maximum in each buttock for an older child or adolescent. Also give IG to unimmunized daycare staff and attendees if one or more cases of HAV have been confirmed in the children or employees, or two cases in two or more households of attendees. In addition, give the first dose of hepatitis A vaccine to all patients >1 year of age. School contacts and healthcare personnel attending to a patient with HAV require only good hand-washing and stool precautions, not immune prophylaxis. When the index patient is known to be infected with HAV, serologic testing of contacts before IG administration is not necessary.

Hepatitis B postexposure prophylaxis

All previously unimmunized persons with direct (perinatal, sexual, or accidental percutaneous or mucosal exposure to blood or body fluids) exposure to an HBsAg-positive source require hepatitis B immune globulin (HBIG). The dose is 0.06 mL/kg IM (0.5 mL/dose for a neonate). Also give the first dose of hepatitis B vaccine, preferably within 24 hours of exposure or birth. Arrange to have the hepatitis B vaccine series completed using the age-appropriate dose and schedule, depending upon the vaccine available. Only the hepatitis B vaccine series is indicated for household contacts of a known HBsAg-positive source or people who have had percutaneous or mucosal exposure to blood or body fluid with unknown HBsAg status.

Hepatitis C postexposure prophylaxis

There is no role for postexposure prophylaxis in the case of hepatitis C exposure.

Follow-up
- Suspected viral hepatitis: primary care follow-up in 1 week
- After HAV or HBV prophylaxis given: primary care follow-up in 2–4 weeks

Indication for admission
- Fulminant hepatitis, with hypoglycemia, coagulopathy, encephalopathy, or vomiting precluding adequate oral intake

Bibliography

Brundage S, Fitzpatrick AN: Hepatitis A. *Am Fam Physician* 2006;73:2162–8.

Committee on Infectious Diseases, *American Academy of Pediatrics: Report of the Committee on Infectious Diseases*, 27th ed.

Elk Grove, IL: American Academy of Pediatrics, 2006, pp. 326–61.

Wasley A, Grytdal S, Gallagher K: Centers for Disease Control and Prevention (CDC): Surveillance for acute viral hepatitis–United States, 2006. *MMWR Surveill Summ* 2008;57:1–24.

Vomiting

Vomiting is the expulsion of gastrointestinal contents through the mouth. Vomiting may be a symptom of a GI illness or a systemic process that is not primarily gastrointestinal in origin. Vomiting may have a protective function in eliminating ingested toxins and infectious agents. Protracted vomiting may lead to complications such as dehydration, metabolic alkalosis, esophagitis, Mallory-Weiss tears, malnutrition, and dental problems.

Clinical presentation

The presentation of vomiting ranges from effortless regurgitation to projectile emesis. Regurgitation is distinguished from vomiting by the lack of forceful abdominal contractions. Vomiting may be associated with fever, abdominal pain, nausea, diarrhea, hematemesis, or other systemic complaints, while bilious emesis may indicate a surgical process. The conditions associated with vomiting are listed in Table 9-23.

Diagnosis

There is a large differential diagnosis for vomiting (Table 9-24). Viral gastroenteritis is the most common cause of vomiting in children and is especially common in the winter months, with rotavirus the most likely viral pathogen in infants.

Differentiate vomiting from regurgitation by the lack of nausea, diarrhea, fever, and forceful abdominal contractions in the latter. Inquire about the feeding pattern, frequency of burping, and history of gastroesophageal reflux. Document the duration and frequency of the vomiting and whether it is projectile. Establish whether the vomiting is bilious.

Inquire about associated fever, abdominal pain, or diarrhea. Ask about headache, diplopia, ophthalmoplegia, personality changes, and, in infants, irritability or lethargy; these findings suggest a CNS lesion.

ED management
Vomiting

Assess the patient's hydration status and compare the current and premorbid weights, if available. Assess vital signs and hemodynamic status and perform thorough physical and neurologic examinations. If intestinal obstruction is suspected, obtain an upright or decubitus abdominal X-ray. If there is bilious emesis, make the patient NPO, and decompress the stomach with a nasogastric tube. Give appropriate IV fluid resuscitation (see pp. 231–233), and consult a pediatric surgeon.

Gastroenteritis (p. 230) usually responds to small sips of sugar-containing clear liquids (oral electrolyte solution, sweetened weak tea, decarbonated soda, fruit juice).

Table 9-23. Conditions associated with vomiting

	Diagnoses
Vomiting characteristics	
Bilious	Obstruction distal to the ampulla of Vater
	Prolonged forceful vomiting
Feculent	Distal GI obstruction, gastrocolic fistula
Bloody	(See Table 9-17: Differential diagnosis of UGI bleeding)
Forceless	Gastroesophageal reflux, overfeeding, rumination
Projectile	Pyloric stenosis, proximal GI obstruction, sepsis, ↑ICP
Chronic small volume	Psychogenic, gastroesophageal reflux, rumination
Relieves abdominal pain	Peptic ulcer disease
Abdominal pain not relieved	Cholecystitis, pancreatitis, appendicitis
Early morning	↑ICP, pregnancy, psychogenic, uremia
During eating	Psychogenic, peptic ulcer disease
Associated sign/symptoms	
Fever	Gastroenteritis, appendicitis, cholecystitis, pancreatitis
	Inflammatory bowel disease
	Infection outside GI tract (otitis, pharyngitis, UTI)
Severe hypotension	Adrenal crisis, sepsis, severe dehydration
Failure to thrive	Congenital adrenal hyperplasia, celiac disease, severe gastroesophageal reflux, metabolic disorder, inflammatory bowel disease
Chronic without weight loss	Psychogenic
Unusual odor	Inborn error of metabolism, DKA, uremia
Jaundice	Hepatobiliary disease, neonate with UTI
Surgical scars	GI obstruction due to adhesions
Scars on knuckles	Bulimia
Mental status change	CNS disease, ingestion, uremia, intussusception, Reye's
Headache	↑ICP, migraine, ↑ intraocular pressure
Diarrhea	Gastroenteritis, food intolerance, intussusception
	Inflammatory bowel disease
RUQ abdominal pain	Cholecystitis, hepatitis, RLL pneumonia
Epigastric pain	Pancreatitis, peptic ulcer disease
High-pitched bowel sounds	GI obstruction

Table 9-24. Differential diagnosis of vomiting

Diagnosis	Differentiating features
Infectious diseases	
Food poisoning	Onset 1–6 h post-ingestion, brief illness
	Diarrhea in one-third of patients, afebrile
Gastroenteritis	Fever (high with bacterial infection), diarrhea, abdominal pain
Sepsis	Toxic-appearing, lethargy, signs of shock
Meningitis/encephalitis	Fever, mental status changes, signs of increased ICP
ENT infection	Pharyngitis, sinusitis, otitis media, URI, labrynthitis
Respiratory infection	Post-tussive emesis
UTI/pyelonephritis	Urinary complaints may be absent in infants
Surgical conditions	
Esophageal stricture	History of caustic ingestion, gradual swallowing difficulty
Foreign body/bezoar	Infant/toddler, developmentally delayed child
Pyloric stenosis	2–8 week-old with projectile vomiting, ↑bicarbonate
Appendicitis	Fever, anorexia, periumbilical then RLQ abdominal pain
Testicular or ovarian torsion	Scrotal or adnexal tenderness, severe pain
GI obstruction	Vomiting may be bilious
Gastrointestinal diseases	
Food intolerance	Related to specific food intake
GER	Infant with forceless vomiting, fussiness, feeding aversion
Peptic ulcer disease	Coffee-ground emesis, vomiting with meals relieves pain
Hepatitis	Hepatomegaly, +/− jaundice with dark urine/acholic stools
Cholecystitis	Low-grade fever, Murphy's sign, pain radiates to scapula
Pancreatitis	Epigastric/RUQ pain radiates to back; high amylase/lipase
IBD	Poor growth, ↑ ESR, guaiac positive stools
CNS conditions	
Increased ICP	Hypertension, bradycardia, VIth nerve palsy
	Focal neurologic exam
Head trauma	Altered mental status, retrograde amnesia, headache
Migraine	Past history, aura, photophobia, motion sickness
Endocrine/metabolic diseases	
Diabetic ketoacidosis	Polyuria/dipsia/phagia, abdominal pain, ketotic breath
Inborn error of metabolism	Poor feeding, hepatomegaly, acidosis, hyperammonemia

Table 9-24. (cont.)

Diagnosis	Differentiating features
Adrenal crisis (CAH)	Hyperkalemia, hyponatremia, hypotensive shock
Hypercalcemia	Confusion, proximal muscle weakness, hyporeflexia
Uremia	Renal failure, pruritus, ammonia breath, encephalopathy
Miscellaneous	
Pregnancy	Missed menses, vomiting may not be limited to morning
Toxic ingestions	Toddler or teen; abuse/suicide-attempt
Nephrolithiasis	Colicky flank pain that radiates to the groin
Anaphylaxis	Multi-system (commonly skin, respiratory, cardiovascular)
Bulimia	Bingeing followed by purging, usually normal or overweight
Rumination	Neurologically impaired child, weight loss
Cyclic vomiting	Onset at 2–5 years, 2–3 day episodes; well in between
Psychogenic vomiting	Associated with anxiety disorder or emotional distress
Munchausen by proxy	Frequent recurrent illnesses without a clear etiology
Overfeeding	Forceless emesis in a thriving infant

Antiemetics are not routinely indicated, but may be used in certain circumstances, such as postoperative vomiting, vomiting associated with chemotherapy, motion sickness, cyclic vomiting, or to prevent electrolyte abnormalities in severe persistent vomiting. Give one oral dose of ondansetron (2 mg 8–15 kg, 4 mg 16–30 kg, 8 mg >30 kg) to children with acute gastroenteritis who do not tolerate oral rehydration in order to limit repeated vomiting and prevent hospitalization. Do not give an antiemetic prior to evaluation for a possible surgical abdomen.

Regurgitation

Most infants and children with regurgitation do not require acute treatment in the ED if there are no associated symptoms. The majority of infants with GER improve by 6 months of age. Instruct the parents to give the infant frequent small feeds and to keep the baby upright after feeds. Thickening the formula with one level tablespoon of rice cereal per 2 ounces may be helpful. Infants and children with GER and associated failure to thrive, pulmonary disease, anemia, or esophagitis require further evaluation; consult a gastroenterologist.

Follow-up

- Tolerating oral fluids and mild or moderate dehydration: primary care follow-up the next day or return to the ED if unable to tolerate clear fluids at home
- Tolerating oral fluids and not dehydrated: primary care follow-up within 1 week

Indications for admission

- Significant ongoing fluid losses and/or inability to tolerate oral fluids
- Severe dehydration or altered mental status
- Suspected surgical abdomen

Bibliography

Chandran L, Chitkara M: Vomiting in children: reassurance, red flag, or referral? *Pediatr Rev* 2008;**29**:183–92.

Freedman SB, Adler M, Seshadri R, Powell EC: Oral ondansetron for gastroenteritis in a pediatric emergency department. *N Engl J Med* 2006;**354**:1698–1705.

Freedman SB, Fuchs S: Antiemetic therapy in pediatric emergency departments. *Pediatr Emerg Care* 2004;**20**:625–33.

Sondheimer JM: Vomiting. In Walker WA, Goulet O, Kleinman RE, et al. (eds). *Pediatric Gastrointestinal Disease*. Ontario: BC Decker, 2004, pp. 203.

Chapter 10

Emergencies associated with genetic syndromes

Robert W. Marion and Joy Samanich

Congenital malformations

Congenital malformations are present in approximately 3% of newborns in the United States. Malformations may occur as isolated conditions, as in the case of a simple cleft lip or palate, or may cluster together in recognizable patterns, or syndromes, such as trisomy 13. Early diagnosis of a specific syndrome provides an explanation for the family, expedites the detection of associated internal anomalies, and facilitates appropriate genetic counseling of the family.

For the physician working in the ED, recognition of a syndromic diagnosis is of special importance. Often, presenting symptoms are due to internal manifestations associated with that syndrome, and early identification of such associated problems can be life-saving. Table 10-1 lists some commonly occurring congenital malformation syndromes and the possible conditions with which affected individuals may present to the ED.

Table 10-1. Emergencies associated with genetic syndromes

Syndrome/genetics	External manifestations	Presentation/possible emergency
Achondroplasia	Short stature	Apnea/SIDS: narrowed foramen magnum (<1 year old)
AD (mutation in FGFR3)	Prominent forehead	Vomiting, irritability: ↑ICP 2° hydrocephalus (<1 year old)
	Proximal limb shortening	"Sciatica": nerve root compression 2° narrow spinal canal (8–18 years old)
Beckwith-Wiedemann	Somatic overgrowth	Hypoglycemia: hyperinsulinism (1st year of life)
Defect of 11p	Omphalocele "Coarse facies"	Abdominal mass, vomiting: Wilms' tumor, hepatoblastoma (occurs in 5–10%, between birth and age 6)
	Large tongue, ear creases	
	Hemihypertrophy	
Craniosynostosis syndromes (including Crouzon, Apert, and Pfeiffer)	Unusual head shape	Obstructive apnea: choanal stenosis (infancy)
Most are AD		

Table 10-1. *(cont.)*

Syndrome/genetics	External manifestations	Presentation/possible emergency
(mutations in *FGFR1, 2* or *3*)	Ocular proptosis	Vomiting, irritability: ↑ICP 2° premature suture closure (infancy)
	Hypertelorism	
	Some with limb defects	
Down syndrome	Hypotonia	Poor feeding, tachypnea: CHF (usually <2 months old)
Trisomy 21 (or robertsonian translocation)	Typical facies	Vomiting: intestinal obstruction 2°duodenal atresia or annular pancreas
	Midfacial hypoplasia	Constipation: Hirschsprung's disease (infancy and early childhood)
	Brachydactyly	Sudden paralysis below neck: cord compression 2° atlantoaxial instability (any age; avoid hyperextension of neck)
	Developmental delay	Failure to thrive, sluggishness: hypothyroidism
		Anemia, bone pain, fever: leukemia
Ectodermal dysplasias	Alopecia	Hyperthermia, febrile seizures: lack of sweat glands
AD, AR, X-linked	Hypodontia/adontia	
	Hypoplastic nails	
Marfan syndrome	Tall, thin body	Sudden chest pain: dissection of ascending aortic aneurysm
AD; mutation in *FBN1*	Long fingers	Sudden decreased vision: lens dislocation or retinal detachment
Myelomeningocele	Spinal defect	Vomiting, irritability: ↑ICP 2° hydrocephalus
Multifactorial	Paraplegia	Stridor, apnea: Arnold-Chiari malformation (neurosurgical emergency)
	Orthopedic abnormalities	Fever, foul-smelling urine: UTI 2° neurogenic bladder
	Hydrocephalus	Fever, irritability, vomiting: ventricular shunt infection
		Deteriorating lower extremity strength, gait, bowel, bladder function: tethering of spinal cord; Anaphylaxis: latex allergy
Neurofibromatosis I	Café-au-lait spots	Gradual vision loss: optic glioma
AD (mutation in *NF1*)	Axillary freckling	Back pain, asymmetry: scoliosis

Table 10-1. (cont.)

Syndrome/genetics	External manifestations	Presentation/possible emergency
	Neurofibromas	Headache, irritability, vomiting: ↑ICP 2° tumor
	Skeletal manifestations	
Neurofibromatosis II	Café-au-lait spots	Hearing loss, tinnitus: acoustic neuromas
AD (mutation in *NF2*)	Neurofibromas	Headache, irritability, vomiting: ↑ICP 2° tumor
	Iris hamartomas	Hypertension: pheochromocytoma, neurofibroma
		Vision loss: cataracts
Noonan syndrome (mutation in PTPN11)	Characteristic face	Cardiac-related symptoms: valvular pulmonic stenosis
	Webbed neck	Bleeding: Factor XI deficiency (in 50%)
	Short stature	Failure to thrive: syndromic short stature
	Pectus excavatum	
Osteogenesis imperfecta	Blue sclerae	Fractures after trivial trauma: osteoporosis (must consider child abuse)
Type I (AD) (mutation in *COL1A1* or *2*)	Bone fragility	Gradual hearing loss: otosclerosis
	± Dentinogenesis imperfecta	± Multiple caries
Osteogenesis imperfecta	White sclerae	Fractures after trivial trauma: osteoporosis (must consider child abuse)
Type IV (AD)	Bone fragility	Gradual hearing loss: otosclerosis
(mutation in *COL1A1* or *2*)	± Dentinogenesis imperfecta	± Multiple caries
	Bowing of some bones	
Pierre-Robin malformation	Micrognathia	Upper airway obstruction: glossoptosis (in infancy)
sequence	U-shaped cleft palate	Often part of another syndrome
	Glossoptosis	
Prader-Willi syndrome (15q11-13 deletion)	Obesity	Polydipsia/uria: diabetes mellitus
	Hypotonia	Upper airway obstruction
	Developmental delay	Severe behavioral disturbance (temper tantrums, usually food related)
	Hypoplastic genitalia	
Sturge-Weber syndrome	Port wine stain overlying dermatome	

Table 10-1. (cont.)

Syndrome/genetics	External manifestations	Presentation/possible emergency
	supplied by deep ophthalmic branch of Vth cranial nerve	Enlarged, hazy cornea, decreased vision: glaucoma 2° hemangioma blocking the angle (infancy)
Usually sporadic		Seizures: "railroad track" calcifications in cerebral cortex
Some AD		
Tuberous sclerosis complex	Hypopigmented macules	Seizures: CNS tumors (cortical tubers, subependymal nodules)
AD (mutation in one of at least two known genes)	"Adenoma sebaceum"	Abdominal pain, hematuria: renal angiomyolipomas
	Shagreen patches	Syncope: cardiac arrhythmia 2° rhadomyoma
	Ungual fibromas	
	± mental retardation	
Turner syndrome (monosomy X)	Female	Hypertension, decreased leg pulses: coarctation of aorta
	Short stature	Fever, dysuria: UTI 2° renal anomaly
	Webbed neck	Poor growth, constipation, obesity: hypothyroidism
	Puffy hands and feet	Failure to enter puberty: gonadal dysgenesis
	Broad chest	
	Characteristic facies	
Williams syndrome (deletion 7q11.2 region)	"Elfin" facies	Constipation, irritability: hypercalcemia (usually <1 year old)
	Short stature	CHF: supravalvular aortic stenosis and other heart lesions (80%)
	Developmental delay	Hypertension: renal artery stenosis
		Chest pain, sudden death: myocardial infarction 2° coronary artery stenosis
		Syncope, weakness: CVA 2° narrowing of cerebral arteries and Moya
		Moya disease
		Failure to thrive: poor feeding, hypothyroidism, syndromic short stature

Bibliography

Jones KL: *Smith's Recognizable Patterns of Human Malformation*, 6th ed. Philadelphia: Elsevier Saunders, 2006.

Levy PA, Marion RW: Section IX: Human genetics and dysmorphology. In Kliegman, Marcdante, Behrman (eds). *Nelson's Essentials of Pediatrics*, 6th ed. Philadelphia: Elsevier Saunders (in press), pp. 217–42.

www.genetests.org.

Genitourinary emergencies

Sandra J. Cunningham

Balanoposthitis

Balanitis is inflammation of the glans penis; posthitis is inflammation of the prepuce. Balanoposthitis, which is inflammation of both sites, occurs in up to 3% of uncircumcised boys. The etiology in most cases is poor hygiene and accumulation of smegma, which can lead to a secondary bacterial infection. In circumcised boys without residual foreskin or glans penis adhesions, balanitis may be secondary to contact dermatitis from urine, laundry soaps, powders, or ointments. In an adolescent with a retractable foreskin, poor hygiene and sexually transmitted diseases are implicated.

Clinical presentation and diagnosis

Balanoposthitis presents with erythema, edema, and pain of the distal phallus, particularly the glans penis. There may be secondary meatitis with resultant dysuria and reluctance to void. The foreskin will be more difficult to retract than it was prior to the onset of illness and a discharge may be present. In severe cases, the cellulitis can extend down the shaft of the penis and onto the lower abdominal wall or the scrotum. Inguinal lymphadenopathy or adenitis is often present.

Recurrent episodes of posthitis can result in phimosis, whereas repeated episodes of balanitis may result in meatal stenosis, with a poor stream and dribbling of urine.

ED management

Acute localized infections usually respond to frequent warm water sitz baths followed by drying of the penis and the application of topical antibiotics (bacitracin tid or mupirocin bid) and topical antifungal cream (nystatin) bid for 2 weeks. Reinforce proper hygiene and the avoidance of forceful retraction of the foreskin. If there is voluntary retention, fever, or cellulitis extending onto the penile shaft, treat with oral antibiotics for 7 days. Use 40 mg/kg per day of either cephalexin (div bid) or cefadroxil (div bid), but if MRSA is a concern, either use clindamycin (20 mg/kg per day div q 6 h) or add trimethoprim-sulfamethoxazole (8 mg/kg per day of TMP div bid) to one of the above regimens.

More severe infections with purulent discharge and widespread cellulitis require admission and treatment with parenteral antibiotics (nafcillin 150 mg/kg per day div q 6 h).

Failure of balanoposthitis to respond to warm soaks and systemic antibiotics may be due to inadequate drainage secondary to phimosis. An urgent incision of the dorsal inner foreskin is indicated if there is a poor urinary stream or dribbling.

Follow-up

- Inability to void: immediate. Otherwise primary care follow-up in 1 week

Indications for admission

- Severe infection
- Urinary retention

Bibliography

Garcia de Freitas R, Nobre YD, Demarchi GT, et al: Topical treatment for phimosis: time span and other factors behind treatment effectiveness. *Pediatr Urol* 2006;2:380–5.

Lawless MR: The foreskin. *Pediatr Rev* 2006;27:477–8.

Leslie JA, Cain MP: Pediatric urologic emergencies and urgencies. *Pediatr Clin North Am* 2006;53:513–27.

Renal and genitourinary trauma

Renal trauma

Blunt trauma, secondary to motor vehicle accidents, falls, or athletic injuries, is the major cause of renal injuries in children. The pediatric kidney is particularly susceptible to injury due to the relative paucity of surrounding fat, its size in relation to surrounding organs, and an immature thoracic cage, which provides inadequate protection. An underlying congenital anomaly, including ureteropelvic junction obstruction, primary obstructive megaureter, or ectopic or solitary kidneys, is found incidentally in up to 20% of cases of traumatic hematuria. Associated intraperitoneal injuries occur in approximately 25% of cases of blunt and 80% of penetrating renal trauma.

Ureteral trauma

Ureteral trauma is relatively uncommon, and when present is usually associated with multiple intraabdominal injuries. Children are at higher risk for avulsion of the ureter at the junction of the renal pelvis (ureteropelvic junction), which is a relatively fixed point in the course of the ureter.

Bladder trauma

The pediatric bladder is particularly susceptible to blunt trauma, especially from motor vehicle accidents. The majority of bladder injuries are associated with pelvic fractures.

Urethral Trauma

Urethral injury is usually the result of blunt trauma to the lower abdomen, a straddle injury to the perineum, or iatrogenic injury from urethral instrumentation.

Clinical presentation

Renal trauma

The patient will commonly present with flank pain, which may be localized or radiate to the ipsilateral groin. There may also be costovertebral tenderness, flank ecchymoses, or a palpable flank mass, if there is extravasation of blood or urine into the perirenal tissues. Associated findings include ipsilateral rib fractures and fractured transverse processes of the vertebral bodies. Either gross or microscopic hematuria is nearly always present, although the degree of hematuria can be variable and does not correlate with the degree of injury. In patients with vascular pedicle injuries, hematuria can be absent.

Ureteral trauma

The early presentation of a ureteral trauma is nonspecific and may be obscured by other associated injuries which are paramount on initial presentation. Hematuria is initially present in only 70% of cases. Later, there may be fever or flank or abdominal pain. A high level of clinical suspicion is required for early diagnosis.

Bladder trauma

The majority of bladder injuries are associated with pelvic fractures. A child's bladder is more susceptible to injury because it sits higher in the abdomen than the adult bladder. Also, a distended bladder is more vulnerable to blunt injury. A patient with a ruptured bladder presents with suprapubic and abdominal pain with tenderness on palpation, hematuria, and, with large tears, inability to void.

Urethral injury

The male urethra is divided into anterior and posterior portions. Posterior urethral injuries are generally caused by severe blunt trauma and are associated with other significant injuries. Lower abdominal and pelvic swelling, tenderness, and ecchymosis are commonly seen, with hematuria and blood at the external meatus. With complete disruption of the urethra, the patient may be unable to void.

Anterior urethral injuries are usually isolated and are caused by direct blunt or penetrating trauma, instrumentation, or a straddle injury. Perineal ecchymosis, usually in a butterfly distribution, and scrotal hematomas may be noted. Bleeding from the meatus is the hallmark of urethral injury and may be associated with an inability to void.

Injuries in females are uncommon due the short length and mobility of the urethra.

Penile and scrotal injuries

Most penile injuries in boys occur as a result of circumcision. The injuries vary from an inappropriate amount of skin removed to complete transection of the penis. Penile injuries due to blunt or penetrating trauma in childhood are rare, but may be associated with urethral injury. Penile and scrotal zipper injuries are common in boys and usually present with skin avulsion, while tourniquet injuries to the penis can occur from hair or other objects forming a tight circumferential band. Scrotal trauma secondary to straddle injuries (biking) or direct trauma (sporting event) can present with acute swelling, bleeding manifesting as ecchymosis or hematocele, and testicular injury with disruption of the tunica albuginea. In severe cases, blood and/or urine extravasates into the upper abdominal wall and into the perineum along the Colles' fascia.

Diagnosis and ED management

Although hematuria is generally present, there is no consistent relationship between the number of red cells and the degree of urinary tract injury, particularly with renal injuries. In fact, the absence of blood does not exclude a major injury, such as a ureteral transection or an injury to the renal vasculature. Therefore, suspect a renal injury in any blunt trauma patient with gross or microscopic hematuria on urinalysis, or with signs or symptoms suggestive of renal injury (flank pain or hematoma, lower rib fracture, shock), particularly with a rapid deceleration as the mechanism of injury. Renal imaging is indicated if the urinalysis has >50 RBCs per high-power field. Always consider the possibility of sexual abuse in a child presenting with trauma to the external genitalia.

Table 11-1. Staging of renal injuries

Grade	Findings	Treatment
1	Contusion with microscopic or gross hematuria	Bed rest
	No intraparenchymal laceration	Serial hematocrits
2	Subcapsular nonexpanding hematoma	Bed rest
	Confined to renal retroperitoneum	Serial hematocrits
	Laceration with a parenchymal tear <1 cm of cortex	
	No involvement of the collecting system	
	No extravasation of urine	
3	Laceration with parenchymal tear >1 cm	Bed rest
	No involvement of the collecting system	Serial hematocrits
	No extravasation of urine	
4	Laceration with extensive parenchymal injury	Ureteral stent
	Involvement of the collecting system	Possible renal exploration with reconstruction or nephrectomy
	Vascular damage to the hilar vessels	
5	Parenchymal destruction (shattered kidney)	Ureteral stent
	Hilar vascular injury with devascularization	Possible renal exploration with reconstruction or nephrectomy

Obtain immediate surgical and urologic consultation for the hemodynamically unstable patient. For the stable patient, arrange for a CT scan with contrast for proper staging of injuries and identification of any other associated intraabdominal injuries.

Renal trauma

If an isolated renal injury is likely, promptly obtain a CT scan of the abdomen and pelvis after administration of IV contrast.

The staging of renal injuries is shown in Table 11-1. Maintain the patient at bed rest with close hemodynamic monitoring and consult a urologist.

Ureteral trauma

If a ureteral injury is suspected, obtain a CT scan (with contrast) of the abdomen and pelvis. Extravasation of the contrast is the hallmark of ureteral injury. Hydronephrosis, ureteral deviation, or lack of visualization of contrast in the distal ureter may also be noted. Consult a urologist to arrange emergent treatment, either intraoperative repair or urinary diversion with a nephrostomy tube. A preoperative retrograde pyelogram may be necessary to delineate the degree of injury.

Bladder trauma

Inability to void, a distended bladder, and gross hematuria suggest a serious bladder injury. Call a urologist immediately, as urethral integrity must be ensured before catheterization is performed. Urethral disruption is suggested by a boggy mass palpated on rectal examination. A retrograde urethrogram is indicated in the male. After evaluation of urethral integrity, obtain a gravity cystogram for all patients. Calculate the age-adjusted bladder capacity before administering the contrast material (in ounces, <2 years: 2 + [age in years × 2]; >2 years: 6 + [age in years]/2). Bladder injuries are classified by extravasation of contrast into either the extraperitoneal, intraperitoneal, or both spaces, particularly with penetrating trauma.

Treat a patient with extraperitoneal extravasation with either a suprapubic or urethral catheter. Intraperitoneal extravasation is an indication for intraoperative repair and suprapubic diversion of urine.

Urethral injury

Blood at the urethral meatus indicates a urethral injury; consult a urologist to perform a retrograde urethrogram. Do not catheterize the patient before urethral integrity is fully evaluated, as catheterization can convert a partial disruption into a complete transection. After the level and degree of urethral injury are ascertained, suprapubic catheter placement is indicated for temporary urinary diversion pending more definitive repair on an emergency or expectant basis.

External genital trauma

Treat penile hair-tourniquet with an ice bag to ease the pain and shrink the swelling. Application of soapy water to the hairs facilitates removal. Wrap any size of penile amputation in saline gauze, put it in a plastic bag, and place it on ice, with pressure and sterile dressings applied to the remaining shaft. Immediate reanastomosis surgery may be successful. If gentle attempts to remove penile skin caught in a zipper are unsuccessful, inject 1% lidocaine (without epinephrine) into the foreskin. Then, the zipper can be closed, cut through at its base, and opened from the base, releasing the entrapped skin.

Treat an amputation or avulsion of scrotal skin with sterile saline-soaked towels and consult a urologist to determine the need for surgery. If there is a urethral foreign body, arrange for cystoscopy and transurethral extraction after percutaneous placement of a suprapubic catheter by a urologist.

Obtain a sonogram for suspected traumatic testicular torsion or testicular rupture.

Indications for admission

- Abnormal CT scan (renal contusion, laceration, collecting system injury, major vessel injury)
- Penile or scrotal amputation
- Bladder or urethral contusion, laceration, or rupture
- Inability to void

Bibliography

Cannon GM Jr, Polsky EG, Smaldone MC, et al: Computerized tomography findings in pediatric renal trauma–indications for early intervention? *J Urol* 2008;179:1529–32.

Lynch T, Martinez-Pinero L, Plas E, et al: EAU guidelines on urologic trauma. *Euro Urol* 2005;47:1–15.

Morey AF, Metro MJ, Carney KJ, Miller KS, McAninch JW: Consensus on genitourinary trauma: external genitalia. *BJU Int* 2004;94:507–15.

Shariat SF, Jenkins A, Roehrborn CG, et al: Features and outcomes of patients with grade IV renal injury. *BJU Int* 2008;102:728–33.

Meatal stenosis

Meatal stenosis is a narrowing of the urethral meatus, usually secondary to recurrent episodes of subclinical meatitis. Etiologies include ammoniacal diaper dermatitis (circumcised boys) and recurrent balanoposthitis (uncircumcised boys). However, acquired meatal stenosis occurs very rarely in uncircumcised boys because the foreskin acts as a protective cover for the meatus. Congenital meatal stenosis is also very rare.

Clinical presentation

Obstructive symptoms occasionally occur, including hesitancy, straining, urgency, frequency, and post-voiding dribbling. An abnormal urinary stream may be seen, with either spraying or upward deflection. There may be pain at the initiation of urination or burning at the meatus, although urinary retention is rare. If there is an associated meatitis, an erythematous, swollen meatus is noted, often with a purulent discharge.

Diagnosis

The diagnosis of meatal stenosis can be made upon direct observation of the urinary stream. However, a narrowed meatus on visual inspection does not constitute a valid diagnosis.

ED management

Treat purulent meatitis with warm water sitz baths and oral antibiotics for 7 days. Use 40 mg/kg per day of either cephalexin (div qid) or cefadroxil (div bid). Refer all patients to a urologist for confirmation of the diagnosis and further evaluation. Immediately consult a urologist for the rare case of acute urinary retention.

Follow-up

• Meatitis without retention: urology follow-up in 1–2 weeks

Indication for admission

• Urinary retention

Bibliography

Bazmamoun H, Ghorbanpour M, Mousavi-Bahar SH: Lubrication of circumcision site for prevention of meatal stenosis in children younger than 2 years old. Urol J 2008;5:233–6.

Leslie JA, Cain MP: Pediatric urologic emergencies and urgencies. Pediatr Clin North Am 2006;53:513–27.

Mahmoudi H: Evaluation of meatal stenosis following neonatal circumcision. Urol J 2005;2:86–8.

Paraphimosis

Paraphimosis is entrapment of the foreskin behind the coronal sulcus of an uncircumcised or inadequately circumcised penis. It occurs when a tight foreskin is retracted proximal to the glans penis then not returned to its normal position. This produces a tourniquet effect with resultant venous congestion and edema of the glans.

Clinical presentation and diagnosis

On examination, there is edema and tenderness of the glans penis with a tight proximal collar of swollen tissue. The glans congestion will progress over time and skin color will change from the normal pink to blue to white (ischemia), with eventual gangrene. The penile shaft is unaffected. The constriction by the foreskin along with resultant edema may lead to urethral obstruction at the coronal level. The patient then complains of difficulty voiding and urinary retention. Direct erosion into the urethra rarely occurs.

ED management

Place an ice bag on the foreskin and administer a topical (EMLA cream) or regional (penile block with lidocaine without epinephrine) anesthetic, and/or sedate the patient (see Sedation and analgesia, pp. 620–70). Reduce the edema by applying manual circumferential compression for several minutes. Then, grasp the penile shaft with the index and third fingers of each hand, with the thumbs on the glans. Firm downward pressure on the glans against counterpressure on the shaft usually advances the foreskin back over the glans. Alternatively, following the application of EMLA cream with an occlusive dressing (30 min to 1 hour), inject 1 mL of hyaluronidase (150Units/mL) into one or more sites in the edematous prepuce. Resolution of the edema is almost immediate, and the foreskin can be gently retracted over the glans. It is critical to attempt to advance the most distal foreskin ring (the portion closest to the coronal margin). If this tight ring can be reduced, then the remainder of the foreskin will follow. Occasionally, there is tearing of the skin with bleeding, which can be controlled by compression. Instruct the patient to avoid retracting his foreskin for several days. Refer the patient to a urologist for follow-up and evaluation of the need for an elective circumcision.

If the paraphimosis cannot be reduced, consult a urologist immediately to perform a dorsal slit to release the constricting ring of tissue.

Follow-up

• Reducible paraphimosis: urology follow-up in 1–2 weeks

Bibliography

Garcia de Freitas R, Nobre YD, Demarchi GT, et al: Topical treatment for phimosis: time span and other factors behind treatment effectiveness. *J Pediatr Urol* 2006; 2:380–5.

Leslie JA, Cain MP: Pediatric urologic emergencies and urgencies. *Pediatr Clin North Am* 2006;53:513–27.

Little B, White M: Treatment options for paraphimosis. *Int J Clin Pract* 2005;59:591.

Phimosis

Phimosis is the inability to retract the tight foreskin over the glans penis. In 50% of uncircumcised boys the foreskin is retractable at 1 year of age, and 90% are retractable by 4 years. The remaining 10% may not become retractable until puberty. If associated infections (local or more proximally in the urinary tract) or voiding difficulties occur, correction may be indicated.

Clinical presentation and diagnosis

Acquired phimosis is a result of poor hygiene with inflammation of the glans. Accumulated smegma may form aggregates that appear as whitish, globular masses under the nonretractile foreskin. Associated inflammatory conditions may coexist, including balano-posthitis (pp. 283–284) and meatitis (p. 288). With severe phimosis, the foreskin may balloon during voiding as the urine collects under it and then dribbles out from the tight opening. The adolescent may complain of pain on erection, secondary to tension on the foreskin from the glandular adhesions.

ED management

Treat accumulated smegma without any associated infection with gentle retraction of the foreskin during bathing. Depending on the patient's age, if there is no infection, refer him to a urologist for consideration of elective circumcision. If there is ballooning of the foreskin with a dribbling urinary stream, or an associated UTI, consult a urologist. Gentle dilatation may be necessary, after which an elective circumcision or preputialplasty (surgical widening of the phimotic ring) is indicated.

Follow-up

- Phimosis without associated difficulty voiding: urology follow-up in 1–2 weeks

Bibliography

MacLellan DL Diamond DA: Recent advances in external genitalia. *Pediatr Clin North Am* 2006;53:499–64.

McGregor TB, Pike JG, Leonard MP: Pathologic and physiologic phimosis: approach to the phimotic foreskin. *Can Fam Physician* 2007;53:445–8.

Ortiz V: Topical treatment for phimosis: time span and other factors behind treatment effectiveness. *J Pediatr Urol* 2006;2:380–5.

Priapism

Priapism is a sustained and painful penile erection that results from either increased arterial flow (high flow) or, more commonly, from decreased venous outflow (low flow). It most frequently occurs as a complication of sickle cell disease (p. 354) with a reported incidence of 30% before the age of 20 years. It may also result from spinal cord injury, leukemic infiltration, medications, or trauma.

Clinical presentation and diagnosis

The patient presents with a sustained, painful erection. Urinary retention may result with a distended bladder palpable on examination. Persistence of the priapism can lead to corporal fibrosis, with resultant erectile dysfunction. In boys with sickle cell disease, other manifestations of the vasoocclusive crisis may be present.

ED management

Initial management includes analgesia or sedation, hydration, and oxygenation. If the patient has sickle cell disease, determine the percent of HgbS. Specific therapy for the sickle cell patient is aimed at reducing the HgbS to 30–35% by exchange transfusion. Consult with a pediatric hematologist to institute HgbS reduction therapy promptly; the goal is to achieve a therapeutic reduction within the first 24 hours. If the priapism persists in spite of adequate reduction of HgbS, consult a urologist to perform aspiration of blood from the corpora cavernosa, followed by irrigation with a dilute epinephrine solution. Most commonly, however, reduction of HgbS is sufficient to effect resolution of the priapism. On occasion, acute bladder drainage with a Foley catheter may be necessary.

Indication for admission

- Priapism

Bibliography

Birnbaum BF, Pinzone JJ: Sickle cell trait and priapism: a case report and review of the literature. *Cases J* 2008;1:429.

Burnett AL: Therapy insight: priapism associated with hematologic dyscrasias. *Nat Clin Pract Urol* 2005;2:449–56.

Mockford K, Weston M, Subramaniam R: Management of high-flow priapism in paediatric patients: a case report and review of the literature. *J Pediatr Urol* 2007; 3:404–12.

Scrotal swellings

A number of conditions can produce an acutely erythematous and tender hemiscrotum. Testicular torsion is the most serious and requires prompt diagnosis and surgical intervention.

Clinical presentation

Testicular torsion

Testicular torsion is caused by twisting of the spermatic cord leading to venous, lymphatic, and eventual arterial occlusion. Although testicular torsion can occur at any age, the peak is 14 years (range 12–18 years). There is another small peak among neonates. About 60% of patients experience the sudden onset of severe testicular or scrotal pain that may radiate to the groin or lower abdomen, often before the boy awakens in the early morning hours. Other symptoms include nausea, vomiting, and a wide-based gait. Younger patients may only complain of abdominal or inguinal pain.

On physical examination, there is hemiscrotal swelling and erythema. The involved testis may be elevated with a horizontal orientation. The hemiscrotal swelling does not transilluminate, elevation of the testicle does not diminish the pain (Prehn's sign), and the ipsilateral cremasteric reflex is absent in nearly all cases. There is no fever or dysuria, and in about half of the cases there is a history of subacute bouts of scrotal pain (previous intermittent torsion).

Torsion of the testicular appendage

The appendix testis is a mullerian duct remnant at the upper pole of the testicle. Torsion on its vascular pedicle can mimic testicular torsion, most often at 7–12 years of age. There is the acute onset of pain and tenderness localized to the superior pole of the testis. At times a characteristic bluish nodule, representing an infarcted appendage, can be seen through the thin scrotal skin (blue dot sign). More often, however, the blue dot is not evident until several days after the surrounding scrotal edema and erythema have resolved. The swelling does not transilluminate, although there may be an associated reactive hydrocele that does. The cremasteric reflex is not affected. Elevation of the testis does not relieve the pain, and there is no fever or urinary symptoms. Previous subacute episodes are uncommon.

Epididymoorchitis

Epididymoorchitis is caused by the spread of an infection from the bladder or urethra to the epididymal and testicular ducts and tubules. It may be confused with a testicular torsion, although it is uncommon in boys <14 years of age. Etiologies in preadolescents include mumps, infectious mononucleosis, varicella, mycoplasma and Coxsackie viruses. When epididymitis occurs in non-sexually active boys, there may be a history of a urinary tract anomaly (ectopic ureter, vesicoureteral reflux), recent urethral instrumentation, or an associated urinary tract infection. In sexually active males, the most common etiologies are *Chlamydia* and *N. gonorrhea*. Noninfectious epididymitis is uncommon.

Symptoms include the gradual onset of localized testicular, and possibly abdominal, pain, nausea, vomiting, fever, and dysuria. On examination, there may be localized testicular or epididymal tenderness, nontransilluminating scrotal swelling, and a thickened epididymis. Manual scrotal elevation often relieves the pain in epididymoorchitis (Prehn's sign), but not in testicular and appendiceal torsions. However, this sign is unreliable in prepubertal boys. The cremasteric reflex is unaffected.

Inguinal hernia

Inguinal hernias are most common in the first year of life, especially among premature infants. The hernias are predominantly indirect, secondary to a patent processus vaginalis, and are more common on the right side. Males are affected ten times more often than females. Typically, recurrent episodes of painless, nonerythematous scrotal and inguinal swelling occur, often when the baby is crying or straining. Bowel sounds may be heard in the scrotum, and transillumination is variable. In females, an ovary may be palpated in the hernia sac. Incarceration within the inguinal ring can occur and presents with acute tenderness, erythema, and induration. Over the course of a few hours, strangulation (vascular compromise) occurs with eventual bowel obstruction and necrosis, causing vomiting, decreased bowel sounds, abdominal distention, and possible fluid and electrolyte imbalances.

Hydrocele

Hydroceles are most common during the first year of life, especially on the right side. The mass transilluminates, and the testicle is usually palpable posteriorly in the scrotum. The swelling generally involves only the scrotum and does not extend into the inguinal canal. Hydroceles are categorized according to whether the processus vaginalis is narrowly patent, permitting passage of peritoneal fluid (communicating) or obliterated (noncommunicating).

Communicating hydroceles typically present with recurrent episodes of painless, nonerythematous scrotal swellings that vary in size. It may be possible to completely reduce the hydrocele fluid by gentle pressure. Noncommunicating hydroceles are usually present at birth, are stable in size without waxing and waning, and are not reducible with gentle pressure.

Varicocele

A varicocele is a collection of dilated spermatic cord veins. They are most commonly found on the left side in adolescents. The patient may complain of a sensation of heaviness or dull ache in the scrotum but more often a varicocele is asymptomatic. Examination in the upright position reveals a nontender, nonerythematous scrotum with a "bag of worms" inside. Varicoceles enlarge with a Valsalva maneuver and decrease in the recumbent position.

Idiopathic scrotal edema

Idiopathic scrotal edema is an uncommon inflammatory condition of unknown etiology causing an erythematous discoloration and swelling of the scrotal wall with a normal underlying testis.

Hematocele

A hematocele can occur after scrotal trauma or in association with a bleeding diathesis. A painful, bluish scrotal swelling is seen. When examination of the ipsilateral testis is difficult, scrotal ultrasound can assess the integrity of the involved testicle.

Testicular tumor

Testicular tumors are unusual in young children, although they are the most common solid tumor in males from 15–35 years of age. There is diffuse or localized unilateral testicular enlargement that is firm or rock-hard, but painless. There can be an associated reactive hydrocele. If the tumor is secondary to leukemic infiltration, the mass can be bilateral.

Diagnosis

Although appendicular torsions and epididymoorchitis may closely resemble a testicular torsion, the diagnosis in patients with acute hemiscrotal pain and swelling is testicular torsion until proved otherwise. If there is any suspicion of torsion, immediately obtain urologic consultation. Arrange for immediate surgery if the clinical signs and symptoms are consistent with testicular torsion. If the diagnosis is uncertain, imaging studies, if available within 1 hour of the patient's presentation, may help differentiate among the causes of an acute hemiscrotum. These include color Doppler ultrasound (decreased blood flow in testicular torsion, increased with appendicular torsion and epididymoorchitis) and radio-isotope scrotal scanning (cold in testicular torsion, normal or hot in appendicular torsion, hot with epididymoorchitis).

With appendicular torsion, pain and swelling may be localized to the superior testicular pole and a blue dot may be seen through the thin scrotal skin. Dysuria with pyuria and possible bacteriuria may occur in epididymoorchitis, along with fever and an elevated white blood cell count.

Inguinal hernias, hydroceles, hematoceles, and varicoceles can usually be distinguished by the clinical findings. If a strangulated inguinal hernia cannot be ruled out, obtain a KUB. Dilated intestinal loops with air–fluid levels may be seen along with a loop of bowel in the scrotum.

ED management

Testicular torsion

All suspected cases must be evaluated immediately by a urologist or general surgeon, as testicular survival depends on the duration and degree of ischemia. The testicular salvage rate approaches 100% if the patient is explored within 6 hours of the onset of symptoms, but it drops to 20% 12 hours after the onset of symptoms and 0% at 24 hours. However, because it is not possible to accurately determine whether the torsion has been intermittent or complete, duration of symptoms for >24 hours is not a reason to defer surgery. The intermittent nature of the torsion increases the chance of survival in spite of the long duration. In preparation for surgery, make the child NPO and obtain a CBC, type and cross-match, and a urinalysis.

In extreme circumstances, when prompt surgical intervention is not possible, manual detorsion may be attempted after administering adequate sedation and analgesia. Two-thirds of cases of testicular torsion occur in the medial direction. Rotate the left testis 180–360° clockwise, or the right counterclockwise ("when in doubt, turn it out") until the torsion is relieved as documented by pain relief, lower position of the testis within the scrotum, or increased blood flow by Doppler. Surgery is still necessary, as retorsion often occurs acutely.

Torsion of appendage testis

Surgery is indicated when testicular torsion cannot be clinically excluded, or if unremitting swelling or pain continue for several days. Otherwise, treat symptomatically with analgesics and bed rest.

Epididymoorchitis

Treat the prepubertal male with antibiotics (trimethoprim-sulfamethoxazole, 8 mg/kg per day of TMP div bid or amoxicillin 40 mg/kg per day div tid) for 10 days, analgesics, bed rest, and scrotal support. The treatment of sexually transmitted epididymitis is detailed elsewhere (pp. 320–325).

Inguinal hernia

An easily reducible hernia requires no acute treatment. Refer the patient to a surgeon so that elective repair can be arranged. The vast majority of incarcerated inguinal hernias can be manually reduced. Manual reduction and elective repair are less hazardous than operating on an incarcerated hernia. If the hernial sac contents cannot be easily pushed back into the abdomen, sedate the patient (pp. 682–691) and place him in the Trendelenburg position, with an ice bag on the hernia. After 30 minutes, attempt to push the hernia back into the abdomen by bimanual reduction. Apply pressure to the internal inguinal ring with one hand, while milking the entrapped gas and fluid of the incarcerated bowel into the intraabdominal intestines with the other hand. This will usually facilitate reduction of the entire bowel. If reduction is successful, refer the patient for prompt elective repair. If reduction is not successful, admit the patient for correction of any fluid and electrolyte imbalances prior to emergency herniorrhaphy.

Hydrocele

Almost all noncommunicating hydroceles spontaneously resolve prior to 12 months of age. Thereafter, refer the patient to a urologist for possible correction. Refer patients with communicating hydroceles for elective surgical repair, and caution the parents about the possible presence of an associated inguinal hernia.

Varicocele

Refer the patient to a urologist for evaluation. There is a 20% risk of subsequent subfertility due to the effect of the varicocele on spermatogenesis. Prompt surgery is indicated in cases of loss of testicular volume.

Idiopathic scrotal edema

No treatment is required, other than rest, analgesia, and antihistamines (diphenhydramine 5 mg/kg per day div qid).

Hematocele

Obtain an ultrasound to rule out rupture of the tunica albuginea, which is an indication for surgical exploration. Otherwise, treat with rest and analgesia. If the patient has a bleeding diathesis, employ appropriate measures (pp. 337–338) and consult with a urologist.

Testicular tumor

If there is any suspicion of a testicular tumor, obtain a scrotal ultrasound. If a mass is detected, obtain serum for βHCG, α-fetoprotein, and LDH, and immediately consult with a urologist.

Follow-up

- Appendiceal torsion: 2–3 days if the pain persists
- Epididymoorchitis, unincarcerated inguinal hernia, idiopathic scrotal edema: primary care follow-up in 7–10 days
- Hematocele: 3–5 days

Indications for admission

- Suspected testicular torsion
- Incarcerated inguinal hernia

Bibliography

Eaton SH, Cendron MA, Estrada CR, et al: Intermittent testicular torsion: diagnostic features and management outcomes. *J Urol* 2005;174:1532.

Gatti JM, Patrick Murphy J: Current management of the acute scrotum. *Semin Pediatr Surg* 2007;16:58–63.

Leslie JA, Cain MP: Pediatric urologic emergencies and urgencies. *Pediatr Clin North Am* 2006;53:513–27.

Undescended testis

Undescended testis (cryptorchidism) occurs in 4% of term and up to 40% of boys born at 30 weeks' gestation. Spontaneous descent occurs in the majority over the first 6–12 months, after which time descent is unlikely. Histologic deterioration begins as young as 1 year of age and affects fertility, even in unilateral cases. Fifty percent of cases are right-sided and approximately 30% are bilateral, predominantly in premature boys. An undescended testis is at higher risk for torsion, trauma, and, possibly, malignant degeneration. Referral to a urologist is warranted by 1 year of age.

Clinical presentation and diagnosis

Eighty percent of undescended testes are palpable in the groin (inguinal canal or in the superficial inguinal pouch) or in an ectopic location. There may be an associated inguinal hernia. Some of these testes are actually retractile and will reenter the scrotum during a warm bath or can be milked into the scrotum without a tendency to spring back up to the groin when released.

Most impalpable testes are ultimately found within the abdomen or on occasion in the groin if atrophic or dysplastic. In the remaining cases there is unilateral or bilateral testicular absence, most commonly, the vanishing testis syndrome.

ED management

Examine the child for other abnormalities, such as hypospadias or hernia. No acute treatment is necessary. Refer an infant <1 year of age to a primary care provider, and instruct the parent to examine the scrotum while the child is in a warm bath. Refer patients at 1 year of age to a urologist. If an inguinal hernia is present, arrange for early surgical correction of the cryptorchidism and the hernia, regardless of the patient's age.

Bibliography

Pettersson A, Richiardi L, Nordenskjold A, et al: Age at surgery for undescended testis and risk of testicular cancer. *N Engl J Med* 2007;356:1835.

Ritzén EM: Undescended testes: a consensus on management. *Eur J Endocrinol* 2008;159 Suppl 1:S87–90.

Wenzler DL, Bloom DA, Park JM: What is the rate of spontaneous testicular descent in infants with cryptorchidism? *J Urol* 2004;171:849.

Urinary retention

Ninety percent of all newborns void within the first 24 hours of life, and 99% do so by 48 hours. Afterwards, urinary retention is defined as the inability to urinate for >12 hours. Acute urinary retention is rare in children.

In the male infant, posterior urethral valves are the most common congenital cause of retention. Other etiologies include a urethral polyp, urethral stricture, urethral diverticulum, meatal stenosis, and fecal impaction. In the female infant, retention is most often secondary to a prolapsing ureterocele, urethral prolapse, labial inflammation and adhesions, or a foreign body. Urinary retention can also be the presenting symptom of tumors (neuroblastoma, Ewing's sarcoma, sacrococcygeal teratoma). Infections (cystitis, urethritis, meatitis), iatrogenic or self-instrumentation, lower urinary tract stones, spinal cord lesions, medications (antihistamines, decongestants, bronchodilator, tricyclic anticholinergics, probantheline), and psychogenic retention are other causes of urinary retention. In addition, urinary retention and dysfunctional voiding may be the presenting symptoms of sexual abuse.

Clinical presentation and diagnosis

Urinary retention in a newborn male presents as dribbling or a poor stream. In the female a bulging introital mass may be seen, representing a ureterocele. In either sex, the bladder may be persistently palpable.

In older patients, urinary retention may present with urgency, hesitancy, frequency, dribbling, a poor stream, and a distended, palpable bladder. Dysuria (cystitis or urethritis), a urethral discharge (urethritis), or an inflamed, swollen urethral meatus (meatitis) may be present. Ensure that uncircumcised males do not have balanoposthitis or phimosis. Ask about a history of recurrent urinary tract infections.

Patients with spinal cord abnormalities usually have a visible deformity of the back (sacral dimple, tuft of hair, sinus). On neurologic examination, there may be altered lower extremity reflexes, decreased anal sphincter tone, a sensory level, or differential responses to sensory testing in the lower extremities compared with the upper extremities.

Psychosomatic retention usually occurs in females with no previous history of voiding abnormalities. The initiating stress factor is often unrecognized by the patient and parents, and no other congenital or acquired etiology can be found.

Consider the possibility of sexual abuse if the history and physical examination are not consistent with any other etiologies for urinary retention.

ED management

Initially provide symptomatic treatment, such as a warm-water bath (if available) or viscous lidocaine for local inflammation. If unsuccessful, catheterize the patient. Obtain blood for BUN and creatinine and urine for urinalysis, and immediately refer all infants with dribbling, poor stream, or failure to void within 48 hours of birth to a urologist.

The management of cystitis (pp. 665–667), urethritis (p. 298), and meatitis (p. 288) is discussed elsewhere.

Treat retention secondary to urinary tract instrumentation with sitz baths tid and phenazopyridine hydrochloride (Pyridium, 12 mg/kg per day div tid, 300 mg/dose maximum, for 1–2 days), but warn the family that the urine will turn orange. Discontinue any medication associated with retention.

If a spinal cord lesion is suspected, consult with a neurologist. However, intermittent catheterization or an indwelling catheter may be required as a temporizing measure.

If psychosomatic retention is suspected, immediately refer the patient to a psychiatrist. Once again, temporary intermittent catheterization or an indwelling catheter may be required. The management of possible sexual abuse is discussed elsewhere (pp. 585–586).

In cases of urinary retention secondary to fecal impaction, rapid treatment of the impaction (see Constipation, pp. 238–240) leads to resolution of the urinary retention.

Indication for admission

- Urinary retention that cannot be relieved in the ED

Bibliography

Asgari SA, Mansour Ghanaie M, Simforoosh N et al: Acute urinary retention in children. Urol J 2005;2:23–7.

Leslie JA, Cain MP: Pediatric urologic emergencies and urgencies. Pediatr Clin North Am 2006;53:513–27.

Urethritis

Urethritis is an inflammation of the urethral mucosa caused by local irritation (chemical, infection, foreign-body insertion). While infectious causes of urethritis are rare in prepubertal children, sexually transmitted infection is the most common etiology in sexually active adolescents.

Clinical presentation and diagnosis

Irritation

Perfumed soaps, bubble bath, or chlorine may cause a chemical irritation of the distal urethral and penile meatus. The patient presents with meatal pain, itching, and dysuria. The urine culture is negative.

Anatomic abnormalities

A prolapsed urethra most commonly occurs in prepubertal African-American females. The prolapsed mucosa is visible as an edematous red or purple doughnut-shaped mass. The initial complaint may be painless bleeding or spotting.

Other abnormalities, such as urethral diverticulum, urethral polyp, and valve of Guérin, are uncommon. They usually present with difficulty voiding, gross hematuria, voiding pain at the dorsal glans penis, and blood spotting on the underpants.

Foreign body

A urethral foreign body causes a bloody urethritis. There may be a clear history of insertion, the object may be palpable in the urethra, or it may be radioopaque.

Posterior urethritis

This is a nonspecific urethral inflammation in boys 5–15 years old. It presents with urethral discharge, urethral bleeding, or terminal hematuria. The physical examination is normal, and routine cultures of the discharge and the urine are sterile.

Sexually transmitted urethritis

In males, gonorrhea, *Chlamydia* or *Ureaplasma* cause dysuria, urethral discharge, and occasionally epididymitis or prostatitis. In females, *Chlamydia* commonly causes the acute urethral syndrome (dysuria, urgency, suprapubic tenderness, pyuria) or pelvic inflammatory disease (pp. 315–316).

Obtain a urinalysis and routine urine culture, and perform a Gram's stain and culture (*Gonococci*, *Chlamydia*) of the urethral discharge.

ED management
Irritation

Discontinue the chemical irritant, if known, and if the symptoms are severe, give phenazopyridine hydrochloride (Pyridium, 12 mg/kg per day div tid, 300 mg maximum dose) for 1 or 2 days, only.

Anatomic abnormalities

Treat a prolapsed urethra with warm compresses or sitz baths, tid. Prescribe a topical estrogen cream bid for 2 weeks and arrange follow-up. Consult a urologist if marked edema causes voiding difficulty. Refer patients with gross hematuria in association with penile voiding pain to a urologist.

Foreign body

Immediately consult a urologist.

Posterior urethritis

Treat with 10 days of antibiotics (<8 years: amoxicillin 40 mg/kg per day div tid; >8 years: trimethoprim-sulfamethoxazole, 8 mg/kg per day of TMP div bid). There is a high rate of recurrence, and bulbar urethral stricture can result. Therefore, refer the patient to a urologist.

Sexually transmitted urethritis

Treat with a single dose of ceftriaxone 125 mg IM, followed by either PO azithromycin 20 mg/kg (1 g maximum) in a single dose, or a 7-day course of oral erythromycin (50 mg/kg per day div q 8 h) or doxycycline 100 mg bid (>8 years of age).

Follow-up

- Urethritis: primary care follow-up in 7–10 days

Indications for admission

- Inability to void
- Urethral foreign body

Bibliography

Leslie JA, Cain MP: Pediatric urologic emergencies and urgencies. *Pediatr Clin North Am* 2006;53:513–27.

Manhart LE, Golden MR, Marrazzo JM: Expanding the spectrum of pathogens in urethritis: implications for presumptive therapy? *Clin Infect Dis* 2007;45:872–4.

Takahashi S, Takeyama K, Kunishima Y, et al: Analysis of clinical manifestations of male patients with urethritis. *J Infect Chemother* 2006;12:283–6.

Chapter 12

Gynecologic emergencies

Dominic Hollman, Elizabeth M. Alderman, and Anthony J. Ciorciari

Breast disorders

Common breast disorders for which emergency care is sought include neonatal hypertrophy, premature thelarche (either alone or with precocious puberty), absence of breast development, asymmetry, breast masses, breast abscesses, and gynecomastia.

Clinical presentation

Neonatal breast hypertrophy

Neonatal breast hypertrophy occurs in up to two-thirds of normal newborns of both genders. It results from maternal hormonal stimulation, and presents as palpable breast tissue, present from birth, in an otherwise healthy infant. Occasionally, in female infants, there is also galactorrhea, clitoral hypertrophy, and a bloody vaginal discharge, also resulting from the effect of maternal hormones. Most cases resolve within a month, although breast hypertrophy may persist for several months.

Premature thelarche

Premature thelarche is defined as breast enlargement in the absence of other signs of puberty in a female <9 years of age, but it is most common in girls <5 years old. At times it is the result of neonatal breast hypertrophy failing to regress. Bilateral breast buds (2–4 cm) are present with no associated nipple or areolar change. The patient will not have nipple discharge, axillary or pubic hair, clitoral enlargement, or acne. She will also not have had a growth spurt. The presence of any of these other findings suggests more significant pathology, including true precocious puberty, CNS disorders, ovarian tumors, and exogenous estrogens.

Absence of breast development

Adolescents may present with a complaint of no breast development. In an otherwise healthy patient with other pubertal signs (pubic hair, pubertal genitalia, menses), it is likely that she has normal breasts, albeit small. However, lack of breast development may be secondary to an absence of glandular tissue (amastia), endocrine issues (congenital adrenal hyperplasia, hypogonadotropic hypogonadism), radiation therapy, or a systemic disorder (Crohn's disease, malnutrition).

Asymmetry

Breast asymmetry is common during puberty and may persist into adulthood. The problem is generally a cosmetic one, although it can cause significant psychosocial stress. Poland syndrome is an uncommon disorder, affecting both females and males, which presents with breast asymmetry due to absence of the sternal head of the pectoralis major muscle and hypoplasia or aplasia of the ipsilateral breast or nipple.

Breast masses

Breast masses are a common source of fear and anxiety in the adolescent female, but most cases are benign, secondary to fibrocystic changes or physiologic breast tissue. While adolescents typically have dense breast tissue at baseline, fibrocystic changes can ensue, appearing as cord-like thickening which may present as "lumps." These "lumps" may become tender and enlarged prior to menses each month.

The most common discrete masses in adolescents are fibroadenomas. These are benign lesions, which present as firm, rubbery, mobile masses with clearly defined borders. Other common benign findings include simple cysts, capillary hemangiomas, and fat necrosis.

Cystosarcoma phyllodes is a rare primary tumor, which is usually, but not always, benign. The tumor is generally large (about 6 cm), and there may be overlying skin changes (tautness, retraction, necrosis). Invasive breast cancer (adenocarcinoma) is exceedingly rare in children and adolescents. A positive family history of breast cancer and prior radiation treatment are risk factors.

Mastitis and breast abscesses

Mastitis (inflammation of the breast) and breast abscesses (a local accumulation of pus in the breast) are infections which can occur in newborns as well as adolescent females. *Staphylococcus aureus* is the most common pathogen in both age groups. In adolescents abscesses are most frequent during lactation, while in nonlactating teenagers the etiology is unclear, but may be due to duct ectasia or metaplasia of the duct epithelium. Trauma or manipulation of the skin can also lead to infection. The abscess presents on the skin adjacent to the areola as a warm, erythematous, tender mass, which may be fluctuant. The patient may be febrile.

Gynecomastia

Nearly 50% of adolescent males undergo benign, usually bilateral, increase in the glandular and stromal tissue of the breast, generally at Tanner stage II–III. It results from an increase in estrogen that is usually part of normal adolescent development.

Gynecomastia resolves within 1–2 years. However, persistence beyond adolescence may be pathologic, secondary to disorders that cause increased estrogen, decreased androgen, or abnormality at the receptors for estrogen or androgen. These include testicular, adrenal, or other hCG-producing tumors. Hypogonadotropic hypogonadism, androgen insensitivity, hyperthyroidism, hyperprolactinemia, liver disease, kidney disease, or obesity can also cause gynecomastia. Drug use, either medical (spironolactone, cimetidine, digoxin) or recreational (marijuana), is another etiology.

Diagnosis

Neonatal breast hypertrophy

A history and physical examination, including a genital exam to assess for other signs of maternal estrogenization, are all that is required.

Premature thelarche

A complete physical examination must be performed to rule out true precocious puberty. Premature thelarche is the diagnosis if no other pubertal changes are present. Note the presence of secondary sexual characteristics, such as pubic hair, estrogenized vaginal mucosa, and clitoral enlargement. The presence of any of these findings is indicative of precocious puberty, not isolated premature thelarche.

Absence of breast development

Examine the patient for evidence of hirsutism or acne, which can indicate a hormone imbalance, such as androgen excess. Inspect the external genitals to assess for clitoromegaly and degree of estrogenization, which can also result from hyperandrogenism.

Asymmetry

Examine the patient in both the upright and supine positions. It is important to rule out a breast mass as the cause of asymmetry. If there is associated breast tenderness, obtain an ultrasound to rule out a breast abscess.

Breast masses

A breast examination is usually sufficient to diagnose fibrocystic changes and to distinguish an abscess from a true breast mass. If a cyst is suspected, schedule the patient to be re-examined after her next menstrual period, as the lesion will often disappear. If a discrete lesion persists, arrange for an ultrasound, which is the imaging modality of choice for evaluating breast masses in adolescents.

Mastitis and breast abscesses

The diagnosis of mastitis is usually evident on inspection of the warm, tender, erythematous breast bud. Neonates may be febrile, although associated symptoms in infant mastitis are uncommon. If the area is fluctuant, presume the child has an associated abscess and arrange for aspiration. This can help confirm the diagnosis and provide a specimen for culture.

Gynecomastia

Gynecomastia can be differentiated from adipose tissue in that gynecomastia presents with a firm, rubbery, discrete mass that is usually <3 cm in diameter. The breast tissue is symmetrically located under the nipple/areolar complex. Although the subareolar nodule may extend beyond the margin of the areola, an asymmetric mass in relation to the areola is not consistent with benign gynecomastia.

In addition, examine the abdomen to evaluate for an adrenal tumor and the testicles to assess testicular volume (or presence of atrophy) and to palpate any masses.

ED management
Neonatal breast hypertrophy

Reassurance, cool compresses, and avoidance of breast massaging are all that is necessary. Refer the infant to a primary care provider.

Premature thelarche/precocious puberty

If there are no other signs of puberty, reassure the patient and family that the condition is not serious and refer the patient to a primary care physician for routine follow-up. However, if other signs of puberty are present, arrange for a pediatric endocrinology visit within one week.

Absence of breast development

If there is no evidence of a pathologic cause for small breast size, reassure the patient and arrange for routine follow-up. Surgical breast augmentation is not an option until the patient has completed pubertal development, and can give informed consent, generally at 18 years of age.

Asymmetry

Reassure the patient that breast asymmetry is common, and it may lessen over time. Surgical intervention may be an option after puberty is complete.

Breast masses

Reassurance is all that is needed for a patient with either physiologic or fibrocystic changes. If a cyst is palpated, arrange for follow-up with the patient's primary doctor after her period. If the lesion persists, or if there is a more concerning finding on examination, obtain an ultrasound and refer to either an adolescent medicine specialist or a surgeon.

Mastitis and breast abscesses

Perform a complete sepsis evaluation (pp. 370–373) and hospitalize neonates <8 weeks old with fever >100.6°F (38.1°C) or a "toxic" appearance. Treat with intravenous nafcillin (150 mg/kg per day div q 6 h), or if MRSA is a concern, clindamycin (40 mg/kg per day q 6 h) for 7–10 days. Prior to instituting antibiotic therapy, perform a needle aspiration if an abscess is suspected and send a specimen for culture to guide further therapy. Also admit infants with mastitis for parenteral antibiotics (as above), even if well-appearing, because of the risk of progression to abscess.

Treat afebrile, well-appearing, older children and adolescents with mastitis with cephalexin or cefadroxil (40 mg/kg per day div q 6 h or q 12 h, respectively) for 7–10 days. If MRSA is a concern, either use clindamycin (20 mg/kg per day q 6 h) or add trimethoprim-sulfamethoxazole (8 mg/kg per day of trimethoprim div bid). Warm compresses four to six times daily are an important adjunctive measure. Follow-up within 24 hours; if the mass enlarges or becomes fluctuant, or if the patient becomes febrile, admit the child for intravenous antibiotics and possible incision and drainage (if an abscess has developed).

Gynecomastia

If the patient has findings consistent with pubertal gynecomastia (duration <2 years, Tanner stage II–III), no laboratory work-up is indicated. If there is concern that this is not benign gynecomastia, or if it has persisted >2 years, obtain a serum testosterone, estradiol, LH, and hCG, and refer the patient to his primary care provider.

Follow-up

- Breast abscess or mastitis in the older child: follow-up with primary care provider in 24 hours

- Breast mass: follow up with adolescent medicine or surgery
- Premature thelarche, asymmetry or gynecomastia: follow-up with primary care provider
- Precocious puberty (premature thelarche associated with other secondary sexual characteristics): pediatric endocrinologist within 1 week

Indications for admission

- Mastitis and breast abscess in the neonate and infant
- Breast abscess in the older child who has fever or is ill-appearing

Bibliography

Arca MJ, Caniano DA: Breast disorders in the adolescent patient. *Adolesc Med Clin* 2004;15:473–85.

Laufer MR, Goldstein DP: The breast: examination and lesions. In Emans SJ, Laufer MR, Goldstein DP (eds), *Pediatric and Adolescent Gynecology*, 5th ed. Philadelphia:

Lippincott Williams and Wilkins, 2005, pp. 729–59.

Lee MC, Rios AM, Aten MF, et al: Management and outcome of children with skin and soft tissue abscesses caused by community-acquired methicillin-resistant Staphylococcus aureus. *Pediatr Infect Dis J* 2004; 23:123–7.

Dysfunctional uterine bleeding

The average age of menarche in the United States is 12.8 years, which is approximately 2 years after breast budding and consistent with Tanner IV stage of pubertal development. The normal interval between periods ranges from 21 to 35 days with 3–7 days of bleeding. With normal menstrual flow, a girl uses 3–6 tampons or pads a day, and the average blood loss is 30–60 mL. Menstrual blood loss of >80 mL is abnormal and can lead to lower hemoglobin, hematocrit, and serum iron levels.

Dysfunctional uterine bleeding (DUB) is irregular, painless bleeding of endometrial origin. Most cases are secondary to anovulation, which is common during the first 2–3 years after menarche. However, up to 20% of females may have anovulatory bleeding 4–5 years after menarche. The etiologies of abnormal vaginal bleeding are listed in Table 12-1.

Clinical presentation

A typical pattern of DUB is prolonged or excessive flow alternating with periods of oligomenorrhea or amenorrhea. Pain, fever, chills, abdominal pain, and vaginal discharge are absent. Below are the definitions of the three clinical stages of DUB. Management is dependent on the severity of vaginal bleeding.

Mild DUB

With mild DUB the menses may be somewhat prolonged or the cycle shortened for 2–3 months. The hemoglobin and hematocrit are normal, >11 g/dL and >35%, respectively.

Moderate DUB

Moderate DUB is characterized by prolonged periods and an increased flow severe enough to cause a decrease in hemoglobin and hematocrit to 9–11 g/dL and 25–35%, respectively.

Table 12-1. Etiologies of dysfunctional uterine bleeding

Complications of pregnancy

Ectopic pregnancy

Implantation bleeding

Spontaneous abortion

S/P termination of pregnancy

Sexually transmitted infections

Acute salpingitis

Cervicitis

Endometritis

Other gynecological causes

Vaginal trauma

First intercourse

Sexual assault

Bleeding disorders

von Willebrand's disease

Factor deficiencies

ITP

Medications

Aspirin

Chemotherapy

Depo-medroxyprogesterone acetate

Oral, patch, and ring contraceptives

Prednisone

Warfarin

Endocrine disorders

Adrenal disorders

Polycystic ovarian syndrome

Thyroid disease

Chronic illness

Inflammatory bowel disease

Chronic renal disease

Liver disease

Severe DUB

Severe DUB results in significant decreases in the hemoglobin and hematocrit, to <9 g/dL and <25%, respectively. Clinical signs of acute blood loss (tachycardia, orthostatic vital sign changes, delayed capillary refill) with a hemoglobin <11 g/dL are also consistent with severe DUB.

Diagnosis

Dysfunctional uterine bleeding is a diagnosis of exclusion. Inquire about the age of menarche, date of last normal menstrual period, length of last menstrual period, frequency and regularity of menses, typical length of flow, the number of pads or tampons used, and when the period before the last menstrual period was and whether it was normal. Ask about other bleeding manifestations such as nosebleeds or easy bruisability, epistaxis, bleeding gums, hematuria, and, rarely, hematochezia. Ask about sexual activity (including genital trauma, history of pregnancy, history of sexually transmitted infections), foreign bodies (tampon use, self-insertion), contraceptive history (particularly oral contraceptives, depo medroxyprogesterone acetate, contraceptive patch or ring), medications used (aspirin, coumadin, antipsychotics, antidepressants, steroids), endocrine disorders (specifically symptoms related to thyroid disease, pituitary adenoma, or androgenizing symptoms such as acne or hirsutism which may be associated with polycystic ovarian syndrome), exposure to diethylstilbestrol (DES) in utero, emotional stress, eating habits (including pica), and chronic illnesses.

Pregnancy (pp. 310–314) is suggested by a history of amenorrhea, but a positive serum hCG confirms the diagnosis. Breast tenderness and an enlarged uterus may be noted. Salpingitis (pp. 314–325) may present with a vaginal discharge, lower abdominal pain, fever, chills, cervical motion tenderness, and/or adnexal tenderness.

On physical examination, the priorities are the vital signs, manifestations of a bleeding diathesis, and the gynecologic examination. Check for orthostatic hypotension, bradycardia (hypothyroidism), tachycardia (hyperthyroidism, significant blood loss), delayed capillary refill (shock), petechiae or ecchymoses (bleeding diathesis), or evidence of a chronic illness such as cachexia or swollen joints.

Inspect the external genitalia to look for signs of trauma or bleeding sources. If the patient is sexually active, perform a speculum exam looking for evidence of trauma, or infection (cervical discharge). Also perform a bimanual examination to check the cervix for tenderness on motion (salpingitis). Palpate the uterus to determine size and tenderness, and examine the adnexae for masses and tenderness. If the patient is not sexually active, but has abdominal pain, perform a rectoabdominal examination assessing for a pelvic mass.

ED management

The management of DUB is almost exclusively based on level of anemia caused by the vaginal bleeding. The goal of the work-up is to exclude other causes of bleeding that may require different ED management.

For all patients, obtain a CBC with platelet count, thyroid function tests (TSH and free T4), pregnancy test, clotting studies (PT, PTT), and a urinalysis. If the patient is sexually active, also obtain a gonorrhea and *Chlamydia* test, RPR, and a quantitative pregnancy test. A type and cross-match is indicated for moderate, severe, or prolonged bleeding or orthostasis. Severe bleeding at menarche warrants a bleeding time, as inherited disorders of coagulations, such as von Willebrand's disease, may not manifest until menarche. If the patient has signs of hyperandrogenism or is obese, or the polycystic ovarian syndrome is suspected, obtain a free and total testosterone, DHEAS, androstenedione, and sex hormone binding globulin, as once a girl begins hormonal treatment, these parameters cannot be accurately assessed. If a pelvic mass is appreciated or ectopic pregnancy suspected, obtain an ultrasound.

Mild DUB

Observation and reassurance are all that are needed. Advise the patient to keep a menstrual calendar. Iron supplementation (325 mg/day of ferrous gluconate or multivitamin with iron) may be necessary, but the majority of these patients spontaneously convert to normal menstrual cycles within several months.

Moderate DUB

Treat with a monophasic oral contraceptive with 35 mcg estrogen/1 mcg progesterone (e.g. Sprintec). Always prescribe the 21-day pill pack, as taking the placebos of the 28-day pack will cause a withdrawal bleed. Give four pills per day for 4 days, then three pills per day for 4 days, then two pills per day for 13–19 days; then one pill a day until follow-up, which should occur within a month of the ED visit. Give the patient or guardian detailed written instructions, as this regimen is complicated, and, if not followed exactly, may result in breakthrough bleeding. Also prescribe an oral antiemetic, such as prochlorperazine (10 mg q 6 h or 25 mg bid) or ondansetron (15–30 kg: 4 mg bid; >30 kg: 8 mg PO bid).

When the patient is at the point of taking one contraceptive pill a day, add ferrous gluconate (325 mg tid) to treat the anemia. Starting the iron while the patient is taking more than one OCP/day may exacerbate the GI side effects. A week after stopping the OCP, begin a new 28-day pill pack and cycle the patient for 6 months. At that time, if the girl is not sexually active, discontinue the pill and observe to see whether her periods are now regular.

Severe DUB

The priority is restoration of adequate perfusion (see Shock, pp. 24–27) with 20 mL/kg boluses of isotonic crystalloid (normal saline or Ringer's lactate). A packed red cell transfusion (10 mL/kg) is indicated if the patient is symptomatic (e.g. tachycardia dizziness), either at rest or standing, after the boluses. To stop the bleeding immediately, give a conjugated estrogen (Premarin), 25 mg IV over 20 minutes, q 4–6 h. This is usually effective after the third dose, but a maximum of 6 doses of Premarin may be given. An antiemetic may be needed (as above). If the bleeding does not subside after the third dose of Premarin or it increases, consult a gynecologist to determine whether a dilatation and curettage is indicated. At the same time as Premarin is started, administer a monophasic 1:35 oral contraceptive, four pills that first day, and follow the regimen outlined for moderate DUB. Admit the patient for both treatment and observation.

Follow-up

- Mild DUB: routine primary care follow-up. Have the patient maintain a menstrual diary. Advise her to call her primary care provider if bleeding continues for another week

- Moderate DUB: 1–2 days, at which time the bleeding should have stopped or slowed significantly. Refer the patient to an adolescent medicine specialist or gynecologist if the bleeding does not stop within 2–3 days of four pills a day

Indications for admission

- Severe DUB
- Moderate DUB with symptoms or signs of inadequate perfusion

Bibliography

Adams Hillard PJ, Deitch HR: Menstrual disorders in the college age female. *Pediatr Clin North Am* 2005; 52:179–97.

Gray SH, Emans SJ: Abnormal vaginal bleeding in adolescents. *Pediatr Rev* 2007;28:175–81.

Grover S: Bleeding disorders and heavy menses in adolescents. *Curr Opin Obstet Gynecol* 2007;19:415–9.

Dysmenorrhea

Dysmenorrhea (painful menstruation) is very common in teenagers and may be a response to elevated levels of prostaglandin. The majority of cases are classified as primary dysmenorrhea, which do not present at menarche and are not associated with significant pelvic pathology. In secondary dysmenorrhea there is pelvic pathology, most often salpingitis, endometriosis, or genital tract obstruction secondary to a congenital malformation of the uterus or vagina.

Clinical presentation

Primary dysmenorrhea

Primary dysmenorrhea usually presents within 6–12 months of menarche. Typically, colicky suprapubic pain begins several hours before or after the start of a period. The pain may radiate to the back or down the thighs. In 50% of patients there may be nausea, vomiting, diarrhea, and migraine headaches. The symptoms can last from a few hours to several days and there is often a family history of dysmenorrhea.

Secondary dysmenorrhea

Secondary dysmenorrhea generally presents years after menarche, although dysmenorrhea with the first menses may be a sign of a congenital anomaly with a gynecologic outflow tract obstruction. As in primary dysmenorrhea, the pain occurs during menstruation. There may be a history of pelvic inflammatory disease, vaginal discharge, abdominal or pelvic surgery, menorrhagia, endometriosis, or IUD use.

Diagnosis

The most important aspect in managing a girl with lower abdominal pain who is perimenstrual is to determine if she has primary or secondary dysmenorrhea. Additionally, nongynecologic causes of lower abdominal pain must be ruled out (see Abdominal pain, pp. 219–222).

Obtain a menstrual history, including age of menarche, last menstrual period, regularity of menses, frequency and severity of the pain and its relation to the periods. Ask about a history of vaginal discharge, sexual activity, IUD use, previous pelvic inflammatory disease, or abdominal/pelvic surgery. Ask about family or personal history of dysmenorrhea.

Table 12-2. Differential diagnosis of dysmenorrhea

Diagnosis	Differentiating features
Congenital anomalies	Cyclical lower abdominal pain at menarche or in an amenorrheic patient
Ectopic pregnancy	Positive hCG
	Unilateral adnexal mass
Endometriosis	Pain starts before bleeding and persists beyond
	Uterus/ovaries tender or enlarged
Imperforate hymen	Bulging vaginal mass with no patent hymen
	Patient is ≥ Tanner III without history of menses
Intrauterine pregnancy	Positive hCG
	Enlarged uterus (> pear or orange size)
Ovarian cyst/tumor	Mass palpated on bimanual or rectoabdominal exam
Salpingitis	Fever, vaginal discharge, cervical motion tenderness
	Adnexal enlargement/tenderness (can be unilateral)

Perform a complete physical examination to exclude any gastrointestinal or urinary causes of lower abdominal pain, such as appendicitis, gastroenteritis, constipation, inflammatory bowel disease, renal colic, or urinary tract infection. Perform an external vaginal examination to assess hymenal patency. If secondary dysmenorrhea is suspected in a girl who is not sexually active, perform a rectoabdominal examination to assess for a pelvic mass, which usually reflects uterine enlargement. If the patient is sexually active, perform a pelvic examination, looking for causes of secondary dysmenorrhea, including cervical motion tenderness, an IUD, and adnexal or uterine enlargement or tenderness. Obtain a pregnancy test for all patients who have had previous menses, or if a girl is Tanner III, or more mature, with no previous menses. See Table 12-2 for the differential diagnosis of dysmenorrhea.

ED management
Primary dysmenorrhea
Oral prostaglandin synthetase inhibitors (nonsteroidal anti-inflammatories) are effective in 70–100% of patients. Use ibuprofen (Motrin, Advil) 400–600 mg q 6 h, naproxen (Anaprox 550 mg first dose, then 275 mg q 12 h; Alleve 440 mg first dose, then 220 mg q 12 h), or mefenamic acid (Ponstel), 500 mg first dose, then 250 mg q 6 h.

Advise the patient to start the medication at the onset of each period. It is best to start with a loading dose and to take the medication with food. If one nonsteroidal anti-inflammatory agent is ineffective, try an alternative. Side effects include nausea, dizziness, dyspepsia, and gastric irritation. These medications are contraindicated in patients with ulcers and aspirin allergy; use with caution in patients taking anticoagulants or with liver or kidney disease. Since patients with primary dysmenorrhea ovulate monthly and therefore have regular cycles, have these patients keep track of their menses with a menstrual calendar or the calendar on their cell phone.

Other treatments that may be helpful include heating pads, exercise, low-salt diet, well-balanced diet, and reduction of stress. Suppression of ovulation by oral contraceptives is effective, but reserve this therapy for the primary care setting, where appropriate follow-up can be arranged.

Secondary dysmenorrhea

Refer the patient to a gynecologist to treat the underlying cause. The management of salpingitis is discussed on pp. 314–325. If endometriosis is suspected, refer the patient to a gynecologist to arrange for laparoscopic confirmation of the diagnosis, followed by hormone therapy.

Follow-up

* Primary dysmenorrhea: primary care follow-up before the next period
* Secondary dysmenorrhea: gynecological follow-up before the next period

Bibliography

French L: Dysmenorrhea in adolescents: diagnosis and treatment. *Paediatr Drugs* 2008;10:1–7.

Mannix LK: Menstrual-related pain conditions: dysmenorrhea and migraine. *J Womens Health (Larchmt)* 2008;17:879–91.

Sanfilippo J, Erb T: Evaluation and management of dysmenorrhea in adolescents. *Clin Obstet Gynecol* 2008;51:257–67.

Pregnancy and complications

Approximately 75 of 1,000 women 15–19 years of age in the United States become pregnant each year. Spontaneous abortions complicate 10–15% of pregnancies, and approximately 2% are ectopic.

Clinical presentation

Knowing whether a patient is pregnant is essential in evaluating her complaints and determining management. The first step is to interview the teenager privately and assure her that the discussion is confidential. Often the pregnant patient presents with vague complaints of "abdominal pain" or "not feeling right" because she does not want her family to suspect the possible pregnancy. The patient may not realize or deny that she is pregnant. Also, she may not volunteer the information that she has missed a period or had unprotected intercourse.

During early pregnancy, a teenager may report "missing" her period or that it was "different" (longer or shorter than usual). Fatigue, dizziness, syncope, nausea and vomiting (especially in the morning), urinary frequency, and weight gain may be noted by 2 weeks. Nipple discharge (colostrum) can occur at 6 weeks.

On examination, the breasts have darkened areolae and enlarged nipples. Often, there is protrusion of Montgomery's glands. Findings on pelvic examination depend on the time elapsed since the first day of the last normal period. At 5 weeks the examination may be normal, at 6–7 weeks there may be softening of the uterus at the junction of the cervix (Hegar's sign), at 8 weeks the cervix and vaginal mucosa may have a bluish tinge due to venous congestion (Chadwick's sign) and the uterus may be soft and slightly enlarged, and by 8–12 weeks the fetal heart may be heard with Doppler. At 12 weeks, the globular uterus can be palpated at the level of the pubic symphysis, at 16 weeks at the midpoint between the symphysis and umbilicus, and at 20 weeks at the level of the umbilicus. However, the best way to estimate gestational age is to use a "pregnancy wheel." This tool will give an approximate gestational age based upon the first day of the patient's last period and the usual interval between her periods.

Threatened abortion

With a threatened abortion, the history is compatible with early pregnancy. There is vaginal bleeding with or without cramps, and the internal cervical os is closed. Patients with threatened abortion usually present with vaginal bleeding and/or pain.

Imminent abortion

With an imminent abortion the cervix is dilated or open. The bleeding and pain are typically more severe than would be expected from a threatened abortion.

Inevitable abortion

An inevitable abortion resembles an imminent abortion, except that there are products of conception protruding from the dilated or open cervix.

Incomplete abortion

In an incomplete abortion, some placental tissue still remains in the uterus. The vaginal bleeding is usually heavy and the patient may complain of severe abdominal pain.

Complete abortion

There is full passage of the products of conception. The patient may be asymptomatic on presentation but will probably have a history of abdominal pain, vaginal bleeding, and passage of tissue.

Missed abortion

A missed abortion is a fetal death in utero before the 20th week, but with the pregnancy retained. If the patient knew she was pregnant, she may report that she does not feel fetal movement. Abdominal pain and/or vaginal bleeding are possible, but unlikely.

Ectopic pregnancy

An ectopic pregnancy occurs when the blastocyst implants in a location other than the uterus; the vast majority are in the fallopian tubes. Major predisposing factors include pelvic inflammatory disease, prior pelvic or abdominal surgery, or prior ectopic pregnancy. However, about half of patients who have an ectopic pregnancy do not have an identifiable risk factor.

The classic presentation is a history of oligomenorrhea, with symptoms of early pregnancy, followed by abdominal pain and mild to moderate vaginal bleeding. A late or missed period occurs in 75% of patients, followed by vaginal spotting or bleeding. Brisk or heavy bleeding is uncommon. The vast majority of patients will complain of abdominal pain, which can be of any severity and in any location in the abdomen or pelvis. Up to 10% of patients may complain of fever.

Physical examination findings include abdominal and pelvic tenderness and cervical motion tenderness. An adnexal mass is found in a minority of patients. If the ectopic pregnancy has ruptured, the patient may present with signs of hypovolemic shock.

Diagnosis

Pregnancy tests detect the presence of hCG in the blood or urine. The standard urine pregnancy test is 99% sensitive and specific, detecting 25 mIUnits/mL of hCG. In normal pregnancies, it may be positive as early as 3–4 days after implantation and virtually always by the expected date of the missed period. However, if the urine is not sufficiently concentrated there may be a false-negative finding.

The serum hCG by radioimmunoassay can be positive within 7 days of conception (before a period has been missed). In most intrauterine pregnancies, the quantitative serum hCG will double every 1.5–2.3 days (about 36–55 hours). The doubling will slow somewhat when the level is >10,000 mIUnits/mL; however, by this time ultrasonography is diagnostic.

With an ectopic pregnancy, the hCG does not rise as fast. However, a single hCG measurement is of limited value, since the exact gestational age is often not known and there is some overlap in the range of hCG levels found in the two conditions. Therefore, obtain serial hCG determinations 2 days apart. Doubling of the hCG within 48 hours suggests an intrauterine pregnancy. A slower doubling time or a rise of less than 66% over 2 days suggests, but does not confirm, an ectopic pregnancy. Up to 15% of normal pregnancies will have an abnormal serum hCG doubling time, and as many as 35% of ectopic pregnancies will have what is considered to be a normal serum hCG doubling time.

The serum progesterone is useful for diagnosing an ectopic pregnancy. In a normal pregnancy, the level is >25 ng/mL, while a level <5 ng/mL is highly associated with an ectopic pregnancy. Values between 5 and 25 ng/mL are indeterminate. In this situation, a diagnostic ultrasound is helpful.

It is not always safe to wait 2 days to confirm the diagnosis. Using transabdominal ultrasound, a normal intrauterine pregnancy can be detected with an hCG >6,500 mIUnits/mL. However, transvaginal ultrasound is far more sensitive (90–95%) and can confirm the presence of a gestational sac at an hCG of 1,000–1,500 mIUnits/mL. The diagnostic and therapeutic approach of ectopic pregnancy is summarized in Figure 12-1.

The differential diagnosis of ectopic pregnancy includes a normal pregnancy with another cause for the abdominal or pelvic pain. These include gynecologic conditions which may complicate pregnancy and can be evaluated by ultrasound, such as an ovarian cyst, ovarian or tubal torsion, or ruptured corpus luteum. Alternatively, the pathology may be nongynecologic, such as an appendicitis or a renal stone.

ED management

The priority is expedient diagnosis and management of an ectopic pregnancy. Suspect an ectopic in any pubertal female with vaginal bleeding and/or lower abdominal pain, especially if her period is late. Perform a pelvic examination; any abnormality suggests the possibility of an ectopic pregnancy. Immediately arrange for gynecologic consultation, obtain blood for hCG, CBC, type and cross-match, insert a large-bore IV, and monitor the patient carefully, with frequent vital signs and serial hematocrits.

If a ruptured ectopic is likely (peritoneal signs, orthostatic vital sign changes, or falling hematocrit associated with a positive hCG), immediate obstetrical consultation is indicated.

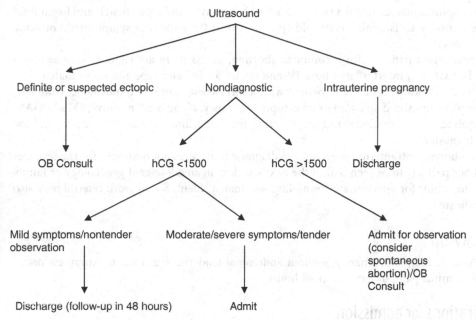

Figure 12-1. Management of suspected ectopic pregnancy.

If a ruptured ectopic is not likely and the patient is not in shock, obtain an ultrasound and hCG and follow the management plan outlined in Figure 12-1. If the ultrasound is nondiagnostic and the hCG is <1,500 mIUnits/mL, admit the patient if the symptoms (abdominal pain, cervical tenderness) are moderate or severe. If the patient has no abdominal tenderness, she may be discharged, if reliable follow-up is guaranteed, for outpatient serial hCG measurements every 48 hours. A normal increase suggests an intrauterine pregnancy, which must be confirmed by transvaginal ultrasound. Obtain obstetrical consultation for all patients with an abnormal hCG rise or no uterine pregnancy on ultrasound.

If the hCG is >1,500 mIUnits/mL and the ultrasound is nondiagnostic, admit the patient for observation (possible spontaneous abortion) and obstetrical consultation. If the ultrasound is not immediately available, admit the patient for close observation, serial hCG measurements, and possible laparoscopy. Culdocentesis is indicated only if transvaginal ultrasound is not available. It is very specific: nonclotting blood in the cul-de-sac mandates surgical exploration. However, sensitivity is poor as "dry taps" can occur and straw-colored fluid excludes only a ruptured ectopic.

Consult a gynecologist to attempt medical management of a confirmed ectopic pregnancy, if the fetus is <4 cm on ultrasound and the patient is hemodynamically stable. Up to 90% of cases will resolve after one dose of methotrexate (50 mg/m^2). Reliable, close follow-up is absolutely necessary.

Manage threatened abortions expectantly, with instructions to return for reevaluation if the bleeding continues for 48 hours or there are worsening symptoms. In such cases, hospitalize the patient and obtain a type and cross-match in case a transfusion becomes necessary (hematocrit <18%; symptoms of hypovolemia not relieved by crystalloid fluid resuscitation).

Admit patients with imminent, inevitable, and incomplete abortions, and consult with a gynecologist for dilatation and curettage. In the ED insert a large-bore IV and obtain a CBC, spun hematocrit, and a type and hold. Order a type and cross-match and begin fluid resuscitation with isotonic crystalloid (pp. 18–19), if the patient is symptomatic of acute blood loss.

Discharge a patient with a complete abortion, unless there are signs of serious blood loss. In that case, insert a large-bore IV and obtain a CBC and type and cross-match.

Check the Rh status for any patient with a threatened, imminent, inevitable, complete, incomplete, or missed abortion or an ectopic pregnancy. If she is Rh negative, IM RhoGAM is required. Give a minidose (50 mcg) during the first trimester; use 300 mcg beyond the first trimester.

If a normal intrauterine pregnancy is diagnosed, make an appointment for the teenager (and her partner) to be seen within the next few days in an adolescent gynecology or family planning clinic for appropriate counseling and management. Social work referral may also be indicated.

Follow-up
• Possible ectopic pregnancy, without abdominal tenderness: at once for dizziness or abdominal pain, otherwise, in 48 hours

Indications for admission
• Ectopic pregnancy (confirmed or probable)
• Ectopic pregnancy unlikely (nondiagnostic ultrasound, hCG <1,500 mIUnits/mL), but follow-up not guaranteed
• Ultrasound nondiagnostic and hCG <1,500 mIUnits/mL, but patient has moderate or severe abdominal pain or cervical motion tenderness
• Ultrasound nondiagnostic and hCG >1,500 mIUnits/mL
• Imminent, inevitable, or incomplete abortion
• Severe acute blood loss

Bibliography
American College of Obstetricians and Gynecologists. ACOG Practice Bulletin No. 94: Medical management of ectopic pregnancy. *Obstet Gynecol* 2008; 111:1479–85.

Goldstein SR: Early pregnancy: normal and abnormal. *Semin Reprod Med* 2008; 26:277–83.

Klein JD: American Academy of Pediatrics Committee on Adolescence: adolescent pregnancy: current trends and issues. *Pediatrics* 2005;116:281–6.

Sexually transmitted diseases
In the United States, one in four teenagers will have a sexually transmitted disease (STD) before graduating from high school. Pelvic inflammatory disease (PID) is a serious complication of STD and is the most common major infection of women aged 16–25. Approximately 85% of infections are spontaneous in sexually active females. The other 15% are secondary to procedures that disturb the integrity of the cervical mucus barrier.

PID is usually a polymicrobial infection caused by bacteria ascending from the vagina and cervix. *Neisseria gonorrhoeae* and *Chlamydia trachomatis* are responsible for most cases, and both can be present in as many as 50% of patients. These organisms can also cause cervicitis, urethritis, epididymitis, or proctitis.

Treponema pallidum, the agent responsible for syphilis, can cause severe systemic disease with long-term sequelae. Herpes simplex virus (HSV) is the agent responsible for the majority of genital ulcers in the United States, and, while treatable, is incurable. Several strains of human papillomavirus (HPV) have been associated with cervical cancer. More commonly in adolescents, certain other strains of HPV cause genital warts. There is now a vaccine which helps prevent infection with four of the most common strains, two of which cause cervical cancer. There is no cure for human immunodeficiency virus (HIV), but treatments continue to evolve. Trichomonas is a protozoan that causes vaginal discharge and inflammation.

Clinical presentation
Cervicitis
Cervicitis can occur with *N. gonorrhoeae* and/or *C. trachomatis* infection. Other pathogens include *Ureaplasma, Mycoplasma, Bacteroides,* and *E. coli.* It is often associated with purulent discharge (especially gonorrhea), though it can be asymptomatic. On examination, the cervix is erythematous and friable, but there is no cervical motion tenderness.

Urethritis
Urethritis is the most common manifestation of STI in males, but it also occurs in females. Commonly, males with urethral infection are asymptomatic, although dysuria and a urethral discharge may occur. Classically, purulent discharge is associated with infection by *N. gonorrhea.* Non-gonococcal urethritis is most often caused by *C. trachomatis,* but many other organisms can be responsible, especially *Ureaplasma* and *Mycoplasma.* In females, chlamydia commonly causes an acute urethral syndrome with dysuria, urgency, suprapubic tenderness, and pyuria without hematuria or bacteriuria.

Orchiepididymitis
Males may present with testicular pain and swelling, associated with epididymitis. This may mimic a testicular torsion. *N. gonorrhea* and *C. trachomatis* are the most common responsible organisms, but it may also occur after a viral infection.

Pelvic inflammatory disease
Pelvic inflammatory disease (PID) is an ascending infection of the upper genital tract. The term PID encompasses the diagnoses of endometritis, salpingitis, oophoritis, tubo-ovarian abscess, and peritonitis. It is often polymicrobial, with *C. trachomatis* and *N. gonorrhea* as the most common causes, although *Mycoplasma, Bacteroides, Peptostreptococcus, Streptococcus,* and *E. coli* are also implicated. However, often no causative organism is identified.

Patients can present with a spectrum of disease, from nonspecific lower abdominal pain to frank peritonitis. Other symptoms often include vaginal discharge, dyspareunia, irregular vaginal bleeding, and nausea and vomiting. Severe cases may present with high fever, shaking chills, and signs and symptoms of possible peritonitis (abdominal pain on cough or ambulating, tenderness to abdominal percussion, abdominal rigidity).

On pelvic examination, at least one of the following are present: cervical motion tenderness, adnexal tenderness, or uterine tenderness. A purulent cervical discharge may be noted, and there may be evidence of acute cervicitis. The WBC, ESR, and C-reactive protein may all be elevated.

Table 12-3. Pelvic inflammatory disease diagnostic criteria

Minimum criteria (one or more must be present)
Cervical motion tenderness
Uterine tenderness
Adnexal tenderness (unilateral or bilateral)
Additional criteria (increases specificity of diagnosis)
Temperature (oral) >101°F (38.3°C)
Abnormal cervical or vaginal mucopurulent discharge
Abundant WBCs on saline microscopy of vaginal secretions
Elevated ESR
Elevated CRP
Laboratory documentation of cervical infection with *N. gonorrhea* or *C. trachomatis*

Note: Consider the patient's risk profile for acquiring STDs when deciding to initiate empiric treatment for PID.
Source: Adapted from Centers for Disease Control and Prevention: Sexually transmitted diseases treatment guidelines, 2006. *MMWR Recomm Rep* 2006;55(RR-11):1–94.

In contrast, a common presentation is less dramatic, with lower abdominal pain and history of vaginal discharge as the only complaints. The patient may be afebrile, without a significant vaginal discharge, and may have relatively normal WBC, ESR, and/or CRP. See Table 12-3 for a summary of diagnostic criteria for pelvic inflammatory disease.

Proctitis

Proctitis occurs most commonly in males who engage in receptive anal intercourse. Patients may present with a history of constipation, anal itching, rectal fullness, pain with defecation, change in bowel habits, or blood in stool. Mild local disease is common and may be accompanied only by an abnormal stool smear (leukocytes present).

Genital herpes

Genital herpes is the most common cause of genital ulcers in the United States. HSV-2 causes 60–70% of genital outbreaks, and HSV-2 infection is more likely than HSV-1 to lead to recurrent outbreaks. The incubation period for primary infections can range from 2 to 12 days. Initially, vesicles appear which then rupture within several days to become small painful ulcers. The patient may complain of dysuria (due to contact of urine with the lesion) in addition to local burning. Inguinal nodes may enlarge and be tender, and about two-thirds of patients complain of a headache, fever, myalgias, and malaise. However, some initial infections present only with the vesicles/ulcers, without the other symptoms. Symptoms may last up to 3 weeks. Recurrent herpes eruptions are less severe and shorter in duration (3–5 days).

Genital or anogenital warts

Condylomata acuminata, or genital warts, are caused by the human papillomavirus (HPV), commonly types 6 and 11. Rarely, they may be caused by autoinoculation if an adolescent has warts on the hand or if a family member of a baby has warts on her hand. Anogenital warts are classically described as cauliflower-like growths, but they may be flat, papular, or pedunculated. Most are asymptomatic, although they can cause itching, burning, pain, or bleeding.

The HPV vaccine protects against types 6 and 11, as well as types 16 and 18, which cause the majority of changes on Pap smears and cervical cancer. However, the presence of warts does not indicate an increased likelihood of cancer.

Trichomoniasis

Trichomoniasis, caused by *Trichomonas vaginalis*, is a common sexually transmitted infection that most commonly causes a vaginitis.

Syphilis

The hallmark of primary syphilis is the chancre, which develops 2–12 weeks after exposure. It appears as a painless ulcer with a smooth clean base, raised indurated borders, and scanty yellow discharge. In males the chancre (usually 3 mm to 3 cm in size) is most frequently seen on the penis, scrotum, anus, lips, or in the mouth. In females, it occurs on the vulva, vagina, cervix, or urethra, lips, or in the mouth. Fifty percent of patients have more than one chancre, and enlarged, firm, painless regional lymph nodes are seen in 60–80% of patients. Untreated, the chancre resolves in 3–7 weeks, and the signs of secondary syphilis may appear 4–10 weeks after the primary lesion appears.

Several skin (and mucous membrane) eruptions are typical of secondary syphilis. Commonly, there are nonpruritic, well-demarcated, brownish red macules, papules, or pustules symmetrically distributed on the trunk and extremities. These are often also found on the palms and soles, which distinguishes them from most other rashes, particularly pityriasis rosea.

Condylomata lata are highly contagious, flat, moist, pink papules that occur in warm, moist intertriginous areas. When the maculopapules involve the mucous membranes in the mouth, they appear as shallow gray ulcers called mucous patches. Other signs of secondary syphilis include "moth-eaten" alopecia and nontender, firm or rubbery lymphadenopathy. Constitutional symptoms, including low-grade fever, headache, fatigue, sore throat, weight loss, arthralgias, and myalgias, occasionally accompany the above findings.

Latent syphilis is an asymptomatic period of varying lengths, which may occur after the symptoms of secondary syphilis resolve. Tertiary syphilis is marked by neurodegenerative changes, blindness, and cardiac, auditory, or gummatous lesions.

Chancroid (haemophilus ducreyi)

Chancroid causes painful genital ulcers. It typically presents as single or multiple lesions, often with ragged edges and tender inguinal nodes. It is relatively uncommon in the United States, usually occurring in outbreaks, but it may be underdiagnosed.

Lymphogranuloma venereum (LGV)

LGV presents with tender inguinal or femoral lymphadenopathy ("buboes"). It is caused by three serotypes of *C. trachomatis* (L1, L2, L3). While it is also associated with ulcers, these are usually transient, and the patient typically seeks medical attention for late sequelae, such as large inguinal nodes or rectal strictures. LGV is rare in the USA and more often seen in males. In Europe, LGV proctitis is seen in men who have receptive anal sex.

Pubic lice

Pediculosis pubis (pp. 120–122) usually presents with itching in the pubic region, or a patient may notice lice or nits (eggs) in the pubic hair.

Diagnosis

In a patient who presents with lower abdominal pain, obtain a thorough adolescent history, without the parent present. Important questions to ask include those regarding sexual activity, including most recent sexual intercourse, number of new partners in last 3 months, number of lifetime partners, types of sexual activity (vaginal, oral, anal), history of previous sexually transmitted infections (STI), and condom use.

Cervicitis

A cervicitis may be diagnosed clinically via visualization of cervical inflammation or mucopurulant discharge from the cervical os, or if there is friability of the cervix on swab collection. In order to distinguish between cervicitis and PID (see below) in symptomatic females, perform a pelvic exam and send a cervical swab to evaluate for gonorrhea and chlamydia. The pelvic exam also allows for direct visualization of the cervix. A bimanual examination can assess for cervical motion or adnexal tenderness. Most often, cervicitis from infection with *N. gonorrhea* or *C. trachomatis* is diagnosed by laboratory testing of either a cervical swab obtained in the context of a pelvic exam, or via screening with a urine nucleic acid amplification test (NAAT).

Urethritis

If available, send a urine nucleic acid amplification test (NAAT) for the diagnosis of gonorrhea (GC) and chlamydia. If possible, ask sexually active males to try to express any discharge, which can then be sent for culture and Gram's stain for gonococcus and chlamydia. Alternatively, insert a urethral swab to obtain specimens for culture and Gram's stain. Obtain a urinalysis and urine culture if there are symptoms of urethritis, although urinary tract infection is rare in adolescent boys who have no urinary tract anomaly. In females, if a pelvic exam is indicated, obtain a cervical swab for GC and chlamydia. With gonococcal urethritis, Gram-negative intracellular diplococci are seen.

Orchiepididymitis

Send a urine NAAT for *N. gonorrhea* and *C. trachomatis*, if available. Alternatively, obtain a urethral swab for detection of the same organisms. Additionally, examine a Gram's stain of urethral secretions. The urine may reveal WBCs or it may be normal and the urine culture is likely to be negative. If the diagnosis is still in question, order an ultrasound looking for increased blood flow to the affected testicle and epididymis.

Pelvic inflammatory disease

The priorities are to identify PID, which is a clinical diagnosis, and to rule out an ectopic pregnancy. A history of new or multiple sexual partners, previous sexually transmitted infections, or a report of inconsistent or absent condom use increases the likelihood of PID as the diagnosis. Ask the patient about her menstrual history, including her last menstrual period, usual interval and duration of menses, and the presence of irregular bleeding. Symptoms beginning within 1–2 weeks of the last period and/or irregular bleeding in a patient who is usually regular suggest PID, though PID can occur at any time during the menstrual cycle.

Perform a careful abdominal exam. Look for evidence of pregnancy and surgical scars on the abdomen. A crucial part of the physical assessment of a patient suspected of having PID is the pelvic examination. An external exam is important to evaluate for evidence of other STIs (herpes, warts). The speculum exam allows the provider to examine the cervix for signs of cervicitis, assess discharge amount and character, and obtain samples for laboratory evaluation. Bimanual examination is a key component; if the patient has cervical motion tenderness, uterine tenderness and/or adnexal tenderness, while other diagnoses can be ruled out, treatment for PID is indicated, regardless of the other findings. Given the morbidity associated with untreated PID (sterility, increased risk of ectopic pregnancy, chronic pelvic pain), it is important to have a low index of suspicion in diagnosing PID in adolescents.

Although PID can be definitively diagnosed via laparoscopy, this is invasive and not routinely indicated. Pelvic ultrasound may be useful to diagnose a tubo-ovarian abscess but may miss endometritis or salpingitis.

In the differential diagnosis of PID, also consider gastroenteritis (diarrhea), inflammatory bowel disease (weight loss, bloody stools, change in bowel pattern), acute appendicitis (right lower quadrant pain and tenderness), urinary tract infection (suprapubic or flank pain, dysuria, bacteruria in association with pyuria), right lower lobe pneumonia (cough, tachypnea, rales, right upper quadrant pain) and, rarely, cholecystitis (right upper quadrant pain). The pelvic exam may be abnormal in any condition that can cause peritonitis. Always consider an ectopic pregnancy when there has been oligomenorrhea or abnormal menses preceding the episode along with a positive pregnancy test.

Fitz-Hugh-Curtis syndrome (perihepatitis) occurs in 20% of patients with PID and presents with right upper quadrant pain, occasionally accompanied by right-sided pleuritic chest and shoulder pain and normal liver function tests. Alternatively but less commonly, a patient may have Fitz-Hugh-Curtis syndrome without symptoms of PID. The causative organisms are the same as those for PID, although *N. gonorrhea* or *C. trachomatis* may or may not be identified on cervical or urine diagnostic testing.

Proctitis

Perform a thorough anal inspection to assess for external lesions (HSV, HPV, hemorrhoids), as well as a rectal examination to assess for tenderness. In addition, send a urine NAAT (or cervical swab) and a rectal swab for gonorrhea, to be plated on chocolate agar, but do not send a rectal specimen for chlamydia. However, cultures are preferred because nonculture test results are difficult to interpret in the presence of stool organisms.

Herpes

Maintain a reasonably high index of suspicion, as herpes lesions may be misdiagnosed as folliculitis, dermatitis, latex allergy, or medical illnesses that present with genital ulcers, such as EBV, Behçet's disease, or Crohn's disease. Viral culture of an active lesion, and not serum testing for HSV-1 and HSV-2 antibodies, is the gold standard for diagnosis, as a positive serology only indicates that an infection has occurred at some time in the past. Swabbing the vesicular fluid, ulcerated lesions, or vesicular scrapings will suffice. Typing HSV has relevance for patient counseling in that HSV-2 is more likely to recur. A Tzanck smear may show multinucleated giant cells and inclusions, but it has relatively poor sensitivity and specificity.

Genital warts

Genital warts are diagnosed by inspection; HPV testing is not recommended. Arrange for a biopsy if the patient is immunocompromised, the diagnosis is in doubt, or there is no response to treatment.

Syphilis

Suspect all genital lesions of being syphilitic. Chancres can be confused with chancroid (multiple soft, tender ulcers; very tender contiguous adenopathy), granuloma inguinale (red, beefy, granulating painless lesion without adenopathy), lymphogranuloma venereum (transient vesicular, papular, or pustular ulceration with markedly enlarged tender nodes), or lichen planus (annular flat-topped papules). Also, rule out herpes (multiple, superficial, painful lesions), pyogenic granuloma (single, painful, erythematous lesion that often looks like hamburger), molluscum contagiosum (grouped, umbilicated, flesh-colored papules, similar lesions elsewhere on body), and condyloma accuminatum (dry, single or clustered, warty lesions). The maculopapular eruption of pityriasis rosea is not present on the palms and soles, although it can otherwise resemble the rash of secondary syphilis. The scaly plaques of psoriasis can be on the penis and elsewhere on the body.

If syphilis is suspected, send a nontreponemal serologic test for syphilis (RPR or VDRL). Approximately 25% of patients with primary syphilis have a negative RPR or VDRL, especially within the first 3–5 weeks after the initial infection. Therefore, if syphilis is likely and the RPR or VDRL is negative, send a treponemal serologic test (FTA-ABS), which has greater sensitivity than the VDRL or RPR. If the VDRL or RPR is positive, follow this with a confirmatory treponemal test (FTA-ABSO or TP-PA), as false-positive nontreponemal tests occur in several medical conditions unrelated to syphilis (measles, chicken pox, mumps, HSV, viral pneumonia, pregnancy, malaria, SLE, hemolytic anemia, HIV).

The nontreponemal antibody titer correlates with disease activity: a four-fold rise in titer (i.e. 1:8 to 1:32) is diagnostic of active infection, while a four-fold drop confirms treatment response. Treponemal tests remain positive throughout life for 75–85% of patients, so they cannot be used to assess treatment response. Samples of tissue or exudates from lesions may also be sent for dark-field microscopy or direct fluorescent antibody (DFA) for the definitive diagnosis of syphilis.

Chancroid and LGV

A high index of suspicion is necessary for making these diagnoses. The diagnosis of chancroid is made clinically by excluding syphilis and herpes, as it is extremely difficult to culture *Haemophilus ducreyi*. LGV is diagnosed by *C. trachomatis* titer.

Pubic lice

The diagnosis of lice is made by inspection. Live lice appear as small (1–4 mm), moving particles resembling dandruff flakes, and nits are firmly attached to the side of hair shafts. Nits fluoresce (white or gray) under a Wood's lamp.

ED management

The antibiotic treatment of STIs is summarized in Table 12-4. Obtain a pregnancy test for all females before initiating any antibiotic treatment.

Table 12-4. Treatment of sexually transmitted diseases

Chlamydia trachomatis: urethritis, cervicitis, and proctitis (for nongonococcal nonchlamydial urethritis, and cervicitis see treatment for pelvic inflammatory disease below)

  Preferred regimen: azithromycin 1 g PO as one dose or doxycycline[a] 100 mg PO bid × 7 days

  Alternative regimen (7-day course): erythromycin 500 mg PO qid

Neisseria gonorrhea[d]: urethral, cervical, or rectal (see treatment for pelvic inflammatory disease below).

  Preferred regimens: ceftriaxone 125 mg IM or cefixime 400 mg PO

  Alternative regimens: Azithromycin 2 g PO

Neisseria gonorrhea[d]: pharyngeal

  Preferred regimen: ceftriaxone 125 mg IM

  Alternative regimens: ceftizoxime 500 mg IM or cefoxitin 2 g IM, administered with probenecid 1 g orally or cefotaxime 500 mg IM

Epididymitis

  Preferred regimen: ceftriaxone 250 mg IM once plus doxycycline[a] 100 mg PO bid × 10 days

  Alternative regimens: ofloxacin[b] 300 mg orally twice a day for 10 days[c] or levofloxacin[b] 500 mg orally once daily for 10 days[c]

Pelvic inflammatory disease: inpatient

  Preferred regimens: cefoxitin 2 g IV q 12 h or cefotetan 2 g IV q 6 h plus doxycycline[a] 100 mg PO or IV q 12 h, until improved; clindamycin 900 mg IV q 8 h plus gentamicin 2 mg/kg IV once, followed by gentamicin 1.5 mg/kg IV q 8 h, until improved

  Alternative regimen: ampicillin/sulbactam 3 g IV q 6 h plus doxycycline[a] 100 mg PO or IV q 12 h, until improved

Once improved on any of these regimens, give doxycycline[a] 100 mg PO bid to complete a 14-day course. Add metronidazole 500 mg PO bid to the above regimens if the patient does not improve in first 48–72 hours. Clindamycin dosing of 450 mg PO qid may provide better anaerobic coverage in the case of tubo-ovarian abscess

Pelvic inflammatory disease: outpatient

  Preferred regimen: ceftriaxone 250 mg IM once, followed by doxycycline[a] 100 mg PO bid × 14 days with or without metronidazole 500 mg PO bid × 14 days

  Alternative regimens:

  Cefoxitin 2 g IM once plus probenecid 1 g PO once, plus doxycycline[a] 100 mg PO bid × 14 days with or without metronidazole 500 mg PO bid × 14 days

  An alternative third-generation cephalosporin (ceftizoxime, cefotaxime) plus doxycycline[a] 100 mg PO bid × 14 days with or without metronidazole 500 mg PO bid × 14 days

Herpes simplex

  First episode: acyclovir 400 mg PO tid × 7–10 days or 200 mg PO 5 times/day × 7–10 days or famciclovir 250 mg PO tid × 7–10 days or valacyclovir 1 g PO bid × 7–10 days

Table 12-4. (cont.)

Recurrent: acyclovir 400 mg PO tid × 5 days or 800 mg PO bid × 5 days or 800 mg PO tid × 2 days or famciclovir 125 mg PO bid × 5 days or 1 g PO bid × 1 day or valacyclovir 500 mg PO bid × 3 days or 1 g PO daily × 5 days

Daily suppressive therapy: acyclovir 400 mg PO bid or famciclovir 250 mg PO bid or valacyclovir 500 mg-1 g PO daily

Genital warts (HPV)

External genital warts: patient-applied

Podofilox 0.5% solution or gel: apply to visible warts bid for 3 days, followed by 4 days of no therapy

May repeat for up to four cycles

Imiquimod 5% cream: apply to warts once daily at bedtime, 3 times a week for up to 16 weeks

Instruct patient to wash with soap and water 6–10 hours later

External genital warts: provider-administered

Podophyllin resin[e] 10–25% in compound tincture of benzoin; apply to wart(s) once weekly and allow to air dry

Trichloroacetic acid (TCA) or bichloroacetic acid (BCA) 80%–90%; apply to wart(s) once weekly and allow to air dry

Cryotherapy with liquid nitrogen or cryoprobe; repeat every 1–2 weeks Surgical removal or intralesional interferon or laser surgery

Vaginal warts: cryotherapy with liquid nitrogen; avoid cryoprobe for risk of vaginal perforation/fistula formation; TCA or BCA 80%-90% (as above)

Anal warts: cryotherapy with liquid nitrogen or TCA or BCA 80%–90% (as above) or surgical removal

Cervical warts: refer to a gynecologist for cervical exophytic warts, as precancerous changes must be ruled out before treatment

Urethral meatus warts

Podophyllin resin[e] 10–25% in compound tincture of benzoin; apply to wart(s) once weekly and allow to air dry

Podofilox 0.5% solution or gel: apply to visible warts bid for 3 days, followed by 4 days of no therapy. May repeat for up to 4 cycles

Imiquimod 5% cream: apply to warts once daily at bedtime, 3 times a week for up to 16 weeks. Instruct patient to wash with soap and water 6–10 hours later

Trichomoniasis

Preferred regimen: metronidazole 2 g PO in one dose

Alternative regimens: tinidazole 2 g PO in one dose or metronidazole 500 mg PO bid × 7 days

Table 12-4. (cont.)

Syphilis

Primary, secondary, and early-latent (<1 year)

   Preferred regimen: benzathine penicillin G 2.4 million units IM as a single dose

   Alternative regimen: doxycycline[a] 100 mg PO bid × 14 days

Late-latent (duration >1 year) and tertiary

   Preferred regimen: benzathine penicillin G 2.4 million units IM weekly × 3 weeks

   Alternative regimen: doxycycline[a] 100 mg PO bid × 4 weeks

Chancroid

   Azithromycin 1 g PO once or ceftriaxone 250 mg IM once or ciprofloxacin[b] 500 mg
   PO bid × 3 days or erythromycin 500 mg PO tid × 7 days

Lymphogranuloma venereum (LGV)

   Preferred regimen: doxycycline[a] 100 mg PO bid × 21 days

   Alternative regimen: erythromycin 500 mg PO qid × 21 days

Pediculosis

   Preferred regimen: permethrin 1% cream (or pyrethrins with piperonyl butoxide): apply to pubic
   area and leave for 10 minutes, then wash out. Wash affected clothing and bedding

   Alternative regimens: malathion 0.5% lotion applied for 8–12 hours and washed off or ivermectin
   250 mcg/kg, repeat in 2 weeks
   Note: If the infestation persists despite the above treatment, use lindane[f] shampoo (apply for
   four minutes)

Notes: [a] Use only if >8 years old and not pregnant.
[b] Quinolones are no longer recommended for uncomplicated gonococcal infections.
[c] For acute epididymitis most likely caused by enteric organisms or with negative gonococcal culture or nucleic acid
   amplification test.
[d] Also give a course of treatment effective against chlamydia.
[e] Limit application to <0.5 ml podophyllin or to an affected area <10 cm^2 per session.
[f] Use only if other treatments fail. Risk of toxicity (seizure, aplastic anemia) is low with the recommended four-minute exposure.

Source: Centers for Disease Control Sexually Transmitted Diseases Treatment Guidelines, 2006 (updated April 12,
2007). MMWR August 4, 2006; Vol. 55 [No. RR-11]. http://www.cdc.gov/STD/treatment/.

Campos-Outcalt; D. Practice alert: CDC no longer recommends quinolones for treatment of gonorrhea. Ceftriaxone is
now the recommended treatment. *J Fam Pract* 2007; **56**: 554–8.

Cervicitis

Treat afebrile patients on an outpatient basis with oral antibiotics. Schedule a follow-up office
visit within 1 week of completing therapy, and emphasize both the avoidance of intercourse
until the patient's partner is cultured and treated (if needed) and the use of condoms to
prevent both future infections and pregnancy. Check local state laws to see whether expedited
partner treatment for chlamydia is permitted.

Urethritis

Treat a male with presumptive or definite urethritis and schedule primary care follow-up
visit in 1 week. The partner(s) must also be treated. Treat females with acute urethral
syndrome for chlamydia urethritis, and schedule a follow-up office visit.

Epididymitis

Treat with an oral outpatient regimen and schedule primary care follow-up visit in 72 hours.

Pelvic inflammatory disease

Since PID is a clinical diagnosis, initiate antibiotic therapy immediately, once the laboratory assessment is completed. Obtain a GC/chlamydia sample via either cervical swab or urine test. Also send a wet preparation to evaluate for trichomoniasis, bacterial vaginosis, and yeast. Obtain an RPR screen for syphilis and a urine hCG, and offer HIV testing. Obtain a CBC, along with either an ESR or CRP, as elevation(s) is indicative, though not specific, for PID. If the patient has RUQ pain consistent with Fitz-Hugh-Curtis, obtain LFTs. Since Fitz-Hugh-Curtis is a perihepatitis, the LFTs will be normal; elevations suggest another diagnosis (hepatitis, gallbladder disease). A pelvic sonogram is indicated if tubo-ovarian abscess is suspected, or if the patient does not improve despite treatment.

Admit the patient for IV therapy if she is ill-appearing, pregnant, vomiting and unable to tolerate food or drink, at high risk of non-compliance, or if she has a tubo-ovarian abscess or has previous failed outpatient therapy. If the diagnosis is in doubt, obtain an adolescent medicine or gynecology consult.

If the patient is to be treated with an outpatient antibiotic regimen, it is important to arrange a follow-up visit within 48–72 hours for re-evaluation via bimanual examination. Also, remind the patient that the sexual partner(s) must be examined and treated. If the patient is not currently using hormonal contraception, this is an opportunity to offer it.

Proctitis

Treat proctitis on an outpatient basis and schedule primary care follow-up visit in 1 week.

Herpes

Treatment of primary herpes will shorten the duration of symptoms, decrease the amount of viral shedding, and prevent the formation of new lesions. It is not curative, nor does it prevent later recurrences. Refer the patient for primary care follow-up in 1 week, at which time suppressive therapy can be discussed.

Genital warts

Treat with patient-applied regimens and arrange for follow-up in 1 week with an adolescent medicine provider, gynecologist, or dermatologist. Alternatively, refer to one of the above physicians for provider-applied treatments, such as podophyllin, trichloroacetic acid, or cryotherapy.

Syphilis

Treat patients with syphilis, and refer them for follow-up with their primary care provider. Arrange for the evaluation and treatment of all sexual partners, and remind the patient to avoid sexual activity until that time. Of note, the Jarisch-Herxheimer reaction may occur within the first 24 hours of treatment for syphilis. It is characterized by fever, headache, myalgia, tachycardia, and mild hypotension, and can occur in the treatment of primary, secondary (most commonly), and early-latent syphilis. In pregnant women, the reaction may cause early labor or fetal distress, but this risk is not a contraindication to treatment.

Chancroid

Clinical response to the treatment of chancroid can be seen within 7 days. Examine and treat any individuals with whom the patient had sexual contact within 10 days preceding the onset of symptoms.

Lymphogranuloma venereum

See Table 12-4.

Pubic lice

See Table 12-4.

Follow-up

- Pelvic inflammatory disease: adolescent medicine, gynecology, or ED follow-up in 48–72 hours for repeat bimanual examination
- Epididymitis: follow-up in 72 hours for re-evaluation
- Cervicitis, proctitis, urethritis, chancroid, primary or recurrent herpes, pubic lice: primary care follow-up in 1 week
- Genital warts: adolescent medicine, gynecology or dermatology follow-up in 1–2 weeks
- Primary or secondary syphilis: 1 month; then serologic testing at 3, 6, 9, 12, and 24 months after treatment

Indications for admission

- Pelvic inflammatory disease: ill-appearance, unable to tolerate oral intake, concurrent pregnancy, tubo-ovarian abscess, uncertain diagnosis, prior treatment failure, high likelihood of non-compliance

Bibliography

Banikarim C, Chacko MR: Pelvic inflammatory disease in adolescents. *Semin Pediatr Infect Dis* 2005;**16**:175–80.

Centers for Disease Control and Prevention: Sexually transmitted diseases treatment guidelines, 2006. *MMWR Recomm Rep* 2006;**55**(RR-11):1–94.

Lewin LC: Sexually transmitted infections in preadolescent children. *J Pediatr Health Care* 2007;**21**:153–61.

Risser WL, Risser JM, Benjamins LJ, Feldmann JM: Incidence of Fitz-Hugh-Curtis syndrome in adolescents who have pelvic inflammatory disease. *J Pediatr Adolesc Gynecol* 2007;**20**:179–80.

Vaginal discharge and vulvovaginitis

Vulvovaginitis is a common problem in prepubertal and pubertal girls. Prepubertal girls are particularly susceptible to vulvovaginitis secondary to irritation by soaps, chemicals, and clothing because of their thin vulvar epithelium and the lack of estrogenic stimulation. In addition, they are also prone to poor hygiene and contamination with bowel flora (due to the proximity of the anus to the vaginal opening). In pubertal girls, sexual activity is the major etiologic factor of vulvovaginitis, and vaginal discharge is a common presenting complaint among adolescents. In both prepubertal and pubertal girls, the wearing of non-absorbent nylon underwear or tights, nylon bathing suits, ballet leotards, or tight-fitting jeans also provides an environment conducive for bacterial infection, particularly in hot weather.

Clinical presentation

Prepubertal girls

Nonspecific vaginitis

Up to 75% of prepubertal vaginitis is nonspecific. This includes chemical vulvovaginitis, most commonly from bubble bath or harsh soaps. These girls present with vulvar and/or vaginal inflammation that is generally low-grade, yet persistent. There may be associated with dysuria, pruritus, and discharge. If there is no obvious etiology for the complaint and a culture is obtained, it will be negative or grow normal flora (lactobacilli, *Staphylococcus epidermidis*).

Bacterial infections

Specific bacterial infections occur most often with respiratory, enteric, or sexually transmitted infections. Group A strep vulvovaginitis can result from self-inoculation from a nasopharyngeal or a skin infection, and causes a distinctive bright red appearance to the vulva and/or perianal areas. *Staphylococcus aureus* can cause a vaginal infection in association with impetigo of the vulva or buttocks. *Haemophilus influenzae* and *Streptococcus pneumoniae* are other common infections of the respiratory tract that can cause vulvovaginitis.

Enteric organisms such as *Shigella* can cause a bloody discharge, usually in a girl who has recently had gastroenteritis. *Escherichia coli* may be found in the flora of asymptomatic prepubertal girls, but it is more common in those with complaints of vulvovaginitis.

Sexually transmitted infections

Infections with *Neisseria gonorrhea* and *Chlamydia trachomatis* present with a copious, green or yellow purulent discharge, which may be associated with labial swelling, dysuria, and genital pruritus. The vagina may be inflamed and excoriated. Suspect child abuse and alert the child protective services whenever a sexually transmitted disease is diagnosed in a prepubertal child. Although there is often no report of sexual contact in these cases, nonsexual acquisition of these organisms is exceedingly rare. Herpes infection of the vulva may be due to autoinoculation from an oral lesion and might not be sexually transmitted. Trichomonas infection is rare in prepubertal girls, but its presence is suspicious for sexual abuse.

Candidal infection

Candida vulvovaginitis is rare in prepubertal girls, unless the child has recently finished a course of antibiotics, has diabetes, is immunosuppressed, or wears diapers.

Foreign body

A vaginal foreign body produces a foul-smelling discharge which can be bloody. Toilet paper remnants are the most common objects found.

Pinworm

Pinworm (*Enterobius vermicularis*) presents with pruritus of the anus and/or vulva. It can also occur in adolescents but is much more common in younger children.

Pubertal girls

In addition to vulvar or vaginal irritation, a discharge is extremely common. It may be associated with pruritus, foul odor, or dysuria, often in association with pyuria. Symptoms of vulvovaginitis may occur with STIs (gonorrhea, chlamydia, trichomonas), infections not usually associated with sexual contact (candida, bacterial vaginosis), or a foreign body, or it may be physiologic.

Gonorrhea and chlamydia

Adolescents may complain of a vaginal discharge, although the infection most often presents as a cervicitis. Abdominal pain along with discharge may indicate pelvic inflammatory disease (see pp. 314–324).

Trichomonas vaginalis

Trichomoniasis is a relatively common sexually acquired infection caused by the motile, flagellated parasite *Trichomonas vaginalis*. A green-gray, thin, malodorous discharge occurs, often associated with pruritus or dyspareunia. There may also be abdominal pain, post-coital bleeding, and/or dysuria.

Candida albicans

Candida is a common cause of vaginitis in the general adolescent population. Diabetes mellitus, immunosuppression, a recent course of antibiotics, pregnancy, obesity, and tight-fitting undergarments are risk factors. Sexual activity rarely plays a role in transmission and partners do not routinely need treatment.

Candida presents with a thick, white, cheesy discharge in association with pruritus, inflammation, and edema of the vulva, which can be associated with dysuria and/or dyspareunia. The discharge may also be thin and watery.

Bacterial vaginosis

Bacterial vaginosis (BV) is a common cause of vaginal discharge and inflammation, caused by a complex alteration of the microbial flora in the vagina. It results from an increase in the concentration (among others) of *Gardnerella vaginalis*, anaerobic organisms such as *Bacteroides* and *Mobiluncus* species, and *Mycoplasma hominus*, in association with a decrease in normal hydrogen peroxide-producing flora such as lactobacillus. BV classically presents with a grayish-white, thin, malodorous discharge. The characteristic "fishy" odor is caused by the overgrowth of the above organisms, resulting in increased vaginal pH and the subsequent production of amines. In addition to discharge, if there is an associated lower abdominal pain, evaluate the patient for possible pelvic inflammatory disease.

Foreign body

In adolescents, a retained tampon is the most common object causing a vaginitis. A foul-smelling, purulent discharge that may be bloody is typically present.

Contact reaction

A contact vaginitis may be caused by soap, bubble bath, douche, perfume, or contraceptive foam or jelly.

Physiologic leukorrhea

Adolescents may sometimes complain of a clear-white or mucoid discharge, either prior to menses or at midcycle. The discharge is nonpathologic, composed of epithelial cells and endocervical mucus. There is no evidence of inflammation.

Psychosocial etiologies

With psychosocial issues, such as sexual molestation and school phobia, the patient's complaints are not consistent with the objective findings.

Diagnosis

Priorities on the physical examination are the breasts (Tanner stage, signs of pregnancy), abdomen (pregnancy, mass, tenderness), and inguinal area (lymphadenopathy). Next, inspect the introitus for Tanner stage, inflammation, swelling, presence of discharge, and signs of trauma.

The vaginal examination of the prepubertal child may be challenging, but most often can be accomplished without sedation or anesthesia. Reassure the child that the examination will not hurt and ask the mother to remain in the room. Have the child lie supine, with her feet together and her knees apart ("frog-leg" position). Alternatively, in an older child, use the lithotomy position. In some children, the examination is more easily performed with the patient lying prone, in a knee-chest position, with the buttocks in the air and the knees 6–8 inches apart. Instruct her to relax and let her belly sag downward (a pillow may be placed below the abdomen), then gently spread the labia to view the vagina.

In an adolescent an external genital exam is necessary. However, if she has complaints of abdominal pain, or has a high-risk history for having acquired a sexually-transmitted disease, a speculum exam is indicated, but defer it if she is virginal. If the discharge is bloody, purulent, or particularly foul-smelling, carefully inspect the vagina for a foreign body. If a foreign body is suspected in a virginal female, palpate the vagina during a rectal exam.

Perform a wet prep on a sample of every vaginal discharge. After the specimen is obtained with a cotton swab, place it in a test tube containing a small amount of room-temperature saline. Place several drops of this solution on a slide, and observe under high power. Budding yeast are seen with candidal infection, with pseudohyphae noted after 10% potassium hydroxide (KOH) is added and the slide gently heated. Trichomonads appear as live, flagellated, motile organisms. Examine the wet prep within 15 minutes of preparation to decrease the chance of trichomonas losing their motility, swelling, or bursting. The wet prep is positive in up to 83% of candidal infections and 70% of trichomonas infections. Bacterial vaginosis is likely if three out of the following four criteria are met:

- presence of a homogeneous white noninflammatory discharge adherent to the vaginal walls
- discharge pH $\geq$4.5
- the odor of the discharge sample becomes fishy or amine-like with the addition of KOH (positive "whiff test")
- the wet prep has clue cells (epithelial cells stippled with dark granules) noted in at least 20% of cells.

See Table 12-5 for a summary of the differences between candidal infection, bacterial vaginosis and trichomoniasis.

Table 12-5. Differential diagnosis of vaginal discharge in pubertal girls

	Discharge	Vaginal pH	Whiff test[a]	WBCs	Wet prep
Candida	"Cottage cheese" Odorless	≤4.5	Absent	Rare to ↑	Pseudohyphae or budding yeast
Bacterial vaginosis	White to gray Malodorous	>4.5	Present	Rare	>20% clue cells
Trichomoniasis	White, gray, green	Often >4.5	Possible	Can be ↑	Motile, flagellated trichomonads

Note: [a]Whiff test: amine odor after the addition of 10% KOH.

Source: Adapted with permission from Sexually Transmitted Infections, in Strasburger VC, Brown RT, Braverman PK, Rogers PD, Holland-Hall C, Coupey S (eds): Adolescent Medicine: A Handbook for Primary Care, Lippincott Williams and Wilkins. Philadelphia, 2006.

If a pelvic examination is indicated, obtain a cervical swab to test for gonorrhea and chlamydia. If no pelvic exam was performed, send a urine sample for gonorrhea and chlamydia.

ED management
Prepubertal girls
Nonspecific vaginitis

Treat with warm water sitz baths once or twice a day. Discuss proper hygiene techniques, such as front-to-back wiping, use of cotton underwear, avoidance of tight-fitting pants, and avoiding wearing wet clothing (such as bathing suits). Recommend applying a small amount of an emollient (petrolatum, A&D) to protect the vulvar skin. If symptoms persist after 2–3 weeks reevaluate the patient for the possibility of a foreign body or infection. Prescribe amoxicillin (40 mg/kg per day div tid) or amoxicillin-clavulanate (45 mg/kg per day of amoxicillin div bid) for 10 days if there is a purulent discharge despite negative cultures. A 5-day course of estrogen-containing cream (Premarin) can thicken the vaginal mucosa and reduce susceptibility to infection.

Gonorrhea and chlamydia

In the prepubertal age group, a positive test for gonorrhea or chlamydia is indicative of sexual abuse. Treat the child with ceftriaxone 125 mg IM (regardless of weight). If the patient has an allergy to beta-lactams, consult with a pediatric infectious disease specialist to determine the appropriate treatment. For chlamydia add erythromycin (<8 years of age: 50 mg/kg per day div qid), azithromycin (1 g orally in a single dose for patients weighing >45 kg) or doxycycline (>8 years of age: 100 mg bid) for 7 days. Report the case to the child protection services.

Other bacterial etiologies

If the culture is positive, treat with a culture-specific antibiotic for 7–10 days.

Foreign bodies

Usually, removal can be accomplished with a forceps. On occasion, sedation or general anesthesia is required.

Pinworms

If pinworms are suspected by a history of rectal itching or characteristic adult thread-like worms seen on the stool, treat with mebendazole (pp. 409–412).

Pubertal girls

Candida albicans

Treat with clotrimazole, miconazole, or terconazole vaginal creams or suppositories for 1 week. The clinical cure rate is about 80%. In complicated patients (immunosuppressed, diabetic, pregnant), prescribe a 10–14 day course. As an alternative, give a single PO dose of fluconazole (150 mg). Advise the patient to avoid pantyhose and tight clothes. Continue treatment during menses and it is not necessary to treat sexual partner(s), unless the patient becomes reinfected quickly.

Trichomonas

Treat with one oral dose of metronidazole (2 g) or tinidazole (2 g). Alternatively, prescribe metronidazole 500 mg PO bid for 7 days. Advise the patient to avoid alcohol during treatment and for 72 hours afterwards, since alcohol consumption while taking metronidazole can lead to nausea, vomiting, flushing, and tachycardia. As trichomoniasis is a sexually transmitted disease, treat all sexual partners.

Bacterial vaginosis

Treat with oral metronidazole 500 mg bid for 7 days and advise against alcohol consumption (as above). Alternative regimens are metronidazole 0.75% gel, one applicator intravaginally daily for 5 days, or clindamycin 2% cream, one full applicator intravaginally nightly for 7 days. It is not necessary to treat sexual partner(s). Oral metronidazole is indicated for symptomatic pregnant women and asymptomatic pregnant women at risk for pre-term delivery.

Foreign bodies

These can usually be removed with a forceps or via warm saline irrigation.

Contact reaction

Avoidance of the offending agent is usually all that is required. Treat severe pruritus with diphenhydramine (25 mg q 6 h) or hydroxyzine (25 mg q 6 h). A low- to mid-potency topical corticosteroid cream (i.e. hydrocortisone 1% or triamcinolone 0.025–0.1%) for 2–3 days and sodium bicarbonate baths (2–4 tablespoons of baking soda in the tub) may also help.

Physiologic leukorrhea

No treatment is necessary, aside from reassurance, although panty liners may be helpful.

Psychosocial etiologies

Have an experienced interviewer speak with the patient to attempt to ascertain whether sexual molestation has occurred. Refer all patients without a definite etiology to a primary care provider.

Follow-up

* Prepubertal girl with nonspecific vaginitis, or culture-proven bacterial vaginitis: primary care follow-up in 7–10 days
* Pubertal girl with vaginitis: primary care follow-up

Indications for admission

* Suspected sexual abuse, if the patient's family is unable to provide the necessary support
* Severe vulvovaginitis with urinary retention or systemic signs (fever, toxicity)

Bibliography

Centers for Disease Control and Prevention: Sexually transmitted diseases treatment guidelines, 2006. *MMWR Recomm Rep* 2006;55(RR-11):1–94.

Lewin LC: Sexually transmitted infections in preadolescent children. *J Pediatr Health Care* 2007;21:153–61.

Woods ER, Emans SJ: Vulvovaginal complaints in the adolescent. In Emans SJ, Laufer MR, Goldstein DP (eds). *Pediatric and Adolescent Gynecology*, 5th ed. Philadelphia: Lippincott Williams and Wilkins 2005, pp. 525–64.

Chapter 13

Hematologic emergencies

Mark Weinblatt

Anemia

Red cell production is determined by oxygen availability to tissues and oxygen requirements, thus varying greatly with age, activity, and environmental circumstances, such as altitude. The lower limits of normal hemoglobin levels range from 9.5 g/dL at 3 months of age to 11 g/dL in the teenager.

Clinical presentation

The signs and symptoms of anemia result from the decreased oxygen-carrying capacity of the blood and depend on the degree of anemia and acuteness of onset. Exercise intolerance, pallor, headache, fatigue, tachycardia, and systolic murmurs may occur with moderate anemia. Severe or rapidly developing anemia can cause nonexertional dyspnea, dizziness, orthostatic vital sign changes, cardiac gallop, syncope, hypotension, and heart failure.

Diagnosis

After determining that a patient is anemic for age with a CBC with red-cell indices, a reticulocyte count, and examination of the peripheral smear, the most expeditious way of narrowing the differential diagnosis is using an algorithm based on the red cell size (see Table 13-1). Microcytic anemias are due to delayed or abnormal hemoglobin formation, with disorders of the iron, globin chain, or porphyrin ring components. These disorders typically have decreased MCV, with a peripheral blood smear revealing hypochromic red cells. To further establish a diagnosis, consider additional testing such as iron and ferritin levels, hemoglobin electrophoresis, and a lead level. The Menser index (MCV in fL divided by the red blood cells [RBC] in millions: MCV/RBC) can help differentiate among the microcytic anemias. If the ratio is less than 11:1, thalassemia minor is likely, while ratios greater than 14:1 suggest iron deficiency, lead intoxication, or anemia of chronic disease.

The uncommon macrocytic anemias with MCV >100 beyond the newborn period result from delayed nuclear maturation or elevated fetal hemoglobin content.

The normocytic anemias comprise the largest differential. Some additional features of the red cells can help establish the diagnosis.

Red cell shape

Variations in shape include sickle cells (both crescent and "box car" shapes); target cells seen in hemoglobinopathies (especially Hgb C disease and the microcytic thalassemia syndromes) and liver disease; burr cells (renal disease, hemolysis); spherocytes (spherocytosis, ABO immune hemolysis); schistocytes (hemolysis).

Table 13-1. Differential diagnosis of anemia

Microcytic

Iron deficiency

Thalassemia

Sideroblastic anemia

Anemia of chronic disease

Copper deficiency

Chronic lead poisoning

Macrocytic

Folic acid deficiency

Vitamin B12 deficiency

Liver disease

Hypothyroidism

Fanconi's anemia

Diamond-Blackfan syndrome

Dyserythropoietic anemia

Normocytic: ↓ reticulocytes

Acquired aplastic anemia

Transient erythroblastopenia

Leukemia

Neuroblastoma

Viral marrow suppression

Drug suppression

Chronic renal disease

Normocytic: ↑ reticulocytes

Acute blood loss

Sickle cell disease

Hemoglobin C disease

Spherocytosis, elliptocytosis

G6PD deficiency

Pyruvate kinase deficiency

Splenic sequestration

Infectious agents (e.g., malaria)

Mechanical or thermal damage

Color

Polychromasia occurs with increased RBC production in association with decreased life span or marrow recovery. This is usually indicative of an elevated reticulocyte count.

Inclusions

There may be Howell Jolly bodies (decreased splenic function); basophilic stippling (thalassemia, lead poisoning, some enzyme deficiencies); or parasites (malaria, babesiosis).

History

A thorough history, including ethnicity, family background and diet, is important in determining the etiology of anemia. Iron-deficiency anemia can be caused by excessive intake of cow's milk in infants or by restricted diets containing no reliable source of iron in older children. A complete lack of fresh vegetables might lead to folate deficiency. Unusual cravings, such as pagophagia and pica, are occasionally seen in patients with iron deficiency, and may further complicate the picture (e.g. causing ingestion of lead-containing paint chips).

A history of recent infections may suggest EBV or mycoplasma-induced hemolysis, or parvovirus suppression of the bone marrow (particularly in patients with chronic hemolytic disorders). Inquire about blood loss, such as irregular menstrual bleeding, hematuria, or gastrointestinal bleeding. A history of unexplained or prolonged bleeding may suggest a hemostatic disorder, such as mild von Willebrand's Disease, that is contributing to anemia. Ask about chronic medical problems and inflammatory disorders, such as rheumatoid arthritis or inflammatory bowel disease. Recurrent episodes of jaundice suggest hemolytic disorders such as G6PD deficiency, hemoglobinopathies, and spherocytosis. A patient with a hemolytic disorder may have a positive family history for anemia, intermittent jaundice, cholecystectomy in a young person, or nontraumatic splenectomy (hereditary spherocytosis, sickle cell disease, and some enzyme deficiencies). Ask about medication use, since many medications can suppress erythropoiesis (e.g. sulfa drugs and anticonvulsants) or trigger hemolysis in patients with G6PD deficiency.

Physical examination

On examination, a healthy, vigorous child is more likely to have mild iron-deficiency anemia, thalassemia trait, or a mild chronic hemolytic anemia. A patient with a malignancy, severe malnutrition, severe chronic disease, or bone marrow infiltration usually appears ill. Jaundice, often accompanied by abdominal pain, splenomegaly and dark urine, is frequently seen in hemolytic processes. Untreated or undiagnosed thalassemia major or intermedia is often associated with frontal bossing, malar prominence, hepatosplenomegaly, and dental malocclusion. Generalized lymphadenopathy and hepatosplenomegaly are frequent features of myeloproliferative disorders and malignancies, especially leukemia and lymphoma. Petechiae, purpura, and multiple ecchymoses can be expected in hemostatic disorders. Orthopedic anomalies may suggest Fanconi's anemia (abnormal radii or thumbs) or Diamond-Blackfan syndrome (triphalangeal or bifid thumbs.)

Iron deficiency

Iron deficiency is the most likely diagnosis in an otherwise well child with mild-to-moderate microcytic, hypochromic anemia. While inadequate dietary intake of iron is the most common cause of iron deficiency in a young child, blood loss is more likely in an older child or adolescent.

ED management
Iron deficiency

Treat with oral ferrous sulfate, 6 mg/kg per day of elemental iron div tid between meals. Give with juice (vitamin C enhances iron absorption), but not with milk, which impairs iron absorption. If there is difficulty with administration, the daily dose can be given on a once-a-day schedule. A rise in hemoglobin and reticulocyte count after 1 week confirms both the diagnosis and adherence to the regimen. Lack of response suggests an incorrect diagnosis, ongoing blood loss, incorrect dose, malabsorption, or noncompliance with medication. Advise the patient or parents that gastrointestinal complaints, particularly constipation and darkening of the stools, may result from iron therapy. For occasional epigastric discomfort, divide the iron doses into smaller volumes at more frequent intervals or administer with food (not milk).

Blood loss

Blood loss, particularly when acute, may require treatment with packed red blood cells, especially if the patient is symptomatic (pronounced tachycardia, orthostatic hypotension, syncope). Do not rely solely on the level of the hematocrit to decide whether a transfusion is necessary, since children often tolerate extremely low red cell counts without exhibiting any symptoms. Consider associated clinical findings, such as resting heart rate and respiratory rate, as well as the likelihood of a further imminent decrease in the hematocrit in bleeding conditions. Other conditions that might warrant a transfusion include disorders associated with decreased erythrocyte production as seen in either bone marrow failure (aplastic anemia, transient erythroblastopenia of childhood, nutritional anemias, and drug-induced marrow suppression) or marrow replacement (leukemia, neuroblastoma, histiocytosis, storage disorders). Consult a pediatric hematologist before giving blood to these patients. (See Transfusion therapy, pp. 341–342)

Autoimmune hemolytic anemia

Initially treat with prednisone (2 mg/kg per day), after consultation with a pediatric hematologist. Packed red-cell transfusions might be required, but this condition can be associated with a high risk of transfusion reactions.

The treatment of most other primary hematologic etiologies of anemia, often requires consultation with a pediatric hematologist.

Follow-up
- Iron-deficiency anemia: 1 week, for a hemoglobin and reticulocyte count; sooner if the initial hemoglobin is extremely low and there is significant tachycardia

Indications for admission
- Significant cardiovascular or cerebral symptomatology (syncope, tachycardia, heart failure)
- Acute blood loss requiring transfusion
- Pancytopenia or suspicion of a malignancy
- Acute Coombs positive or extrinsic hemolytic anemia with hemoglobin <8 g/dL

- Chronic hemolytic disease with acute reticulocytopenia and significant fall in hematocrit (aplastic crisis seen in sickle cell disease and spherocytosis)
- Severe glucose-6-phosphate dehydrogenase (G6PD) deficiency with exposure to oxidant stress (e.g. infections, mothballs, sulfonamides, antimalarials)
- Hemoglobin <6 g/dL

Bibliography

Borgna-Pignatti C, Marsella M: Iron deficiency in infancy and childhood. *Pediatr Ann* 2008;37:329–37.

Oski FA, Brugnara C, Nathan DG: A diagnostic approach to the anemic patient. In Nathan DG, Oski FA (eds), *Hematology of Infancy and Childhood*, 6th ed. Philadelphia: WB Saunders, 2003, pp. 409–18.

Pearson HA, Dallman PR: Anemia: diagnosis and classification. In Rudolph CD, Rudolph AM (eds), *Rudolph's Pediatrics*. New York: McGraw-Hill, 2003, pp. 1523–47.

Hemostatic disorders

Thrombocytopenia involves a decrease in the number of circulating platelets secondary to underproduction, as in marrow failure (aplasia, infections, or drugs) or marrow replacement (leukemia, storage disorders, histiocytosis); increased peripheral destruction (immune thrombocytopenic purpura [ITP], hypersplenism, infections, hemangiomas); ineffective production (myelodysplasia); or microangiopathic processes (hemolytic-uremic syndrome, disseminated intravascular coagulation [DIC]).

Platelet dysfunction can also cause bleeding manifestations. These disorders of platelet function can be acquired (uremia; ingestion of aspirin or nonsteroidal anti-inflammatory medications) or inherited (von Willebrand's disease, storage pool disorder).

Coagulation factors are necessary for the formation of fibrin strands at bleeding sites. Hemorrhage can occur when any of these proteins are either decreased in amount or dysfunctional. Factor activity is decreased in inherited deficiencies (hemophilia [factor VIII], von Willebrand's disease [Factor IX]), vitamin K deficiency (normal newborns, sodium warfarin [Coumadin] therapy, prolonged oral antibiotic therapy), liver failure, and DIC. Abnormal proteins with markedly diminished or absent function, as in hemophilia and dysfibrinogenemia, are less common causes.

The endothelium is responsible for the production of factor VIII and prostacyclin (a platelet inhibitor) and the insulation of coagulation factors and platelets from exposure to underlying collagen. Dysfunction of the endothelial system is observed in vasculitis (lupus, Henoch-Schönlein purpura) and infections (meningococcemia, *Rickettsia*).

Clinical presentation

The presenting complaint of hemostatic disorders may vary greatly, depending on the location, acuity, and severity of bleeding. Platelet abnormalities are commonly associated with petechial or mucosal bleeding that occurs immediately after the trauma and will often respond to local pressure. With ITP, skin and mucosal bleeding often follow a benign viral illness or measles vaccination. Patients with coagulation factor abnormalities, particularly the hemophilias, may have delayed, posttraumatic deep tissue hemorrhages into muscles and joints. In the first few weeks of life, a coagulopathy may present with delayed, persistent bleeding from the circumcision site or the umbilical stump. Abrasions and tooth extractions respond poorly to local pressure and can continue to ooze and bleed for days. Bleeding secondary to vasculitis (such as Henoch-Schönlein purpura) usually presents as palpable purpura.

Diagnosis

Suspect a bleeding disorder in a child who presents with a history of bruising or bleeding that is out of proportion to the level of trauma, bleeding in unusual locations, spontaneous hemorrhage, and prolonged or recurrent bleeding. Ask about a family history of inherited hemorrhagic disorders, such as hemophilia A and B (X-linked), factor XI deficiency (autosomal recessive), and von Willebrand's disease (usually autosomal dominant), or unexplained significant bleeding, particularly if a blood transfusion was necessary. A seriously ill child may have leukemia (pallor, fever, fatigue, hepatomegaly, lymphaden-opathy), hemolytic-uremic syndrome (lethargy, diarrhea, oliguria), liver disease (vomiting, jaundice, hepatomegaly, dark urine, acholic stools), or DIC.

The diagnosis can be facilitated by a few simple screening tests. Platelet count and prothrombin time (PT) or International Normalized Ratio (INR) test the extrinsic clotting system (factor VII, plus the factors in the common pathway [I, II, V, X]); partial thrombo-plastin time (PTT) tests the intrinsic system (factors VIII, IX, XI, XII, plus the factors in the common pathway [I, II, V, X]). Bleeding time, which assesses the platelet-endothelium interaction (normal: 8 min) is rarely used these days. See Tables 13-2 (Differential diagnosis of bleeding) and 13-3 (Differential diagnosis of thrombocytopenia).

ED management

For the patient with vitamin K deficiency who is actively bleeding, give 5–10 mg of vitamin K by slow intravenous infusion. Correction of coagulation factor levels begins within hours, with marked improvement by 24 hours. Treat severe bleeding with an infusion of fresh frozen plasma to rapidly correct the deficiencies. If there is a history of warfarin ingestion, a repeat administration of vitamin K might be necessary.

Treat thrombocytopenic conditions with local pressure to superficial bleeding sites. If this is unsuccessful, or the platelet count is <50,000/mm³, obtain a type and cross-match and consult a pediatric hematologist. Treat patients with documented ITP and serious, life-threatening bleeding with high-dose intravenous gamma-globulin (0.25–0.5 g/kg over 4–5 hours) or high-dose corticosteroids (methylprednisolone 20–40 mg/kg over 1 hour), while awaiting consult-ation with a hematologist. A patient who is Rh positive can also be treated with WinRho at a dose of 50 mcg/kg. For patients with thrombocytopenia caused by decreased production (leukemia, other marrow failure syndromes), transfuse single-donor apheresis platelets (see Transfusion therapy, pp. 341–342). Replace deficient clotting factors as soon as possible to avoid complications. As a general rule, 1 unit/kg of factor VIII will raise a patient's factor level by 2%. Always consult with a hematologist before treating a coagulopathy patient with factor replacement, as the selection and dose of the factor product vary greatly. Factor VII concentrate will often treat a variety of coagulopathies. Avoid giving aspirin and other medications that can inhibit proper platelet function to any child with a bleeding diathesis.

Obtain a CT scan of the head for a patient with a hemostatic disorder who has a moderate or severe headache or any neurologic symptoms (irritability, lethargy, vomiting, ataxia, loss of consciousness) after head trauma.

Follow-up

- Patient with ITP: repeat platelet count in 1–3 days, depending on the initial platelet count
- Patient treated with factor VIII: next day

Table 13-2. Differential diagnosis of bleeding disorders

Platelet count[a]	Prothrombin time[a]	Partial thromboplastin time[a]	Diagnoses
Normal	Prolonged	Normal	Coumadin ingestion
			Factor VII deficiency
			Mild liver disease
			Mild vitamin K deficiency
Normal	Normal	Prolonged	Circulating antibodies
			Factor VIII, IX, XI, or XII deficiency
			Heparin effect
			von Willebrand's disease
Decreased	Prolonged	Prolonged	Congenital heart disease
			DIC
			Severe liver disease
Decreased	Normal	Normal	Thrombocytopenia
Normal	Prolonged	Prolonged	Dysfibrinogenemia
			Factor II, V, or X deficiency
			High-dose heparin or warfarin therapy
			Moderate liver disease
			Vitamin K deficiency
Normal	Normal	Normal	Child abuse and trauma
			Connective tissue disease
			Factor XIII deficiency
			Henoch-Schönlein purpura
			Platelet dysfunction (inherited and acquired)
			Scurvy
			von Willebrand's disease

Note: [a]Normal values: platelet count: 150,000–300,000/mm^3; PT: <13 s or within 2 s of control or INR <1.2; PTT: <35–39 s or within 5 s of control.

Indications for admission

- Massive bleeding that causes hypovolemia or requires transfusion of packed red blood cells
- Suspected or proven intracranial, intrathoracic, or abdominal hemorrhage
- Hemophiliacs or patients with other severe hemostatic disorders who sustain significant head trauma (e.g. lethargic, skull fracture, abnormal neurologic finding, or loss of consciousness)

Table 13-3. Differential diagnosis of thrombocytopenia

Diagnosis	Differentiating features
Drug induced	Taking antibiotics for 1-2 weeks
Epstein-Barr virus	Fever, pharyngitis, fatigue, splenomegaly
Fanconi's anemia	Short stature, abnormal thumbs, café au lait spots, macrocytosis
Gaucher's disease	Family history; bone pain, pathologic fractures, splenomegaly
Histiocytosis	Eczema, chronic otitis, bone lesions, hepatosplenomegaly
HIV	Adenopathy, recurrent infections, bruising, pallor, lymphopenia
HUS	Bloody diarrhea, lethargy, oliguria, pallor, jaundice
ITP	Extensive bruising and petechiae in a well-appearing child
	↑MPV; RBCs and WBCs are normal
Kasabach-Merritt syndrome	Enlarged portions of extremities, bleeding
Leukemia	Fever, bruising, pallor, adenopathy, abnormal white cells
Malaria	High fever, jaundice, splenomegaly, foreign travel
May-Hegglin anomaly	Family history of bruising and petechiae
	↑↑MPV, WBC inclusions
Meningococcemia	Fever and toxicity; palpable purpura, hypotension
Neuroblastoma	Fever, lower extremity weakness, abdominal mass
Osteopetrosis	Infant with severely impaired vision; bruising, splenomegaly,
Thrombocytopenia-Absent radii	Bleeding from birth, abnormal forearms
Wiskott-Aldrich syndrome	Infant boy with eczema, frequent infections, ↓MPV

- Significant hematemesis, hematochezia, or hematuria
- Newly diagnosed thrombocytopenia (platelet count $<15,000/mm^3$) in a young child
- Severe inherited coagulopathy with gross hematuria, large laceration, or severe abdominal pain
- Clinical features suspicious for marrow replacement, DIC, hemolytic-uremic syndrome, or hepatic failure
- Generalized petechial or purpuric eruption in an acutely ill febrile child

Bibliography

Franchini M: Advances in the diagnosis and management of von Willebrand's disease. *Hematology* 2006;11:219–5.

Schafer AI: Approach to bleeding. In Loscalzo J, Schafer AI (eds), *Thrombosis and*

Hemorrhage, 3rd ed. Philadelphia: Lippincott Williams & Wilkins, 2003, pp. 315–29.

Stasi R, Evangelista ML, Stipa E, et al: Idiopathic thrombocytopenic purpura: current concepts in pathophysiology and management. *Thromb Haemost* 2008;99:4–13.

Thrombophilia

There are a number of inherited disorders that may present in childhood and predispose patients to thrombosis and abnormal clot formation. Three important proteins, protein C, protein S, and antithrombin III, are important in preventing abnormal clot formation; inherited and acquired deficiencies are significant risk factors for thrombosis. DNA mutations, including the factor V Leiden and prothrombin mutations, are important causes of thrombosis. Consider the antiphospholipid syndrome in any patient presenting with thrombosis.

Thrombocytosis can occur with a variety of conditions, as the platelet count often behaves as an acute-phase reactant. Thrombocytosis may be seen in children with recent infections, major physical stress, or as a "rebound" phenomenon after a period of bone marrow suppression. Underlying disorders associated with thrombocytosis include malignancies (chronic myelogenous leukemia, neuroblastoma), Kawasaki syndrome, sarcoid, chronic inflammatory disorders (inflammatory bowel disease), chronic hemolytic disorders, and iron deficiency. Primary idiopathic thrombocytosis is a rare condition that can sometimes be a precursor to leukemia. A platelet count $>1,000,000/mm^3$ may require treatment because of the risk of thrombosis.

Clinical presentation

Patients will often present with swelling and pain in an extremity, most commonly a leg. Occasionally a distinct firm "cord" can be palpated, but more commonly there will be painful swelling, sometimes with overlying erythema. The swelling can be significant, with a marked asymmetry when comparing both extremities. A pulmonary embolus presents with sudden onset of respiratory distress and tachypnea, typically with chest pain and areas of decreased breath sounds on auscultation. A possible sinus thrombosis is suggested by persistent severe headaches with a history of inflammation or infection in the head and neck area. A patient with acute onset of neurologic symptoms and a CT scan that demonstrates an infarct requires an evaluation for thrombophilia. A patient with swelling, numbness and a cold upper extremity is highly suspect for thoracic outlet syndrome. Radiographic studies are necessary to identify mechanical obstruction to flow from compression of the major vessels.

Diagnosis

If there is a suspicion of thrombophlebitis of an extremity, a Doppler study can assess patency of the vasculature. On occasion, MRI of the vessels can add more detail to the evaluation, particularly for thrombosis of deep veins. For the patient with respiratory symptoms, particularly if there is also suspicion of a thrombus in an extremity, a CT scan of the chest will usually demonstrate the affected area. Ventilation/perfusion scans can add more information and help clarify the clinical picture. D-dimers are usually elevated in patients with thrombosis; they can be markedly elevated with pulmonary embolism.

Ask about any history of indwelling catheters, particularly in the neonatal period or in patients with PICC lines or indwelling central venous catheters. Dehydration, birth control pills, and prolonged periods of immobilization can lead to localized stasis and thrombosis.

To evaluate the patient for a possible underlying predisposition, obtain a CBC, PT, PTT, anticardiolipin antibodies; factor VIII activity; lupus anticoagulant; protein C, protein S panels, antithrombin III panels; factor V Leiden, prothrombin mutation, MTHFR DNA studies, and homocysteine levels.

ED management

The presence of a thrombus warrants rapid intervention to prevent propagation and worsening symptoms. For patients with elevated platelet counts, give antiplatelet medications to reduce the risk of thrombus formation, including aspirin (often just 1 baby aspirin every other day) and dipyridamole (50–75 mg bid-tid). If a thrombus of the lower extremity is detected, institute anticoagulation promptly, preferably with low molecular weight heparin (1 mg/kg q 12 h). Thrombolysis is another option, particularly for life-threatening pulmonary emboli and large deep-vein thromboses, but this should be undertaken by vascular surgeons and interventional radiologists experienced in dealing with these situations.

Indications for admission

- Suspicion or confirmation of venous thrombosis
- Suspicion or confirmation of pulmonary embolus

Bibliography

Gerotziafas GT: Risk factors for venous thromboembolism in children. *Int Angiol* 2004;23:195–205.

Revel-Vilk S, Massicotte P: Thromboembolic diseases of childhood. *Blood Rev* 2003;17:1–6.

Tormene D, Gavasso S, Rossetto V, Simioni P: Thrombosis and thrombophilia in children: a systematic review. *Semin Thromb Hemost* 2006;32:724–8.

Transfusion therapy

Criteria for transfusions vary, depending on the underlying condition, the desired effect, and the risks of transfusion versus the anticipated benefits. Each 1 mL/kg of packed cells raises the hematocrit approximately 0.7%. If the patient has a slowly evolving moderately severe anemia requiring red cell transfusion, appropriate compensatory mechanisms, and a normal blood pressure, transfuse a maximum volume of 10–15 mL/kg of packed red cells slowly, slowly, over 2–3 hours. For very severe, chronic, or well-compensated anemias, administer the blood in smaller 5 mL/kg aliquots, with several hours between transfusions to allow for the vascular compartment to remove excess fluid. A diuretic, such as furosemide (0.5 mg/kg IV), may be required between transfusions to prevent volume overload and heart failure. When treating acute or ongoing blood loss, particularly if there is hypovolemia or hypotension, administer the blood rapidly. This situation includes splenic sequestration crises in patients with chronic hemolytic anemias, such as sickle cell disease and spherocytosis.

For multiply transfused patients or patients who have experienced prior febrile, non-hemolytic transfusion reactions, use leukocyte-depleted RBCs to decrease the likelihood of transfusion reactions. Request irradiated red cells for any immunodeficient patient, including neonates, patients with malignancies or immunodeficiency diseases, bone marrow transplant candidates, and patients on immunosuppressive therapy. Irradiation destroys lymphocytes that might cause serious graft-versus-host disease in the recipient.

Premedicate with acetaminophen (15 mg/kg) to decrease the risk of febrile nonhemolytic transfusion reactions. For patients with a history of frequent reactions, particularly if urticarial, give diphenhydramine (1 mg/kg PO or 0.5 mg/kg IV). Give corticosteroids (hydrocortisone 1 mg/kg PO or IV) to patients with more significant or frequent prior allergic reactions. A patient with an autoimmune hemolytic anemia who requires transfusions poses additional difficulties. It may be impossible to find a completely compatible donor unit, so the least reactive unit is often the only alternative. If a cold antibody is present, infuse the red blood cells through an intravenous fluid warmer to decrease the amount of hemolysis. Because of the high risk of reactions, administer high-dose steroids (hydrocortisone 1–1.5 mg/kg IV) prior to and every 3–4 hours during the transfusion.

Platelet transfusions can help stop bleeding in a thrombocytopenic patient who is not producing platelets (leukemia, aplastic anemia) but are of little value in patients with ITP, unless severe internal bleeding develops. Generally, use single-donor apheresis platelets to expose the patient to fewer donors with a lessened risk of antibody sensitization and possible infection. Always premedicate the patient since reactions to platelet transfusions are more common than those associated with transfused red blood cells.

Bibliography

Bell MD: Consultation with the specialist: red blood cell transfusions. *Pediatr Rev* 2007;28:299–304.

Fasano R, Luban NL: Blood component therapy. *Pediatr Clin North Am* 2008;55:421–45.

Radhakrishnan KM, Chakravarthi S, Pushkala S, Jayaraju J: Component therapy. *Indian J Pediatr* 2003;70:661–6.

The abnormal CBC

See Table 13-4.

Table 13-4. The abnormal CBC

Finding	Diagnoses
RBC abnormalities	
Microcytic	Iron deficiency, the thalassemias, sideroblastic anemias (including lead poisoning), porphyrias, the anemia of chronic inflammation
Normocytic	Marrow failure or replacement, immune and extrinsic hemolysis, acute blood loss, hemoglobinopathies, membrane disorders, enzyme deficiencies
Macrocytic	Vitamin B12 and folic acid deficiencies, liver disease, hypothyroidism, inherited aplastic anemia or pure red cell hypoplasia
Platelet abnormalities	
Increased size	Immune thrombocytopenic purpura, Bernard-Soulier syndrome, May-Hegglin anomaly
Decreased size	Wiskott-Aldrich syndrome, leukemias
Absence of color	Storage pool disorders
White cell abnormalities	
↑ mature granulocytes	Infections, inflammation, stress reactions
↑ immature cells	Leukemia
Leukopenia	Viral infections, overwhelming bacterial infections, drug suppression, marrow failure or marrow replacement
Atypical lymphocytes	Viral infections (EBV, CMV)
Increased eosinophils	Parasitic infection, allergic disorders
Basophilia	Chronic myelogenous leukemia
Inclusions (Döhle bodies)	Serious infections, May-Hegglin anomaly

Bibliography

Segel GB, Halterman JS: Neutropenia in
pediatric practice. *Pediatr Rev* 2008;29:12–23.

Wagelie-Steffen A, Aceves SS: Eosinophilic
disorders in children. *Curr Allergy Asthma Rep* 2006;6:475–82.

Infection and the immunocompromised host

The hallmark of an immunocompromised patient is an increased susceptibility to infection, including increased frequency, duration, and severity, as well as infection caused by unusual pathogens.

Clinical presentation

Although symptoms will vary with the organism and site of infection, immunocompromised patients often have recurrent respiratory infections and repeated severe bacterial illnesses (sepsis, pneumonia, meningitis). Persistent lymphadenopathy and hepatosplenomegaly are common findings in these disorders. Many patients have chronic diarrhea with some form of malabsorption and failure to thrive (IgA deficiency, exocrine pancreatic insufficiency). A variety of skin lesions are seen, including eczema (Wiskott-Aldrich syndrome), pyoderma (cyclic neutropenia, Kostmann's syndrome, Job syndrome), and diffuse dermatitis (chronic granulomatous disease).

HIV infection presents in a variety of ways: lymphadenopathy, hepatosplenomegaly, and failure to thrive in an infant with maternal risk factors; a hemophiliac or multiply transfused child with interstitial pneumonitis; or a child with poorly responsive immune thrombocytopenic purpura.

Although most children with sickle cell disease are identified early in life by newborn hemoglobinopathy screening, a Caucasian child of Mediterranean background with unsuspected sickle cell disease may present with frequent bouts of unexplained bone pain, leukocytosis, and a chronic hemolytic anemia.

Lymphoma in an adolescent can cause adenopathy, fever, weight loss, splenomegaly, and herpes zoster or prolonged varicella infection.

Diagnosis

Prior to proceeding with an extensive immunologic evaluation, try to differentiate the immunodeficient child from one with frequent colds and normal immunologic function. Children can have 8–10 respiratory infections in any given year, but these are usually mild, self-limited, occasionally accompanied by fever, but with complete recovery between bouts. Allergy is more likely in children with repeated or persistent infections limited to the upper respiratory tract. An incompletely treated sinusitis or enlarged tonsils/adenoids are frequent underlying causes of recurrent upper respiratory infections. Likewise, infections limited to a particular organ suggest specific disease entities: cystic fibrosis, foreign body, collagen vascular diseases, or bronchiectasis with recurrent pneumonia; cow's milk sensitivity, celiac disease, and inflammatory bowel disease with chronic diarrhea and failure to thrive. Many chronic diseases predispose patients to frequent infections (rheumatic disorders, chronic renal disease, sickle cell disease, diabetes, nutritional deficiencies, malignancies). Finally, a history of blood product administration to the patient or parent, intravenous drug abuse, or high-risk sexual activity raises the possibility of HIV infection.

ED management

If the child has had either two or more serious infections (pneumonia, meningitis, sepsis, osteomyelitis) in a short period of time or an infection with an unusual pathogen, obtain a CBC with differential and platelet count, ESR, and quantitative immunoglobulins. In addition, evaluate cell-mediated immunity by measuring T-cell subsets and consider skin testing (*Candida*, streptokinase-streptodornase, mumps, and purified protein derivative [PPD]). Assume that any patient with a history of treatment with chemotherapeutic drugs for malignancy or autoimmune disorders, or with immunosuppressive medications (including corticosteroids for disorders such as asthma or inflammatory bowel disease) is at high risk for infections. Consult a pediatric hematologist or immunologist for further evaluation with specific definitive tests.

When a patient with a known immunodeficiency or neutrophil disorder presents with a fever (>38.6°C, 101.5°F), a conservative approach is mandatory. Obtain a CBC and cultures of the blood, urine, and any wounds prior to initiating treatment. If there are central nervous system symptoms, perform a lumbar puncture with additional fluid to evaluate for unusual organisms (mycobacteria, India ink stain for *Cryptococcus*) in addition to the standard culture, cell count, glucose, and Gram's stain.

Treat an ill-appearing neutropenic patient with a combination of an aminoglycoside such as tobramycin or gentamicin (6 mg/kg per day IV div q 8–12 h) and either a semisynthetic penicillin (piperacillin/tazobactam 250 mg/kg per day IV div q 6 h) or ceftazidime (100 mg/kg per day IV div q 8 h) for adequate *Pseudomonas* coverage. Cefepime (100 mg/kg per day IV div q 12 h) can be used for monotherapy in a patient who does not appear seriously ill or unstable.

Treat a child with defective cell-mediated immunity who has fever and respiratory symptoms with trimethoprim-sulfamethoxazole (20 mg/kg per day of TMP div q 6 h) along with broad-spectrum antibiotics, as listed above. Treat patients with splenic dysfunction with ceftriaxone or cefuroxime (100 mg/kg per day). If the patient has a very high fever or a toxic appearance, add vancomycin (60 mg/kg per day div q 6 h) to cover for resistant *Pneumococcus*. Consult a hematologist for patients with neutrophil disorders who have serious infections, as granulocyte transfusions or granulocyte colony stimulating factor (G-CSF), 5 mg/kg per day, may be indicated. With the advent of more resistant organisms such as vancomycin-resistant enterococcus and methicillin-resistant *S. aureus*, other antibiotic combinations often need to be explored with an infectious disease expert or hematologist.

Follow-up

- Immunocompromised patient with low-grade fever not treated with antibiotics: next day, if still febrile

Indications for admission

- Fever (>38.6°C, 101.5°F) in a patient with a granulocyte count <500/mm^3, a documented phagocytic defect, or other immunodeficiency
- Immunocompromised patient with pneumonia, an abscess, or localized infection (e.g. otitis, cellulitis) not responding to initial antibiotic therapy
- Patient with sickle cell disease under 2 years old with fever >38.3°C (101°F); older patient with high fever (>38.9°C, 102°F)

- Suspected malignancy
- Immunocompromised patient with a toxic appearance, regardless of the temperature
- Varicella or herpes zoster infection in a child with defective cell-mediated immunity

Bibliography

Ahmed N, El-Mahallawy HA, Ahmed IA, et al: Early hospital discharge versus continued hospitalization in febrile pediatric cancer patients with prolonged neutropenia: a randomized, prospective study. *Pediatr Blood Cancer* 2007;49:786–92.

Corapcioglu F, Sarper N, Zengin E: Monotherapy with piperacillin/tazobactam versus cefepime as empirical therapy for febrile neutropenia in pediatric cancer patients: a randomized comparison. *Pediatr Hematol Oncol* 2006;23:177–86.

Härtel C, Deuster M, Lehrnbecher T, Schultz C: Current approaches for risk stratification of infectious complications in pediatric oncology. *Pediatr Blood Cancer* 2007;49:767–73.

Leukemia and lymphoma

The most common pediatric malignancy is acute lymphoblastic leukemia (ALL); lymphomas are second only to brain tumors in frequency of solid tumors.

Clinical presentation

Leukemia

The presenting symptoms of ALL usually result from the absence of normal hematopoietic elements, along with the proliferation and accumulation of abnormal cells. Clinical findings are related to the degree of anemia (pallor, fatigue, light-headedness, palpitations), thrombocytopenia (petechiae, purpura, epistaxis), and neutropenia (infections). Other signs and symptoms include joint or bone pain, hepatosplenomegaly, lymphadenopathy, skin nodules, and gingival hypertrophy. CNS involvement can be asymptomatic; alternatively, there can be symptoms related to elevated intracranial pressure (headache, vomiting, irritability, visual disturbances) or unusual constellations of findings such as an isolated cranial nerve paresis or the "hypothalamic syndrome" (marked hyperphagia with weight gain, personality changes). Leukemic infiltration in organs such as the testes, kidneys, and ovaries can lead to firm, painless enlargement.

Hodgkin's disease

Hodgkin's disease in children and adolescents most commonly presents with either firm, nontender, asymptomatic lymphadenopathy (particularly the cervical, supraclavicular, mediastinal or para-aortic nodes) or, less commonly, with constitutional symptoms (fever, night sweats, cough, weight loss). Pruritus rarely occurs in children, and complications such as jaundice and superior vena cava obstruction are uncommon. There may be a history of prolonged varicella or herpes zoster.

Non-Hodgkin's lymphomas

The non-Hodgkin's lymphomas may also present with isolated, nontender, firm lymphadenopathy, but children more frequently have widespread disease. A primary mediastinal mass may cause dyspnea, cough, pleural effusion, and superior vena cava obstruction (respiratory distress; distended veins in neck and arms). Children can have primary tumors in Waldeyer's ring, presenting with tonsillar involvement misdiagnosed as a peritonsillar abscess. Primary gastrointestinal lymphomas (Peyer's patches of the distal ileum) can cause asymptomatic abdominal distention, vomiting and diarrhea, intussusception, or intestinal obstruction. Burkitt's lymphoma can present with retroperitoneal or mesenteric tumors and occasionally with involvement of the maxillary sinus, but jaw masses are uncommon in the United States.

Diagnosis

In addition to cytopenia, the hallmark of leukemia is the presence of large numbers of primitive leukocytes (blasts) in the blood and bone marrow. While metastatic neuroblastoma may also replace the bone marrow with malignant cells, these cells do not appear in the peripheral blood.

Most often confused with leukemia and lymphomas are infectious mononucleosis and mono-like syndromes (cytomegalovirus, toxoplasmosis), which can present with fever, lymphadenopathy, hepatosplenomegaly, cytopenias, and immature leukocytes on blood smear. However, these cells can usually be distinguished from leukemic blast cells. Pertussis can induce a profound leukocytosis ($>100,000/mm^3$) and neutropenia, but the cells are mature and anemia is not usually present. Children with ITP do not appear chronically ill, the platelets are usually large, and cytopenia of other cell lines is absent. Storage disorders (Gaucher's disease) may present with hepatosplenomegaly and pancytopenia, necessitating DNA testing, enzyme assays, and, less commonly, a bone marrow examination or liver biopsy for confirmation.

A lymphoma-like picture can be seen with sinus histiocytosis, diphenylhydantoin therapy, and, rarely, in Kawasaki syndrome. A node biopsy is indicated if there is weight loss or supraclavicular lymphadenopathy, or the node is nontender, firm, and progressively enlarging.

ED management

If leukemia or lymphoma is suspected, obtain a CBC with differential, platelet count, reticulocyte count, heterophile antibody or monospot test, electrolytes, liver function tests, lactic dehydrogenase, uric acid, a blood culture, and chest X-ray. Consult with a pediatric hematologist-oncologist.

Follow-up

- Asymptomatic patient with lymphadenopathy: 7–10 days
- Mild pancytopenia: repeat CBC in 3–4 days

Indications for admission

- Blasts on peripheral smear
- Lymphadenopathy that meets the criteria for biopsy
- Newly diagnosed or suspected malignancy
- Pancytopenia
- Suspicion of mass pressure on a vital structure

Bibliography

Gross TG, Termuhlen AM: Pediatric non-Hodgkin's lymphoma. *Curr Oncol Rep* 2007 9:459–65.

Pui CH, Robison LL, Look AT: Acute lymphoblastic leukaemia. *Lancet* 2008;371:1030–43.

Lymphadenopathy

Palpable lymph nodes are a common finding and may be normal or a sign of minor or life-threatening disease. Lymph nodes are not usually palpable until a few months of age. Afterward there is a steady increase in the body's normal lymphoid tissue, so that by puberty nearly 100% of children will have at least some palpable nodes, most commonly in the cervical and inguinal areas. A variety of factors must be considered when deciding whether to pursue a work-up for enlarged nodes.

Clinical presentation

Generalized lymphadenopathy

Generalized lymphadenopathy is defined as enlargement in at least three noncontiguous lymph node regions. It is always abnormal, and usually nonlymphoid features of the primary disease process are evident (fever, rash, pharyngitis, arthritis, arthralgia, bruising, pallor, hepatosplenomegaly, etc.). The most common etiology is infection, particularly viral disease such as infectious mononucleosis or mono-like illnesses (cytomegalovirus, toxoplasmosis). Other infectious etiologies include the exanthematous viral infections of childhood (measles, rubella, varicella), enteroviruses (echo, Coxsackie), tuberculosis, hepatitis B, syphilis, malaria, and HIV. Noninfectious causes include rheumatoid diseases (idiopathic juvenile arthritis, systemic lupus erythematosus), serum sickness, drug reactions (diphenylhydantoin), sarcoidosis, storage diseases, and eczema. Malignancies and related disorders to consider include leukemia, lymphoma, and histiocytosis.

Localized lymphadenopathy

Reactive adenopathy

Localized lymphadenopathy is most often a response to a regional infection. The location often suggests the underlying infection. Reactive cervical enlargement is most common, frequently secondary to a viral upper respiratory infection. Occipital lymphadenopathy occurs in response to scalp conditions such as seborrhea, tinea capitis, and pediculosis; preauricular enlargement can be secondary to conjunctivitis and acne; and submandibular and submental nodes may enlarge with infection of the gingiva, teeth, buccal mucosa, and tongue. Axillary lymphadenopathy can be caused by cat scratch fever, rat bite fever, or a recent immunization, while inguinal involvement occurs with venereal diseases (syphilis, gonorrhea, lymphogranuloma venereum, chancroid) and lower extremity infections. Since the supraclavicular nodes drain from the lungs and mediastinum, enlargement here is always a concern. Etiologies include infections (tuberculosis, histoplasmosis, coccidioidomycosis), neoplasms (lymphomas), and sarcoidosis. For any node site, a nearby cellulitis, dermatitis, or local pyogenic infection will cause reactive enlargement.

Adenitis

A second category of local lymphadenopathy is primary infection of the node, or adenitis. Most often this is bacterial in origin. The most common organisms are *Staphylococcus aureus* and group A *Streptococcus*, although anaerobes, tuberculosis, atypical mycobacteria, and HIV are other etiologies to consider.

Diagnosis

A complete history and physical examination are necessary to locate a primary infection, document a local adenitis, or diagnose a disease causing generalized lymphadenopathy. Note any fever, weight loss, rash, jaundice, arthritis, arthralgias, bruising, pallor, pharyngitis or upper respiratory symptoms, hepatosplenomegaly, contact with contagious diseases, history of a cat scratch or rat bite, and sexual activity. When examining the involved node(s) there are six features to consider.

Location

Significant generalized lymphadenopathy always warrants further investigation, as does supraclavicular or axillary adenopathy. Isolated cervical, inguinal, and occipital nodes are less commonly pathologic.

Size

Generally, consider nodes > 1 cm in diameter to be abnormal. However, particularly in the cervical area, nodes may be 2–3 cm without indicating serious underlying disease.

Rate of enlargement

Rapid enlargement is most commonly caused by an infection, either an adenitis or a reactive hyperplasia. Slow growth suggests a malignancy or a systemic disease.

Mobility

A node fixed to adjacent structures or matted to other nodes suggests an infiltrative disease that demands further evaluation. A freely mobile node is generally benign.

Consistency

Soft, shotty nodes are usually normal or represent reactive enlargement. Adenitis causes fluctuance, while malignancy is associated with hard, rubbery nodes.

Overlying skin

Bacterial adenitis causes erythema and warmth of the overlying skin. Adherence of the skin to the node occurs in cat scratch fever and atypical mycobacterium infection. A reactive node does not affect the overlying skin.

While abnormality of any one of these characteristics might not be worrisome, multiple abnormalities (e.g. a firm, fixed, supraclavicular node) are suspicious for an underlying serious disorder, particularly a malignant disease, and require further investigation. See Table 13-5 for the differential diagnosis of lymphadenopathy.

ED management

Generalized lymphadenopathy

If infectious mononucleosis is suggested by the clinical findings (fever, fatigue, pharyngitis, hepatosplenomegaly), obtain a CBC with differential (to look for atypical lymphocytosis or monocytosis) and a monospot or heterophile antibody test to confirm the diagnosis. However, since the heterophile is likely to be negative in a child <6 years old with active mononucleosis, obtain EBV serology, including IgM. Treatment is supportive (bed rest,

Table 13-5. Differential diagnosis of lymphadenopathy

Diagnosis	Differentiating features
Cat scratch	Fever, history of contact with kitten
	Localized lymphadenopathy proximal to scratch wound
Epstein-Barr virus	Pharyngitis, fatigue, splenomegaly, atypical lymphocytes
	Generalized lymphadenopathy
Enterovirus	Summertime; fever, petechia, hand-foot-mouth rash, aseptic meningitis
HIV	Opportunistic infections, bruising, lymphopenia
Histoplasmosis	Fever, flu-like illness, cough, chest pain
Hodgkin's disease	Rubbery nodes, fever, night sweats
IRA	Fever, joint pains, fleeting rash
	Elevated ESR/CRP, anemia
Kawasaki disease	Strawberry tongue, conjunctivitis
	Thrombocytosis
Langerhans histiocytosis	Fever, chronic otitis, hepatosplenomegaly, eczema
Leukemia	Fever, bone pain, pallor, bruising, hepatosplenomegaly, anemia, abnormal white cells
Lyme disease	Fever, "bullseye" rash, joint pains, headaches
Neuroblastoma	Abdominal mass, fever, bone pain
RMSF	Tick bite, fever, rash on distal extremities, splenomegaly
Rubella	Maculopapular rash, joint pains
SLE	Adolescent girl with facial rash, joint pains
Streptococcus	Fever, headache, cervical adenopathy
Tuberculosis	Fever, cough, weight loss, pulmonary lesions
Tularemia	Animal contact; fever, chills, skin ulceration, tender nodes

acetaminophen as needed). Instruct the patient to avoid contact sports if there is significant splenomegaly because of the risk of splenic rupture. Admission and steroid therapy (prednisone 2 mg/kg per day div bid) are indicated for neurologic symptoms, respiratory distress, massively enlarged tonsils, or cytopenias.

For other situations, the clinical picture guides the evaluation, although in general a CBC with differential, ESR, liver function tests, VDRL, hepatitis B antigen, heterophile antibody, PPD, and chest X-ray are often indicated. If any risk factors are present, obtain HIV serology.

Localized lymphadenopathy

Reactive adenopathy

In most cases a contiguous infection will be found and reactive adenopathy diagnosed. Treat the primary infection appropriately. The reactive node(s) will shrink as the infection resolves.

Adenitis

Treat an adenitis with cefadroxil (40 mg/kg per day div bid), cephalexin (40 mg/kg per day div qid), erythromycin (40 mg/kg per day div qid), cefprozil (20 mg/kg per day div bid), clarithromycin (15 mg/kg per day div bid), or azithromycin (12 mg/kg per day). Warm compresses applied for 15–30 minutes every 3–4 hours are an important adjunct. Reevaluate the patient in 48–72 hours. If there has been a response, continue the antibiotic for a full 10-day course. If there has been no change in the node in an otherwise asymptomatic child, change the antibiotic to clindamycin (20 mg/kg per day div qid) or amoxicillin-clavulanate (875/125 formulation, 45 mg/kg per day of amoxicillin div bid) and follow up in two days. However, if there is no improvement and the patient appears ill, or if the node continues to enlarge, obtain a CBC and blood culture and admit for further evaluation (including surgical consultation) and parenteral antibiotics (nafcillin 150 mg/kg per day div q 6 h, ceftriaxone 100 mg/kg per day div q 12 h, clindamycin 40 mg/kg per day div q 6 h, or cefazolin 75 mg/kg per day div q 8 h). Add vancomycin (40 mg/kg per day div qid) if MRSA is a concern. If malignancy is suspected at any time because of a change in the nature of the node, unresponsiveness to treatment, or associated physical or laboratory findings, request an immediate oncology consultation for node biopsy and/or other definitive diagnostic procedures.

Follow-up

• Adenitis treated with oral antibiotics: 2 days

Indications for admission

• Systemic toxicity
• Suspicion of a malignancy or AIDS, to facilitate the work-up and management
• Adenitis unresponsive to oral antibiotics

Bibliography

Leung AK, Robson WL: Childhood cervical lymphadenopathy. *J Pediatr Health Care* 2004;18:3–7.

Oguz A, Karadeniz C, Temel EA, Citak EC, Okur FV: Evaluation of peripheral lymphadenopathy in children. *Pediatr Hematol Oncol* 2006;23:549–61.

Yaris N, Cakir M, Sözen E, Cobanoglu U: Analysis of children with peripheral lymphadenopathy. *Clin Pediatr (Phila)* 2006;45:544–9.

Oncologic emergencies

Aggressive chemotherapy has dramatically increased the response and cure rates for malignancies, but is associated with significant adverse effects. While these complex treatment regimens are usually administered by pediatric oncologists, patients often present to the ED with complications. It is crucial for the ED staff to recognize potential and existing problems related to the cancer therapy.

Chemotherapeutic agents share many common side effects, including myelosuppression, nausea, and alopecia, but each drug has the potential for specific toxicities (Table 13-6). Consult a pediatric oncologist during the evaluation of a patient receiving treatment for a malignancy who presents to the ED with possible side effects.

The most common serious problems are fever, acute neurologic symptomatology, superior vena cava obstruction, respiratory distress, metabolic derangements, and intestinal perforation.

Table 13-6. Side effects of chemotherapy

Drug	Potential adverse effects
Asparaginase	Allergic reactions, anaphylaxis, pancreatitis, fever, coagulopathy, hepatotoxicity
Avastin	Abdominal pain, headache, GI bleeding, nausea, diarrhea, neuropathy, epistaxis
Bleomycin	Fever, chills, allergic reactions, vomiting, pulmonary fibrosis, mucositis
Busulfan	Myelosuppression, pulmonary fibrosis, glossitis, skin darkening
Carboplatin	Myelosuppression, nausea and vomiting, ototoxicity, fatigue, nephrotoxicity
Carmustine (BCNU)	Myelosuppression, vomiting, nephrotoxicity, mucositis, phlebitis, fever, pulmonary fibrosis
Chlorambucil	Myelosuppression, nausea and vomiting, diarrhea, pulmonary fibrosis, skin rash
Cisplatin	Nausea and vomiting, nephrotoxicity, neurotoxicity, hypomagnesemia, ototoxicity, hepatotoxicity
Clofarabine	Myelosuppression, fever/chills, diarrhea, nausea and vomiting, hepatotoxicity
Cyclophosphamide	Myelosuppression, vomiting, SIADH, hemorrhagic cystitis, immunosuppression, cardiotoxicity, skin darkening
Cytosine arabinoside	Myelosuppression, vomiting, hepatotoxicity, mucositis, conjunctivitis, fever, neurotoxicity
Dacarbazine	Myelosuppression, vomiting, hepatotoxicity, blistering
Dactinomycin	Myelosuppression, vomiting, hepatotoxicity, mucositis, blistering
Daunorubicin	Myelosuppression, cardiotoxicity, blistering, mucositis, diarrhea
Dexamethasone	Weight gain, hypertension, diabetes, moodiness
Doxorubicin	Myelosuppression, vomiting, cardiotoxicity, blistering, mucositis, diarrhea
Etoposide	Myelosuppression, vomiting, hypotension, hepatotoxicity
Fludarabine	Myelosuppression, vomiting, diarrhea, blurred vision, mucositis, fatigue
5-Fluorouracil	Myelosuppression, vomiting, diarrhea, mucositis, headache, dermatitis
Gemtuzumab	Vomiting, chills, fever, mucositis, headache, hepatotoxicity, hypotension
Hydroxyurea	Myelosuppression, nausea and vomiting, mucositis, diarrhea
Idarubicin	Myelosuppression, vomiting, cardiotoxicity, blistering, diarrhea
Ifosfamide	Myelosuppression, vomiting, nephrotoxicity, neurotoxicity, hemorrhagic cystitis
Irinotecan	Myelosuppression, vomiting, severe diarrhea, abdominal pain, headache
Lomustine (CCNU)	Myelosuppression, vomiting, hepatotoxicity, nephrotoxicity, anorexia
Mechlorethamine	Myelosuppression, vomiting, blistering, phlebitis, diarrhea, mucositis
Melphalan	Vomiting, mucositis, pulmonary fibrosis

Table 13-6. (cont.)

Drug	Potential adverse effects
6-Mercaptopurine	Myelosuppression, vomiting, hepatotoxicity
Methotrexate	Myelosuppression, vomiting, mucositis, hepatotoxicity, neurotoxicity, nephrotoxicity
Mitoxantrone	Myelosuppression, cough, GI bleeding, mucositis, diarrhea, headache
Prednisone	Weight gain, hypertension, diabetes, moodiness
Procarbazine	Myelosuppression, vomiting, diarrhea, neurotoxicity, fever, mucositis, myalgias
6-Thioguanine	Myelosuppression, vomiting, hepatotoxicity, mucositis
Thiotepa	Myelosuppression, mucositis, neurotoxicity
Topotecan	Myelosuppression, vomiting, abdominal pain
Tretinoin	Abdominal pain, muscle pain, constipation, anorexia
Vinblastine	Myelosuppression, vomiting, blistering
Vincristine	Peripheral neuropathy, SIADH, constipation, seizures
Vinorelbine	Myelosuppression, neuropathy, anorexia, constipation

Clinical presentation

Since malignant diseases and their treatments are associated with immunodeficiency and neutropenia, patients are particularly susceptible to infectious complications, typically manifested by fever $>38.6°C$ (101.5°F). The immunodeficient patient with pneumonia might be suffering from an opportunistic infection (*Pneumocystis*, *Aspergillus*, *Candida*, Legionnaire's disease). An absolute neutrophil count $<500/mm^3$ places the patient at risk for Gram-negative and fungal infections. Indwelling central venous catheters increase the risk of staphylococcal and streptococcal infections. Cultures are most important since the range of infection is very broad.

Acute neurologic symptomatology may result from spinal cord or nerve root compression (back pain, lower extremity weakness and sensory loss, and bladder and bowel dysfunction). Headache, vomiting, and isolated cranial nerve paresis can result from intracranial involvement.

A patient with lymphoma or leukemia who presents with a mediastinal mass is at risk for superior vena cava obstruction with dyspnea, edema of the head and neck, and prominence of the superficial veins on the upper body. Mediastinal masses may also compress the tracheobronchial tree and cause respiratory distress.

A patient who develops mucositis, particularly in combination with prolonged neutropenia, is at risk for intestinal perforation. The possibility increases with superimposed diarrhea and steroid use. Because of the decreased inflammatory response and neutropenia, a perforation may present without the classic physical findings of peritoneal irritation, although there may be abdominal pain, fever, and distention.

A patient with a large tumor burden and rapidly proliferating disease is at risk for significant metabolic derangements, including hyperuricemia (oliguria), hyperkalemia (muscle weakness; peaked T waves, PR prolongation, and QRS widening on the ECG), and hypocalcemia (tetany, laryngospasm, carpopedal spasm, seizures).

Diagnosis and ED management

For all febrile (>38.6°C, 101.5°F) oncology patients, obtain a CBC with differential, urinalysis, chest X-ray (if there are respiratory symptoms or chest pain), and cultures of the throat, blood, urine, and wound (if any). If there is granulocytopenia (<1,000/mm^3), consult the oncologist and consider admitting the patient for IV antibiotics pending culture results. The ultimate choice of antibiotic is best determined after checking the sensitivities of the local hospital flora. Give combination IV antibiotic therapy with an aminoglycoside such as tobramycin or gentamicin (6 mg/kg per day div q 8–12 h) and either a semisynthetic penicillin (piperacillin/tazobactam 250 mg/kg per day div q 6 h) or ceftazidime (100 mg/kg per day div q 8 h). Cefepime (100 mg/kg per day div q 12 h) can also be used as a single agent. If an interstitial pneumonia is found, add trimethoprim-sulfamethoxazole (20 mg/kg per day of TMP div q 6 h). If the patient has a central venous catheter with erythema surrounding any part of the catheter or port, add vancomycin (40 mg/kg per day div q 6 h).

The treatment of varicella exposure in a patient with a negative history (and negative varicella titers) is zoster-immune globulin (VZIG), 1 vial/10 kg (5 vials maximum) given within 4 days of exposure. There is no benefit of VZIG if the patient is seen 4 or more days after the exposure. Regardless of VZIG treatment, if clinical varicella develops, admit the patient and treat with IV acyclovir (500 mg/m^2 IV q 8 h) or valacyclovir.

If spinal cord compression is suspected, obtain plain films of the spine and consult the oncologist and neurologist immediately. Definitive diagnosis usually requires an MRI scan or, rarely, a myelogram. A patient with signs of intracranial involvement requires an emergency CT or MRI. If a mass lesion is found, immediately consult with a neurologist and an oncologist. Urgent treatment is required with some combination of radiation therapy, dexamethasone, and surgical intervention.

The diagnosis of superior vena cava obstruction is confirmed by finding an anterior mediastinal mass on chest film or chest CT. Obtain a CBC with differential, platelet count, and serum creatinine while awaiting consultation with an oncologist. Secure IV access in a lower extremity to avoid aggravating the condition with intravenous fluids directed toward the superior vena cava. The treatment is chemotherapy, steroids, and possibly radiation.

Treat elevation of uric acid (>5 mg/dL) with hydration (twice maintenance) and allopurinol (250 mg/m^2 per day); add alkalinization of the urine with sodium bicarbonate (1–2 mEq/kg) if there is greater concern about tumor lysis. If the uric acid is >8 mg/dL, treat with rasburicase (0.15 mg/kg per day). Treat hyperkalemia > 6 mEq/L with kayexalate enemas (1 g/kg). If the hyperkalemia is associated with ECG changes (peaked T waves), give insulin (0.1 units/kg IV) and glucose (0.5 g/kg IV). If there is an associated QRS widening or PR lengthening, also give calcium chloride (20 mg/kg IV over 3–5 min). Dialysis is indicated for a serum potassium > 7.5 mEq/L. Treat hypocalcemia (p. 182) <7.5 mEq/L with 75 mg/kg per day of elemental oral calcium, div q 6 h, and amphojel 500 mg PO to lower the phosphorus.

If intestinal perforation is suspected, obtain an upright or right and left lateral decubitus films of the abdomen looking for free air. A CT scan often confirms the diagnosis. Immediately treat with broad-spectrum antibiotics (as for febrile patient, see above), including additional anaerobic coverage (metronidazole 30 mg/kg per day, div q 6 h or piperacillin/tazobactam 250 mg/kg per day div q 6 h). Carefully monitor the blood pressure, since these patients can rapidly develop both hypovolemia and septic shock. Treat hypotension expeditiously with isotonic fluid and packed red cell transfusions, along with vasopressors. Consult a surgeon to arrange for possible emergency laparotomy.

Indications for admission

- Fever (>38.6°C, 101.5°F) and granulocytopenia (<1,000/mm^3), pneumonia, or evidence of any serious infection
- Clinical varicella
- Spinal cord compression, CNS leukemia, superior vena cava obstruction, airway obstruction
- Significant complication of therapy or serious metabolic derangement (uric acid >10 mg/dL; potassium >6 mEq/L; calcium <7.5 mEq/L)
- Suspected intestinal perforation

Bibliography

Balis FM, Holcenberg JS, Poplack: General principles of chemotherapy. In Pizzo PA, Poplack DG (eds), *Principles and Practice of Pediatric Oncology*, 3rd ed. Philadelphia: JB Lippincott-Raven, 1997, pp. 215–72.

Haut C: Oncological emergencies in the pediatric intensive care unit. *AACN Clin Issues* 2005;16:232–45.

Higdon ML, Higdon JA: Treatment of oncologic emergencies. *Am Fam Physician* 2006;74:1873–80.

Sickle cell disease

The sickle cell syndromes are inherited disorders characterized by a chronic hemolytic anemia of variable severity, as well as recurrent obstruction of the microvasculature.

Clinical presentation

Children with sickle cell disease (SCD) may present with a constellation of signs and symptoms, termed crises.

Vasoocclusive crisis

The most frequent complication of sickle cell disease is the vasoocclusive crisis, which is secondary to obstruction of blood flow caused by sickled red blood cells in capillaries and small veins. Multiple organ systems are frequently involved, with severe pain, fever, and symptoms that can mimic many infectious and inflammatory disorders. A common finding is bone pain in multiple sites, particularly the extremities and back. Other presentations may include priapism, pneumonia, limp, hematuria, acute hemiplegia (stroke), acute visual impairment caused by retinal vein occlusion or proliferative retinopathy, and leg ulcers. Right upper quadrant pain and jaundice occur in older children secondary to cholelithiasis from chronic hemolysis. In children under 2 years of age, vasoocclusive crises often take the form of dactylitis, or the "hand-foot" syndrome, with pain and swelling in the hands, feet, fingers, and toes.

Aplastic crisis

Aplastic crises are manifested by worsening anemia and reticulocytopenia. These crises, lasting 7–10 days, usually follow viral infections (particularly parvovirus B19) that transiently suppress the bone marrow. Patients present with fatigue, light-headedness, tachycardia, and palpitations. With parvovirus B19 infection, the patient may have a prodrome of fever, malaise, and myalgias, but the characteristic rash is usually absent.

Sequestration crisis

Splenic sequestration crises, with pooling of red blood cells in a rapidly enlarging spleen, are most often seen in young patients doubly heterozygous for HbS and another abnormal hemoglobin, such as β-thalassemia (S-Thal) or hemoglobin C (S-C disease). The patient may present with cold clammy skin, marked tachycardia, extreme pallor and profound hypotension, as well as a large left-sided abdominal mass (spleen). If unrecognized, deterioration can be rapid with a fatal outcome.

Hyperhemolytic crisis

A hyperhemolytic crisis, with a falling hematocrit, increasing jaundice, and markedly elevated reticulocyte counts (>20%), is rare and may in reality be the resolving phase of an aplastic crisis. Increased hemolysis with a rise in bilirubin can also be seen in patients with concurrent G6PD deficiency.

Megaloblastic crisis

A megaloblastic crisis, due to folate depletion, is rare and may be diagnosed by finding hypersegmented neutrophils and pancytopenia.

Infection

Infections account for many of the serious problems in patients with SCD. Hyposplenism (initially functional, then anatomic) in conjunction with decreased antibody production, decreased serum-opsonizing activity, vasoocclusion, and defective neutrophil function places these children at risk for fulminant overwhelming sepsis, particularly with encapsulated organisms such as *Streptococcus pneumoniae*. They are also at increased risk for meningitis, pneumonia, pyelonephritis, and osteomyelitis (particularly *Salmonella*). While the polyvalent pneumococcal vaccine does not reliably prevent serious pneumococcal infections in children under 2 years of age, Prevnar conjugate vaccine is very effective in young infants and decreases the incidence of life-threatening pneumococcal disease.

Diagnosis

Most children with sickle cell disease are diagnosed in the neonatal period with mandatory newborn hemoglobinopathy screening tests. However, test an undiagnosed child who presents with any of the classic sickle cell symptomatology noted above for SCD. Confirm the screening test with hemoglobin electrophoresis to determine the particular form of the disease (S-S, S-C, S-Thal). Suspect the diagnosis in an asymptomatic patient whose peripheral blood picture reveals anemia, sickle cells, and reticulocytosis (>5%). In addition, the smear will often contain target cells, "helmet" cells, polychromasia, and Howell-Jolly bodies.

A major diagnostic problem in children with SCD is in determining the cause of certain symptomatology, in particular differentiating between infection and infarction. A vasoocclusive crisis is always a diagnosis of exclusion. Leukocytosis (>18,000–25,000/mm^3)

is typical in SCD, and fever may not be helpful in distinguishing the different entities. Particular difficulties are seen with the symptoms described below.

Bone pain

Differentiating between bone infarcts and osteomyelitis can be very difficult, particularly when only one site is involved. Plain films and bone scans are often unreliable, necessitating needle aspiration to obtain a specimen for culture. An elevated ESR and an increased number of bands (>10% of the total WBC) on peripheral smear may indicate an infection, but are by no means foolproof. Aseptic necrosis of the head of the femur or humerus presents with bone pain and, in most cases, abnormal radiographs of the affected limb. An MRI scan is often necessary to detect early osteonecrosis.

Right upper quadrant abdominal pain

Consider hepatitis (especially for patients on chronic transfusion therapy), hepatic infarction, and cholelithiasis in patients with severe right upper quadrant pain, fever, and elevated bilirubin. With hepatic infarcts, abnormal liver chemistries, as a rule, return to baseline in a much shorter amount of time (days) than with hepatitis, while an abdominal sonogram usually detects biliary stones. Right lower lobe pneumonia, rib infarcts, intestinal wall infarcts, and renal disorders (pyelonephritis and papillary necrosis) can all cause pain in the same location, other physical and laboratory findings, including urinalysis and radiographs, help to differentiate among these conditions.

Chest pain and respiratory distress (acute chest syndrome)

Patients with acute chest syndrome can deteriorate rapidly and occasionally require assisted ventilation. The major differential is between vasoocclusion (pulmonary infarct) and infection (pneumonia). Fever, leukocytosis, and similar radiographic and auscultatory findings occur with both diseases. In addition, the two conditions can coexist and one can lead to the other, so it is prudent to treat for both entities. A ventilation-perfusion scan may differentiate between the two, although generally therapy will not be any different regardless of the results and this test is not usually necessary. Finally, chest pain can be secondary to rib infarcts and abdominal disorders.

ED management

Vasoocclusive crisis

Hydroxyurea is currently used for selected patients to increase the fetal hemoglobin level and thus prevent sickling. However, since there is no safe, effective antisickling agent to abort acute crises, therapy consists of treatment of the triggering event and potentiating factors, and supportive care including the following.

Vigorous hydration

The patient often presents with decreased plasma volume secondary to fever, vomiting, and chronic hyposthenuria. In addition to ad lib oral intake, administer several hours of intravenous hydration at a twice-maintenance rate, except for a patient with a pulmonary infarct (use no more than maintenance fluids since these patients can rapidly develop pleural effusions and worsening respiratory status). The type of fluid is controversial, but $D_5\frac{1}{2}NS$ or $D_5\frac{1}{4}NS$ is satisfactory.

Sodium bicarbonate

Add sodium bicarbonate (1 mEq/kg) to the solution only if marked acidosis is present (pH <7.20).

Analgesics

For mild vasoocclusive crises, give aspirin (15 mg/kg), ibuprofen (10 mg/kg), or acetaminophen (15 mg/kg) with codeine (0.5 mg/kg). For a teenager, 5 mg oxycodone plus 325 mg acetaminophen (Percocet) q 3–4 h is an alternative. Ketorolac (0.5 mg/kg q 6 h), a potent non-narcotic analgesic that is less likely to cause respiratory depression, is another excellent alternative. Occasionally, a single injection of morphine (0.1 mg/kg) in conjunction with a few hours of vigorous hydration can prevent hospital admission.

Antipyretics

Fever leads to further dehydration and sickling, so treat with aspirin (15 mg/kg q 4 h), ibuprofen (10 mg/kg q 6 h), or acetaminophen (15 mg/kg q 4 h).

Bed rest

Muscular activity can produce lactate and worsen the acidosis.

Radiograph

If the patient is limping, a radiograph of the hip must be obtained to rule out aseptic necrosis of the femoral head. If positive, immediately institute bed rest and consult with an orthopedist.

Oxygen

Oxygen therapy has not been shown to be of benefit for the management of most painful crises, and in fact may be detrimental since there can be a "rebound" crisis with an outpouring of sickle cells from the bone marrow after oxygen administration is discontinued. Indications for supplementary oxygen include severe anemia, pneumonia, or pulmonary infarction, (particularly if there is documented hypoxia), and shock from infection or splenic sequestration.

Aplastic crisis

If the patient has not yet begun to recover, as manifested by a brisk reticulocytosis, follow the hemoglobin closely; these patients often have little reserve. A transfusion is usually necessary if the hematocrit is <15% with a reticulocyte count <1%.

Sequestration crisis

Rapid intravenous boluses of dextrose or saline can sometimes cause pulmonary edema, and are not the preferred treatment. Therefore, if the patient is hypotensive, immediately infuse plasmanate (10–20 mL/kg), followed by a transfusion of packed red cells (5–10 mL/kg) if the hematocrit is <15%. This is one instance where rapid red cell transfusion can be life-saving.

Megaloblastic crisis

If the hematocrit is >20%, the absolute granulocyte count >1,000/mm^3, and the platelet count >50,000/mm^3, administer folic acid 1 mg/day. Repeat the blood count in 4–7 days. For more pronounced cytopenia, the dose can be increased up to 5 mg/day.

Fever

For a patient >2 years of age in no distress, with a temperature <38.9°C (102°F), and no obvious source for the fever, obtain a blood culture, CBC, ESR, and a urinalysis. Obtain a urine culture if the patient has symptoms of dysuria, frequency or urgency, or if the urinalysis is suspicious for a UTI. If there is no marked left shift and the absolute band count is <3,000/mm^3, send a non-ill-appearing patient home to take oral antibiotics (<15 years: cefaclor 40 mg/kg per day div tid; >15 years penicillin VK 250 mg qid). Give one dose of ceftriaxone (50 mg/kg IM) and observe for several hours before discharge from the ED. Arrange for follow-up in 24 hours, or sooner if the temperature goes higher.

Admit the patient with a temperature >38.9°C (102°F). Also admit a toxic-appearing patient and a child younger than 2 years with a temperature >38.3°C (101°F). Treat with IV ceftriaxone (100 mg/kg per day div q 12 h). For a patient taking hydroxyurea (which can cause neutropenia), broad-spectrum antibiotic coverage is indicated (p. 394) if the absolute neutrophil count is <500/mm^3.

In addition to the basic fever work-up, if there are any respiratory symptoms or chest pain, obtain a chest X-ray, regardless of the auscultatory findings. Admit and treat any sickle cell patient with a pulmonary density as having a possible pneumonia. Administer ceftriaxone (100 mg/kg per day div q 12 h), oxygen if hypoxic, and a red cell transfusion, and if the patient is >5 years of age, add azithromycin (10 mg/kg, once on day 1, followed by 5 mg/kg q day on days 2–5) for possible mycoplasma infection. If there is any suspicion of an osteomyelitis (fever, swelling, point tenderness of a single bone), consult an orthopedist and arrange for a needle aspiration for Gram's stain, cell count, and culture. Indications for a lumbar puncture include a febrile irritable infant <2 years of age and a lethargic older patient with a temperature >39.2°C (103°F) and no fever source.

Acute chest syndrome

Monitor the oxygen saturation and give supplemental oxygen and a packed red blood cell transfusion to a hypoxic patient. For milder episodes, pain medication and incentive spirometry are useful to prevent deterioration.

Follow-up

- Vasoocclusive crisis: next day
- Megaloblastic crisis: 4–7 days
- Patient > 2 years old with temperature < 38.9°C (102°F): 24 hours, or sooner if the temperature goes higher

Indications for admission

- Serious symptoms, including acute hemiplegia, gross hematuria, acute visual disturbance, severe right upper quadrant pain, or acute chest syndrome
- Splenic sequestration or aplastic crisis with hematocrit <15%

- Patient younger than 2 years with temperature >38.3°C (101°F), older child with sudden temperature >38.9°C (102°F) with or without an identifiable source
- Severe or prolonged vasoocclusive crisis with pain unresponsive to usual therapeutic measures
- Irritable infant with hand-foot syndrome
- Clinical pneumonia or any newly discovered pulmonary density on chest film
- Severe megaloblastic crisis (hematocrit <20%, platelet count <50,000/mm³, or granulocyte count <1,000/mm³)

Bibliography

Caboot JB, Allen JL: Pulmonary complications of sickle cell disease in children. *Curr Opin Pediatr* 2008;20:279–87.

Frei-Jones MJ, Baxter AL, Rogers ZR, Buchanan GR: Vaso-occlusive episodes in older children with sickle cell disease: emergency department management and pain assessment. *J Pediatr* 2008;152:281–5.

Redding-Lallinger R, Knoll C: Sickle cell disease-pathophysiology and treatment. *Curr Probl Pediatr Adolesc Health Care* 2006;36:346–76.

Splenomegaly

A palpable spleen tip that is slightly below the costal margin is a frequent finding on routine physical examination in normal infants up to 1 year of age, as well as in patients with fevers or colds. However, a spleen that extends 2 cm below the costal margin or persists for more than 2 months warrants further investigation. Most often, a viral infection (Epstein-Barr virus, adenovirus, cytomegalovirus) is implicated, but a more serious, nonmalignant or malignant condition may be the etiology (Table 13-7).

Clinical presentation

Associated clinical findings depend on the primary disease. Regardless of etiology, massive splenomegaly can cause anemia (pallor, tachycardia, weakness), leukopenia, and thrombo-cytopenia (petechiae, purpura, frank bleeding).

Diagnosis

Inquire about risk factors for HIV infection in the patient or parents, recent travel to endemic areas of disease (malaria, Leishmania, histoplasmosis), and a family history of inherited disorders (thalassemia, sickle hemoglobinopathies, Gaucher's disease, Hurler's syndrome), or splenectomy (thalassemia, hereditary spherocytosis). Ask about fevers (infection, inflammation, malignancy), easy bruising or bleeding (leukemia, lymphoma, marrow replacement), hematemesis (cirrhosis), and transfusions (hemoglobinopathy).

On physical examination, look for evidence of infection (adenopathy, exanthem, pharyngitis), storage disorders (asymptomatic organ enlargement), malignancy (weight loss, bruising, bleeding, adenopathy, hepatomegaly, fever), or connective tissue disorders (arthritis).

Although generalized adenopathy and hepatomegaly might be significant findings, they are associated with splenomegaly of many etiologies, and therefore are usually not helpful in making the diagnosis. One of the most common constellations is fatigue, fever, pharyngitis, generalized adenopathy, and hepatosplenomegaly consistent with infectious mononucleosis, a mono-like syndrome (cytomegalovirus), and, rarely, a more serious illness (leukemia).

Table 13-7. Differential diagnosis of splenomegaly

Diagnosis	Differentiating features
Infections	
Adenovirus	URI symptoms, bronchitis, bronchiolitis, conjunctivitis
Cytomegalovirus	Jaundice, fevers, pharyngitis
EBV	Generalized lymphadenopathy, fever, pharyngitis, hepatomegaly
Histoplasmosis	Travel to endemic area
HIV	Opportunistic infections, bruising, lymphopenia
Malaria	Travel to endemic area, fever; parasites seen on thick smear
RMSF	Tick bite, fever, rash on distal extremities, headache
SBE	Fever, murmur, Roth spots, splinter hemorrhages
Syphilis	Firm adenopathy, sexual history, lesion on penis or labia; congenital infection
Tuberculosis	Fevers, cough, weight loss, pulmonary lesions; positive skin test
Neoplasms	
Leukemia	Anemia, thrombocytopenia; blasts on smear
Lymphomas	Rubbery nodes, fever, night sweats
Storage and inflammatory diseases	
Gaucher's disease	Bone lesions, hepatosplenomegaly; usually asymptomatic (Type I)
Hurler's syndrome	Coarse facial features, hydrocephalus, umbilical hernia, sleep apnea, growth retardation
Langerhans histiocytosis	Bone lesions, fever, chronic otitis, hepatomegaly, eczema
Sarcoid	Fatigue, weight loss, adenopathy, cough, hoarseness, mediastinal adenopathy
Other	
Benign cyst	Radiographic appearance of cystic density in spleen
Extramedullary hematopoiesis	Usually some anemia with abnormal morphology
Hemolytic disorder	Fragmented or abnormally shaped red blood cells
IRA	Joint pains, fevers, elevated ESR, fleeting rash, anemia
Outflow obstruction	Heart murmur or established cardiac disease
Serum sickness	Fevers, joint pain
SLE	Adolescent girl with facial rash, joint pains

ED management

In general, laboratory examination is not immediately necessary for an infant or child who appears well and has a palpable spleen tip. Follow the patient and repeat the abdominal examination. Undertake further evaluation if the spleen remains palpable for more than 2 months, enlarges to >2 cm below the costal margin, or becomes associated with other signs or symptoms.

If the patient presents with fatigue, upper respiratory congestion, and pharyngitis, obtain a CBC and EBV titers, to confirm the diagnosis of infectious mononucleosis. Obtain thin and thick smears if a febrile patient has been in a region that is endemic for malaria.

A more thorough laboratory evaluation is indicated for the child who has a history of weight loss or persistent splenomegaly, or exhibits any serious signs and symptoms, such as pallor, ecchymoses, arthritis, or a toxic appearance. Admit the patient and obtain a CBC with differential, platelet and reticulocyte counts, an ESR, CRP, blood chemistries, and a chest X-ray, and place a 5 TU PPD. If the clinical picture is suggestive of an infection, obtain a blood culture and specific antibody titers. Obtain a sonogram or CT scan to determine the consistency and size of the spleen, although sometimes scans can exaggerate the size.

Isolated splenomegaly usually does not cause significant problems, except for cytopenias and rupture following trauma. The patient may attend school (if otherwise well) but caution about participating in contact sports and other activities that increase the risk for abdominal injury. Otherwise, management depends on the underlying etiology.

Follow-up

- Well child with palpable spleen tip: primary care follow-up in 2–4 weeks

Indications for admission

- Suspected malignancy
- Splenomegaly and neutropenia (<1,000/mm^3) with associated fever, thrombocytopenia (<40,000/mm^3), or hematemesis
- Massive, unexplained splenomegaly for evaluation
- Splenomegaly with anemia and abdominal pain, particularly with a history of abdominal trauma

Bibliography

Miller D, Ladisch S: Disorders of the spleen and monocyte-macrophage system. In Miller DR, Baehner RL (eds), Blood Diseases of Infancy and Childhood. Philadelphia: CV Mosby, 1995, pp. 805–16.

Pearson HA. The spleen and disturbances of splenic function. In Nathan DG, Oski FA (eds), Hematology of Infancy and Childhood, 5th ed. Philadelphia: WB Saunders, 1998, pp. 1051–68.

Infectious disease emergencies

Glenn Fennelly and Michael Rosenberg

Contributing authors
Ellen F. Crain: Evaluation of the febrile child
Christina M. Coyle: Parasitic infections

Botulism

Botulism is a paralyzing disease caused by a neurotoxin elaborated by *Clostridium botulinum*, a Gram-positive, spore-forming, obligate anaerobe whose natural habitat is the soil. Botulinum toxin is tasteless, odorless, and extremely toxic. It acts by irreversibly blocking the release of acetylcholine in peripheral somatic and autonomic synapses as well as at the motor end plates. Raw, home canned, or inadequately prepared foods may be contaminated with the toxin, which is heat labile. Heating food to the boiling point destroys the toxin, but the bacterial spores are resistant to heat and may survive the home canning process. Canned fish, vegetables, and potatoes have been implicated in outbreaks of botulism.

In children, botulism usually occurs after the ingestion of preformed toxin in spoiled food. Since infants lack the *Clostridium*-inhibiting bile acids and protective bacterial flora found in the normal adult intestinal tract, ingested botulism spores can germinate in the intestinal tract. There are approximately 100 cases of infant botulism annually in the United States, with a peak incidence between 2 and 4 months of age; honey consumption is a significant risk factor. Botulism has been implicated in some cases of sudden infant death syndrome.

In wound botulism, *C. botulinum* grows in the injured tissue and produces toxin. Most cases in the United States occur either in intravenous drug users or in children with compound extremity fractures.

Clinical presentation

Symptoms of food-borne botulism begin within 12–36 hours of ingestion of contaminated food. The patient develops blurred vision, diplopia, ptosis, ophthalmoplegia, dysarthria, and dysphagia. Autonomic signs include constipation, dry mouth, postural hypotension, urinary retention, and pupillary dilatation with a sluggish or absent light reflex. Nausea and vomiting may occur in one-third of patients. A descending weakness follows, which, in severe cases, may involve the respiratory muscles. Weakness is usually bilateral, but may be asymmetric. The sensory nerves and mentation are notably spared.

Infantile botulism begins gradually, 2–4 weeks after ingestion of the spores. Breast-fed infants are infected later than formula-fed infants, and breast feeding may moderate the severity of the illness. Constipation is often the first symptom, followed by a weak cry, weak suck, drooling, difficulty feeding, dysphagia, loss of head control, signs of descending cranial nerve palsies, and hypotonia. Progressive paralysis can lead to respiratory failure.

After a 4–14 day incubation period, the presentation of wound botulism is similar to food-borne botulism. There may be fever, but not nausea and vomiting. The wound may exhibit no signs of infection.

Diagnosis

Other causes of paralysis include Guillain-Barré syndrome (ascending paralysis with an elevated CSF protein), poliomyelitis (asymmetric involvement, fever, CSF pleocytosis), myasthenia gravis (muscle fatigability, reversal of ptosis with Tensilon), spinal muscular atrophy (severe weakness, absent DTRs, tongue fasciculations), and tick paralysis (rapidly progressive generalized paralysis, absent DTRs, normal CSF protein, possible dysethesias). In a febrile infant who is lethargic and feeding poorly, consider bacterial sepsis or meningitis. Metabolic causes of acute weakness include hypokalemia, hypo- and hyper-calcemia, and hypo- and hyperthyroidism. The diagnosis can be confirmed by analyzing suspected food, serum, gastrointestinal contents, or wound exudates for evidence of toxin or organisms.

ED management

Admit the patient to an ICU for monitoring, as respiratory arrest can occur at any time. Antitoxin is available from the CDC for older children but is not recommended for infants because it is of equine origin and is associated with hypersensitivity reactions. Antibiotics are not necessary to eradicate the bowel colonization of infants. If sepsis cannot be excluded, obtain a CBC, blood culture, and lumbar puncture, and start age-appropriate antibiotics (see pp. 371–373). However, aminoglycosides are contraindicated because they may potentiate the effects of the toxin. In infants and children, recovery takes about 4 weeks and is generally complete.

Indication for admission

• Suspected botulism

Bibliography

American Academy of Pediatrics. Botulism and infant botulism. In Pickering LK, Baker CJ, Kimberlin DW, Long SS (eds), *Red Book: 2009 Report of the Committee on Infectious Diseases*, 28th ed. Elk Grove Village, IL: American Academy of Pediatrics, 2009: pp. 259–62.

Brook I: Botulism: the challenge of diagnosis and treatment. *Rev Neurol Dis* 2006; 3:182–9.

Underwood K, Rubin S, Deakers T, Newth C: Infant botulism: a 30-year experience spanning the introduction of botulism immune globulin intravenous in the intensive care unit at Childrens Hospital Los Angeles. *Pediatrics* 2007;120:e1380–5.

Cat scratch disease

Cat scratch disease (CSD) is caused by *Bartonella henselae*, a Gram-negative bacillus whose reservoir is the cat flea. The disease is associated with scratches or bites by cats. Although there is no evidence that fleas transmit the disease directly to humans, the precise mechanism of cat to human transmission is unclear. Approximately 22,000 cases are reported each year, with most occurring in the southern states, Hawaii, and California. The disease occurs more often in the fall and winter months, and clusters occur in families with new pets. Sixty percent of cases occur in children.

Clinical presentation

Typical CSD is benign and self-limited and is characterized by regional lymphadenopathy occasionally associated with fever. However, infections can be accompanied by focal or diffuse inflammatory responses (atypical CSD) involving the liver and spleen, as well as the nervous, lymphatic, or skeletal systems. During a 7–12 day incubation period, one or more erythematous papules may erupt at the site of inoculation and persist for from 1 to 7 weeks (median 12 days), after which proximal lymphadenopathy develops. In 50% of cases only a single node is affected. In other cases, several nodes draining the site of inoculation become involved, including the axillary, cervical, submandibular, preauricular, epitrochlear, femoral, or inguinal lymph nodes. The infected node is usually tender and swollen, and the overlying skin may become erythematous, warm, and indurated. Lymph nodes remain enlarged for 2–4 months and may be associated with fever (38–39°C; 100.4–102.2°F), malaise, anorexia, fatigue, and headache in 30% of patients. An evanescent, polymorphic, maculopapular rash may occur early in the course of the disease. If the primary inoculation site is near the eye, Parinaud oculoglandular syndrome may ensue, with mild to moderate conjunctivitis and preauricular lymph node involvement.

Encephalitis is a rare complication of CSD, occurring in 1–7% of cases and typically develops 2–6 weeks after classic onset of lymphadenopathy. CSD can cause encephalitis, with high fever and convulsions. Other uncommon complications include osteolytic bone lesions, granulomatous hepatitis, mesenteric lymphadenitis, pneumonia, arthralgia, subacute iritis, chorioretinitis, optic neuritis, urethritis, lymphedema, thyroiditis, and endocarditis.

Diagnosis

Suspect CSD if a patient with persistent regional lymphadenitis (>3 weeks) has a history of contact with a cat and an identifiable inoculation site. More than 90% of patients with CSD will have a history of recent contact with a cat or kitten. Indirect immunofluorescence and enzyme immunoassay serologic tests for *B. henselae* are available. The differential diagnosis of cat scratch disease includes most causes of lymphadenopathy (see pp. 347–350).

ED management

Localized CSD is usually self-limited over 2–4 months, so only symptomatic therapy is necessary.

Reserve antibiotic therapy (trimethoprim-sulfamethoxazole, 40 mg/kg per day div bid; azithromycin, 12 mg/kg q day; ciprofloxacin 500 mg bid; erythromycin 40 mg/kg per day div tid or qid) for a patient with severe systemic symptoms, hepatomegaly, large painful adenopathy, or immunocompromise. The systemic symptoms usually resolve in 2 weeks, and the prognosis for neurologic complications is good. Consult with a pediatric infectious disease specialist to determine appropriate therapy based on organ involvement as well as disease severity. Surgical excision of affected nodes is unnecessary, although needle aspiration of painful, suppurative nodes may relieve symptoms.

Indication for admission

- Cat scratch disease with encephalitis, seizures, severe liver disease

Bibliography

American Academy of Pediatrics. Cat-scratch disease. In Pickering LK, Baker CJ, Kimberlin DW, Long SS (eds), *Red Book: 2009 Report of the Committee on Infectious Diseases*, 28th ed. Elk Grove Village, IL: American Academy of Pediatrics, 2009, pp. 249–50.

English R: Cat-scratch disease. *Pediatr Rev* 2006;27:123–8.

Florin TA, Zaoutis TE, Zaoutis LB: Beyond cat scratch disease: widening spectrum of Bartonella henselae infection. *Pediatrics* 2008;121:e1413–25.

Dengue viruses

Dengue viruses are transmitted to humans by certain species of *Aedes* mosquitoes. Most dengue cases in the United States are contracted during travel to tropical and subtropical areas outside the continental USA, although transmission has been documented in Texas and Hawaii. The incidence of travel-associated dengue has increased dramatically during the past decade due to epidemics in tropical regions, including in the Western hemisphere. However, most persons with dengue infections in endemic areas are asymptomatic or have a mild self-limiting, acute, febrile illness.

Clinical presentation

After an incubation period of 4–7 days (range 3–14 days), manifestations can range from mild, undifferentiated fever to severe disease that includes hemorrhage and shock. The manifestations of classic dengue include the sudden onset of fever, headache, retro-orbital pain, abdominal pain, and fatigue along with severe muscle, joint and bone pain (so-called "breakbone fever"). Other manifestations include macular or maculopapular rash (50% of patients), flushed facies, lymphadenopathy, conjunctivitis, and mild respiratory and gastrointestinal symptoms. Common associated laboratory abnormalities include thrombocytopenia, leukopenia with lymphopenia, hyponatremia, and mild-to-moderate AST/ALT and LDH elevations.

Severe manifestations that occur with dengue reinfection include dengue hemorrhagic fever (DHF) and dengue shock syndrome (DSS). DHF begins 4–7 days after the onset of typical disease and may be heralded by abdominal pain, vomiting, altered mental status, hypothermia, and profound thrombocytopenia. It is characterized by fever, bleeding manifestations, thrombocytopenia (platelets $\leq 100,000/mm^3$), and evidence of increased vascular permeability with hemoconcentration (hematocrit $\geq 20\%$ above baseline), pleural or abdominal effusions, or hypoproteinemia.

Twenty to thirty percent of DHF cases progress to DSS, which is manifested by signs of circulatory failure, including narrow pulse pressure (≤ 20 mmHg) and hypotension. There is a fatality rate of approximately 10% if not treated. Other rare complications include myocarditis, hepatitis, and neurologic abnormalities (encephalopathy and neuropathies)

Diagnosis

Consider dengue in any patient with fever and a history of travel to tropical areas within 2 weeks before symptom onset.

The WHO DHF case definition includes the four following criteria:

- fever
- hemorrhagic tendencies: positive tourniquet test (>20 petechiae in a 1 square inch); petechiae, ecchymoses, purpura, or bleeding from the GI tract, mucosal surfaces, or injection sites

- platelets $<100,000/mm^3$
- evidence of increased vascular permeability: absolute increase in hematocrit $>20\%$ above baseline value, pleural effusion, ascites, or hypoproteinemia.

The WHO DSS case definition is: all four DHF criteria plus rapid, weak pulse (pulse pressure < 20 mmHg), and profound hypotension.

Obtain both acute-phase (0–5 days after symptom onset) and convalescent-phase (preferably 1–2 weeks after the first sample) serum samples for detecting anti-dengue antibody or send acute-phase serum for culture. Forward the serum samples through state or territorial health departments to the CDC's Dengue Branch, Division of Vector-Borne Infectious Diseases, National Center for Infectious Diseases, 1324 Calle Cañada, San Juan, Puerto Rico 00920–3860; telephone, 787–706–2399. Additional information regarding dengue case reporting and instructions for specimen shipping are available at http://www.cdc.gov/ncidod/dvbid/dengue/dengue-hcp.htm.

ED management

No specific therapy exists for mild dengue. Treat with bed rest, oral fluids, and acetaminophen (15 mg/kg q 4 h), as aspirin and other nonsteroidal anti-inflammatory drugs are contraindicated because of their anticoagulant properties. Avoid IM injections which may cause hematomas.

If DHF or DSS is suspected, give a bows of IV Ringers lactate or normal saline at 10–20 mL/kg. Avoid fluid overload, which can cause pulmonary edema. Treat anemia and DIC with packed RBCs and fresh frozen plasma (10 mL/kg).

Follow-up

- Patients who are not dehydrated, have stable vital signs and are tolerating fluids: daily in order to promptly recognize impending DHF

Indication for admission

- Possible DHF or DSS

Bibliography

American Academy of Pediatrics. Arboviruses. In Pickering LK, Baker CJ, Kimberlin DW, Long SS (eds), *Red Book: 2009 Report of the Committee on Infectious Diseases*, 28th ed. Elk Grove Village, IL: American Academy of Pediatrics, 2009, pp. 214–20.

Centers For Disease Control And Prevention (CDC). Travel-associated dengue–United States, 2005. *MMWR Morb Mortal Wkly Rep* 2006;55:700–2.

Wilder-Smith A, Schwartz E: Dengue in travelers. *N Engl J Med* 2005; 353:924–32.

Encephalitis

Encephalitis is characterized by inflammation of the brain. Approximately 20,000 cases occur in the United States each year, most of which are mild. Causes of sporadic encephalitis in the United States are the herpes simplex viruses (HSV 1 and 2) and the rabies virus. Other viral etiologies include arthropod-borne viruses (St. Louis encephalitis, California encephalitis, eastern, western, Venezuelan equine encephalitis and West Nile virus [WNV]), other herpesviruses (Epstein-Barr, cytomegalovirus, varicella zoster), and enteroviruses (enterovirus, echovirus, Coxsackie viruses) that occur in summer/fall epidemics.

Bacterial causes include *Haemophilus influenzae, Neisseria meningitides, Streptococcus pneumoniae*, and *Mycobacterium tuberculosis*, although these organisms more often cause meningitis (see pp. 401–405). Spirochetal infections include *Treponema pallidum, Leptospira* species, and *Borrelia burgdorferi* (Lyme disease). Other nonviral causes of encephalitis include *C. pneumoniae, Mycoplasma pneumoniae, M. hominis*, and *Coccidiodes immitus*. Additionally, *Toxoplasma gondii, Cryptococcus neoformans* and *Listeria monocytogenes* can cause encephalitis in an immunocompromised patient.

Postinfectious encephalitis is thought to be an autoimmune phenomenon initiated by viral (influenza, varicella, measles) or bacterial (mycoplasma) pathogens in children with symptoms of CNS inflammation in the absence of an acute bacterial or fungal infection. Characteristically, there is a latent phase between the acute illness and the onset of neurologic symptoms.

Clinical presentation

Encephalitis most commonly begins as an acute systemic illness with fever and headache. Most patients have diffuse disease with behavioral or personality changes, altered level of consciousness, or generalized seizures. Some patients may have localized findings, such as ataxia, cranial nerve defects, hemiparesis, or focal seizures. Alternatively, there may be high fever, convulsions with bizarre movements, and hallucinations alternating with periods of clarity. Nuchal rigidity, if present, is less pronounced than with meningitis.

Herpesvirus

Herpes can affect newborns, as well as older children and adults. CNS involvement occurs in approximately 50% of newborns with HSV infection. Morbidity and mortality depend on whether the infant has isolated CNS involvement or disseminated disease. The mortality rate with antiviral therapy is 60%, and approximately 40% of survivors have neurologic impairment. Encephalitis in an older child or adolescent is usually secondary to HSV-1. Fever, focal or generalized seizures, focal neurologic signs, and altered level of consciousness can occur. Therapy improves survival; however, more than 50% of patients progress to significant neurologic impairment or death. Epstein-Barr virus encephalitis causes a focal encephalopathic disease in conjunction with fever, pharyngitis, lymphadenopathy, atypical lymphocytosis, and a positive heterophile test. Recovery is usually complete. Varicella encephalitis follows the distinctive exanthem and may lead to nystagmus, dysarthria, and cerebellar ataxia.

Arthropod-borne

The responsible agents are transmitted by mosquitoes and ticks, and outbreaks occur primarily during the summer and fall seasons. Cases of human WNV illness were first documented in the United States in the New York City area in 1999 and now are reported throughout the continental United States. Mosquitoes that prey on birds and humans are the principal vectors. After an incubation period of 3–6 days, there is the abrupt onset of a febrile, flu-like illness with headache, sore throat, myalgias, and fatigue. In addition, there may be conjunctivitis, retrobulbar pain, and a maculopapular rash that spreads from the trunk to the extremities and head. In contrast to adults, CNS involvement is rare in children. However, cases have been reported in infants as young as 1 month of age. Other severe complications of WNV include hepatitis, pancreatitis, myocarditis, and hepatosplenomegaly. Recovery is usually complete in children.

Enteroviral

Enteroviral infection usually occurs in the summer. Following a prodrome of fever and upper respiratory tract symptoms, the patient develops acute neurologic findings such as confusion, altered level of consciousness, or irritability. Neurologic manifestations are usually global rather than focal, although flaccid paralysis may occur. Other possible manifestations include photophobia and a macular or petechial rash.

Rabies

Rabies has an average incubation period of 4–6 weeks (range from 5 days to 6 years). Rabies infection is transmitted by the bite of an infected animal and is fatal. Clinically, there is anxiety, dysphagia, and hydrophobia (see Rabies, p. 726).

Postinfectious

A patient with measles parainfectious encephalitis presents during recovery from the acute illness with the abrupt onset of fever, neurologic symptoms, and altered mental status. Neurologic sequelae occur in most survivors and may include intellectual, motor, psychiatric, epileptic, visual, or auditory defects. Approximately 50% of patients have seizures.

Diagnosis

Obtain a detailed history, including whether there has been any antecedent viral infection, systemic symptoms, ill contacts, or exposure to mosquitoes, ticks, or animals. Inquire about the immunologic status of the patient, recent travel or immunizations, and the possibility of accidental exposure to heavy metals or pesticides. Perform a thorough physical examination looking for rashes, enanthems, lymphadenopathy, focal neurologic abnormalities, cerebellar signs, and evidence of increased intracranial pressure (including fundoscopy).

The differential diagnosis for a patient with fever, fatigue, stiff neck, headache, nausea and vomiting, and myalgias includes hepatitis viruses B and C, as well as zoonotic infections such as leptospirosis, brucellosis, tularemia, hantavirus, dengue, Colorado tick fever, plague, rickettsial infections, ehrlichiosis, psittacosis, *Bartonella henselae*, and Q fever. With a history of rural freshwater exposure, consider infection with hepatitis A, salmonellosis, toxoplasmosis, and naegleria meningitis.

Consider metabolic diseases such as hypoglycemia, uremia, or hepatic encephalopathy, and inborn errors of metabolism (disorders of glucose or ammonia metabolism), toxic disorders (drug ingestion, Reye's syndrome), and mass lesions (tumor or abscess). Also consider vascular (subarachnoid hemorrhage from an arteriovenous malformation or aneurysm and embolic lesions from bacterial endocarditis) or purulent parameningeal (sinusitis, with associated cavernous venous thrombosis or subdural or epidural empyema) etiologies. Acute demyelinating disorders, including multiple sclerosis, acute hemorrhagic leukoencephalitis, and status epilepticus, are also possible diagnoses. Postinfectious conditions including Guillain-Barré syndrome and Miller-Fisher syndrome, brainstem encephalitis, and acute cerebellar ataxia are also in the differential diagnosis of encephalitis.

ED management

Perform an immediate lumbar puncture to exclude bacterial meningitis unless there are focal neurologic signs or evidence of increased intracranial pressure. In such a case, give first doses of IV ceftriaxone (50 mg/kg) plus vancomycin (15 mg/kg), depending upon local pneumococcal susceptibility patterns, and immediately arrange for a CT scan of the head prior to performing the lumbar puncture. HSV is associated with hemorrhagic inflammation of the temporal lobe and sylvian fissure; MRI findings in children with acute disseminated encephalomyelitis include multifocal white matter lesions characterized by perivenous demyelination.

Send the CSF for Gram's stain, cell count, protein, glucose, culture, rapid antigen identification test, viral culture, and, if tuberculosis is a possibility, acid fast stain, culture and/or PCR for *Mycobacterium*. The CSF in viral encephalitis is usually clear, and the leukocyte count can range from none to several thousand with a polymorphonuclear predominance early in the course. The protein is normal to moderately elevated, and the glucose is initially normal.

Obtain a CBC, platelet count, electrolytes, BUN, creatinine, glucose, blood culture, and a urinalysis. If specific viral etiologies are being considered, send urine, stool, CSF, and throat swabs for viral diagnostic tests and sera for viral titers (repeat the titer in 2–4 weeks). In particular, if HSV or enterovirus is a possibility send CSF for PCR, which is about 98% sensitive and 94% specific. In several states, the Department of Health offers additional CSF testing for a PCR panel (along with serological testing) of most likely pathogens for cases of encephalitis with additional testing (arbovirus or West Nile serology), as the history warrants.

Admit patients with encephalitis for close observation of vital signs and fluid status. Treat for bacterial meningitis with vancomycin and ceftriaxone (as above) and add doxycycline (4 mg/kg div q 12 h; 200 mg/dose maximum) for *Bartonella* and *Mycoplasma*.

Better outcomes after neonatal HSV infection are strongly associated with a shorter interval between diagnosis and initiation of treatment. Have a high index of suspicion for neonatal HSV infection in an acutely ill infant <28 days of age. If herpes is suspected, treat with acyclovir, 60 mg/kg per day div q 8 h for 21 days (for children ≤12 years of age).

Isolate the patient until a specific agent is identified. If rabies is suspected, immediately initiate passive and active immunization for personnel whose mucous membranes or open wounds may have contacted the patient's saliva, CSF, or brain tissue.

During enteroviral epidemics in the summer and fall, a patient >6 years of age who develops presumed meningitis without encephalitis (mild to moderate headache that responds to acetaminophen or ibuprofen, nontoxic appearance, CSF with a monocytic pleocytosis and normal chemistries) may be sent home for bed rest, fluids, and antipyretic therapy. Admit any patient with nuchal rigidity, unresponsive moderate to severe headache, or lethargy.

Follow-up

- Nontoxic patient with probably enteroviral infection: daily

Indication for admission

- Encephalitis or meningoencephalitis

Bibliography

Silvia MT, Licht DJ: Pediatric central nervous system infections and inflammatory white matter disease. *Pediatr Clin North Am* 2005;52:1107–26.

Tunkel AR, Glaser CA, Bloch KC, Sejvar JJ, et al: Infectious Diseases Society of America: The management of encephalitis: clinical practice guidelines by the Infectious Diseases Society of America. *Clin Infect Dis* 2008;47:303–27.

Whitley RJ: Therapy of herpes virus infections in children. *Adv Exp Med Biol* 2008;609:216–32.

Evaluation of the febrile child

During the evaluation and management of the febrile child, decisions are based on clinical impression and physical examination, reinforced by the results of selectively ordered laboratory tests.

Fever is one of the most common causes for a visit to the emergency department. It is defined here as a rectal temperature >38.1°C (100.6°F). It may be the presenting sign for a viral illness, a minor bacterial infection, or a life-threatening bacterial process. While fever most typically indicates the presence of an infection, on rare occasions it may be the presenting sign of poisoning (aspirin, phenothiazines), collagen vascular disease, or malignancy. Although a patient can have sepsis without fever, it is more likely that a seriously ill child has some elevation in temperature.

Clinical presentation

Clinical impression is a component of every strategy for evaluating febrile infants and young children. The best-known tool is the Yale Observation Scale (YOS), an objective scoring system based on the child's alertness, playfulness, interaction with the environment, color, state of hydration, quality of cry, and ability to be consoled. The older the patient, the more reliable the clinical impression becomes as a predictor of serious underlying illness. In addition, an older child is more likely to have specific localizing signs of illness.

A young infant (<8 weeks) may have bacterial sepsis without many clinical findings. The YOS has been shown to be neither sensitive nor specific for identifying which young febrile infant is at risk for serious bacterial infection.

There may be a history of excessive crying, irritability, lethargy, or decreased feeding. Unfortunately, an infant is at highest risk for sepsis in the first few days of life, when there has been little time for behavior patterns to develop. Therefore, the history is often not helpful. However, a history of a cyanotic episode or a seizure in an infant with fever is extremely worrisome and mandates a full evaluation for sepsis.

On physical examination, the young infant may be pale or mottled, tachypneic, tachycardic, with weak cry and grunting respirations. Alternatively, the infant may simply be sleeping and difficult to arouse. Focal infections typically do not present with localized findings. Meningeal signs may be absent despite the presence of meningitis, and there may be no ear tugging with otitis media. The infant with a urinary tract infection (UTI) may only have a fever, perhaps accompanied by vomiting or diarrhea.

Beyond 8 weeks of age, clinical impression becomes more accurate, at least when applied to young, febrile children with serious bacterial infections such as pneumonia or meningitis. The child with sepsis does not smile and is rarely interested in the surroundings. The parent often reports that there is a definite change in the child's behavior. Moreover, localized infections are often associated with focal complaints. The older child (toddler age) with meningitis usually has nuchal rigidity and positive Kernig's or Brudzinski's signs.

The widespread use of the conjugate pneumococcal vaccine has invalidated previously published management guidelines for the evaluation of nontoxic-appearing febrile children aged 3 months to 3 years for "occult" bacteremia. Regardless, the risk for occult bacteremia is extremely low in children with temperatures <38.9°C (102°F) but increases as the temperature rises above 39°C (102.2°F). The patient may have symptoms of an upper respiratory infection or pharyngitis but no other detectable etiology for the fever. Despite efforts to develop reliable methods for diagnosis, these children may be clinically indistinguishable from children with self-limited viral diseases, and they may have no localizing signs whatsoever.

A temperature >41.1°C (106.0°F) is unusual. However, these children have the same risk of a serious bacterial infection (SBI) as patients with temperatures between 38.5 and 41.1°C (101.3 and 106°F).

Diagnosis and ED management

The priority is the identification of the child with an SBI. Clinical impression and physical examination are the mainstays of diagnosis. Certain laboratory tests may help predict the risk of serious infection when the results of the clinical evaluation are equivocal. A WBC >15,000/mm^3, band-to-neutrophil ratio >0.2 (in infants 0–2 months of age), an ESR >30 mm/h or a CRP >5 have been shown to correlate with SBI or a risk of OB. However, because of the low prevalence of bacteremia, the positive predictive value of any single test remains very low.

The management of febrile infants and children is summarized below. These guidelines may need to be modified if unusual pathogens are suspected (immunocompromised host, cerebrospinal fluid shunt, recent course of antibiotics).

Under 8 weeks of age

Since clinical impression is considered unreliable in young infants, perform a full evaluation for sepsis including CBC with differential count, blood and urine cultures, urinalysis, and lumbar puncture for cell count, glucose, protein, Gram's stain, and culture. Obtain urine by catheter insertion or suprapubic aspiration (not clean-catch bag). A chest radiograph is indicated only if there are respiratory signs or symptoms. The following criteria have been used to identify infants at low risk for sepsis:

- well appearance
- no identifiable source of infection on physical exam
- no known immunodeficiency
- urinalysis with ≤10 WBC per high-power field and no bacteria
- CSF with <8 WBC/mm^3 and no bacteria on Gram's stain
- WBC <15,000/mm^3
- ESR <30 mm/h, a band:neutrophil ratio <0.2, or a CRP <1
- if the infant has diarrhea, the stool is heme negative and there are ≤5 WBC per high-power field
- normal chest radiograph. (if indicated)

Under 4 weeks of age

Admit the infant to the hospital and treat with ampicillin (<1 week of age: 100 mg/kg per day, div q 12 h; >1 week of age: 200 mg/kg per day, div q 6 h) and cefotaxime (<1 week:

100 mg/kg per day, div q 12 h; 1–4 weeks: 150 mg/kg per day, div q 8 h). If meningitis is suspected, increase the cefotaxime dose to 200 mg/kg per day div q 6 h.

Four to 8 weeks of age

Infants in this age group who meet the criteria for low risk for SBI may be managed as outpatients, without expectant antibiotic therapy. However, admit an infant who appears clinically ill, has evidence of SBI, or meets high-risk criteria for SBI regardless of appearance and treat with ceftriaxone (100 mg/kg per day div q 12 h). Obtain all cultures, including a lumbar puncture, before starting antibiotics unless the infant is in shock or has evidence of respiratory distress.

Eight weeks to 6 months of age

Clinical impression is more reliable in this age group. After ensuring that the patient is comfortable, carefully observe the infant, preferably being held by the parent. If no fever source can be found, examine and culture the urine. Obtain a chest radiograph if there are any respiratory signs, including tachypnea. Administer appropriate therapy for focal infections such as otitis media, suspected UTI, and pneumonia, and admit an infant <3 months of age with presumed bacterial pneumonia (pp. 629–633) or UTI (pp. 664–667).

The most important aspects of care are careful and frequent follow-up and parental vigilance for clinical deterioration. One of the true arts of pediatrics is the ability to distinguish irritability associated with hunger, colic, otitis media, or nonspecific viral febrile illness from that associated with meningitis or sepsis. Give a dose of acetaminophen (15 mg/kg) or ibuprofen (10 mg/kg) to a patient who seems irritable, but has normal vital signs and is not lethargic, and reevaluate in one-half hour. Admit a patient who appears toxic (lethargic, inconsolable, poor perfusion, grunting), but discharge the patient who is alert, consolable, and feeds well in the ED. Arrange for a follow-up examination the next day.

Six months to 36 months of age

With the widespread use of pneumococcal vaccine, the risk of occult bacteremia is probably <1–2% in a child with a temperature $\geq 39.5^\circ$C (103°F). When evaluating (at a follow-up visit) a patient with documented *S. pneumoniae* bacteremia, obtain a repeat blood culture if the child is still febrile or afebrile for <24 hours. Admit the patient if ill-appearing or febrile, complete the work-up for sepsis, and treat with IV penicillin G (100,000 units/kg per day div q 6 h). Because of emerging patterns of resistant *S. pneumoniae*, check local antibiotic sensitivities and use a third-generation cephalosporin plus vancomycin (10–15 mg/kg q 8 h) if resistance is a concern. If a patient with *S. pneumoniae* bacteremia has been afebrile for >24 hours and is well-appearing, treat as an outpatient with oral penicillin (50 mg/kg per day div qid) for 7 days. Give the parents specific guidelines for temperature control (15 mg/kg of acetaminophen q 4 h) and for assessing the child at home (increased irritability or lethargy, decreased PO intake) and provide for a follow-up visit within 24–48 hours, or sooner, if the patient seems worse to the parents.

Over 36 months of age

Localized findings are generally reliable. Look for meningeal signs, evidence of focal infection, or petechiae.

All infants and children with fever without a source

When there is no identified source of the fever, management includes the following.

- Perform a lumbar puncture if there is any suspicion of sepsis or meningitis. Admit and treat any toxic-appearing child.
- Obtain a urinalysis and urine culture in boys <1 year of age and girls <2 years of age with persistent fever, particularly in the absence of URI signs and symptoms. Infants and young children still in diapers are unable to give a midstream sample; obtain urine by suprapubic aspiration or catheter insertion. Approximately 8% of uncircumcised boys <1 year of age and 16% of white girls ≤2 years of age with fever without a source will have a UTI. The Gram's stain is 99% sensitive for UTI, although only a culture can prove or exclude an infection.
- The chest radiograph is usually negative in a child without signs or symptoms of respiratory illness, although a patient beyond the newborn period can have an "occult pneumonia." Usually the child will have persistent fever, dehydration, chest pain or discomfort, or decreased breath sounds. A chest radiograph is indicated in any child with tachypnea unresponsive to antipyretic therapy or persistent cough. Pneumonia may be diagnosed clinically in the febrile child with rales.
- Send a stool culture if the patient has bloody diarrhea or >5 WBC per high-power field on a stool smear. Obtain a blood culture and begin antibiotic therapy in a febrile infant with a stool culture positive for *Salmonella* (see Diarrhea, pp. 240–245). An older child with *Salmonella* enteritis rarely needs antimicrobial therapy.

Follow-up

- 4–8 weeks: daily, until cultures are negative
- 8 weeks – 6 months: daily, until afebrile
- 6–36 months: 24–48 hours
- >36 months: 2–3 days, if still febrile

Indications for admission

- All infants <4 weeks of age with a temperature > 38.1°C (100.6°F) or the local institutional temperature cutoff
- Most infants <3 months of age with focal bacterial infection other than otitis media
- Toxic appearance regardless of age or degree of fever.
- Patient recalled for a positive blood culture who is ill-appearing, febrile, or afebrile for <24 hours

Bibliography

Herz AM, Greenhow TL, Alcantara J, et al: Changing epidemiology of outpatient bacteremia in 3- to 36-month-old children after the introduction of the heptavalent-conjugated pneumococcal vaccine. *Pediatr Infect Dis J* 2006;25:293–300.

Ishimine P: Fever without source in children 0 to 36 months of age. *Pediatr Clin North Am* 2006;53:167–94.

McCarthy P: Fever without apparent source on clinical examination. *Curr Opin Pediatr* 2005;17:93–110.

HIV-related emergencies

Human immunodeficiency virus (HIV) is transmitted horizontally, via sexual contact, exposure to contaminated blood or blood products (e.g. transfusions, used needles), and vertically from mother to fetus. Combination antiretroviral treatment and improved medical and obstetrical management of HIV-infected pregnant women have reduced vertical transmission rates to an estimated 1–4% nationwide. In addition, potent combination antiretroviral therapy (cART) has been shown to slow disease progression and reduce the risk of opportunistic infections, so that in some children immune reconstitution has occurred. At this time, perinatally infected infants and children constitute the largest group of pediatric AIDS patients and, as the HIV epidemic enters its third decade, greater numbers of adolescents and young adults with severe immunodeficiency and its attendant complications are presenting for care. Victims of rape or sexual abuse and teenagers engaging in unprotected sex may also present to the ED for HIV counseling, testing, and post exposure chemoprophylaxis.

Clinical presentation and diagnosis

Children and adolescents with HIV can experience the same spectrum of acute illnesses as uninfected patients. However, because of HIV-induced immunodeficiency, the presentation, clinical course, and response to therapy may differ.

Acute fever

HIV-infected children with fever may have otitis media, a viral infection, or a serious bacterial or opportunistic infection. They develop bacteremia with the same organisms that affect other children, such as pneumococci, meningococci, and Gram-negative bacilli (*Salmonella, Pseudomonas*). In addition, patients with indwelling catheters or soft tissue infections are prone to bacteremia with *S. aureus* or other coagulase-negative staphylococci. Prolonged courses of antibiotics predispose patients to infections by multiple drug-resistant bacteria (e.g. penicillin-resistant pneumococci, Gram-negative bacilli) and fungi, especially *Candida* species.

The sexually active teenager with signs and symptoms suggestive of a mononucleosis-like illness, including fever, malaise, headache, pharyngitis, rash, and generalized lymphadenopathy, may have acute HIV infection (acute retroviral syndrome, or ARS), which can result in clinical syndromes indistinguishable from classic EBV-induced mononucleosis.

Chronic fever

Fever lasting >2 weeks may be due to undiagnosed or untreated HIV infection or may be secondary to an occult abscess, opportunistic infection, or malignancy. Disseminated *Mycobacterium avium-intracellulare* (MAI) infection may cause chronic fevers. It is often associated with anemia due to bone marrow infiltration. In contrast, tuberculosis is far more common among HIV-positive adults than among HIV-infected children.

Skin and soft tissue infections

HIV-infected children with common cutaneous disorders such as impetigo or cellulitis may have a more extensive and rapid spread of infection. Also, scabies may present with a generalized papulosquamous eruption or with diffuse areas of crusting and scale, indicating severe infestation.

Exanthematous diseases

Viral exanthems are common. In some cases of chickenpox, the lesions either do not resolve or take a much longer period of time to heal than in immunocompetent children. Complications include dehydration secondary to poor fluid intake from severe mucous membrane involvement, and visceral dissemination to the lung, liver, pancreas, or brain. Herpes zoster presents with characteristic lesions in a dermatomal distribution usually involving the trunk. Secondary dissemination involving multiple dermatomes and viscera can occur.

EENT infections

Acute otitis media, chronic suppurative otitis media with perforation, conjunctivitis, sinusitis, and pharyngitis are common. Bacterial sinusitis is second to pneumonia as the most frequent clinically diagnosed infection. Oropharyngeal candidiasis, mucosal ulcerations, and esophagitis can develop in patients with advanced immunosuppression. HIV-infected children are more prone to gingivitis and periodontitis, and, in cases of poor dental hygiene, dental abscesses. Parotid infiltration or adenopathy increases the risk for bacterial superinfection, which then can present with erythema, warmth, tenderness, induration, and fluctuation. Although uncommon, consider suppurative parotitis, caused by *S. aureus* or oral streptococci, in a patient presenting with fever, toxicity, and tender parotid enlargement. On exam, frank pus can often be expressed from Stensen's duct.

Pulmonary

Respiratory problems are a common cause of morbidity and mortality. Reactive airway disease and community-acquired pneumonia are the most prevalent conditions encountered in the ED. *Pneumocystis jiroveci* (formerly *carinii*) pneumonia (PCP) is the most common opportunistic infection, but is becoming increasingly rare due to the widespread provision of PCP prophylaxis and the dramatic decrease in the number of infected infants. It usually occurs in children <18 months of age and is associated with rapid onset of respiratory distress, with tachypnea, fever, and dry cough. In older children, it can present in an insidious fashion with wheezing, mild cough, and progressive dyspnea. The pulmonary examination reveals wheezing, diminished breath sounds, and occasionally rales. Hypoxia ($pO_2 < 70$ mmHg) is common, with an A–a O_2 gradient >30 mmHg. The typical radiologic finding is a diffuse interstitial process; occasionally there is a pattern suggestive of adult respiratory distress syndrome, with complete opacification of the lung fields. Rarely, the chest radiograph may show clear lungs, slight hyperinflation, or cystic changes. Serum lactate dehydrogenase (LDH) levels are often markedly elevated (>500 IU/L); a normal LDH level is strong evidence against PCP.

The etiology and presentation of bacterial pneumonia is the same as for immunocompetent patients, although HIV-infected children are particularly susceptible to encapsulted pathogens, such as the pneumococcus. In addition, *Moraxella*, *Legionella*, and *Nocardia* pneumonia can occur. Patients receiving antibiotics or who have recently been hospitalized are at risk for antibiotic-resistant Gram-positive and Gram-negative bacterial pneumonias.

Cardiac

Wheezing unresponsive to bronchodilators can be due to heart failure secondary to HIV cardiomyopathy. Heart failure usually occurs in older children with advanced HIV disease and presents with tachypnea, rales, decreased activity, or wheezing. Hepatomegaly is often found, although it is not specific. Radiographic examination shows an enlarged cardiac silhouette, but definitive diagnosis may require an echocardiogram. Consider infective endocarditis in a patient who presents with fever, toxicity, and a new cardiac murmur.

Gastrointestinal

Nausea, vomiting, and diarrhea (acute and chronic) are common complaints in HIV-infected children. In addition to the usual viral causes of acute gastroenteritis, these patients are susceptible to unusual gastrointestinal pathogens. *Cryptosporidium*, a protozoan, can cause intractable watery diarrhea associated with abdominal pain and vomiting. The diagnosis is made by staining the stool with a modified acid fast stain. *Isospora belli* may cause a similar syndrome. Diagnosis is made by identification of oocytes in the stool. Disseminated *Mycobacterium avium* complex (MAC) can cause a multisystem disease characterized by wasting, recurrent fevers, night sweats, abdominal pain, and diarrhea. MAC organisms can be isolated from the blood, liver biopsy, lymph node, bone marrow, or the GI tract of infected patients. Cytomegalovirus (CMV) colitis can also present with bloody diarrhea; diagnosis of this disorder usually requires histologic verification.

Salmonella gastroenteritis causes fever, vomiting, and malaise, in addition to watery or bloody diarrhea. It is a common cause of bacteremia and can lead to sepsis, septic arthritis, and meningitis. These complications can develop weeks to months after recovery from the acute enteritis.

Medications are often responsible for causing gastrointestinal symptoms. Liquid protease inhibitors such as ritonavir and lopinavir can cause nausea and vomiting, while nelfinavir can cause loose stools. Owing to mitochondrial toxicity, stavudine and didanosine can trigger a potentially fatal lactic acidosis syndrome and severe steatohepatitis. Didanosine has been associated with pancreatitis, but this complication is uncommon in children.

Hematologic

Hematologic complications are common. Medications, infections, nutritional deficiencies, and HIV itself can cause bone marrow dysfunction and result in a spectrum of mild to severe cytopenias. Undiagnosed HIV infection occasionally presents with asymptomatic thrombocytopenia. Bleeding is rare in these circumstances, but the risk of potentially catastrophic intracranial hemorrhage increases as the platelet count falls below 10,000/mm^3. These cytopenias may resolve with potent antiretroviral therapy, or growth factors such as G-CSF and erythropoietin.

Genitourinary/renal

The incidence and clinical manifestations of urinary tract infections are not influenced by the presence of HIV infection. African-American children with advanced disease are at higher risk of developing HIV nephropathy, a condition characterized by nephrotic-range proteinuria and eventual progression to renal failure. The protease inhibitor indinavir can cause nephrolithiasis which may remain asymptomatic or present with flank pain, hematuria, and crystalluria. Tenofovir, a nucleotide reverse transcriptase inhibitor, can cause proximal renal tubular dysfunction and induce a Fanconi-like syndrome characterized by impaired tubular electrolyte reabsorption, glycosuria, and acidosis.

Neurologic

Bacterial meningitis and most aseptic meningitis syndromes are not more common or virulent in asymptomatic HIV-infected children than in seronegative controls. In addition to HIV-related encephalopathy, children with low T cell counts ($<$50–100 cells/mm^3) are susceptible to opportunistic CNS infections such as cryptococcal meningitis, progressive multifocal leukoencephalopathy (PML), and cerebral toxoplasmosis. CNS lymphoma can also occur, but is rare.

ED management

Fever

Occult bacteremia is of particular concern in HIV patients, although the period of susceptibility is beyond 3 years of age. Take a history and perform a careful examination, focusing on any possible localized infection.

Well-appearing

If the patient appears well but has a fever $>$39°C (102.2°F), obtain a CBC and blood culture, and if the child is still in diapers, obtain urine for analysis and culture. Obtain a urine culture if there are any urinary complaints, CVA tenderness, irritability, or an abnormal urinalysis. If there are any respiratory findings, including isolated tachypnea or cough, or an elevated WBC count with a left shift, obtain a chest radiograph. Baseline CBCs are helpful in evaluating these children since many of them are leukopenic. If such data are not available, use a WBC $>$15,000/mm^3 as abnormal. If no obvious focus of infection is found, treat with ceftriaxone (50 mg/kg per day IM) pending culture results. Alternatively, prescribe a beta-lactamase-stable antibiotic such as amoxicillin-clavulanic acid (875/125 formulation, 45 mg/kg per day div bid), or an oral second-generation cephalosporin such as cefuroxime axetil (30 mg/kg per day div bid). Schedule a follow-up visit for the next day, but advise the family to return if symptoms worsen or if the patient becomes lethargic.

Ill-appearing

Obtain cultures of the blood, urine, and, stool, if indicated. If there is meningismus, altered mental status, or an underlying abnormal mental status which makes evaluation unreliable, perform a lumbar puncture (unless the child is unstable). Start an IV and give ceftriaxone (one 75 mg/kg dose followed by 100 mg/kg per day div q 12 h). Add vancomycin (60 mg/kg per day div q 6 h) for suspected bacterial meningitis.

If the patient has recently been taking antibiotics or has an indwelling catheter, administer broad-spectrum IV antibiotics such as either pipericillin-tazobactam (240 mg/kg per day div q 6 h) or vancomycin (40 mg/kg per day div q 6 h) and ceftazidime (150 mg/kg per day div q 8 h).

Chronic fever

The goal of the ED evaluation is to rule out possible bacterial infection. Obtain a CBC, ESR or CRP, urinalysis, chest and sinus X-rays, and blood, urine, and stool cultures. Also obtain a blood culture for MAI (use culture bottles that are specific for the isolation of mycobacteria, e.g. Bactec 13A system). If there is no obvious source of infection and the laboratory evaluation is negative, admit the patient to begin a diagnostic work-up for fever of unknown origin.

Skin, soft tissue, and HEENT infections

Obtain a CBC, blood culture, and wound culture. Treat a well-appearing child with a well-circumscribed infection as an outpatient. For parotitis, prescribe an antibiotic active against *S. aureus* and oral streptococci, such as amoxicillin-clavulanic acid (875/125 formulation, 45 mg/kg per day div bid), cefadroxil 40 mg/kg per day div bid. Use clindamycin (30 mg/kg per day div tid) or trimethoprim-sulfamethoxazole (10 mg/kg TMP-50 mg/kg SMX div bid) for suspected cases of "community-associated MRSA" (CA-MRSA). Frequent warm-water rinses are a useful adjunctive measure. Treat cellulitis due to a break in the skin with the same antibiotics as above. For a dental abscess, use clindamycin (30 mg/kg per day div tid). Reevaluate the child within 48 hours, and if there is no improvement, admit for parenteral antibiotics. Also admit any child who appears toxic, has a large area involved, or whose infection impinges on important structures (e.g. the airway) for parenteral antibiotic therapy.

Varicella zoster virus (VZV) infection

Carefully evaluate the child's hydration, mental, and respiratory status and order a chest X-ray if the patient is tachypneic. Admit all patients with low CD4+ ($<500/mm^3$) counts and primary VZV infection for IV acyclovir ($1500 \, mg/m^2$ q 8 h). Give oral acyclovir (80 mg/kg per day div qid) for the treatment of mild infections in patients with good immune function. Treat children with localized zoster as outpatients with oral acyclovir (80 mg/kg per day div qid). Newer antiviral agents with greater bioavailability such as famciclovir (1500 mg per day div tid) and valacyclovir (3,000 mg per day div tid) are approved for the treatment of zoster in adults and may be useful in older children and adolescents who can swallow pills. Instruct the caretaker to bring the child back if the rash starts to disseminate. Reevaluate the patient within 48 hours, and if there is no improvement, admit for IV acyclovir. For an unimmunized patient who has not had chickenpox or shingles and reports an exposure to varicella, administer VariZIG (1 vial/10 kg, 5 vials maximum) within 4 days of exposure. If VariZIG is not available, give either a single dose of IVIG or chemoprophylaxis with oral acyclovir (80 mg/kg per day div qid for 7 days). Patients already receiving monthly infusions of IVIG or who have had chicken pox or varicella vaccine in the past do not require any specific intervention for subsequent exposure.

Pneumonia

If pneumonia is suspected, obtain a CBC, blood culture, chest radiograph, and either an ABG or an oxygen saturation (pulse oximetry). Obtain a serum LDH to help differentiate PCP from a bacterial process. If the child is over 1 year of age, not in respiratory distress, taking fluids well and has an arterial oxygen saturation >95% and an X-ray consistent with bacterial pneumonia, treat as an outpatient with cefuroxime (30 mg/kg per day div bid) if <5 years old or a macrolide such as azithromycin (12 mg/kg per day for 5 days) if >5 years of age. Use a fluoroquinolone, such as levofloxacin (500 mg once daily) or moxifloxacin (400 mg once daily), for a patient >18 years of age. Schedule a follow-up visit within 24 hours, and instruct the guardian to bring the child back to the ED if his or her condition worsens at any time. If PCP is suspected start TMP-SMZ (20 mg/kg per day of TMP div q 6 h) and prednisone (2–4 mg/kg per day div q 6 h).

Admit a child with pneumonia who appears ill, is hypoxic, or <1 year of age. Treat suspected bacterial pneumonia with IV cefuroxime (100 mg/kg per day div q 8 h) or ceftriaxone (100 mg/kg per day div q 12 h); add vancomycin (40 mg/kg per day div q 6 h) for necrotizing pneumonia consistent with *S. aureus* infection. Suspect PCP if the chest X-ray shows a diffuse interstitial pattern or ARDS, the LDH is >500 IU/L, or if the child has an A–a gradient >30 mmHg. Admit for IV TMP-SMZ (20 mg/kg per day of TMP div q 6 h). Treat patients with profound hypoxia (pO_2 <70 mmHg) with prednisone (2 mg/kg per day) or the IV equivalent. Do not delay antibiotic therapy until definitive diagnosis can be made by bronchoalveolar lavage. PCP does not resolve rapidly; clinical improvement within 24–48 hours suggests a bacterial etiology for the pneumonia.

Consider an atypical organism (*Mycoplasma, Chlamydia, Legionella*) if there is an interstitial pneumonitis without a significant increase in the LDH. Treat with azithromycin (12 mg/kg per day for 5 days) or with a fluoroquinolone, such as moxifloxacin (400 mg q day for 7 days).

If an older patient with a history of bronchiectasis presents with an exacerbation of the underlying lung disease (worsening cough and sputum production, fever, persistent rales), give an anti-pseudomonal antibiotic such as ciprofloxacin (20–30 mg/kg per day div bid), moxifloxacin (400 mg q day), or pipericillin-tazobactam (240 mg/kg per day div qid).

Wheezing

The treatment of wheezing is the same as for HIV-negative children (see pp. 606–612). Discharge a patient who responds well to bronchodilator therapy, has a respiratory rate <40/minute, an oxygen saturation >95%, and is taking fluids well. Prescribe the usual medications for asthma, including a short course of prednisone, if it would otherwise be indicated for an immunocompetent child with reactive airway disease. Obtain a chest X-ray if the patient has a temperature >39°C (102.2°F) to help determine whether a pneumonia is present.

A child <6 months of age who presents with wheezing for the first time most likely has bronchiolitis, which can be treated in the usual manner (pp. 614–616). However, PCP can present with wheezing, so the infant must have a normal oxygen saturation (>95%) in room air prior to discharge home. Otherwise, obtain a chest X-ray and serum LDH, and admit the patient. If PCP is suspected, give TMP-SMZ (as above) in addition to broncho-dilator therapy, consult a pulmonologist, and arrange for bronchoalveolar lavage to confirm the diagnosis.

Heart failure

Prior to admission, obtain a chest X-ray to assess cardiac size, an ABG or pulse oximetry, electrolytes, and LFTs. Therapy is the same as for an immunocompetent patient (see pp. 56–59).

Diarrhea

The ED treatment of diarrhea is similar to that for immunocompetent patients. Focus on the history of possible exposures, recent infections, the duration and severity of symptoms, and fluid intake. Note the patient's state of hydration, and perform a careful physical examination. Test the stool for blood and order a stool culture and smear for PMNs.

A patient who appears well hydrated and has no blood or PMNs in the stool can be treated symptomatically with dietary management and close follow-up visits. However, if examination of the stool shows either blood or >5 PMN per high-power field, treat with oral TMP-SMZ (10 mg/kg per day of TMP div bid) for possible *Salmonella* infection. Treat confirmed *Campylobacter* enteritis with a macrolide, such as erythromycin (40 mg/kg per day div qid) or azithromycin (10 mg/kg per day) for 5–7 days. If the child attends day-care, instruct the caretaker to keep the child at home until the illness resolves and the culture is negative. Arrange for follow-up with the patient's primary care provider. Admit the child with diarrhea who appears ill or dehydrated for IV hydration and empiric antibiotic therapy.

If diarrhea with negative bacterial cultures is unresponsive to dietary therapy and/or has persisted for >2 weeks, order an examination of the stool for ova and parasites, and send a stool sample (not a swab) to test for *Clostridium difficile* toxin. Treat *C. difficile* infection with metronidazole (15–35 mg/kg per day div tid). Do not use oral vancomycin for *C. difficile* due to the increasing prevalence of vancomycin-resistant enterococci (VRE).

Bleeding

If a child presents with evidence of bleeding (e.g. petechiae, bruising, mucosal bleeding), obtain a medication history, perform a careful physical exam, and obtain a CBC and PT/PTT. In patients with HIV-related thrombocytopenia and platelet counts >50,000/mm^3, no intervention is required. When severe bleeding episodes such as intracranial or internal hemorrhage occur, admit the patient for urgent platelet transfusions and supportive therapy. In milder cases of immune thrombocytopenia, (platelet count 20–50,000/mm^3), treat with IVIG (1–2 g/kg) and consult with an HIV specialist and a pediatric hematologist.

Seizures, meningismus, altered mental status

Knowledge of the patient's past medical history, current immune function, and medications (especially those for opportunistic infection prophylaxis) may be helpful in excluding certain CNS disorders associated primarily with advanced immunodeficiency, e.g. cryptococcal meningitis, toxoplasmosis, lymphoma, PML, and cerebral vasculitis syndromes. A CT or MRI scan of the neuraxis may be necessary to demonstrate bleeding, edema, infarction, space-occupying lesions, or other pathology. Although extremely rare in children, if cryptococcal meningitis is suspected, send serum and CSF for cryptococcal antigen determination and ask the lab to perform a CSF India ink preparation to confirm the diagnosis. In unusual cases, or those associated with fastidious or non-culturable pathogens (e.g. JC virus of PML, CMV encephalitis, VZV-associated vasculitis), collect and refrigerate an extra tube of CSF. In these situations the saved CSF can later be analyzed using molecular tests such as PCR to aid in making a definitive diagnosis and guide treatment.

Indications for admission

- Ill appearance with or without fever
- Soft tissue infection involving a large area, not well circumscribed, impinging on important structures, or unresponsive to oral antibiotics
- Suspected PCP
- Pneumonia in a patient <1 year old
- Persistent respiratory distress despite appropriate ED management (tachypnea, oxygen saturation <95% or 5% below patient's baseline, retractions, or flaring)
- Inadequate oral intake
- Varicella or disseminated zoster
- Uncontrolled or excessive bleeding, CNS hemorrhage
- New-onset seizures
- Altered mental status

Universal precautions

Human immunodeficiency virus has been isolated from all body fluids; blood, semen, and cervical secretions are most often associated with viral transmission. Transmission has not been shown to occur through tears, saliva, urine, stool, sweat, or via casual contact. The risk to healthcare workers, therefore, comes largely from contact with blood, either from needle stick injuries or onto abraded skin or mucous membranes. The risk of seroconversion following needle stick injuries involving blood of infected patients is approximately 1 in 300.

Compliance with the CDCs "universal precautions," which follow, will help prevent transmission of HIV to healthcare workers in the ED setting:

- Wear gloves for all procedures that involve touching blood or body fluids, mucous membranes, or non-intact skin.
- Wash hands immediately after removing gloves or if contaminated by blood or body fluids.
- Do not recap needles. Dispose of them in puncture-resistant containers, which should be located near all work areas.
- Minimize the need for mouth-to-mouth resuscitation by keeping ventilation devices available in areas where they are likely to be needed.
- Wear glasses or goggles and a mask when performing procedures which may cause blood or bodily fluids to splash (e.g. irrigating a wound).

Guidelines for managing blood and body fluid exposures

General considerations

The efficacy of HIV post exposure prophylaxis (HIV PEP) following sexual assault/ abuse, accidental needle stick injuries, and human bites in non-occupational settings is unknown and has led to a lack of consensus among public health authorities. Therefore, emergency consultation with a pediatric infectious diseases, immunology, or HIV specialist may be required. In contrast, the management of occupational exposures is clear: After notification of the employee health department immediate evaluation and treatment is indicated.

The per-episode risk of infection following sexual exposure is difficult to define, but it is highest with unprotected receptive anal intercourse (0.8–3.2%), followed by receptive vaginal intercourse (0.05–1.5%), and insertive vaginal intercourse (0.03–0.09%). Although no per-contact estimates of risk with insertive anal intercourse or with oral sex have been published, seroconversion as a result of such an exposure has been documented. In comparison, the estimated risk following a percutaneous occupational exposure is 0.3% and that following sharing of a needle is 0.67%. Accidental needle stick injuries following exposure to discarded needles, such as in parks or alleyways, are associated with a negligible risk for HIV exposure. Other types of exposure among children that carry an unknown, but probably minimal risk, are bites and sports-related injuries resulting in exposure to blood or blood-tinged secretions.

Recommendations

General considerations and specific elements necessary for a rational and consistent approach to HIV PEP after potential HIV exposure in children and adolescents are outlined

Table 14-1. HIV postexposure prophylaxis (PEP): general considerations

Consideration	Comments
Assessment of HIV risk	See Tables 14-2 and 14-3
Timing of HIV PEP	Initiate as soon as possible after exposure
	Limited efficacy if started past 72 hours
Choice of antiretrovirals	Offer a dual drug regimen composed of zidovudine and lamivudine, or, if indicated, the co-formulated product Combivir
	Consult with an HIV expert for the addition of nelfinavir (<13 years old) or tenofovir (>13 years old) for high-risk exposures
	See Table 14-4 for age-specific drug dosages
	Duration of PEP: 4 weeks
Evaluation for PEP toxicity	See Table 14-4 for drug-related side effects and toxicities
Baseline laboratory testing	HIV serologies, liver function tests, CBC, and hCG (if indicated)
Psychosocial counseling	Medical social worker or psychiatric nurse familiar with crisis intervention
Involvement of parents or legal guardian	Parent or legal guardian must sign informed consent to allow HIV testing of the patient (unless an emancipated minor)
Established follow-up	Initial follow-up: 24–72 hours, in person or over the telephone, with a physician comfortable with the use of antiretroviral drugs in children.
	Assess medication compliance, side effects, and financial barriers.
	Follow-up visit with physician: within 1 week
Other considerations	Forensic evidence collection
	Hepatitis B and C evaluation
	PEP for other sexually transmitted diseases, emergency contraception, wound care, assessment of tetanus immunization status

Source: Adapted with permission from Babl FE, Cooper ER, Damon B, et al: HIV postexposure prophylaxis for children and adolescents *Am J Emer Med* 2000;18:282–7.

in Tables 14-1 through 14-4. The various HIV diagnostic tests are summarized in Table 14-5. In cases involving no to low-risk exposures, reassure the caregiver that the child will not contract HIV infection and that postexposure chemoprophylaxis is not necessary. For an individual presenting to the ED more than 72 hours following an exposure, chemoprophylaxis is not indicated; exceptions may be made for high-risk exposures. Consult an HIV expert, especially when the selection of alternative prophylactic drug regimens is indicated. If local expertise is not available, advice may be obtained 24 hours a day from the National Clinicians' Consultation Center PEP line at 1–888-HIV-4911. Federal, state, and local HIV PEP guidelines are subject to modification based upon the epidemiology of HIV in your community, resource availability, and the continued advancement of knowledge in this complex area.

Table 14-2. Risk assessment for providing sexual PEP

PEP recommended

1. The HIV exposure is high-risk, specifically:

    a. Unprotected receptive anal or vaginal intercourse

    b. Unprotected insertive anal or vaginal intercourse

    c. Unprotected receptive fellatio with ejaculation

2. The patient's partner is known to be either HIV-infected or in an HIV risk group (gay or bisexual man, IV drug user, sex worker)

3. The exposure is isolated or the patient has made a commitment to safer sex in the future. If the unsafe practices are expected to continue, PEP is not indicated

4. The exposure occurred ≤72 hours ago; if patient presents to ED >72 hours after exposure, PEP may still be offered in exceptional circumstances where risk of HIV exposure/infection significantly outweighs PEP drug toxicity risk. Consult state and local guidelines as acceptable intervals between exposure and provision of PEP may vary anywhere from 36–72 hours

PEP not recommended

1. After other sexual exposures, including:

    a. Cunnilingus

    b. Receptive fellatio without ejaculation

2. Exposure occurred >72 hours ago

Source: Adapted with permission from Katz MH, Gerberding JL: Care of persons with recent sexual exposure to HIV. *Ann Intern Med* 1998;128:306–12.

Table 14-3. Risk assessment for providing HIV PEP following accidental needle stick injuries and human bites

Needle stick injuries

Characteristics of injury

    Penetrates the skin (more than a scratch)

    Large hollow bore needle

    Visible blood on needle

    Needle placed directly in vein/artery of source

Other factors

    Source patient with known HIV risk factors

    Prevalence of HIV infection among local IV drug users

Human bites

Bite recipient

    Break in the skin

    Presence of bleeding gums or other lesions facilitating admixture of blood and saliva

    Known HIV risk factors in bite inflictor

Bite inflictor

    Exposure to blood of bite wound victim with known HIV risk factors

    Presence of oral/mucosal lesions

Table 14-4. PEP following non-occupational exposure including sexual assault

<13 years of age and/or unable to swallow pills

Zidovudine (retrovir syrup, 10 mg/mL): 9 mg/kg bid (300 mg dose maximum), plus

Epivir (lamivudine syrup, 10 mg/mL) 4 mg/kg bid (150 mg dose maximum), plus

Kaletra (lopinavir/ritonavir elixir, 400/100 mg per 5 mL): use a dose that is equivalent to 10 mg/kg per dose of lopinavir PO bid (400/100 mg dose maximum)

≥13 years of age

Combivir (zidovudine 300 mg + lamivudine 150 mg): 1 tab PO bid, plus

Viread (tenofovir disoproxil 300 mg) 1 tab PO q day

Source: Adapted with permission from New York Department of Health AIDS Institute. *HIV PEP Regimen Following Non-Occupational Exposure Including Sexual Assault.* Albany, NY: NYDOH AI, 2008. Available at: http://www.hivguidelines.org

Table 14-5. Spectrum of tests for the diagnosis and monitoring of HIV-1 infection

Assay	Other names	Comments
Routine serology	HIV antibody test	Gold-standard for diagnosis of established HIV infection
	HIV serologies	Informed consent required
	HIV enzyme	Rapid testing (blood, saliva) results available ~20 minutes
	(a) Immunoassay (EIA)	If EIA is positive, must confirm with WB
	(b) Western blot (WB)	Seroconversion detectable 6–12 weeks following infection
	Rapid HIV test (various commercial assays)	95% of infected patients seropositive by 6 months
		Serology not useful in HIV-exposed infant <18 months old
OraSure Test	Salivary test	Salivary collection device to collect IgG for EIA and WB
	Saliva HIV test	Sensitivity/specificity comparable to standard blood tests
	HIV spit test	
	Rapid HIV	
Calypte 1	Urine HIV test	EIA test to detect HIV antibodies in urine
	Urine test	Must be administered by physician
		Positive result must be verified by serology
DNA PCR	DNA-PCR test	Used to detect cell-associated proviral DNA
	Virus DNA test	Requires confirmation

Table 14-5. (cont.)

Assay	Other names	Comments
	Virus test	Test of choice for diagnosis of neonatal HIV infection
		Usually positive by 2–4 weeks of age
Quantitative	Viral load	
HIV-RNA	HIV RNA-PCR (Roche)	Quantification of plasma viral RNA using reverse transcription and
	bDNA assay (Chiron)	amplification by PCR
	NASBA (Organon)	Results reported as copies/mL
		Dynamic range varies according to assay used
		Can measure between 20 and 10,000,000 copies/mL
		Used to monitor response to antiretroviral therapy
		Not FDA-approved for diagnosis of established HIV infection
		Acute HIV associated with high viral loads and lack of HIV antibodies (window period).
		Consider this test in settings of recent, high-risk HIV exposure, especially in adolescents presenting with mononucleosis-like syndrome
CD4 cell count	T cell count	Number of CD4+ T lymphocytes circulating in blood
	T cell subsets	Target cell depleted during course of HIV infection
	T helper cell count	Marker of host's current immune status
	CD4+ T cell count	Presented as percentage or absolute number of CD4 cells:
		>25% considered normal in children
		≤15% indicates profound immunosuppression

Bibliography

American Academy of Pediatrics. Human immunodeficiency virus infection. In Pickering LK, Baker CJ, Kimberlin DW, Long SS (eds), *Red Book: 2009 Report of the Committee on Infectious Diseases*, 28th ed. Elk Grove Village, IL: American Academy of Pediatrics, 2009, pp. 380–400.

McKellar MS, Callens SF, Colebunders R: Pediatric HIV infection: the state of antiretroviral therapy. *Expert Rev Anti Infect Ther* 2008;6:167–80.

New York Department of Health AIDS Institute: *HIV Post-Exposure Prophylaxis for Children Beyond the Perinatal Period*. Albany, NY: NYDOH AI, 2004. Available at: http://www.hivguidelines.org.

Read JS: Committee on Pediatric AIDS, American Academy of Pediatrics: Diagnosis of HIV-1 infection in children younger than 18 months in the United States. *Pediatrics* 2007;120:e1547–62.

Infectious mononucleosis and mononucleosis-like illnesses

Infectious mononucleosis (IM) is a clinical syndrome consisting of prolonged fever, pharyngitis, and lymphadenopathy. Epstein-Barr virus (EBV) causes approximately 90% of cases of IM. Other infections that produce a mononucleosis-like syndrome include, in the order of their frequency, human herpesvirus 6 (HHV-6), CMV, HSV-1, group A strep, *Toxoplasma gondii*, HIV, and adenovirus. Additional diseases with presentations suggestive of IM include connective tissue disorders (sarcoidosis, SLE), malignancies (Hodgkin's disease, non-Hodgkin's lymphoma), infections (diphtheria, enteroviruses, hepatitis A or B virus, rubella), and drug reactions (carbamazepine, minocycline, phenytoin).

EBV is a ubiquitous herpesvirus that replicates in epithelial cells and B-lymphocytes. It infects children and young adults primarily. By adulthood 90% of people worldwide have serologic evidence of prior EBV infection. The incidence of symptomatic disease is 30-times higher in whites than in African-Americans, with no known gender differences. There is no obvious seasonal pattern of EBV infection.

Transmission occurs primarily through exposure to oropharyngeal secretions, although transmission via blood products has also been reported. Despite the fact that the virus has been found to be present in cervical mucosa and semen, sexual transmission has not been demonstrated. The virus infects oral epithelial cells and spreads to B-lymphocytes, triggering a robust but self-limited immunologic response. This includes the characteristic formation of atypical lymphocytes, which represent activated cytotoxic T lymphocytes directed against specific viral antigens expressed within the infected B cells. The infection causes polyclonal B cell stimulation and results in the production of antibodies against EBV antigens as well as unrelated antigens (heterophile antibodies, HetAb). Like other herpesviruses, such as CMV, VZV, and HSV, EBV remains in the body for life.

Clinical presentation

Clinical manifestations of IM are age related. After an incubation period that can range from 30 to 50 days, a young child (<4 years old) is usually asymptomatic or has mild nonspecific symptoms, such as a URI, tonsillopharyngitis (without exudate), or a prolonged febrile illness with or without lymphadenopathy. This age group has a higher frequency of organomegaly. The older child or teenager is more likely to develop the classic triad of fever, sore throat, and lymphadenopathy. The patient may have a prodromal illness consisting of 1–2 days of malaise, anorexia, fatigue, headache, and high fever (40°C, 104°F), before the onset of sore throat and lymphadenopathy. Alternatively, there may be the abrupt onset of focal symptoms. Pharyngitis is often most severe in the first 3–5 days, and 30% of patients have exudative pharyngitis. There may also be palatal petechiae.

An enlarged spleen is palpated in 17% of patients, but splenomegaly has been documented on ultrasound in 100% of patients. Bilateral, nontender, posterior and anterior cervical lymphadenopathy often occurs. Less common clinical features include upper airway compromise, abdominal pain, hepatomegaly, jaundice, and periorbital edema.

Rash occurs in 5% and may be macular, petechial, scarlatiniform, urticarial, or erythema multiforme-like. In about 90% of patients, a non-allergic maculopapular, pruritic rash develops 7–10 days after starting a beta-lactam antibiotic.

The duration of illness is variable. Symptoms peak at 7 days after onset and fade over the next 1–3 weeks. Fever can last 1–2 weeks, splenomegaly usually resolves within 4 weeks of the onset of symptoms, but fatigue can persist for months.

Table 14-6. Interpretation of Epstein-Barr antibodies

Infection status	Antibody test		
	VCA IgG	VCA IgM	EBNA
No current or prior infection	–	–	–
Acute primary infection	+	+	–
Recent (<6 months ago) infection	+	+/–	+/–
Past infection	+	–	+

Note: VCA, viral capsid antigen; EBNA, EBV nuclear antigen.

Complications include thrombocytopenia (25–50%), upper airway obstruction (<5%), hemolytic anemia (3%), and splenic rupture (<0.5%). Neurologic complications occur in 1–5% of cases, and include meningoencephalitis, Guillain-Barré syndrome, transverse myelitis, encephalitis, and cranial nerve palsies. An "Alice in Wonderland" syndrome, characterized by metamorphopsia (distortion of sizes, shapes, and spatial relations of objects), has been reported.

Diagnosis

Although the diagnosis of IM is clinical, laboratory testing is useful for confirming the diagnosis, especially when the presentation is atypical. Specifically, the diagnosis is proven if there is a lymphocytosis ($\geq$50%) with 10% or more atypical forms, or a positive heterophile titer or monospot test. The percentage of patients with acute EBV infection who have heterophile antibodies increases relative to the time since onset of symptoms but may be negative in up to 50% of patients <4 years old. EBV titers are indicated for a patient with an atypical presentation or negative heterophile antibody test, or who is severely ill or immunocompromised. In such cases, obtain serum for viral capsid antigen (VCA) IgG and IgM and for EBV nuclear antigen (EBNA) IgG. See Table 14-6 for the interpretation of EBV serology.

Other laboratory abnormalities associated with IM include a two- to three-fold increase in hepatic transaminase levels (90% of cases) and abnormalities on urinalysis, including proteinuria, pyuria, and microscopic hematuria.

ED management

Treatment for IM is supportive. Perform a rapid test to rule out strep pharyngitis, and treat, if positive (pp. 154–156). Encourage rest and fluids and recommend acetaminophen (15 mg/kg q 4 h) or ibuprofen (10 mg/kg q 6 h), for symptomatic relief from sore throat or headache.

Admit a patient with significant upper airway obstruction (stridor). Continuously monitor the oxygen saturation and treat with elevation of the head of the bed, IV hydration, humidified air, and systemic corticosteroids (prednisone 2 mg/kg per day div bid, 60 mg/day maximum). However, steroids have not been proven to provide significant or reproducible benefit for lymphadenopathy or hepatosplenic involvement. More than half of all splenic ruptures occur in patients without a palpable spleen. Therefore, advise the patient to not participate in contact sports or strenuous activities for approximately 4 weeks.

Follow-up

- Primary care follow-up in 2–4 weeks. Instruct the family to return immediately for stridor or inability to swallow (persistent drooling)

Indications for admission

- Upper airway obstruction
- Inadequate fluid intake
- Neurologic complications

Bibliography

Ebell MH: Epstein-Barr virus infectious mononucleosis. *Am Fam Physician* 2004;70:1279–87.

Hurt C, Tammaro D: Diagnostic evaluation of mononucleosis-like illnesses. *Am J Med* 2007;120:911.e1–8.

Kutok JL, Wang F: Spectrum of Epstein-Barr virus-associated diseases. *Annu Rev Pathol* 2006;1:375–404.

Infectious disease associated with exanthems

Illnesses with cutaneous manifestations are caused by a variety of agents including viruses, *Chlamydiae, Rickettsiae, Mycoplasma*, bacteria, fungi, and protozoa. Today, enteroviruses are the leading cause of exanthematous diseases. Although most exanthematous illnesses are benign, the differential diagnosis is important because skin involvement may be an early sign of potentially fatal bacterial and rickettsial diseases, emerging viruses (West Nile, dengue), and reemerging vaccine-preventable viral infections (measles, mumps) in returning travelers.

Clinical manifestations

Viral infections

Nonspecific viral exanthems

The most common etiologies of nonspecific viral exanthems are enteroviruses (Coxsackie viruses, echovirus, enterovirus) and respiratory viruses (adenovirus, rhinovirus, parainfluenza virus, respiratory syncitial virus, influenza virus). Most summertime exanthems are due to enteroviruses, while the respiratory viruses predominate during the colder months. The typical nonspecific viral exanthem presents as blanching erythematous macules and papules, distributed diffusely on the trunk and extremities, with occasional facial involvement. Associated symptoms can include fever, headache, upper respiratory tract or gastrointestinal symptoms, myalgias and fatigue.

Coxsackie viruses

Coxsackie A4 causes fever and herpangina (1–5 mm vesicles and ulcers of the posterior pharynx). An erythematous, maculopapular exanthem can develop after the patient defervesces. In some patients, the lesions become vesicular, spread to the extremities including the palms and soles, then regress to a brownish discoloration in 1–2 weeks. Fever and an erythematous rash that starts on the face and neck, then spreads to the trunk and extremities, characterize Coxsackie A9.

Coxsackie A16 virus causes hand-foot-mouth syndrome which presents with a mild fever, anorexia, malaise, and a sore mouth, followed by a vesicular eruption on the hands and/or feet associated with herpangina-like intraoral lesions. The rash associated with Coxsackie B5 virus is usually maculopapular, but it can be petechial at times. Rarely, there may be concomitant aseptic meningitis or myocarditis.

Echovirus 9 and enterovirus 71

These can be associated with aseptic meningitis. The rash of echovirus 9 is usually rubelliform or petechial, whereas the rash associated with enterovirus 71 varies from erythematous maculopapular to vesicular. Enteroviral infection may cause meningitis (in particular Coxsackie 19, A16, and B5; and enterovirus 9 or 71) or myocarditis (Coxsackie B5). Severe fatal enterovirus 71 meningitis infections are increasingly common in certain parts of the world.

Dengue virus

Dengue (pp. 365–366) causes a diffuse maculopapular rash and petechiae. It occurs almost exclusively among returning travelers from Latin America, the Caribbean, or SE Asia.

West Nile virus

West Nile (pp. 366–370) presents with a maculopapular rash and MS changes, usually in older adolescents or adults.

Measles (rubeola)

Although vaccination has greatly reduced the incidence of measles in the United States, outbreaks continue to occur, primarily during the winter and spring, and are increasingly linked to contact with travelers returning from the Europe, the Middle East, Africa, and Asia. Measles is spread by direct contact with infectious droplets or by air-borne spread, with a subsequent incubation period of 8–12 days. Measles classically presents with the "three C's": cough, coryza, and conjunctivitis, usually associated with a high fever (up to 40°C; 104°F). During the prodrome, pathognomonic Koplik's spots appear. They consist of small white spots with a red background on the buccal mucosa. Koplik's spots disappear within 48 hours of the onset of exanthem, which typically appears on the fourth day of the illness. Nonpruritic erythematous macules and papules appear first on the face and spread to the trunk and extremities. The rash fades in the same order as it appeared. Complications include pneumonia, otitis, bronchitis, encephalitis, and myocarditis.

Two other types of measles are now recognized, modified measles and atypical measles. Modified measles occurs in a partially immunized patient, presenting with a shorter prodrome, a less severe rash, and the possible absence of Koplik's spots. Atypical measles occurs most often in patients who become infected after receiving the killed measles vaccine, although it has been reported rarely among patients who received the live attenuated vaccine. Atypical measles presents with abrupt onset of high fever, myalgias, and cough. In contrast to typical measles, the rash begins on the extremities 2–5 days later and spreads centrally. Lobar pneumonia is frequently present.

Erythema infectiosum (Fifth disease)

This infection is caused by parvovirus B19. It is most common in the spring, primarily affecting 4–10-year-olds. Transmission is by respiratory droplets, followed by an incubation period of 6–14 days. Some patients have a mild prodrome of headache, low-grade fever, malaise, pharyngitis, joint pain, and gastrointestinal symptoms before the onset of the rash. The eruption begins with the sudden appearance of "slapped cheeks" (erythematous patches on the cheeks). It then progresses to the trunk and extremities, where it appears as erythematous macules and papules, before developing into a lacy reticular pattern. Arthralgia and arthritis can be present in 10% of patients. Parvovirus can suppress the bone marrow, so that patients with shortened RBC life spans (sickle cell disease, thalassemia, hereditary spherocytosis, pyruvate kinase deficiency) are at risk for a transient aplastic crisis. Parvovirus infection during pregnancy can cause fetal hydrops and death.

Roseola infantum

Roseola, thought to be caused by human herpesvirus-6, is transmitted by respiratory droplets. It affects children between 6 months and 2 years of age, with a peak incidence at 6–7 months. It is generally a self-limited, benign illness characterized by 3–5 days of high fever (39–40.5°C; 102.2–104.9°F), which peaks in the evening. Other symptoms are rare, but can include mild respiratory symptoms, irritability, and malaise. The fever ends abruptly, followed by the rash within 24–48 hours. The eruption is characterized by pink, blanching, discrete macules and papules over the trunk. The rash is rarely pruritic and usually fades over 1–2 days.

Rubella

Prior to the rubella vaccine, the peak incidence of infection was in children 5–14 years of age, but the disease is now seen in nonimmune older children and adults. After a 14–21 day incubation period, rubella presents with an upper respiratory infection. The rash of rubella is variable, beginning on the face, then spreading to other areas. It starts as maculopapules, which may become pinpoint papules, similar to those seen in scarlet fever. Mild pruritus may be present and resolution usually occurs within 72 hours. Rose-colored macules may develop on the soft palate immediately preceding the rash, and the patient may have tender retroauricular, posterior cervical, and occipital lymphadenopathy. Rubella can cause a severe fetal infection if a susceptible pregnant woman is exposed.

Varicella (chicken pox)

Once an exceedingly common childhood disease, varicella is now seen much less frequently, as a result of the vaccine. It is a highly contagious disease with an incubation period of 11–21 days. The patient presents with fever, malaise, headache, anorexia, and abdominal pain. After 24–48 hours an intensely pruritic rash appears on the face, scalp, or trunk and spreads peripherally. It begins as erythematous macules, which evolve into papules, and then vesicles containing serous fluid. The vesicles spontaneously rupture and develop into crusts, before resolving. Subsequent crops of lesions develop over 4–6 days, so that the presence of lesions in different stages is characteristic of varicella. The patient is infectious from the beginning of the prodromal illness (about 2 days before the rash erupts) until each pox has a crust, about 7–10 days. Complications include bacterial superinfection of the skin (which may rarely progress to necrotizing fasciitis), pneumonia, thrombocytopenia, arthritis, hepatitis, cerebellar ataxia, encephalitis, meningitis, and glomerulonephritis. The virus establishes latency in the dorsal root ganglia during primary infection, and reactivation results in herpes zoster (shingles).

Herpes zoster

Herpes zoster is caused by reactivation of the varicella virus. Pain and tenderness along a dermatome precede the eruption of classic chicken pox lesions clustered within one to three continuous dermatomes. Pain, tenderness, and localized lymphadenopathy persist while the skin lesions are present (1–2 weeks).

Herpes simplex

Primary HSV gingivostomatitis (p. 82) causes fever, irritability, and lesions involving the gingival and mucous membranes of the mouth. Genital herpes (p. 117), characterized by vesicular lesions, is most common in adolescents. Consider sexual abuse if genital herpes is seen in a prepubertal child. Reactivation of the latent virus causes "cold sores," single or grouped vesicles in the perioral region, but not inside the mouth, or as lesions on the external genitalia. Neonatal HSV can present as a focal or systemic infection (pp. 116–118), presenting any time from the day of birth until 4–6 weeks of life.

Bacterial infections

Meningococcemia

N. meningitides is a Gram-negative diplococcus which is carried in the upper respiratory tract in up to 25% of adolescents. Disease occurs more commonly in the winter and early spring, and the majority of cases are seen in children <2 years of age. The disease can progress extremely rapidly, presenting with a range of severity from self-resolving bacteremia to meningitis to septic shock and coma. The rash usually presents with nonblanching petechiae and purpura, classically described as asymmetric gunmetal gray palpable purpura of the extremities. However, maculopapular, bullous, and pustular lesions can also occur.

Scarlet fever

Scarlet fever is caused by group A beta hemolytic streptococci. After an incubation period of 1–7 days, the illness presents with fever, vomiting, headache, and pharyngitis. The tonsils are hyperemic and edematous and may be covered with exudates, there may be palatal petechiae, and the tongue may have a strawberry appearance (pp. 154–156). The rash is usually erythematous, punctate, or finely papular, with the texture of sandpaper. It appears in the axillae, groin, and neck first and generalizes within 24 hours. Accentuation in the flexion creases (Pastia's lines) and circumoral pallor are common. Desquamation begins on the face at the end of the first week and proceeds over the trunk and then to the hands and feet.

Diagnosis

An assessment of possible exposure, season of the year, and travel history, along with an awareness of the incubation period of various infections are important in diagnosing patients with a rash. Inquire about exposure to a similar illness, and immunization and medication histories. The appearance, progression, and distribution of the rash can be very helpful, as can the time elapsed between the exposure and the current illness.

The age of the child and season of the year can provide clues for determining the diagnosis. Certain diseases occur more commonly in particular age groups. Roseola infantum occurs primarily in 6–36-month-olds, erythema infectiosum in 2–12-year-olds, and scarlet fever in school-age children. Some diseases have seasonal predilection, such as scarlet fever in the late winter and early spring and enteroviruses during the summer and fall.

The time elapsed between the onset of fever and the appearance of the rash provides an important clue to the diagnosis. The rash in rubella occurs simultaneously with the fever. A patient with scarlet fever is generally febrile for 12–24 hours prior to the onset of the rash, while a patient with roseola has 3–5 days of fever, and then defervesces, prior to the onset of the rash. While these relationships are not absolute, they represent the norm and are therefore valuable adjuncts in determining the diagnosis.

The appearance, progression, and distribution of the rash can also be very helpful in determining the diagnosis. Maculopapular rashes are the most common and are usually associated with enteroviral infections. Vesicular exanthems present either as single or localized lesions (herpes simplex, herpes zoster), generalized lesions (varicella), or in a peripheral distribution (hand-foot-mouth disease).

Pertinent physical findings include the patient's appearance, presence of regional or generalized lymphadenopathy, conjunctivitis, hepatomegaly, or gastrointestinal involvement. Children who are very ill-appearing may have meningococcemia, Rocky Mountain spotted fever, Kawasaki disease, dengue fever, or measles.

Adenopathy is particularly important when considering the diagnosis of rubella (post-auricular and suboccipital adenopathy) and infectious mononucleosis (generalized with hepatosplenomegaly). Koplik's spots on the buccal mucosa suggest measles prior to the appearance of the exanthem in a febrile child.

The differential diagnosis of these diseases includes many of the infectious illnesses with fever and rash. The first phase of erythema infectiosum resembles scarlet fever, but the patient appears well and there is no evidence of streptococcal infection. Infection may be confirmed, if necessary, by serum B19-specific antibody. A roseola-like illness has been ascribed to an enterovirus. Many children with the prodromal fever of roseola are given antibiotics, so the rash is occasionally diagnosed as a drug allergy or amoxicillin rash.

Measles can be confused with scarlet fever (cough and coryza absent), Kawasaki disease (stomatitis, rash does not spread down the body), and rubella (shorter prodrome and rash duration, patient appears much less sick). In none of these are Koplik's spots seen. Diagnosis can be confirmed by viral isolation from nasopharyngeal secretions, conjunctiva, blood, and urine during the febrile phase or by comparing paired acute and convalescent sera. Some laboratories can detect measles-specific IgM antibody with a single serum sample. The diagnosis of rubella can be confirmed by IgM-specific antibody or virus isolation from nasal secretions, throat swab, blood, urine, or CSF.

Varicella has a typical appearance. However, mild eruptions can be confused with bullous impetigo and insect bites, although these lesions do not erupt in crops or go through a series of stages. Zoster may resemble a contact dermatitis in which pruritus is more common than pain.

The rash of meningococcemia can be confused with other causes of bacterial sepsis, viral infections, idiopathic thrombocytopenic purpura, and Rocky Mountain spotted fever. Unroofing a skin lesion and Gram's staining the contents may reveal the pathognomonic Gram-negative intracellular diplococci. The diagnosis is confirmed by a positive blood culture.

If diagnostic confirmation of an enterovirus is needed the organism can be isolated from the throat and rectum. A polymerase chain reaction (PCR) assay may be available for serum viral identification.

ED management

There is no specific treatment for many of these diseases. Therapy consists largely of reassurance and supportive care. Treat fever with acetaminophen (15 mg/kg q 4 h) or ibuprofen

(10 mg/kg q 6 h). Assess the hydration status and give intravenous fluids when appropriate. Generally, blood tests and cultures are not necessary unless the patient appears seriously ill.

Measles

Treatment is supportive. Admit a patient with pneumonia (for antibiotic therapy), and perform a lumbar puncture if the child presents with lethargy, excessive irritability, or nuchal rigidity. Obtain serum for measles IgM (available through most public health or commercial laboratories) and notify public health officials of any suspected case of measles so that appropriate community measures can be instituted. Vitamin A decreases the morbidity and mortality of measles in children with vitamin A deficiency; give vitamin A (50,000 U/day) to children 6 months to 2 years hospitalized with complications of measles. Institute appropriate prophylaxis, either measles vaccination (within 72 hours) or immune globulin (0.25 mL/kg within 6 days) for unvaccinated or immunosuppressed contacts.

Rubella

Treatment is supportive. If rubella is suspected, refer pregnant contacts to their obstetricians immediately for titers.

Varicella

Treat pruritus with antihistamines (diphenhydramine 5 mg/kg per day div qid or hydroxyzine 2 mg/kg per day div tid) and oatmeal baths. Do not use aspirin because it is associated with an increased risk of Reye's syndrome. Oral acyclovir is not routinely recommended in otherwise healthy children with varicella. Possible indications include an exposed patient >12 years of age who does not have a history of varicella, a child with chronic cutaneous or pulmonary disorders, a patient receiving long-term salicylate therapy, and a patient receiving glucocorticoids, including short, intermittent, or aerosolized courses. Give 80 mg/kg per day div qid for 5 days (3,200 mg/day maximum).

Give postexposure immunization to a susceptible patient within 72 hours and possibly up to 120 hours after varicella exposure. A newborn whose mother develops varicella within 5 days before delivery or up to 48 hours after delivery, a patient with varicella pneumonia, or an immunocompromised patient with zoster has a serious risk of overwhelming infection. Admit these patients and consult with an infectious disease specialist regarding antiviral therapy.

Varicella zoster immune globulin (VZIG) or immune globulin intravenous (IGIV) is recommended if significant exposure (5–60 minutes of face-to-face play, residing in the same household) occurs in an immunocompromised patient who does not have a history of chicken pox, susceptible pregnant women, and newborns whose mothers develop chicken pox within 5 days before to 48 hours after delivery. Give VZIG, one vial (125 units) IM for each 10 kg of body weight (five vials maximum, one vial minimum) or IGIV (400 mg/kg) within 96 hours of exposure (preferably within 48 hours). Consult with a pediatric infectious disease specialist to determine the need for prophylaxis as well as whether IGIV is an acceptable alternative to VZIG in complicated cases.

If a patient with varicella is hospitalized, implement air-borne and contact precautions for a minimum of 5 days after the onset of the rash, and as long as the rash remains vesicular.

Herpes zoster

Treatment is supportive and includes analgesia for these painful lesions (acetaminophen with codeine, 1 mg/kg per dose). Consult with a pediatric infectious disease specialist to determine the need for therapy.

Herpes simplex

The treatment of primary and recurrent herpes is summarized on pp. 116–118. Consult an ophthalmologist if there is ocular involvement (pp. 533–535). Treat suspected neonatal HSV infection with IV acyclovir (60 mg/kg per day div tid for 21 days).

Meningococcemia

If meningococcemia is suspected, immediately obtain a blood culture and initiate antibiotic therapy with IV cefotaxime (200 mg/kg per day div q 6 h) or ceftriaxone (100 mg/kg per day div q 12 h). Perform a lumbar puncture if there are meningeal signs or altered consciousness (see Meningitis, pp. 401–405). If meningococcemia is confirmed, treat with IV penicillin (250 000 units/kg per day in six divided doses) or cefotaxime (as above). Give prophylactic rifampin (10 mg/kg bid, 600 mg/day maximum, for 2 days), IM ceftriaxone (<12 years: 125 mg; >12 years: 250 mg), or ciprofloxacin (500 mg once) to household, day care or nursery school contacts, and persons having direct contact with the patient's secretions (kissing, shared toothbrush, eating utensils), as well as any medical provider who has had close contact with the patient's secretions (unprotected mouth-to-mouth resuscitation, intubation, suctioning).

Scarlet fever

The treatment is the same as for streptococcal pharyngitis (pp. 154–156).

Follow-up

- Return immediately for altered consciousness, respiratory distress, inability to take adequate fluids
- Possibly susceptible pregnant patient in the third trimester exposed to varicella: obstetrical follow-up immediately
- Possibly susceptible pregnant patient in the first trimester exposed to rubella or parvovirus: obstetrical follow-up within 2–3 days
- Herpes zoster: 2–3 days

Indications for admission

- Measles pneumonia or encephalitis
- Varicella or suspected HSV in immunocompromised patients and newborns
- Suspected meningococcemia
- Dehydrated patients requiring IV fluid therapy.

Bibliography

American Academy of Pediatrics. Human herpesvirus 6 (including roseola) and 7. In Pickering LK, Baker CJ, Kimberlin DW, Long SS (eds), *Red Book: 2009 Report of the Committee on Infectious Diseases*, 28th ed. Elk Grove Village, IL: American Academy of Pediatrics, 2009, pp. 378–9.

Dyer JA: Childhood viral exanthems. *Pediatr Ann* 2007;**36**:21–9.

Middleton J, Lee BE, Fox JD, Tilley PA, Robinson JL: Comparison between the clinical and laboratory features of enterovirus and West Nile virus infections. *J Med Virol* 2008;**80**:1252–9.

Rebora A: Life-threatening cutaneous viral diseases. *Clin Dermatol* 2005;**23**: 157–63.

Kawasaki syndrome

Kawasaki syndrome (KS) is an acute, self-limited, multiorgan vasculitis. It predominately affects young children, with a peak incidence between 6 and 12 months of age. More than 50% of patients are younger than 2 years, and 80% are younger than 4 years; KS rarely occurs in children older than 8 years or younger than 3 months. In the United States an estimated 3,000 children are hospitalized each year with KS. The etiology of KS is unknown, but it is believed to be due to an infectious agent with activation of the immune system playing a role in its pathogenesis. Epidemics are most common in the spring and fall.

Clinical presentation

There are three distinct stages of the illness. The acute stage (days 1–10) is characterized by an abrupt onset of high fever, typically over 40°C (104°F), without prodrome, for at least 5 days. The fever persists for a mean of 12 days if untreated. Within 2–5 days of the onset of fever, the patient develops other characteristic features of the illness including at least four out of the following five:

- conjunctival injection without exudate
- erythema of the mouth and pharynx, a strawberry tongue, and cracked, red lips
- erythematous rash of almost any pattern
- induration of the hands and feet with erythematous palms and soles
- isolated, unilateral cervical lymphadenopathy (>1.5 cm), typically seen on the first day of fever.

Cardiac manifestations in the first stage may include tachycardia (60%), myocarditis with associated pericardial effusion (30%), and ECG changes such as prolongation of the PR interval (first-degree heart block).

In the subacute stage (days 11–24), the fever, rash, and lymphadenopathy resolve, and periungual and perineal desquamation occur during the second to third week of the illness. Patients may remain irritable and anorectic after defervescence. Cardiac complications, including coronary artery aneurysms, coronary obstruction and thrombosis, and myocardial and endocardial inflammation occur in as many as 20–25% of patients. Males and infants are at highest risk.

In the final stage (after day 24) there is resolution of the external findings. The cardiovascular complications either resolve or progress to myocardial infarction or chronic myocardial ischemia.

Other clinical features of KS include arthralgias and arthritis, involving the small joints during the acute phase and later the large, weightbearing joints. Myringitis, urethritis with sterile pyuria, aseptic meningitis, and, rarely, hydrops of the gallbladder may be present. Other features include diarrhea, vomiting, abdominal pain, cranial nerve palsies, and thrombosis.

Atypical presentations, often termed incomplete Kawasaki disease, are increasingly common, especially among infants <12 months of age. Patients may have fever and fewer than four of the principal diagnostic features. Infants with KS are more likely to develop coronary artery aneurysms than older patients, emphasizing the importance of timely diagnosis and treatment.

Cardiac sequelae occur in up to 25% of patients with untreated KS. Males under 6 months of age are at greatest risk of coronary involvement. Myocardial infarction and subsequent heart failure are the most likely clinical sequelae from previous KS. Young children with an MI rarely present with chest pain but instead with shock, vomiting, and excessive or "hard" crying.

Laboratory abnormalities, which persist for 6–10 weeks, include leukocytosis with a predominance of neutrophils, anemia, thrombocytosis, elevated liver transaminases, and increased bilirubin and alkaline phosphatase. Additionally, there may be elevated levels of acute-phase reactants, such as the ESR and CRP.

Diagnosis

Strongly suspect KS if a patient has fever for >5 days in association with four of the five other major manifestations. Consider KS likely if the patient has fever and three of these features. Obtain a CBC with differential, platelet count, ESR, CRP, blood culture, urinalysis, throat culture, chest radiograph, and ECG. During the first 2 weeks of illness the ESR and CRP are elevated, and a platelet count > 450,000 is typical after the first week. The early performance of an echocardiogram is recommended by some experts.

The differential diagnosis of KS includes staphylococcal or streptococcal toxic shock syndrome (hypotension, renal involvement with elevated BUN and creatinine), rheumatic fever, scarlet fever (pharyngitis, Pastia's lines, no conjunctivitis), staphylococcal scalded skin syndrome (desquamation early with positive Nikolsky's sign), Rocky Mountain spotted fever (petechial and purpuric rash, no enanthem), and leptospirosis (icterus, proteinuria). It also includes viral illnesses (less sick-appearing, no or dissimilar extremity involvement) such as adenovirus, measles (Koplik's spots, different progression of exanthem), influenza, and Epstein-Barr virus infections. Non-infectious diseases include Stevens-Johnson syndrome, erythema multiforme, adverse drug reactions (use of presumptive agent), and IRA.

ED management

Management in the acute phase is aimed at reducing inflammation in the myocardium and coronary artery wall and at preventing thrombosis. The mainstays of therapy are aspirin (80–100 mg/kg per day div qid) plus high-dose IV immunoglobulin (2 g/kg IVSS over 10–12 hours), but defer initiating treatment to the inpatient setting. Admit the patient because of the high rate of cardiac complications during the subacute stage and consult a pediatric cardiologist.

Indication for admission

- Suspected Kawasaki syndrome

Bibliography

Ashouri N, Takahashi M, Dorey F, Mason W: Risk factors for nonresponse to therapy in Kawasaki disease. *J Pediatr* 2008;153:365–8.

Baker AL, Newburger JW: Kawasaki disease. *Circulation* 2008;118:e110–2.

Freeman AF, Shulman ST: Kawasaki disease: summary of the American Heart Association guidelines. *Am Fam Physician* 2006; 74:1141–8.

Leptospirosis

Approximately 100–200 cases of leptospirosis are reported annually in the United States. Fresh water may be contaminated with *Leptospira* shed in the urine of infected animal reservoirs such as rodents, wild ungulates, and livestock. Humans are infected upon ingestion of contaminated water and inhalation of aerosolized droplets, or through skin abrasions or direct contact with animal reservoirs. Leptospirosis is treatable, but may progress rapidly with severe sequelae.

Clinical presentation

After an incubation period of 5–14 days (range 2–30 days), there is the acute onset of a nonspecific febrile illness with chills, headache, nausea, vomiting, and a transient rash resulting from generalized vasculitis. More distinctive clinical features are myalgias of the calf and lumbar regions (80% of cases) and nonpurulent conjunctivitis (30–40% of cases). The disease is self-limited in approximately 90% of cases. This initial "septicemic" phase usually lasts for 3–7 days and can be followed by a second "immune-mediated" phase, with fever, aseptic meningitis, conjunctival suffusion, uveitis, muscle tenderness, adenopathy, and purpuric rash. Approximately 10% of patients will have a potentially fatal (5–40%) illness with jaundice and renal failure (Weil syndrome), hemorrhagic pneumonitis, cardiac arrhythmias, or circulatory collapse. Elevated creatinine, mild hepatitis, and a normal WBC count are typical. The overall duration of symptoms for both phases of disease varies from less than 1 week to several months.

Diagnosis

Consider leptospirosis in a febrile patient with a history of freshwater recreation, even in states with a low reported incidence of infection. Obtain a CBC, urinalysis, liver function tests, and creatinine and perform a lumbar puncture if there are meningeal signs.

ED management

Early in the course of infection doxycycline (4 mg/kg per day div q 12 h, 200 mg/dose maximum) usually leads to complete recovery. For severely ill patients, intravenous penicillin G (250,000–400,000 Units/kg in 4–6 doses; 24 million Units/day maximum) is the treatment of choice, although it may precipitate a Jarisch-Herxheimer reaction, an acute febrile reaction accompanied by headache, myalgia, and an aggravated clinical picture lasting <24 hours. Ceftriaxone (80–100 mg/kg per day div q day or bid, 4 g/day maximum) is an alternative.

Follow-up

• Patient with mild disease: immediately for worsening symptoms, such as recrudescence of fever with signs of jaundice

Indication for admission

• Severe disease that may include jaundice, impending renal failure, arrhythmias or circulatory collapse

Bibliography

American Academy of Pediatrics. Leptospirosis. In Pickering LK, Baker CJ, Kimberlin DW, Long SS (eds), *Red Book: 2009 Report of the Committee on Infectious Diseases*, 28th ed. Elk Grove Village, IL: American Academy of Pediatrics, 2009, pp. 427–8.

Meites E, Jay MT, Deresinski S, et al: Reemerging leptospirosis, California. *Emerg Infect Dis* 2004;10:406–12.

Table 14-7. Signs and symptoms of Lyme disease

	Early localized	Early disseminated	Late
Skin	Erythema migrans (1 lesion)	+/− Multiple erythema migrans lesions	Acrodermatitis chronica atrophicans
Lymphadenopathy		Regional or generalized	
Musculoskeletal	+/− Arthralgias	Arthralgias	Chronic/recurrent arthritis
	+/− Myalgias	Oligo/polyarthritis Migratory polyarthritis	
Neurologic		Meningitis VIIth nerve palsy	Chronic encephalomyelitis
Cardiac			Peripheral neuropathy
Cardiac			Radiculopathy
Cardiac			Myo- or pericarditis AV block
Constitutional	+/− Fever, +/− malaise	Fever, malaise, fatigue	Chronic fatigue

Lyme disease

Lyme disease, caused by the spirochete *B. burgdorferi*, is the most common vector-borne illness in the United States. The most important vector is the *Ixodes* (deer) tick, which has a 2-year life cycle, including larval, nymph, and adult forms. The tiny nymphs are most prevalent in the spring and summer and feed on white-footed mice. White-tailed deer are the preferred hosts of mature ticks, which feed throughout the fall, winter, and early spring. Both nymphs and mature ticks may attach to humans and transmit the spirochete.

Although cases have been reported from all parts of the country, the Northeast, Mid-Atlantic States, Northern Midwest, and Pacific Northwest are endemic areas. In the East and Midwest the majority of infections are acquired between May and August; in the West between January and May. However, infection may occur from early spring to late fall in endemic areas.

Clinical presentation

The disease is categorized into two stages: early and late infection (see Table 14-7). Early Lyme disease is further subdivided into localized or disseminated disease. Early localized infection is characterized by erythema migrans (EM), which is found in over 90% of cases of pediatric Lyme disease. It is a distinctive skin lesion which usually appears between 2 and 32 days after a tick bite. EM typically appears at the site of the bite as an erythematous macule that enlarges (to >5 cm) over several days to weeks. Most often, as the lesion evolves over days, there is central clearing, so that it resembles a ring or target. EM is usually asymptomatic, although pruritus, tenderness, or warmth can occur. If left untreated, it will resolve spontaneously over several weeks. However, it is not a transient rash that will disappear within hours or a few days.

The onset of early disseminated infection is several weeks to months after the tick bite. Manifestations include multiple lesions of erythema migrans, fever, headache, myalgias, arthralgias, arthritis, cardiac involvement (most commonly AV block or bundle branch block), meningitis, cranial nerve palsy, or acute radiculopathy. Gastrointestinal and respiratory symptoms are rare. Acute arthritis is usually monarticular, most often involving large joints, especially the knee. The typical "Lyme knee" is swollen and tender, but erythema and warmth are notably absent. Migratory arthritis and polyarthritis may also occur. Twenty percent of patients have neurologic involvement, including meningoencephalitis, seventh nerve palsy, and peripheral radiculoneuropathy. Cardiac manifestations, such as AV block, myocarditis, and pericarditis are seen in up to 10% of patients. Conjunctivitis, hepatitis, nonexudative pharyngitis, microscopic hematuria, and proteinuria can also occur.

Late Lyme disease, characterized by persistent or relapsing symptoms, is relatively uncommon in children. Chronic and recurrent episodes of arthritis and chronic encephalo-myelitis occur most frequently. The cutaneous manifestation, acrodermatitis chronica atrophicans, is seen far more commonly in Europe than in North America. It is a progressive lesion, presenting with hyperpigmentation and swelling, followed by hypopigmentation and atrophy of the skin on an extremity. In addition, during the late Lyme stage, many patients will complain for months, even after treatment, about recurrent arthralgias, headaches, and malaise. However, these symptoms do not reflect active disease, but rather represent a self-limited immune response. Prolonged or repeated antibiotic courses are not necessary to treat these symptoms.

Diagnosis

A history of a tick bite or travel to an endemic area is helpful, but absence of this information does not eliminate the possibility of Lyme disease.

EM can resemble an insect bite reaction, nummular eczema, tinea corporis, cellulitis, and rarely erythema marginatum or erythema multiforme. However, erythema migrans typically is asymptomatic and macular without scaling, and it enlarges over days or weeks into a ringlike lesion (see Table 5-7, the Differential diagnosis of annular lesions, p. 114).

The generalized systemic symptoms may also occur in influenza and enteroviral infections, and acute and chronic EBV infection. Viral syndromes are far more likely to cause vomiting, diarrhea, and hepatosplenomegaly. In endemic areas, consider Lyme disease for all patients with flu-like illnesses occurring outside flu season.

Septic arthritis, trauma, transient synovitis, and rheumatologic diseases (ARF, JRA, SLE, Crohn's disease) can all resemble Lyme disease. Acute joint swelling with fever always raises the concern of septic arthritis, which presents with a hot, red, tender joint. With Lyme arthritis, however, the joint may be swollen and tender, but warmth and erythema are absent.

Ehrlichiosis and anaplasmosis (pp. 416–420) are relatively uncommon tick-borne illnesses caused by organisms that can also be transmitted by *Ixodes* ticks. They can present with an abrupt flu-like syndrome (fever, headache, myalgias), similar to early Lyme disease. In addition, there may be anorexia, nausea, abdominal pain, vomiting, and acute weight loss. About 1 week into the illness, a maculopapular or petechial rash develops on the extremities, but the palms and soles are usually spared. Thrombocytopenia along with leukopenia and elevation of liver transaminases are often present. Co-infection with *B. burgdorferi* may occur.

Babesiosis is caused by a protozoon, *Babesia microti*. Most cases are reported from the Northeastern states, as well as Minnesota and Wisconsin. Babesiosis is similar to Lyme disease and anaplasmosis, in that it is transmitted by the deer tick and the typical symptoms are nonspecific, including fever, headache, and myalgias. However, a malaria-like picture can develop with hemolytic anemia and thrombocytopenia. This is more severe in immuno-compromised or asplenic patients. As with malaria, diagnosis requires identification of the parasite on thick smear.

Also consider Lyme disease in the differential diagnosis of a peripheral facial nerve palsy (pp. 502–503). CSF changes in Lyme meningitis are similar to the findings in viral meningitis (pleocytosis with normal glucose and mild protein elevation), though the pleocytosis found with Lyme is less marked (CSF WBC <100 cells/mm^3).

Early localized disease

The accurate and expeditious diagnosis of early Lyme disease requires clinical recognition of erythema migrans. Antibodies against *B. burgdorferi* are usually not detectable during the first few weeks after infection, while some patients who receive antibiotics for early Lyme disease never develop antibodies. In addition, serologic screening may yield false-positive results as a result of cross-reacting antibodies directed against spirochetes in normal oral flora, other spirochetal infections (syphilis, leptospirosis, relapsing fever), certain viral infections (varicella, Epstein-Barr virus), or autoimmune diseases (systemic lupus erythematosus).

Early disseminated and late disease

Virtually all patients will develop antibodies against *B. burgdorferi* that may persist for life. For these patients, the diagnosis requires that the results of serologic tests be interpreted with careful consideration of the clinical setting and the quality of the testing laboratory.

Use a two-step approach for serologic testing, by obtaining a sensitive screening test (either an enzyme immunoassay [EIA] or immunofluorescent assay [IFA]) in association with a Western immunoblot. Specimens that yield negative results by EIA or IFA do not require immunoblot testing. However, if early Lyme disease is strongly suspected, repeat the testing in 2–4 weeks. In contrast, confirm all positive or borderline results of EIA or IFA testing by Western immunoblot. For patients early in the disease (<4 weeks duration of symptoms) interpret both the IgM and IgG tests, but use only the IgG for later disease, since false-positive results may occur with the IgM immunoblot.

ED management

If Lyme disease is suspected, but typical EM is not present, obtain blood for a Lyme titer, CBC, and ESR or CRP. If the patient has a flu-like illness obtain EBV titers or a heterophile; obtain radiographs of any arthritic joints (see Arthritis, pp. 671–675). If the patient has meningeal signs or a change in mental status, perform a lumbar puncture and send the CSF for Lyme serology. An ECG is indicated if the patient has disseminated disease. Do not withhold antibiotic therapy while awaiting the confirmatory titer results in patients with suspected early disseminated or late disease.

Ticks attach themselves by secreting a chemical, as well as screwing themselves into the skin in a clockwise direction. To remove an attached tick intact, rub a cotton ball or gauze soaked in a warm soapy water solution directly over the tick, in a counter-clockwise circular motion to dissolve the chemical attachment and "unscrew" them from the skin.

Amoxicillin (50 mg/kg per day div tid, 3 g/day maximum, for 21 days) is the treatment for early disease in children <8 years of age. Give older children doxycycline (100 mg bid) or amoxicillin. Cefuroxime (30 mg/kg per day div bid, 500 mg bid maximum) is an acceptable alternative. Macrolides, including erythromycin and azithromycin, are not as effective and are indicated only for patients who are allergic to amoxicillin, doxycycline, and cefuroxime. Once antibiotic therapy is initiated, symptoms usually resolve within the first few days or week.

Treat Lyme meningitis, carditis, and polyarthritis with systemic toxicity with IV ceftriaxone, 100 mg/kg per day div q 12 h (2 g/day maximum). Bell's palsy without meningitis and monarticular arthritis may be successfully treated with oral antibiotics for 28 days. Use the IV regimen for patients who have not responded to oral therapy.

Ticks probably need to be attached for at least 24 hours to transmit the disease. In addition, not all deer ticks are infected. Even in endemic areas, only 1–4% of deer tick bites result in transmission of infection. Although recent evidence suggests that two doses of doxycycline 200 mg given 12 hours apart following removal of an engorged deer tick may be effective in preventing Lyme disease in adults, currently prophylactic administration of antibiotics following tick bites is not recommended for children.

Follow-up
- Early disease: 3–5 days

Indications for admission
- Meningitis
- Third-degree AV block
- Arthritis with systemic toxicity

Bibliography
American Academy of Pediatrics. Lyme disease. In Pickering LK, Baker CJ, Kimberlin DW, Long SS (eds), *Red Book: 2009 Report of the Committee on Infectious Diseases*, 28th ed. Elk Grove Village, IL: American Academy of Pediatrics, 2009, pp. 430–35.

DePietropaolo DL, Powers JH, Gill JM, Foy AJ: Diagnosis of lyme disease. *Am Fam Physician* 2005;72:297–304.

Feder HM Jr: Lyme disease in children. *Infect Dis Clin North Am* 2008;22:315–26.

Meningitis
Meningitis is an inflammation of the membranes surrounding the brain and spinal cord. It is caused by a wide variety of agents, most commonly bacteria and viruses. Fungi and parasites can be etiologies in immunosuppressed patients. Widespread use of the HIB conjugate vaccine in the United States has led to a dramatic reduction in *Haemophilus influenza* type B meningitis. Similarly, since the introduction of PCV7 for routine infant immunization in 2,000, the incidence of all invasive pneumococcal infections has decreased by 80% for children <2 years of age and approximately 90% for infections caused by vaccine-related serotypes. However, there has been an increase in invasive disease caused by serotypes not contained in PCV7 (serotype replacement).

Meningitis case-specific morbidity and mortality rates have not changed substantially in the last 20 years. Up to 20% of neonates and 5–10% of infants and children die from meningitis, and sequelae occur in 25–50% of survivors. The etiology of meningitis varies by age and immunologic status.

Neonates

The most common bacterial agents are group B *Streptococcus, Escherichia coli*, and *Listeria monocytogenes*. Congenital syphilis presents rarely as aseptic meningitis during the first few weeks of life. Viral etiologies include herpes simplex virus, enteroviruses, and, less commonly, cytomegalovirus.

One to 3 months

The most common bacterial agents in this age group are *Streptococcus pneumoniae* and *Neisseria meningitides*. Group B *Streptococcus* and *E. coli* meningitis may occur in infants up to 3 months of age. Viral pathogens are the same as for neonates.

Three months to 3 years

The principal bacterial causes of meningitis in this age group are *Streptococcus pneumoniae* and *Neisseria meningitides*, although universal vaccination is changing the epidemiology. However, also consider HIB meningitis in recent immigrants from parts of the world where the vaccine is not routinely used. Viral pathogens include the enteroviruses, arboviruses, and herpesviruses.

Three to 21 years

Viral pathogens (see Encephalitis, pp. 366–370) account for most of the cases of meningitis in this age group. Less common viral etiologies include Epstein-Barr virus, human herpesvirus 6, and influenza A and B viruses. Common bacterial causes are *S. pneumoniae* and *N. meningitides*. Extension from frontal sinusitis into the cranium can occur in adolescents, particularly males.

Immunocompromised patients (including patients with cancer undergoing systemic or intrathecal chemotherapy, brain surgery and/or bone-marrow transplantation) are also susceptible to meningitis caused by a variety of pathogens including *Cryptococcus* and other fungi, *Toxoplasma gondii*, tuberculosis, acanthamoeba, *Bacillus cereus, Stomatococcus* and *Listeria monocytogenes*. The frequency of Gram-positive meningitis infections among individuals with cancer appears to be increasing.

Clinical manifestations

Meningitis presents with fever, headache, neck pain and stiffness, nausea, vomiting, photophobia, and irritability. However, these signs and symptoms are often absent in immunocompromised patients. Young infants may exhibit irritability, somnolence, bulging fontanel, and low-grade fever. Nuchal rigidity in older children may be elicited by a positive Kernig's sign (while the hip and knee are flexed 90° degrees, passive knee extension produces spasm and/or pain) and Brudzinski's sign (passive neck flexion causes hip flexion). Seizures occur in 20–30% of patients, and the syndrome of inappropriate antidiuretic hormone (SIADH) occurs in 30–60%.

Table 14-8. Typical cerebrospinal fluid findings

	WBC/ mm³	%PMN	Protein mg/dL	Glucose mg/dL	RBC/ mm³
Infant <2 weeks	0–30	<60	<170	30–115	0–2
Child	0–6	0	20–30	40–80	0–2
Bacterial meningitis	>1,000	>50	>100	<30	0–10
Viral meningitis	100–500	<40	50–100	>30	0–2
Herpes meningitis	10–1000	<50	>75	>30	10–500
Tuberculous meningitis	100–500	<30	50–80	<40	–

Viral meningitis can mimic bacterial meningitis. During summertime enterovirus epidemics, older children with viral meningitis can have fever, headache, photophobia, myalgias, meningeal signs, and occasionally an exanthem that can be petechial. *Herpes simplex* virus can cause meningitis or encephalitis (pp. 366–370), particularly in newborns, frequently without skin lesions. HSV infection in a neonate (birth to 4 weeks of age) can present with irritability and seizures. Meningitis with milder, self-limited findings, usually associated with HSV-2, occurs in older infants and children. There may be an associated Bell's palsy, atypical pain syndromes, or trigeminal neuralgia.

Diagnosis

In bacterial meningitis, the CSF has a pleocytosis with a PMN predominance, decreased glucose, and elevated protein (Table 14-8). Immunocompromised individuals often have a muted CSF inflammatory response. Latex agglutination and immunoelectrophoresis may help identify the etiologic agent, particularly if the patient has received antibiotics before the lumbar puncture. Gram's stain and culture of the CSF remain the standard for establishing the etiologic diagnosis of bacterial meningitis. In viral meningitis, the spinal fluid has a normal glucose, slightly elevated protein, and a mononuclear predominance, although early in the course there can be a predominance of PMNs.

The bacterial meningitis score (BMS) is a simple multivariable model that uses the following objective parameters to distinguish bacterial meningitis from aseptic meningitis in patients ranging from 29 days to 19 years of age: Gram's stain of CSF showing bacteria, CSF protein ≥ 80 mg/dL, peripheral absolute neutrophil count $\geq 10,000$ cells/mm³, CSF absolute neutrophil count $\geq 1,000$ cells/mm³, and seizure prior to or at time of presentation. The BMS attributes 2 points for a positive Gram's stain and 1 point for each of the other variables. The negative predictive value of a score of 0 for bacterial meningitis is 100% (95% confidence interval: 97–100%), so that outpatient management may be considered for patients in the low-risk (BMS = 0) group. In contrast, a BMS ≥ 2 predicts bacterial meningitis with a sensitivity of 87% (95% confidence interval: 72–96%). Note that the widespread use of conjugate pneumococcal vaccination may further decrease the prevalence of pneumococcal meningitis and affect BMS post-test probability.

Table 14-9. Empiric antibiotic therapy for suspected bacterial meningitis

Age	Antibiotics
Neonates	
0–1 week	
<2 kg	Ampicillin 100 mg/kg per day div q 12 h *plus* cefotaxime 100 mg/kg per day div q 12 h
>2 kg	Ampicillin 150 mg/kg per day div q 8 h *plus* cefotaxime 150 mg/kg per day div q 8 h
1–4 weeks	Ampicillin 200 mg/kg per day div q 6 h *plus* cefotaxime 150 mg/kg per day div q 6 h
Older patients[a]	
4–8 weeks	Ampicillin 200 mg/kg per day div q 6 h *plus*:
	Ceftriaxone 100 mg/kg per day div q 12 h *or* cefotaxime 200 mg/kg per day div q 6 h
>8 weeks	Ceftriaxone 100 mg/kg per day div q12 h *or* cefotaxime 200 mg/kg per day div q 6 h

Note: [a]Give initial combination therapy with vancomycin (60 mg/kg per day div q 6 h, 1 g/day maximum) and cefotaxime or ceftriaxone to all patients >8 weeks of age with definite or probable bacterial meningitis, because of the increased prevalence of *S. pneumoniae* resistant to penicillin, cefotaxime, and ceftriaxone.

ED management

Maintain a high index of suspicion in a patient with any of the presenting signs and symptoms. One of the most important early features of meningitis is a subtle change in the patient's affect or state of alertness, which may be noted only by the parent. In an infant, check for a bulging fontanel; in any febrile child, check for meningeal signs, irritability, or lethargy. If meningitis is suspected, perform a lumbar puncture as quickly as possible. The only contraindications are increased intracranial pressure, impending respiratory failure, or extreme toxicity with inability to tolerate the procedure. Obtain a CT scan prior to lumbar puncture in the presence of papilledema, focal neurologic signs, or if frontal sinusitis is suspected (to exclude intracranial empyema or brain abscess with mass effect), but give antibiotics (Table 14-9) before obtaining the CT scan.

CSF analysis must include Gram's stain, protein, glucose, cell count with differential, and culture. Gram's stain of a CSF smear can be performed quickly, and is very helpful. Other important diagnostic tests include blood cultures, urinalysis and urine culture, CBC, platelet count, electrolytes, and liver enzymes. If viral meningitis is suspected, send CSF and throat and fecal swabs for viral culture. Also obtain serum and CSF for viral PCR, if available.

Monitor the patient for SIADH (pp. 186–189), which is characterized by hyponatremia, low serum osmolality, and high urine specific gravity. If the patient is not in shock or dehydrated, restrict IV fluids to two-thirds maintenance. However, give sufficient IV fluids to maintain a normal systolic blood pressure in order to preserve cerebral perfusion pressure.

Because of the increased prevalence of resistant *S. pneumoniae*, start with combination therapy with vancomycin (60 mg/kg per day div q 6 h) and cefotaxime or ceftriaxone to all patients ≥1 month of age with definite or probable bacterial meningitis. Give dexamethasone (0.6 mg/kg per day div q 6 h, 2 g/day maximum) before the first dose of antibiotics only if HIB is suspected. See p. 394 for the treatment of herpes.

Indications for admission
- Severely ill patients with meningitis of any etiology
- Suspected bacterial meningitis

Bibliography

American Academy of Pediatrics. Meningococcal infections, Pneumococcal infections. In Pickering LK, Baker CJ, Kimberlin DW, Long SS (eds), *Red Book: 2009 Report of the Committee on Infectious Diseases* 28th ed. Elk Grove Village, IL: American Academy of Pediatrics, 2009, pp. 455–63, 524–35.

Nigrovic LE, Kuppermann N, Macias CG, et al: Clinical prediction rule for identifying children with cerebrospinal fluid pleocytosis at very low risk of bacterial meningitis. *JAMA* 2007;297:52–60.

Safdieh JE, Mead PA, Sepkowitz KA, Kiehn TE, Abrey LE: Bacterial and fungal meningitis in patients with cancer. *Neurology* 2008; 70:943–7.

Mycoplasma pneumoniae infections

M. pneumoniae can infect people of any age. It is transmitted by respiratory droplets during close contact with a symptomatic person. Community-wide epidemics occur every 4–7 years, and there is no seasonal predilection. Because of its long incubation period, *M. pneumoniae* can spread within households for many months.

Clinical manifestations

M. pneumoniae is a leading cause of pneumonia in school-age children and adolescents but is uncommon in patients <5 years of age. After an incubation period of 2–3 weeks (range 1–4 weeks), the most common clinical syndromes in children are acute bronchitis and URIs, including pharyngitis and, occasionally, otitis media or myringitis. In approximately 10% of patients, pneumonia with cough and diffuse rales develops within a few days and lasts for 3–4 weeks. The cough is nonproductive initially but later may become productive, particularly in older children and adolescents. Approximately 10% of children with pneumonia also develop a rash, most often maculopapular. Malaise, fever, and occasionally headache are other nonspecific manifestations of infection. Abnormalities detected on radiography vary, but bilateral, diffuse infiltrates are common and focal abnormalities, such as consolidation, effusion, and hilar adenopathy, may occur.

Severe pneumonia with pleural effusion can develop in patients with predisposing conditions, including Down syndrome, immunodeficiencies, chronic cardiorespiratory disease, and sickle cell anemia. A substantial proportion of acute chest syndrome and pneumonia associated with sickle cell disease is attributable to *M. pneumoniae*.

Uncommonly, there may be CNS involvement, including aseptic meningitis, encephalitis, demyelinating disease, cerebellar ataxia, transverse myelitis, and peripheral neuropathy. *M. pneumoniae* encephalitis presents with fever, lethargy, and altered consciousness, while gastrointestinal and respiratory symptoms are less common. Other rare complications include myocarditis, pericarditis, erythema multiforme (that may progress to Stevens-Johnson syndrome), hemolytic anemia, and arthritis.

Diagnosis

Suspect that any school-age patient with pneumonia has *M. pneumoniae*. In contrast to pneumococcal pneumonia, the fever may be lower, auscultatory findings commonly will be diffuse (versus localized), and the patient may be hypoxic.

There is no readily available, rapid method for confirming an acute *M. pneumoniae* infection. Culture involves a special enriched broth or agar media and requires up to 21 days. Also, isolation of the *M. pneumoniae* may not indicate acute infection, because respiratory tract excretion of the organism may occur for several weeks after acute infection despite appropriate therapy. Serum cold hemagglutinin titers of >1:32 can be detected in about 50% of patients with *M. pneumoniae*-associated pneumonia by the beginning of the second week of illness. Therefore, a negative test result for cold agglutinins does not exclude the diagnosis. Immunofluorescence tests and enzyme immunoassays to detect *M. pneumoniae*-specific IgM and IgG antibodies are now widely available in commercial laboratories. Although the presence of IgM against *M. pneumoniae* confirms recent infection, these antibodies persist in serum for several months and may not necessarily indicate current infection; false-positive test results also occur.

Serologic confirmation of an acute infection requires a four-fold or greater increase in complement fixation antibody titer between acute and convalescent serum specimens. The antibody titer peaks at approximately 3–6 weeks and persists for 2–3 months after infection. Because *M. pneumoniae* antibodies may cross-react with some other antigens, interpret the results of these tests cautiously when evaluating febrile illnesses of unknown origin. Sensitive and specific PCR tests for *M. pneumoniae* appear to be superior to serology for diagnosis, although they are not widely available.

ED management

Acute bronchitis and upper respiratory tract illness caused by *M. pneumoniae* generally are mild and resolve without specific antimicrobial therapy. Treat pneumonia in children >5 years of age with erythromycin (40 mg/kg per day div qid, 1 g/day maximum), azithromycin (10 mg/kg, once on day 1, followed by 5 mg/kg q day on days 2–5), or clarithromycin (15 mg/kg div bid, 1 g/day maximum). Tetracycline (25–50 mg/day div tid or qid, 1 g/day maximum) and doxycycline (4 mg/kg per day div q 12 h, 200 mg/dose maximum) also are effective for use in patients ≥8 years of age. There is no evidence that treatment of nonrespiratory tract disease is beneficial.

Promptly institute therapy if a household contact of a patient with acute infection develops compatible lower respiratory tract illness. Although antimicrobial prophylaxis for exposed contacts is not recommended routinely, tetracycline and azithromycin for prophylaxis have been shown to decrease symptomatic diseases and reduce rates of transmission within families and institutions. Offer prophylaxis to people who are exposed intimately to a person acutely ill with *M. pneumoniae* and live in a house with a person who has an underlying condition that predisposes to severe *M. pneumoniae* infection, such as children with sickle cell disease.

Follow-up
- Every 48 hours until it is certain that the patient is not worsening or developing post-tussive emesis

Indications for admission
- Severe pneumonia
- Encephalitis or other severe complications of *Mycoplasma pneumoniae* infection

Bibliography

American Academy of Pediatrics. *Mycoplasma Pneumoniae* infections. In Pickering LK, Baker CJ, Kimberlin DW, Long SS (eds), *Red Book: 2009 Report of the Committee on Infectious Diseases*, 28th ed. Elk Grove Village, IL: American Academy of Pediatrics, 2009, pp. 473–5.

Atkinson TP, Balish MF, Waites KB: Epidemiology, clinical manifestations, pathogenesis and laboratory detection of *Mycoplasma pneumoniae* infections. *FEMS Microbiol Rev* 2008;32:956–73.

Christie LJ, Honarmand S, Talkington DF, et al: Pediatric encephalitis: what is the role of *Mycoplasma pneumoniae*? *Pediatrics* 2007;120:305–13.

Nontuberculous mycobacteria diseases

Nontuberculous mycobacteria (NTM) species are ubiquitous in nature and are found in soil, food, water, and animals. Although many people are exposed to NTM, only a small proportion develop chronic infection or disease. NTM species that most commonly cause infection in children in the United States are *Mycobacterium avium* complex or MAC (includes *Mycobacterium avium* and *Mycobacterium intracellulare*), *Mycobacterium fortuitum*, *Mycobacterium abscessus*, and *Mycobacterium marinum*. Other mycobacterial species that typically are not pathogenic have been associated with the presence of a foreign body. There is no definitive evidence supporting person-to-person transmission of NTM.

Clinical manifestations

The usual portals of entry of NTM infections are abrasions in the skin (e.g. cutaneous lesions caused by *M. marinum* after exposure to fresh or salt water in fish tanks, surgical incisions (especially for central catheters), oropharyngeal mucosa (the presumed portal of entry for cervical lymphadenitis), and respiratory tract (including tympanostomy tubes for otitis media). Most infections remain localized at the portal of entry or in regional lymph nodes.

NTM cause several syndromes in otherwise healthy children, most often cervical lymphadenitis and, less commonly, cutaneous infections, osteomyelitis, otitis media, and central catheter infections. MAC-associated pulmonary disease and, rarely, mediastinal adenitis and endobronchial disease can occur in otherwise healthy children, and have been linked to hot-tub use. Disseminated disease with MAC is a marker for an underlying immunodeficiency, usually HIV infection (pp. 374–380) or congenital immune deficiency.

Diagnosis

Definitive diagnosis of NTM disease requires isolation of the organism. Recovery of NTM from sites that usually are sterile (CSF, pleural fluid, bone marrow, blood, lymph node aspirates, middle ear or mastoid aspirates), surgically excised tissue, or from draining sinus tracts is the most reliable diagnostic test. Since these organisms are ubiquitous, contamination of cultures or transient colonization is common, particularly for specimens obtained from nonsterile sites (gastric washing specimens, a single expectorated sputum specimen, urine). Therefore, consult the mycobacteriology laboratory to ensure that culture specimens are handled and incubated correctly. MAC, *M. kansasii*, and *M. simiae* grow rapidly and typically can be recovered and identified in the laboratory within 3–7 days. Most other NTM, as well as *Mycobacerium tuberculosis*, often require weeks before sufficient growth occurs.

Because the purified protein derivative preparation (derived from *M. tuberculosis*) shares certain antigens with NTM species, patients with NTM infection can have a positive tuberculin skin test (TST) result (usually ≤ than 10 mm of induration, but can measure ≥15 mm).

ED management

Only limited controlled trials of antituberculous drugs have been performed in patients with NTM infections. Many NTM are relatively resistant in vitro, although this does not necessarily correlate with clinical response, especially with MAC infections. Whenever possible, remove any infected foreign bodies and debride localized lesions. In deciding the timing and choice of empirical treatment, consider the likely causative species, the site(s) of infection, the patient's underlying disease (if any), and the urgency of beginning treatment for presumptive tuberculosis while awaiting culture results. Consult with an infectious diseases expert in order to make the best choice of drugs, dosages, and duration of therapy.

For NTM lymphadenitis (most commonly associated with MAC) in otherwise healthy children, complete surgical excision almost always is curative. If surgical excision is incomplete, or for children with recurrent disease, consult with an infectious diseases expert. Therapy with clarithromycin combined with ethambutol or rifabutin may be beneficial, although these agents have not been studied in clinical trials.

Follow-up

- NTM adenitis (for resolution)

Indication for admission

- Severe pulmonary or disseminated NTM infections

Bibliography

Heyderman RS, Clark J: Clinical manifestations of nontuberculous mycobacteria. *Adv Exp Med Biol* 2006;**582**:167–77.

Jarzembowski JA, Young MB: Nontuberculous mycobacterial infections. *Arch Pathol Lab Med* 2008;**132**:1333–41.

Johnson MM, Waller EA, Leventhal JP: Nontuberculous mycobacterial pulmonary disease. *Curr Opin Pulm Med* 2008; **14**:203–10.

Parasitic infections

As many as 20% of Americans are infected with nematodes, and outbreaks of other parasitic infections are frequently reported. Immigrants from regions where parasites are endemic have high rates of infection, and travelers to endemic areas can become infested with a number of organisms.

Clinical presentation

Pinworms

Pinworm (*Enterobius vermicularis*) is the most common parasite in North America. Pinworms are acquired from ingestion of eggs, which hatch in the duodenum and migrate to the cecum, where they mature. Gravid adult females migrate to the perineum, where they lay eggs. The eggs are infective within 6 hours, and person-to-person transmission occurs. Anal pruritus is the most common complaint, although pinworms can be asymptomatic. Vaginal discharge and vulvar itching can rarely occur if a worm has migrated into the vagina. There is no tissue migration of the larvae and no eosinophilia.

Roundworms

Roundworm (*Ascaris lumbricoides*) infection, or ascariasis, is usually asymptomatic while the worm inhabits the intestine. Roundworms enter the body through ingestion of eggs, which hatch in the small intestine, releasing larvae that migrate by lymphatics or venules into the portal circulation, and then travel to the liver, right side of the heart, and lungs. The larvae penetrate the capillaries, enter the airways, travel over the glottis to the esophagus, and mature in the small intestine. Larval migration through the lungs can cause fever, cough, malaise, and eosinophilia. Other less common complications are intestinal obstruction, blockage of the bile or pancreatic ducts, appendicitis, intussusception, and volvulus. Ascaris can also affect the nutritional status of infected children by causing malabsorption of fats, proteins, and carbohydrates.

Hookworms

Hookworm (*Necator americanus* and *Ancyclostoma duodenale*) disease is found in the southern United States and tropical regions. The infection is acquired through exposure of skin to moist soil infested with larvae. Penetration of the soles of the feet by the larvae causes a papulovesicular dermatitis sometimes referred to as "ground itch." Pruritis and burning can occur and are most intense at the site of host entry, usually on the hands and feet. The larvae migrate through the lungs, enter the alveoli, and ascend the respiratory tree. This is usually associated with wheezing, dyspnea, and a nonproductive cough. The larvae can also migrate to the intestinal mucosa, causing mild abdominal pain, nausea, and anorexia. Blood loss occurs secondary to parasite-mediated destruction of capillaries in the intestinal mucosa; *A. duodenale* causes more blood loss than *N. americanus*. The subsequent blood loss leads to a hypochromic, microcytic anemia that can be accompanied by hypoalbuminemia. Eosinophilia is common.

Threadworms

The life cycle of the threadworm (*Strongyloides stercoralis*) involves parasitizing the human small intestine, where eggs are laid in the intestinal mucosa. These then hatch into rhabiditiform larvae which are shed in the stool. Some rhabditiform larvae transform into invasive filariform larvae before being excreted, enabling them to reinfect the host by invading the intestinal wall or the perianal skin.

There is a spectrum of illness due to *Strongyloides stercoralis*. Acute strongyloides can present with a local reaction at the site of larval entry, which can occur almost immediately and may last up to several weeks. Pulmonary symptoms such as a cough and tracheal irritation occur as larvae migrate through the lungs several days later. Gastrointestinal symptoms (diarrhea, anorexia, abdominal pain) begin about 2 weeks after infection, with larvae detectable in the stool after 3–4 weeks. Chronic infection is most often asymptomatic, but has been associated with intermittent vomiting, diarrhea, constipation, and recurrent asthma.

Hyperinfection is a syndrome of accelerated autoinfection generally secondary to immunocompromise, most commonly with HTLV-1 infection and corticosteroid use. Patients may have diarrhea, abdominal pain, ileus, or small bowel obstruction. Massive larvae penetration through the lungs results in pulmonary hemmorrhage and infiltrates on chest X-ray. Meningitis can occur and is usually due to enteric organisms. Hyperinfection is often complicated by bacteremia with gut organisms such as *Escheriachia coli*, *Klebsiella pneumoniae*, *Proteus mirabilis*, *Pseudomonas* spp. and *E. faecalis*.

Whipworms

Whipworm (*Trichuris trichuria*) infections are usually asymptomatic, although heavy infections can cause nausea, vomiting, diarrhea, abdominal distention and tenderness, rectal prolapse, and occasionally intestinal bleeding.

Giardia lamblia

Giardia lamblia is transmitted by oral ingestion of the cyst form of the parasite. Transmission can be water-borne, oral–fecal, and food-borne. Outbreaks of giardia have been associated with recreational water activities, drinking stream or lake water in mountainous areas of the United States, and day-care center attendance. Disease can range from asymptomatic passage of cysts to chronic diarrhea, malabsorption, and weight loss. However, most symptomatic patients experience a fairly characteristic syndrome of diarrhea with foul-smelling stools and gas, bloating, and abdominal cramps. Eosinophilia does not occur, fever is uncommon, and symptoms usually persist for days, but can linger for months. A syndrome of chronic malabsorption can occur with weight loss, protuberance of the abdomen, and anemia.

Entamoeba histolytica

Entamoeba histolytica infection is usually asymptomatic, although there can be a spectrum of disease. Patients with amebic colitis typically present with a several-week history of gradual onset of abdominal pain and tenderness, diarrhea, and bloody stools. Fever is usually absent or low grade. The presentation may mimic inflammatory bowel disease. Patients with liver abscesses are usually young males from endemic regions. Signs include right upper quadrant pain and fever, generally without a colitis. Spread to the lungs, pleura, and skin can occur by direct extension.

Malaria

Malaria is caused by *Plasmodium falciparum*, *P. vivax*, *P. ovale*, and *P. malariae*. The infection is usually transmitted by an infected mosquito, with an incubation period ranging from 6 to 30 days, depending on the *Plasmodium* species. *P. falciparum* is the most commonly seen malarial infection in the United States. Unless properly treated, *P. vivax* and *P. ovale* persist in a dormant stage ("hypnozoites") for several months to 5 years and can cause periodic relapses. Untreated *P. malariae* infection can also persist subclinically for more than 30 years with periodic recrudescence.

Malaria is a common cause of fever in tropical countries. Headache, fatigue, and abdominal discomfort can be followed by fevers. The classic malarial paroxysms, in which fever spikes, chills, and rigors occur at regular intervals, are unusual and suggest infection with *P. vivax* and *P. ovale*. Uncomplicated *P. falciparum* malaria carries a mortality rate of approximately 0.1%; however, once there is end-organ involvement or the parasitemia rises above 3%, mortality increases greatly. Cerebral malaria is a diffuse encephalopathy. If coma is present the mortality rises to 15% for children.

Hypoglycemia is a common complication of severe malaria in pregnant women and children. Quinine and quinidine can induce the release of insulin, thereby worsening hypoglycemia. Acidosis is a major feature of severe malaria and an important cause of death.

Diagnosis

The diagnosis of most parasitic infections can only be made if the possibility is considered. Recent travel to or emigration from endemic areas makes infestation likely. A history of chronic or bloody diarrhea, dysentery, weight loss, or cutaneous eruptions suggests the possibility of a parasitic infection. Eosinophilia suggests roundworms, hookworms, threadworms, and whipworms. Occasionally the patient or parent will report seeing a worm in the stool, vomitus, sputum, or perianal region. Often the physical examination is not helpful in determining the diagnosis.

A history of anal pruritus is virtually diagnostic of pinworm infestation. If confirmation is necessary, use the cellotape (unfrosted Scotch tape) test to demonstrate parasite eggs. The eggs adhere to the tape and can then be visualized under the microscope. The sensitivity of the test increases when performed in the morning prior to the first bowel movement and if multiple samples are collected on different days.

The diagnosis of other parasitic infections can be confirmed by microscopic examination of a fresh stool specimen ("stool for ova and parasites"). Ninety percent of infections will be detected by the collection of samples on three successive mornings. Refrigerate stool that cannot be examined within 1 hour.

Ascaris, Strongyloides, Trichuris, and hookworms are diagnosed by finding eggs in the stool. Stool identification requires patience and experience and is best performed by trained laboratory personnel. In addition, sputum may demonstrate the filariform or rhabditiform larvae and, occasionally, the eggs of *Strongyloides*. The diagnosis of chronic threadworm infection is made by serology. The diagnosis can be established by performing a direct stool examination, although this is negative in up to 50% of cases. A rapid detection ELISA test is available and is highly sensitive and specific.

Entamoeba is diagnosed by either a positive serology or needle aspiration. The IHA test for antiamebic antibody is 70% sensitive early in the illness and >95% sensitive during convalescence for the diagnosis of amebic liver abscess. Findings associated with a liver abscess include fever, leukocytosis, increased alkaline phosphatase, an elevated right hemidiaphragm, and a defect on CT scan.

Suspect malaria in any febrile patient returning from an endemic area, even if prophylaxis was taken. Order thick and thin blood smears or a rapid antigen detection test. It is important to determine the density of parsitemia, particularly for *P. falciparum* infections. Rapid, simple, sensitive, and specific antibody-based diagnostic stick or card tests (RDTs) can detect *P. falciparum*-specific histidine-rich protein (HRP) 2 or lactate dehydrogenase antigens. These tests can remain positive for weeks.

ED management

Although a pinworm infection may be treated on the presumptive evidence of rectal itching in the absence of local pathology, treat other parasitic infections only if positive identification is available. Otherwise, arrange for the collection of specimens and refer the patient for primary care follow-up.

Parasitic infections can now be treated with safe, effective, broad-spectrum medications. For additional information, consult with an infectious disease specialist or the *Red Book*. Appropriate follow-up includes repeated stool cultures 1–2 weeks after the completion of therapy.

Pinworms

Treat with a single dose of mebendazole (100 mg), pyrantel pamoate (11 mg/kg), or albendazole (400 mg); repeat in 2 weeks after the initial dose. If arranging for family members to be screened is difficult, provide simultaneous single-dose therapy for all household residents. Advise the parents to pay careful attention to hand hygiene, trimming of fingernails, and washing of bedclothes and underwear. When *Dientameba fragilis* is isolated from a stool specimen, a follow-up Scotch tape test is indicated to rule out concurrent pinworm infection.

Roundworms

Treat with a single dose of albendazole (400 mg), mebendazole (500 mg), or ivermectin (150–200 mcg/kg). Manage intestinal obstruction medically, but surgery is indicated if there are signs of peritonitis. Medical treatment may be effective for biliary tract complications.

Hookworms

Treat with a single dose of albendazole (400 mg) or mebendazole (500 mg), or a 3-day course of pyrantel pamoate (11 mg/kg per day).

Threadworms

The treatment of choice for acute or chronic strongyloides for patients weighing >15 kg is ivermectin (200 mcg/kg per day × 2 days). An alternative is a 7-day course of albendazole (400 mg bid). Consult with a pediatric infectious disease expert to arrange treatment for patients with hyperinfection syndrome.

Whipworms

Treat with a 3-day course of mebendazole (100 mg bid), albendazole (400 mg/day), or ivermectin (200 mcg/kg). Arrange for follow-up stool examination 6–8 weeks after treatment.

Giardia

Use metronidazole (15 mg/kg per day div tid × 5–7 days), tinidazole (50 mg/kg once), or nitazoxanide (1–3 years: 100 mg q 12 h × 3 days; 4–11 years: 200 mg q 12 h × 3 days; >12 years: 500 mg q 12 h × 3 days).

Amoebiasis

Treat asymptomatic colonization with a luminal agent, such as iodoquinol (30–40 mg/kg per day div tid × 20 days), paromomycin (25–35 mg/kg per day div tid × 7 days), or

Table 14-10. Prevention of malaria

	Drug	Dose
All Plasmodium *species in chloroquine-sensitive areas*		
Drug of choice	Chloroquine phosphate	5 mg/kg base once per week (300 mg base maximum)
All Plasmodium *species in chloroquine-resistant areas*		
Drug of choice	Atovaquone/proguanil	5–8 kg: ½ peds tab/day
		9–10 kg: ¾ peds tab/day
		11–20 kg: 1 peds tab/day
		21–30 kg: 2 peds tabs/day
		31–40 kg: 3 peds tabs/day
		>40 kg: 1 adult tab/day
or	Doxycycline	2 mg/kg per day (100 mg/day maximum)
or	Mefloquine	5–10 kg: ⅛ to ¼ tab/week
		11–20 kg: ¼ tab/week
		21–30 kg: ½ tab/week
		31–45 kg: ¾ tab/week
		>45 kg: 1 tab/week
Alternative	Primaquine phosphate	0.6 mg/kg base daily
Prevention of relapses		
Drug of choice	Primaquine phosphate	0.6 mg base/kg per d × 14 days

Source: Adapted with permission from Drugs for parasitic infections. *Med Lett* 2007 (Suppl), pp. 1–15.

diloxanide furoate (20 mg/kg per day div tid × 10 days). For invasive amebiasis (colitis, liver abscess), use metronidazole (35–50 mg/kg per day div tid × 7–10 days) plus either iodoquinol or paromomycin (as above). Liver abscess responds within 3–4 days, but larger cysts or cysts not responding to therapy may require drainage.

Malaria

Consult with an infecious diseases specialist or the *Red Book* for the treatment of malaria. For *P. falciparum* acquired in resistant areas use quinine sulfate (30 mg/kg per day div tid) for 3 or 7 days (treat patients from Southeast Asia for 7 days) plus doxycycline (4 mg/kg per day div bid) or clindamycin (20 mg/kg per day div tid). For severe *P. falciparum* give a loading dose of IV quinidine gluconate (10 mg/kg), followed by an infusion (0.02 mg/kg per min) until oral treatment can be started.

Treat *P. vivax* acquired in resistant areas with malarone or mefloquine, followed by primaquine phosphate.

Malaria prophylaxis is summarized in Table 14-10. For *P. vivax, P. malariae, P. ovale* and chloroquine-sensitive *P. falciparum* use chloroquine phosphate (5 mg/kg base once/

week). Patients with *P. vivax* and *P. ovale* also need primiquine phosphate (0.6 mg base/kg per day × 14 days) to prevent relapses. Patients with G6PD deficiency are at risk of hemolyzing if given primiquine; therefore, obtain a G6PD level prior to treatment. For this reason, do not give pregnant woman primiquine phosphate. For uncomplicated case of *P. falciparum* acquired in areas of chloroquine resistance use malarone (atovaqune/progguamil).

Follow-up
• Primary care follow-up at the completion of therapy

Indications for admission
• Dehydration or severe weight loss
• Extraintestinal amoebiasis
• Strongyloidiasis in immunocompromised patients
• Malaria with infection of greater than 5% of blood cells or any systemic complication

Bibliography
American Academy of Pediatrics. Drugs for parasitic infections. In Pickering LK, Baker CJ, Kimberlin DW, Long SS (eds), *Red Book: 2009 Report of the Committee on Infectious Diseases*, 28th ed. Elk Grove Village, IL: American Academy of Pediatrics, 2009, pp. 783–816.

Ashley E, McGready R, Proux S, Nosten F: Malaria. *Travel Med Infect Dis* 2006;4:159–73.

Cancrini G: Human infections due to nematode helminths nowadays: epidemiology and diagnostic tools. *Parassitologia* 2006;48:53–6.

Moon TD, Oberhelman RA: Antiparasitic therapy in children. *Pediatr Clin North Am* 2005;52:917–48.

Pertussis

Pertussis (whooping cough) is a highly communicable disease of the respiratory tract caused by *Bordatella pertussis*, for which humans are the only known host. The disease occurs worldwide and affects all age groups, but is recognized primarily in children and is most serious in young infants. Between 1993 and 2004, 86% of hospitalizations, 95% of cases requiring mechanical ventilation, and all fatalities were in infants <3 months of age.

Transmission occurs by droplets from a coughing patient and is most likely early in the illness. Pertussis is most common in the summer and fall and epidemics occur in 2–5 year intervals, suggesting that early childhood immunization does not prevent transmission of the organism. Unrecognized infection in adults (commonly manifested as a cough persisting for >2 weeks) is an important reservoir of infection for susceptible unimmunized or partially immunized child household contacts, in whom attack rates range from 70 to 100 percent. The safety and efficacy of Tdap against diphtheria, tetanus and pertussis have been demonstrated in individuals from adolescence through age 64.

Clinical presentation

The clinical presentation of pertussis varies by age. In older children, adolescents, and adults symptoms are milder, so that the diagnosis of pertussis is often not entertained.

After an incubation period of 7–10 days, the classic illness occurs in children 1–10 years old and consists of three stages: catarrhal, paroxysmal, and convalescent. The catarrhal stage lasts 2 weeks and resembles a URI with rhinorrhea, conjunctival injection, low-grade or no fever, and a mild cough that gradually worsens. In the paroxysmal stage, coughing increases in frequency and severity over a 2–4 week period. Repetitive, forceful coughs in a series of 5–10 occur during a single exhalation. These paroxysms are followed by a massive inspiratory effort producing the characteristic whoop, as air is inhaled forcefully through a narrowed glottis. Most young infants are unable to generate sufficient respiratory effort to whoop, so they are mistakenly diagnosed with a respiratory virus. Posttussive emesis, cyanosis, and apnea may occur. The paroxysms are exhausting and the patient may appear dazed and apathetic. The convalescent stage is characterized by less frequent coughing spells and decreased severity of episodes over a 1–2 week period.

Common complications associated with pertussis include pneumonia and otitis media. Others include seizures, activation of latent tuberculosis, ulceration of the frenulum of the tongue, epistaxis, melena, subconjunctival hemorrhages, subdural hematomas, rupture of the diaphragm, umbilical or inguinal hernia, rectal prolapse, dehydration, meningoencephalitis, the syndrome of inappropriate antidiuretic hormone secretion, apnea, and nutritional disturbances. The most important, but rare, systemic complication of pertussis is encephalopathy, whose cause is not known but is probably explained by hypoxia associated with coughing paroxysms.

Diagnosis

Whooping does not occur in all children, especially infants <6 months of age. In infants <2 months, coughing or choking, along with cyanosis and rhonchi upon initial ED evaluation, strongly predicts pertussis.

Suspect pertussis in any patient with coughing spasms and vomiting (especially posttussive), especially if the primary DTaP vaccination series has not been completed. Obtain a CBC to look for a leukocytosis with a lymphocytosis. The chest radiograph is usually normal, but may have some perihilar, lobar, and diffuse or patchy infiltrates. Definitive diagnosis is made by nasal culture or specific antibody studies. Alert the laboratory that you will be sending a nasal culture for pertussis, as they have to prepare the Bordet-Gengou medium and plate the specimen promptly. Obtain the specimen using a Dacron or calcium alginate swab. PCR testing on these specimens, or serology, can be used to diagnose an infection later in the course of the disease when culture results are often negative.

A pertussoid illness can be caused by adenovirus and B. parpertussis, but confirming an etiologic diagnosis is not crucial to proper management. Chlamydia pneumoniae presents with a staccato cough in an afebrile, tachypneic infant younger than 12 weeks of age (pp. 629–632). Rhinorrhea is usually absent, but eosinophilia and bilateral infiltrates on chest X-ray are characteristic. Also consider bronchiolitis (pp. 614–616), bacterial pneumonia, cystic fibrosis, tuberculosis (pp. 423–427), and an airway foreign body.

ED management

Prompt isolation of infants presumed to have pertussis may decrease the transmission of pertussis to other patients and hospital staff. Treatment consists of supportive therapy, avoidance of stimuli that trigger coughing attacks, maintenance of hydration and nutritional needs, and antibiotics.

Erythromycin (40–50 mg/kg per day div q 6 h for 14 days) reduces infectivity and, if started during the catarrhal stage, may reduce the severity of the illness. Azithromycin (10 mg/kg [maximum 500 mg] on day 1; 5 mg/kg [maximum 250] qd on days 2–5) may also be effective. If erythromycin is given, inform parents about the risks and signs of pyloric stenosis. Treat close contacts with either erythromycin or azithromycin, irrespective of immunization status. If the contact is unimmunized, or has had fewer than four doses of pertussis vaccine, begin or continue immunization according to the standard schedule. Also give a vaccine dose to a patient who received the third dose >6 months prior to exposure. If a patient <7 years of age has had four doses of pertussis vaccine, give a booster dose of DTaP, unless a dose has been given within the last 3 years.

Admit a patient who is under 6 months of age, as well as a patient of any age with cyanosis or respiratory distress. Isolate hospitalized patients with droplet precautions for 5 days after the initiation of treatment.

Follow-up
- Patient >6 months of age: immediately for cyanosis, otherwise every other day until the disease is no longer progressing

Indications for admission
- Cyanosis, respiratory distress, or feeding difficulties
- Suspected pertussis in an infant less than 6 months old

Bibliography

American Academy of Pediatrics. Pertussis. In Pickering LK, Baker CJ, Kimberlin DW, Long SS (eds), *Red Book: 2009 Report of the Committee on Infectious Diseases*, 28th ed. Elk Grove Village, IL: American Academy of Pediatrics, 2009, pp. 504–19.

Guinto-Ocampo H, Bennett JE, Attia MW: Predicting pertussis in infants. *Pediatr Emerg Care* 2008;24:16–20.

Munoz FM: Pertussis in infants, children, and adolescents: diagnosis, treatment, and prevention. *Semin Pediatr Infect Dis* 2006;17:14–19.

Rickettsial diseases

The rickettsial infections, Rocky Mountain spotted fever (RMSF), ehrlichiosis, Q fever, and the typhus fevers are infections that occur worldwide and throughout the United States. Since the signs and symptoms are variable, a high index of suspicion is needed to properly diagnose and manage these patients. The clinical manifestations and geographic distributions of ehrlichiosis and RMSF overlap. Ideally, these infections will be recognized early in their clinical course when antibiotic therapy is most effective. The absence of a history of a tick bite should not discourage considering a diagnosis of RMSF or ehrlichiosis. Signs and symptoms of rickettsial diseases are variable; therefore a high index of suspicion is needed to diagnose and manage patients appropriately.

Clinical presentation
Rocky Mountain spotted fever

RMSF is the most prevalent rickettsial disease in the USA. The principal vectors are the wood tick in the Western United States, the dog tick in the East, and the lone star tick in the

Southwest. About 600 cases are reported annually, most between April and September. Two-thirds of patients are younger than 15 years old. Although antibiotic therapy is effective treatment, the overall case fatality rate is 3.9%.

RMSF infection causes a systemic, small vessel vasculitis characterized by a rash, severe headache, confusion, and myalgias. The disease usually occurs 2–8 days after an infected tick bite and the onset may be either gradual or abrupt. Fever tends to be high (40–40.6°C; 104–105°F) and may oscillate. The rash appears on the second or third day of the illness, as small blanching erythematous macules which progress to become maculopapular and petechial and, in untreated patients, may become hemorrhagic and confluent. The rash appears peripherally first and then spreads to the trunk, with involvement of the palms and soles characteristic. Rarely, the rash may be absent. The patient may appear restless, irritable, apprehensive, and may become confused or comatose. Other neurologic symptoms include nuchal rigidity, photophobia, seizures, ataxia, spastic paralysis, VIth nerve palsy, and deafness. Congestive heart failure and arrhythmias are common. Occular manifestations include blindness, retinal edema, papilledema, and retinal hemorrhages and cotton wool spots. Other signs include edema of the hands and face, and gastrointestinal symptoms including nausea, vomiting, diarrhea, and abdominal pain.

Ehrlichiosis

Human ehrlichiosis, a tick-borne rickettsial disease, is caused by at least three distinct pathogens: *Ehrlichia chaffeensis* (human monocytotrophic ehrlichiosis [HME]), *Anaplasma phagocytophilum* (human granulocytotrophic anaplasmosis [HGA], formerly *Ehrlichia phagocytophila*), and *Ehrlichia ewingii* (ehrlichia ewingii ehrlichiosis). Although symptomatic ehrlichiosis tend to occur in much older individuals (>40 years of age), recent seroprevalence data suggest that *E. chaffensis* infection may be common in children. Most human infections occur between April and September (peak from May through July) yet cases may occur year-round. The incidence of reported cases seems to be increasing. Most human *E. chaffeensis* infections occur in the southeastern and south central United States. Infections caused by *E. chaffeensis* and *E. ewingii* are typically associated with the bite of the lone star tick (*Amblyomma americanum*), although cases have occurred beyond the geographic distribution of *A. americanum*, suggesting transmission by *Dermacentor variabilis* or other tick species. *Anaplasma phagocytophilum* is transmitted by the black-legged or deer tick (*Ixodes scapularis*), which also is the vector of *Borrelia burgdorferi* (the agent of Lyme disease), and most recognized HGE cases have originated from states with high rates of Lyme disease, particularly Connecticut, Minnesota, New York, and Wisconsin. Coinfections of anaplasmosis with Lyme disease and other tick-borne diseases, including babesiosis, have been reported. The mammalian reservoirs for the agents of human ehrlichiosis include white-tailed deer, white-footed mice, and Neotoma woodrats. In the western United States, *Ixodes pacificus* is the main vector for A. *phagocytophilum*.

Following an incubation period of 5–10 days after a tick bite (median, 9 days), all three infections cause acute, systemic, febrile illnesses accompanied by headache, chills or rigors, malaise, myalgia, arthralgia, nausea, vomiting, anorexia, and/or acute weight loss that are similar clinically to Rocky Mountain spotted fever except for (1) leukopenia, absolute lymphopenia, and neutropenia in HME; (2) neutropenia in HGA; (3) anemia; (4) hepatitis; (5) absence of vasculitis; and (6) rash less commonly. Diarrhea, abdominal pain, cough, or change in mental status are less frequent. A rash (variable in location and appearance, either macular, maculopapular, or petechial) typically develops approximately 1 week after onset of illness in approximately 60% of children with reported *E. chaffeensis* infection and <10% of people with *A. phagocytophilum* infection. *E. chaffeensis* characteristically causes more severe illness than *A. phagocytophilum*. More severe manifestations include pulmonary infiltrates, bone marrow hypoplasia, respiratory failure, encephalopathy, meningitis, disseminated intravascular coagulation, spontaneous hemorrhage, and renal failure. Anemia, hyponatremia, thrombocytopenia, increased serum hepatic transaminase concentrations, and cerebrospinal fluid abnormalities (i.e. pleocytosis with a predominance of lymphocytes and increased total protein concentration) are common. Characteristic cytoplasmic inclusion bodies (morulae) can sometimes be seen in the leukocytes. Whereas recovery typically occurs without sequelae after 1 to 2 weeks of symptoms, neurologic complications may occur in some children after severe disease, and fatal infections have been reported. Secondary or opportunistic infections may occur in severe illness, resulting in possible delayed recognition of ehrlichiosis and appropriate antimicrobial treatment. People with underlying immunosuppression are at greater risk of severe disease.

Q fever

This disease, caused by *Coxiella burnettii*, primarily infects animals. Close contact with infected animals and consumption of raw milk are risk factors, while epidemics occur when infected animals are slaughtered. The disease has been diagnosed in an increasing number of children younger than 3 years old, usually beginning abruptly with chills, high fever, malaise, myalgias, and intractable headache, 9–20 days after exposure to the organism. Pneumonia, with cough and chest pain, occurs in 50% of cases. Hepatosplenomegaly is common and gastroenteritis may also be present, but there is no rash. Complications include endocarditis and hepatitis.

Typhus fevers

Three rare diseases make up this group, louse-borne typhus, Brill-Zinsser disease and murine flea-borne typhus. The first two are transmitted by the louse and the third by the rat flea. Symptoms of louse-borne typhus occur 1–2 weeks after a bite by an infected louse. High fever, headache and a rash occur, with a rash that appears on the trunk and spreads peripherally. Complications are uncommon but include myocardial and renal failure, gangrene, parotitis, pleural effusion, and pneumonia. Brill–Zinsser disease is a relapse of louse-borne typhus occurring years after the initial episode. Murine typhus is a disease of rats that is accidentally transmitted to humans by a rat flea bite. The symptoms are similar to those of louse-borne typhus but usually are milder.

Diagnosis
RMSF

Consider RMSF if the patient has "flu in the summertime." The diagnosis can be confirmed by a four-fold change in titer between paired acute and convalescent serum specimens (indirect immunofluorescence antibody, enzyme immunoassay, compliment fixation, latex agglutination, indirect hemagglutination, or microagglutination tests). These tests are seldom diagnostic before the seventh day of the illness. Other nonspecific laboratory findings that can suggest the diagnosis earlier include a normal or low WBC, thrombocytopenia, and hyponatremia. Anemia and elevated liver enzymes and BUN may also be present. Definitive diagnosis can also be made by fluorescent or peroxidase tagged antibody testing of a skin biopsy of the rash.

Consider measles (characteristic rash, conjunctivitis, cough, coryza) and meningococcemia (central petechial rash), typhoid fever (headache, malaise, anorexia, abdominal pain, hepatosplenomegaly, rose spots), leptospirosis (fever, chills, myalgias, conjunctival suffusion, contact with infected mammals), rubella (characteristic rash), scarlet fever (sandpaper rash, Pastia's lines, circumoral sparing, fever, pharyngitis), disseminated gonococcal disease (migratory arthritis, maculopapular rash), infectious mononucleosis (fever, exudative pharyngitis, lymphadenopathy, hepatosplenomegaly, atypical lymphocytosis), secondary syphilis (maculopapular rash including the palms and soles, condyloma, lymphadenopathy, fever, splenomegaly, headache, arthralgias), rheumatic fever, enteroviral infections, ITP, TTP, immune complex vasculitis, and hypersensitivity reactions.

Ehrlichiosis

As with RMSF, consider ehrlichiosis if the patient has "flu in the summertime." The diagnosis can then be documented by a four-fold increase in antibody titer by indirect immunofluorescence assay between paired acute and convalescent serum samples, PCR, detection of morulae seen on peripheral smear, or a single high serum antibody titer.

Ehrlichia or *Anaplasma* organisms can be cultured from blood or cerebrospinal fluid. Acute and convalescent serum specimens (ideally collected 2–3 weeks apart) can be submitted for indirect immunofluorescent antibody (IFA) assay. Alternatively, PCR amplification of specific DNA from a clinical specimen (in particular, peripheral blood of patients in the acute phase of ehrlichiosis) seems sensitive, specific, and promising for early diagnosis. These tests are available in reference laboratories, in some commercial laboratories and state health departments, and at the CDC. A single positive serum IFA antibody titer ($\geq$1:64) in conjunction with the detection of intraleukocytoplasmic microcolonies of bacteria (morulae) in a patient with a consistent history is considered diagnostic. New techniques, including enzyme immunoassays using recombinant ehrlichial antigens and multiplex fluorescence-detection PCR, are under investigation. Nonspecific laboratory abnormalities include mild leukopenia, anemia, thrombocytopenia, hyponatremia, and elevated liver enzymes.

Q fever

Diagnosis of Q fever is made by immunofluorescent enzyme immunoassay, complement fixation, and immune adherence hemagglutination antibody tests using paired serum samples.

Typhus

The typhus fevers can be diagnosed by a four-fold change in antibody titer between paired serum specimens obtained during the acute and convalescent phases. PCR may also be useful, if available.

ED management

Rickettsial infections may be severe or fatal in untreated patients, and initiation of therapy early in the course of disease helps minimize complications of illness. Patient outcome is best if therapy is started before day 5 of illness (before paired antibody titer results are available). Therefore, do not delay treatment while waiting for a diagnosis. If a presumptive diagnosis of rickettsial diseases is made, immediately treat all patients, regardless of age, with doxycycline (4 mg/kg per day div bid, 100 mg bid maximum). Despite concerns regarding dental staining with tetracycline-class antimicrobial agents in young children, doxycycline provides superior therapy for this potentially life-threatening disease. Available data suggest that courses of doxycycline for <14 days do not cause significant discoloration of permanent teeth. Because tetracyclines are contraindicated in pregnancy, rifampin has been used successfully in a limited number of pregnant women with documented HGE. Treatment of RMSF, ehrlichiosis and Q fever should continue for at least 3 days after defervescence for a minimum total course of 5–10 days. Q fever may relapse and require repeated courses. Treat louse-borne typhus until the patient is afebrile for 72 hours (usually 7–10 days) and flea-borne typhus with a single dose of doxycycline. Restrict fluids to two-thirds maintenance if hyponatremia develops.

Follow-up

• Tick-borne disease: 2–3 days

Indications for admission

• Suspected RMSF
• Severely ill patient with ehrlichiosis, Q fever, or one of the typhus fevers

Bibliography

American Academy of Pediatrics. *Ehrlichia* and *Anaplasma* infections (human ehrlichiosis). In Pickering LK, Baker CJ, Kimberlin DW, Long SS (eds), *Red Book: 2009 Report of the Committee on Infectious Diseases*, 28th ed. Elk Grove Village, IL: American Academy of Pediatrics, 2009, pp. 284–7.

Chapman AS, Bakken JS, Folk SM, et al: Tickborne Rickettsial Diseases Working Group; CDC: Diagnosis and management of tickborne rickettsial diseases: Rocky Mountain spotted fever, ehrlichiosis, and anaplasmosis–United States: a practical guide for physicians and other health-care and public health professionals. *MMWR Recomm Rep* 2006;55(RR-4):1–27.

Razzaq S, Schutze GE: Rocky Mountain spotted fever: a physician's challenge. *Pediatr Rev* 2005;26:125–30.

Toxic shock syndrome

Staphylococcal toxic shock syndrome (SaTSS) and streptococcal TSS (SpTSS) are clinically overlapping acute febrile illnesses caused by a group of specific toxins (superantigens) produced by *Staphylococcus aureus* and invasive group A streptococci, respectively. Initially SaTSS was almost exclusively seen with high-absorbency tampon use during menses; such "menstrual cases" still account for about one-half of all SaTSS cases.

Following the withdrawal of certain tampon brands, "non-menstrual" cases of SaTSS became more widely recognized. These are most commonly associated with surgical and postpartum wound infections, cutaneous and subcutaneous lesions (especially of the extremities, perianal area, and axillae), and respiratory infections following influenza.

SpTSS usually develops in the setting of deep skin and soft tissue group A strep infections and has been associated with primary varicella and NSAID use. However, widespread varicella vaccination has virtually eliminated this risk factor. Mortality rates for children with SpTSS and SaTSS are 5–10% and 3–5%, respectively. Early recognition is critical to prevent significant morbidity and mortality.

Clinical presentation

For SaTSS, the onset of the illness is usually abrupt. Initial symptoms can include headache, fever, chills, malaise, conjunctival hyperemia, sore throat, myalgias, muscle tenderness, fatigue, vomiting, diarrhea, abdominal pain, orthostatic dizziness, syncope, and rash. Progression to multiple organ involvement and shock can occur. In the first 1–2 days, diffuse erythroderma, severe watery diarrhea, decreased urine output, and cyanosis and edema of the extremities may be present. Somnolence, confusion, irritability, agitation, and hallucinations may occur as a result of cerebral ischemia or edema or toxin-mediated CNS effects.

Diffuse macular erythroderma and mucosal erythema usually develop, and within 1–2 weeks desquamation occurs, especially on the fingers, palms of the hands, toes, and soles of the feet. In menstrual TSS, edema and erythema of the inner thighs and perineum may occur. In postoperative TSS, which occurs within 12–48 hours following surgery, there may be little or no inflammation of the surgical wound.

Mild episodes of SaTSS may occur, particularly in menstruating women who use tampons. These women may develop fever, headache, sore throat, diarrhea, vomiting, orthostatic dizziness, syncope, and myalgias. Recurrences can occur and are associated with either inadequate treatment and/or impaired toxin-specific antibody responses by the patient.

While the clinical characteristics of SpTSS (fever, profound hypotension, shock, and multiorgan failure) are similar to those found with SaTSS, the two differ in several respects. The onset of SpTSS often spans several days and there is no vomiting, diarrhea, or significant encephalopathy as seen in SaTSS. Severe diffuse or localized pain which usually precedes tenderness or physical findings of soft tissue infection is the most common initial symptom in SpTSS. Skin involvement is variable, and presents as an extremely painful sandpaper-like rash, rather than erythroderma.

Diagnosis

The diagnosis of both staphylococcal and streptococcal TSS is made on the basis of clinical criteria and presentation. The case definition of SaTSS is based on the following major diagnostic criteria from the CDC:

1. Fever $\geq$38.9°C (102°F)
2. Rash: diffuse macular erythroderma
3. Desquamation: 1–2 weeks after onset of illness, particularly of palms, soles, fingers, and toes
4. Hypotension: systolic BP <90 mmHg for adults; <5th percentile by age for children <16 years old; orthostatic drop in diastolic BP $\geq$15 mmHg; orthostatic syncope or dizziness
5. Involvement of three or more of the following organ systems:
   a. gastrointestinal: vomiting or diarrhea at onset of illness
   b. muscular: severe myalgias or CPK level > twice the upper limit of normal
   c. mucous membranes: vaginal, oropharyngeal, or conjunctival hyperemia
   d. renal: BUN or serum creatinine greater than twice the upper limit of normal or $\geq$5 WBC/hpf in the absence of a urinary tract infection.
   e. hepatic: total bilirubin, AST or ALT > twice the upper limit of normal

   f. hematologic: platelets $<100,000/mm^3$
   g. central nervous system: disorientation or alteration in consciousness, without focal neurologic signs, when fever and hypotension are absent
6. Negative results on the following tests: blood, throat, or CSF cultures (although blood cultures may be positive for *S. aureus* in 5% of cases) and, if obtained, serologic tests for RMSF, leptospirosis, or measles.

A probable case of SaTSS is defined by having five of the six clinical findings described above. A confirmed case is defined by having all six clinical findings unless the patient dies before desquamation can occur.

Laboratory abnormalities include a CBC differential with >90% neutrophils, thrombocytopenia, anemia, prolongation of the PT and PTT, sterile pyuria, elevated BUN and creatinine, elevated AST or ALT, profound hypocalcemia, hypoproteinemia, and an elevated CPK. The majority of these tests will return to normal within 7–10 days of disease onset. A major difference between the two syndromes is the fact that blood cultures are frequently positive in SpTSS (60%) but negative in SaTSS (95%).

More than 80% of patients with menstrual TSS will have *S. aureus* cultured from the cervix or vagina. The same proportion of patients with nonmenstrual TSS will have *S. aureus* cultured from the focus of infection. Since 10–20% of healthy individuals may have *S. aureus* isolated from the anterior nares or vagina and approximately 10% of such strains can produce TSS toxin 1, the identification of toxin-producing *S. aureus* is only presumptive evidence of infection. Moreover, although methicillin-sensitive *S. aureus* (MSSA) are most commonly isolated in these cases, community-acquired strains of methicillin-resistant *S. aureus* (CA-MRSA) have also been found to produce superantigen toxins and cause TSS. In contrast, most nosocomial strains of MRSA do not produce these toxins.

The differential diagnosis of TSS includes clinical entities in which rapid onset of fever, rash, hypotension, and multisystem involvement occur. Septic shock, particularly meningococcemia, is often associated with a petechial or purpuric rash. Consider streptococcal and staphylococcal scarlatiniform eruptions (normotensive, sandpaper-like rash), Kawasaki disease (normotensive, no erythroderma, nonpurulent conjunctivitis), and conditions associated with particular exposure histories and clinical findings, such as leptospirosis (animal urine, conjunctival suffusion), RMSF (tick bite, petechial or purpuric rash of distal extremities), typhoid fever (travel, indolent course, hepatosplenomegaly, leukopenia), dengue hemorrhagic fever/shock syndrome (travel, mosquito bite, hepatomegaly, encephalopathy, hemoconcentration), and measles (travel, unimmunized, cough, coryza, conjunctivitis),

ED management
If TSS is suspected, provide oxygen, assist with ventilation as needed, and establish IV access with a large-bore cannula. Begin volume replacement and vasopressors, if necessary. Give 20 mL/kg of NS or lactated Ringer's solution immediately, and repeat the fluid bolus as needed until the vital signs return to normal (see Shock, pp. 24–27). The patient may require large amounts of fluid replacement. Continue close monitoring of vital signs and fluid status in the intensive care unit for moderately or severely ill patients.

Obtain blood for CBC, platelets, electrolytes, BUN, creatinine, liver transaminases, PT and PTT, CPK, and blood cultures. Order a urinalysis and obtain cultures of the throat, stool, and urine. If there is an alteration in the level of consciousness, perform a lumbar puncture (if the patient can tolerate the procedure).

For empiric TSS therapy, treat with both an anti-staphylococcal antibiotic such as nafcillin (150 mg/day div q 6 h) to eradicate the focus of toxin-producing *S. aureus* and *S. pyogenes* and clindamycin (40 mg/kg per day div q 6 h) to reduce toxin production. In areas with a high prevalence of community-associated MRSA, use vancomycin (40 mg/day div q 6 h) instead of nafcillin. For documented SpTSS, use the combination of penicillin and clindamycin.

Remove any vaginal tampons or wound packing. Explore and drain infected wounds, even if there are no obvious signs of inflammation; immediate surgical consultation may be required for more extensive infections such as necrotizing fasciitis. Obtain cultures of the cervix, vagina, or incisional wounds.

Indication for admission

*   Suspected toxic shock syndrome

Bibliography

American Academy of Pediatrics. Staphylococcal infections, group A Streptococcal infections. In Pickering LK, Baker CJ, Kimberlin DW, Long SS (eds), *Red Book: 2009 Report of the Committee on Infectious Diseases*, 28th ed. Elk Grove Village, IL: American Academy of Pediatrics, 2009, pp. 601–15, 616–28.

Byer RL, Bachur RG: Clinical deterioration among patients with fever and erythroderma. *Pediatrics* 2006;118:2450–60.

Young AE, Thornton KL: Toxic shock syndrome in burns: diagnosis and management. *Arch Dis Child Educ Pract Ed* 2007;92:ep97–100.

Tuberculosis

Tuberculosis (TB) is caused by *Mycobacterium tuberculosis*, an acid fast microorganism with the ability to infect humans and then persist in a dormant state for many years. It can also cause active disease within a few months, particularly in infants or immunocompromised hosts. About 4–6% of the population of the United States (15 million people) is infected, compared to a rate of 20–45% worldwide. Risk factors include immigration from high-risk countries, lower socioeconomic status, HIV infection, drug use, homelessness, travel to high-risk areas, history of incarceration, and employment in healthcare facilities.

Children exposed to adults in any of the high-risk groups are at increased risk of infection. In recent years, foreign-born children living in the United States have had more than a ten-fold higher infection rate compared to US-born patients. Patients born in Mexico, the Philippines, Vietnam, Somalia, Haiti, Russia, and the newly independent states of the former Soviet Union account for almost two-thirds of all foreign-born children with TB in the United States.

Mycobacterium bovis is being recognized increasingly as a cause of pediatric tuberculosis in the United States, particularly among children who travel from or who consume unpasteurized dairy products imported from Mexico. *M. bovis* infections also account for a significant proportion of all cases of extrapulmonary TB in children.

The major route of transmission of TB is respiratory. For children, household contacts are the most likely source, with infection rates around 20%, while short, casual contact is usually not sufficient for infection. Children <12 years old are generally not contagious, despite having active disease, because they tend not to develop pulmonary cavities (that contain a high concentration of tubercle bacilli) and lack the adult tussive force to expel infectious droplets.

With latent tuberculosis infection, tubercle bacilli establish an infection, usually in the lung, but there is no clinical or radiologic evidence of disease, despite a positive PPD. These individuals are not contagious.

Five to ten percent of individuals with latent tuberculosis infection will progress to tuberculosis disease during their lifetime. Tuberculosis disease is usually manifested by clinical symptoms and/or radiologic findings, most often (75%) pulmonary in children. Extrapulmonary disease may occur in any part of the body, with 70% of cases presenting as lymphatic disease.

Clinical presentation

Primary tuberculosis

Most childhood TB is primary. The hallmark is the Ghon complex, consisting of a primary pulmonary focus (site of initial seeding), lymphangitis, and regional (hilar or paratracheal) lymphadenopathy. There is no typical clinical presentation of primary TB, which is most often subtle despite significant radiographic changes. When symptoms do occur, there may be low-grade fever, cough, anorexia, weight loss, irritability, malaise, or fatigue. The cough in childhood TB is typically mild and nonproductive. Infrequently, primary TB may progress rapidly and mimic bacterial pneumonia, with sudden onset of high fever, cough, and respiratory distress, with or without pleural effusions. Infants may have wheezing and respiratory distress, or develop a purulent pneumonia from bronchial obstruction secondary to enlarged hilar nodes.

Chronic pulmonary tuberculosis

Reactivation disease is the most common form of TB in adults and occurs most commonly during adolescence. It results from activation of latent bacilli in untreated individuals with latent tuberculosis infection. Manifestations include a cough that may become productive with blood-streaked sputum, fever, weight loss, night sweats, and malaise.

Lymphadenitis

Tuberculous lymphadenitis presents with discrete, painless, usually bilateral cervical lymph node enlargement that is indistinguishable from other causes of lymphadenitis. The nodes may become matted, develop a sinus tract, or become fluctuant. In contrast to suppurative adenitis, the nodes are usually not warm.

Meningitis

Most cases of TB meningitis occur within 6 months of the onset of pulmonary disease, particularly in children 4 months to 6 years of age. Unlike bacterial meningitis, the initial course is indolent, with nonspecific symptoms such as headache, poor feeding, low-grade fever, and apathy. The CSF has a mononuclear predominance with an elevated protein and low glucose. If untreated, signs of increased intracranial pressure develop later in the course. The chest radiograph is positive in 50% of cases.

Miliary tuberculosis

The patient initially is febrile and may appear toxic, although there may be no localizing signs. Later, diffuse lymphadenopathy and hepatosplenomegaly develop. The chest radiograph, which may initially be negative, displays mottling within 1–3 weeks of presentation.

Congenital tuberculosis

Congenital disease occurs rarely and only in infants whose mothers have disseminated tuberculosis (e.g. miliary or meningitis). The infant presents with failure to thrive, jaundice, anemia, hepatosplenomegaly, ear discharge, cough, or respiratory distress during the first few weeks of life.

Other infections

Tuberculosis can also involve bones, eyes, ears, skin, kidneys, adrenals, or the genitourinary or gastrointestinal tracts.

Diagnosis

The tuberculin skin test (TST), containing 5 tuberculin units (TU) of purified protein derivative (PPD), administered intradermally, is the only practical tool for diagnosing tuberculosis infection in asymptomatic patients. However, there is emerging evidence that T-SPOT.TB and QuantiFERON-TB Gold blood-based assays may have higher specificity than the tuberculin skin testing, particularly for older children who are close contacts of adult TB cases. If a patient has pneumonia, persistent cough, pleural effusion, failure to thrive, persistent fever for more than 2 weeks, meningitis, or cervical lymphadenitis, place a 5 TU PPD (intermediate strength, 0.1 ml) intradermally, to raise a wheal, on a nonhairy surface of the forearm. Also place a TST on recent contacts of an individual with active TB. Arrange for a health professional to read the PPD in 48–72 hours. Note the amount of induration, not erythema, in millimeters that develops.

A negative TST result does not exclude latent tuberculosis infection or tuberculosis disease. TST reactivity cannot be demonstrated initially in approximately 10% to 15% of immunocompetent children with culture-documented disease. Factors such as young age, poor nutrition, immunosuppression, certain viral infections (especially measles, varicella, and influenza), recent tuberculosis infection, and disseminated tuberculosis disease can diminish TST reactivity. Measles vaccination causes suppression of the skin test reaction 48–72 hours after vaccination, but the vaccine may be given at the same time as the skin test. Many children and adults co-infected with HIV and *M. tuberculosis* have diminished or no reactivity to a TST. However, control skin tests to assess cutaneous anergy are no longer routinely recommended.

Greater than 5 mm

Consider positive if the patient is immunocompromised, had recent contact with a case of active TB, or has a chest X-ray consistent with TB.

Greater than 10 mm

Consider positive in children >4 years of age, immigrants from high-prevalence countries in Asia, Africa, and Latin America, residents or employees of nursing homes, correctional facilities, and homeless shelters. Also consider positive in intravenous drug users, healthcare workers, and patients with Hodgkin's disease, lymphoma, diabetes, renal failure, malnutrition, or those who are taking chronic steroids or other immunosuppressive agents.

Greater than 15 mm

Consider positive in children >4 years without any risk factors.

False-positive reactions to TST may occur in patients sensitized to nontuberculous mycobacteria and in patients previously vaccinated with BCG. These reactions tend to be <10 mm, and can be useful in diagnosing atypical mycobacterial infections. Individuals with a true-positive TST will remain reactive for life; do not administer repeat TSTs.

Obtain a chest X-ray for all patients with a positive TST. Individuals with latent tuberculosis infection have no findings. Patients with active disease often have hilar or paratracheal adenopathy, perihilar hazy densities, and/or pleural thickening. Alveolar densities, atelectasis, and effusion may be present. Apical lesions and, rarely, cavitation may be present in individuals with chronic TB.

In children able to produce sputum, collect three samples for culture on consecutive mornings to identify *Mycobacterium tuberculosis* and to determine drug susceptibility. The AFB smear is rarely positive in children with TB disease and laboratory findings are nonspecific (elevated ESR, anemia, and a CBC with a high percentage of monocytes). In infants and young children unable to produce sputum, obtain gastric washings early in the morning, to prevent swallowing large amounts of saliva and tears, which may dilute the sample.

Thoracocentesis may be useful to provide relief from dyspnea, tachypnea, or hypoxia caused by a large pleural effusion or to obtain fluid for analysis. Although pleural fluid rarely yields a positive TB culture, tuberculosis is characterized by a high protein and LDH and several hundred WBC/mm^3 (lymphocyte predominance).

Tuberculous adenitis is usually firm and nontender, unlike suppurative adenitis, which is usually warm and tender. Children with nontuberculous mycobacteria (NTM) adenitis usually have TST reactivity <10 mm and a negative chest X-ray. However, since therapy for TB and NTM differs, obtain tissue for mycobacterial culture either by fine-needle aspiration or whole-node excisional biopsy to differentiate between TB and NTM.

ED management

Consider local susceptibility patterns and the likelihood of infection with a multi-drug-resistant (MDR) strain when deciding upon the empiric therapy for TB. MDR TB is more likely in individuals who are urban residents; Asian, African, or Hispanic immigrants; homeless; HIV-positive; or who have a history of prior antituberculosis chemotherapy. When isoniazid (INH) is used, supplement with pyridoxine if the patient is poorly nourished, pregnant, or a breast-fed infant. Routine liver function testing is unnecessary unless there is concurrent hepatic disease, liver tenderness, jaundice, an INH dosage >10 mg/kg per day is used in combination with rifampin, or there is disseminated (miliary or meningeal) disease.

Since children with primary TB are rarely infectious, respiratory precautions and hospital isolation are not always necessary. However, use AFB precautions, and place the patient in a single room with use of a mask until the sputum AFB smear (or culture, in cases of multi- or extensively drug-resistant TB) is documented and the cough abates for children (particularly adolescents) with AFB smear-positive sputum or with a productive cough. Instruct all symptomatic adult household members who accompany the patient to wear a mask, undergo immediate chest radiograph screening (when possible), and be isolated if they are symptomatic. Immediately refer all close contacts of a TST-positive patient for evaluation for TB.

Positive TST, negative chest radiograph

Treat with INH (10 mg/kg per day, 300 mg maximum) for 9 months. If there is a known contact with INH-resistant TB, give rifampin (10–20 mg/kg per day, 600 mg maximum). Give pyridoxine supplementation (25–50 mg/day) to breast-fed infants, pregnant adolescents, symptomatic HIV-positive children, and children on meat- and milk-deficient diets.

Positive chest radiograph

Admit the patient and arrange for drainage of a symptomatic effusion. Begin three-drug therapy with INH, rifampin, and pyrazinamide (PZA, 20–40 mg/kg per day, 2 g maximum) for 2 months, followed by 4 months of INH and rifampin by directly observed therapy for presumed drug-susceptible TB. If drug resistance is possible, add ethambutol (15–25 mg/kg per day) or streptomycin (20–40 mg/kg per day) until susceptibilities of the patient or index case are known. For drug-susceptible *M. bovis* inherently resistant to pyrazinamide, treat with INH and rifampin for 9 months.

Extrapulmonary TB

Signs of CNS involvement mandate a head CT and lumbar puncture. For bone and joint disease, miliary TB, and TB meningitis, give 12 months of therapy with INH, rifampin, PZA, and either ethambutol (substitute ethionamide for meningitis, due to superior CNS penetration) or streptomycin. Also give corticosteroids for TB meningitis.

Lymphadenitis with a positive TST

Obtain a chest radiograph and initiate therapy as for pulmonary TB, along with antibiotics for staphylococcal coverage because superinfection is common with TB adenitis. Excisional biopsy and culture are frequently necessary.

Recent contacts of a known case

Place a TST, obtain a chest radiograph, and begin prophylactic therapy (as for positive TST negative chest radiograph) at the initial visit, if the contact is <35 years old. Continue therapy despite a negative skin test, and repeat the PPD 10 weeks after discontinuation of contact with the index case. If it is again negative, discontinue therapy. If the TST is positive, treatment depends on the result of the chest radiograph and index case susceptibilities.

Pediatric dosing

Avoid INH suspension because of gastrointestinal side effects; crushed pills given with semisolid food are better tolerated. Rifampin is available in capsules that a pharmacist can make into a suspension, but do not give with food.

Follow-up

- TB infection without disease: primary care follow-up in 1–2 weeks

Indication for admission

- Suspected active TB disease

Bibliography

American Academy of Pediatrics. Tuberculosis. In Pickering LK, Baker CJ, Kimberlin DW, Long SS (eds), *Red Book: 2009 Report of the Committee on Infectious Diseases*, 28th ed. Elk Grove Village, IL: American Academy of Pediatrics, 2009, pp. 680–701.

Marais BJ, Pai M: Recent advances in the diagnosis of childhood tuberculosis. *Arch Dis Child* 2007;**92**:446–52.

Molicotti P, Bua A, Mela G, et al: Performance of QuantiFERON-TB testing in a tuberculosis outbreak at a primary school. *J Pediatr* 2008;**152**:585–6.

Diseases transmitted by exposure to animals (zoonoses) or arthropod vectors

Zoonotic infections are transmitted from animals to humans by direct contact, scratch, bite, inhalation, contact with urine or feces, and ingestion of contaminated food, water, or feces. In addition, bites from arthropod vectors may cause severe or life-threatening infection in children. Consider zoonoses in patients who interact with pets, wild rodents, and other animals, after certain environmental or recreational exposures, or after international travel. They are caused by a wide variety of pathogens, including viruses, *Rickettsia*, bacteria, fungi, and parasites. Salmonellosis, campylobacteriosis and shigellosis (see pp. 241–243), the most frequently encountered zoonotic infections in children, are transmitted most often by food, but can also be acquired from pets, wildlife, or infected humans.

Selected zoonoses encountered in North America and Hawaii and that can cause severe or fatal disease include those linked to animal (Table 14-11) and arthropod vectors. Certain of these diseases that are related to exposure to wildlife (rabies, p. 726) or wild rodents

Table 14-11. Zoonoses associated with animals

Disease	Transmission	Clinical findings	Diagnosis and treatment
Brucellosis (*Brucella* species)	Inhalation of or contact with contaminated birth products, ingestion of dairy products through skin wounds	Fever, sweats, malaise, headache, myalgias. Complications: meningitis, endocarditis, osteomyelitis	Diagnosis: culture of blood or bone marrow, acute and convalescent serum Treatment: doxycycline and rifampin Use TMP-SMX if <8 years old
Avian influenza (H5N1)	Contact with infected chickens, birds or swine Aerosols (markets, slaughter houses)	Initially: high fever and influenza-like symptoms Occasional: diarrhea, vomiting, abdominal pain, chest pain, bleeding from the nose and gums Rapid progression to acute respiratory distress or multiorgan failure (kidney and	Diagnosis: contact the CDC Influenza Branch (800-CDCINFO; axk0@cdc.gov) Treatment: http://www.who.int/ csr/disease/ avian_influenza/ guidelines/ ClinicalManagement07. pdf

Table 14-11. (cont.)

Disease	Transmission	Clinical findings	Diagnosis and treatment
		heart) within 6 days (range 4–3) Lymphopenia, leukopenia, ↑ALT/AST, ↓platelets	Use appropriate respiratory and isolation
Leptospirosis (*Leptospira* species)	Contact with or ingestion of water, food, or soil contaminated with urine from rodents, other animals Sporadic common-source outbreaks throughout the US and Hawaii	Acute onset of fever with chills, headache, nausea, vomiting, nonpurulent conjunctivitis, myalgias, transient rash Self-limited (approximately 90%) May progress to severe illness with jaundice and renal failure (Weil syndrome), cardiac arrhythmias, hemorrhagic pneumonitis, or circulatory collapse (fatality rate 5–40%)	Diagnosis: culture of blood, CSF or urine, acute and convalescent serum, immunohistochemical techniques or PCR Treatment: mild – doxycycline; severe – penicillin IV (alternative: ceftriaxone)
Plague (*Yersinia pestis*)	Bites of rodent fleas Direct contact with infected animals: rodents, cats, squirrels, prairie dogs Pneumonic: person-to-person Most common in western third of United States	Abrupt onset of fever, chills, headache, myalgias, malaise Bubonic: acute onset of fever and painful swollen regional lymph nodes (buboes), most commonly inguinal Bioterrorism-related plague would manifest chiefly as pneumonic When left untreated, plague often will progress to over-whelming sepsis with renal failure, acute respiratory distress syndrome, hemodynamic instability, DIC	Diagnosis: Culture (observe biosafety precautions) Immunofluorescent or Gram's stain of blood, sputum, or node aspirates Acute and convalescent serum for antibody PCR and immunohistochemical staining (if available) Treatment: streptomycin or gentamycin Alternatives: tetracycline, doxycycline, TMP-SMX chloramphenicol (preferred for meningitis)
Psittacosis (*Chlamydophila psittaci*)	Inhalation of aerosols from feces of infected pet birds and poultry	Acute febrile respiratory tract infection with fever, dry cough,	Diagnosis: acute and convalescent serum, PCR, or respiratory tract

Table 14-11. (cont.)

Disease	Transmission	Clinical findings	Diagnosis and treatment
		headache, and malaise Radiographic findings: severe interstitial pneumonia more severe than expected from clinical findings Rarely: pericarditis, myocarditis, endocarditis, hepatitis	culture (observe biosafety precautions) Treatment: tetracyclines; use macrolides for patients <8 years
Q fever	See pp. 419–420		
Rabies	See pp. 368–369		
Rat-bite fever (*Streptobacillus moniliformis*)	Bites and ingestion of food, water, or milk contaminated by rodents, cats, and weasels	Fever, chills, rash (maculopapular or petechial), arthritis (nonsuppurative, migratory in approximately 50%), arthralgias, myalgias, vomiting, headache, and adenopathy Regional adenopathy without ulceration at bite site Complications: soft tissue and organ abscesses, pneumonia, myocarditis, endocarditis, meningitis	Diagnosis: culture of blood, synovial fluid, abscesses, or bite lesion Treatment: penicillin G IV/IM; doxycycline or streptomycin for penicillin-allergic patients. Addition of streptomycin may be useful
Severe acute respiratory syndrome coronaviruses (SARS-CoVs)	Contact with civet cats or potentially other animal species Possible person-to-person Travel in an area where SARS is known to be occurring	Early: fever, malaise, and myalgias Later: cough and/or shortness of breath, often in the absence of upper respiratory tract symptoms Diarrhea in ≥25% Pneumonia or acute respiratory distress syndrome (ARDS) in nearly all infected adults (10% case:fatality ratio) Children <12 years of age: shorter, less severe course, with rare progression to ARDS and death	Diagnosis: guidance is available at the CDC web site www.cdc. gov/ncidod/sars/. Treatment: no proven effective or recommended treatment for SARS-CoV Steroids may decrease mortality of ARDS Observe strict air-borne, droplet, contact precautions

Table 14-11. (cont.)

Disease	Transmission	Clinical findings	Diagnosis and treatment
Tularemia (*Francisella tularensis*)	Tick or deerfly bite Contact with infected animal:wild rabbits, voles, muskrats, moles, sheep, cattle or cats Bites or scratch from cats Aerosolization of tissues or excreta.	Abrupt onset of fever, chills, myalgias, headache Several tularemic syndromes: ulceroglandular (most common), pharyngeal, oculoglandular, and typhoidal forms	Diagnosis: acute and convalescent serology DFA or PCR in ulcer exudate or aspirate material Culture: blood, skin, ulcers, lymph node drainage, gastric washings, or respiratory tract secretions Observe biosafety precautions Treatment: streptomycin, gentamycin, or amikacin
Typhus	See pp. 419–420		
Yersiniosis (*Yersinia enterocolitica* and *pseudotuberculosis*)	Ingestion of food, water or milk contaminated by various animal species Person-to-person fecal-oral (rare)	*Y. enterocolitica*: fever and diarrhea in young children Pseudoappendicitis in older children and adults Bacteremia occurs most often in children <1 year of age and immunocompromised older children *Y. pseudotuberculosis*: fever, scarlatiniform rash, and pseudoappendiceal abdominal pain Ultrasound of edema in the terminal ileum and cecum can help to distinguish pseudoappendicitis from appendicitis Stool often contains leukocytes, blood, and mucus	Diagnosis: culture (stool, throat swabs, and blood) and serum antibody Treatment: treat patients with septicemia, extra-intestinal infections and immunosuppression Usually susceptible to TMP-SMX, aminoglycosides, cefotaxime, fluoroquinolones, and tetracyclines Clinical benefit uncertain for patients with enterocolitis, or pseudoappendicitis syndrome

(plague) are rare. Others related to pet exposure (cat scratch disease, pp. 363–365) or ticks (Lyme disease, pp. 398–401) are common. Included in the table are infections that are most commonly acquired abroad (Q fever, pp. 419–420; brucellosis), including those increasingly reported during the past few years (dengue, pp. 365–366) and those that have not yet been reported in the United States, but could potentially be introduced or imported (H5N1 and SARS).

Bibliography

American Academy of Pediatrics. Diseases transmitted by animals (zoonoses) In Pickering LK, Baker CJ, Kimberlin DW, Long SS (eds), *Red Book: 2009 Report of the Committee on Infectious Diseases*, 28th ed. Elk Grove Village, IL: American Academy of Pediatrics, 2009, pp. 864–70.

Lieberman JM: North American zoonoses. *Pediatr Ann* 2009;38:193–8.

Rabinowitz PM, Gordon Z, Odofin L: Pet-related infections. *Am Fam Physician* 2007;76:1314–22.

Chapter

15

Ingestions

Stephen M. Blumberg and Carl Kaplan

Contributing author
Katherine J. Chou: Carbon monoxide

Evaluation of the poisoned patient

Acute pediatric poisonings generally present in preschool-age children or in adolescents. Children under five typically ingest a household product or pharmaceutical accidentally, while adolescents may ingest medications or illicit substances recreationally or in the context of a suicide attempt.

Clinical presentation

Young children often present to the emergency department without symptoms, so it is important to differentiate exposures (e.g. found in an area with pills available) from actual ingestions. Ingestions in this age group usually involve a single medication or household product. Toddlers often taste objects that appear attractive and may share them with a younger companion. Many medications are remarkably similar in color, size, and shape to candy. With liquids, parents may report children taking a single or multiple swallows of a substance before spitting it out. Estimate the volume of a swallow to be approximately 0.25 ml/kg. Occasionally, previously well children may present with an acute change in mental status or a clinical decompensation. A high level of suspicion is required to discover and manage a surreptitious ingestion in these cases.

Adolescent ingestions are generally non-accidental. The ingestions may be impulsive whether stemming from recreational use or psychiatric disorders (mood disorders, schizophrenia, substance abuse), and the history may be unclear at the time of presentation. These ingestions often involve multiple medications, illicit drugs, and alcohol, and frequently result in symptoms. It is also important to consider that the patient may be despondent over an unwanted pregnancy or attempting to self-induce an abortion. The patient rarely shares this information, so obtain a pregnancy test in all female overdoses.

If the toxin is known, the physician must assess the likelihood of toxicity. Most household products (Table 15-1A) and plants (Table 15-1B) are nontoxic. However, some common plants are toxic (Table 15-1C), and several medications can be fatal to infants in very small amounts (Table 15-2). In addition, several specific medications may cause delayed toxicity (Table 15-3).

Symptoms may develop from toxins that are ingested, inhaled, or absorbed through the skin. This is especially important when evaluating neonates or infants. Their relatively large body surface area to mass ratio is such that toxicity from dermal or mucosal absorption of solvents, alcohols, topical anesthetics, and pesticides is more likely.

Diagnosis

In most instances, the diagnosis may be made based on history. In adolescents, and occasionally in toddlers, the parent or child may intentionally conceal the diagnosis or the ingestion may not be known. In these cases, the diagnosis requires a high index of

Table 15-1A. Readily available products with limited toxicity

Abrasives	Fertilizer
Adhesives	Fish food
Air fresheners	Glowsticks
Aluminum foil	Glues and pastes
Antacids	Golf ball (core may cause mechanical injury)
Antibiotics (few exceptions)	Gum
Antiperspirants	Greases
Ash, fireplace	Gypsum
Baby product cosmetics	Hand lotions and creams
Ballpoint pen inks	Hydrogen peroxide (medicinal 3%)
Bath oils	Incense
Bathtub floating toys	Indelible markers
Battery (dry cell)	Ink (without aniline dyes)
Bath oil (castor oil and perfume)	Lip balm
Bleach (<5% sodium hypochlorite)	Lipstick
Bubble bath soaps (detergents)	Lubricant
Calamine lotion	Lubricating oils
Candle (beeswax or paraffin)	Magic markers
Caps (toy pistols)	Makeup (eye, liquid facial)
Chalk (calcium carbonate)	Mineral oil
Charcoal briquettes	Motor oil
Cigarette or cigar ashes	Newspaper
Clay (modeling)	Paraffin
Cosmetics	Pencil (lead-graphite, coloring)
Crayons (marked AP or CP)	Perfumes
Dehumidifying packets (silica or charcoal)	Petroleum jelly (Vaseline)
Detergents (phosphate type, anionic)	Phenolphthalein laxatives (Ex-Lax)
Deodorants	Photographs
Deodorizers (spray and refrigerator)	Plaster
Elmer's glue	Plastic
Erasers	Play-Doh
Etch-A-Sketch	Porous-tip ink marking pens
Eye makeup	Putty (<60 g)
Fabric softeners	Rouge

Table 15-1A. (cont.)

Rubber cement	Styrofoam
Saccharin	Sunscreen preparations
Shampoos	Sweetening agents (saccharin, cyclamate, aspartamine)
Shaving creams and lotions	Teething rings
Sheetrock	Thyroid hormone
Shoe polish (most do not contain aniline dyes)	Toilet water
Silica gel	Toothpaste (without fluoride)
Silly putty (99% silicones)	Wallboard
Soap (handsoap only)	Watercolor paints
Soil	Wax
Spackles	Zinc oxide ointment

suspicion. Consider a poisoning in any previously well child with change in mental status, lethargy, hallucinations, delirium, seizures, dysrhythmia, or coma.

In the critically ill child, symptomatic care must be initiated immediately with the history obtained at the same time. The first priority in the critically ill child is the ABCs, including, IV/IO access and monitoring. Empiric therapy for common disorders, such as dextrose for hypoglycemia and naloxone for opioid toxicity, can then be considered. After assessment of vital signs and initiation of therapy, the specific toxin may be determined by physical findings and/or laboratory data, and specific care may be rendered.

In less acute situations, or after stabilization, a thorough physical examination focusing on vital signs, mental status, pupillary responses, bowel sounds, and skin and mucosal findings may lead to identification of a specific exposure.

The unconscious patient

1. Assess the patient's respirations and oxygen saturation. If they are not adequate, perform a jaw lift, insert a nasopharyngeal or oral airway (if tolerated), and suction any secretions. If necessary, initiate bag-mask ventilations while preparing to intubate the patient, preferably with a cuffed endotracheal tube.
2. Secure one or more large-bore IV lines or an intraosseous line.
3. Measure the blood pressure and pulse. If there are clinical signs of hypoperfusion (poor capillary refill, pallor, cool extremities), give a rapid bolus (20 mL/kg) of normal saline or Ringer's lactate (may be repeated twice), and if possible place the patient in the Trendelenburg position.
4. Obtain an ECG, and initiate continuous cardiorespiratory monitoring.
5. Although it may be clear that the patient is an overdose or ingestion victim, assess the level of alertness, pupillary responses, gag reflex, muscle tone, deep tendon reflexes, and examine the head and neck carefully for evidence of injury while maintaining the cervical spine in neutral position.

Table 15-1B. Household plants with limited toxicity

African violet (*Saintpaulia ionantha*)	Lipstick plant (*Aeschynanthus lobbianus*)
Aluminum plant (*Pilea*)	Inch plant (*Tradescantai*)
Aralia, false (*Dizygotheca elegantissima*)	Magnolia bush
Baby's tears	Monkey plant (*Ruellia makoyana*)
Begonia (botanical name)	Moses-in-a-boat (*Rhoea spathacea*)
Bloodleaf plant (*Iresine*)	
Boston fern (*Nephrolepsis exata*)	Palm
Bridal veil	Parlor palm (*Chamaedorea elegans*)
Cattail (*Acalypha hispida*)	Patient Lucy
Chinese evergreen	Peacock plant (*Calathea makoyana*)
Christmas cactus (*Zygocactus truncatus*)	Peperomia (botanical name)
Coleus (botanical name)	Piggy-back plant (*Tolmiea menziesiti*)
Corn plant (*Dracaena*)	Pilea (botanical name)
Creeping Charlie (*Pilea nummularifolia* or *Plectranthus australis*)	Pink polka dot plant (*Hypoestes sanguinolenta*)
Crocus (spring blooming) *Crocus* spp.	Plectranthus (botanical name)
Dandelion (*Taraxacum officinale*)	Prayer plant (*Maranta leuconeura kerchoveana*)
Devil's walking stick (*Aralia*)	Primula
Donkey tail (*Sedium morganianum*)	Rattlesnake plant (*Calathea insignis*)
Dracaena spp. (corn plant)	Rose (*Rosa* species)
Dusty miller (*Cineraria*)	Rose begonia (*Begonia semperflorens*)
Dwarf cactus	Rose of Sharon
Dwarf palm (*Chamaedorea elegans*)	Rubber plant (*Ficus elastica*)
Emerald ripple	Sensitive plant (*Mimosa pudica*)
Gardenia	Snake plant (*Sanservieria*)
Geranium (*Pelargonium*)	Snapdragon (*Antirrhinum*)
Grape hyacinth	Spider plant (*Anthericum* or *Chlorophytum cosmosum*)
Hawaiian Ti (*Cordyline terminalis*)	String of hearts (*Creopegia woodii*)
Hens and chicks (*Echeveria* or *Sempervivum tectorus*)	Swedish ivy (*Plectranthus australis*)
Hibiscus	Umbrella plant (*Brassaia actinophylla*)
Honeysuckle (*Lonicera*)	Violets (*Saintpaulia ionantha*)
Impatiens	Wandering Jew (*Zebrina pendula*)
Jade plant (*Crassula argentea*)	Wax plant (*Hoya*)
Kalanchoe (pregnant plant)	Weeping fig (*Ficus benjamina*)
Lady's slipper	Zebra plant (*Aphelandra squarrosa*)
Lilac (*Syringa*)	

Table 15-1C. Common poisonous plants

Plant	Poisonous part
Indoor plants	
Aroids (*Dieffenbachia, Monstera*)	Leaves
Aroids (*Philodendron, Spathiphyllum*)	Leaves, stems
Mistletoe (*Phoradendron serotinum*)	Berries
Poinsettia (*Euphorbia pulcherrima*)	Milky sap
Outdoor plants – trees	
Black cherry (*Prunus serotina*)	All, except ripe fruit flesh
Black locust (*Robinia pseudoacacia*)	Seeds, leaves, inner bark
Mulberry (*Morus* spp.)	Unripe fruits and milky sap
Outdoor plants – shrubs and bedding plants	
Azalea (*Rhododendron* spp.)	All parts
Boxwood (*Buxus* spp.)	Leaves
Caladium (*Caladium* spp.)	All parts
Cardinal flower (*Lobelia cardinalis*)	All parts
Castor-bean (*Ricinus communis*)	Seeds
Heavenly-bamboo (*Nandina domestica*)	Berries (potentially)
Hollies (*Ilex* spp.)	Berries, when eaten in quantity
Hydrangea (*Hydrangea* spp.)	Bark, leaves, flower buds
Jimson weed (*Datura stramonium*)	All parts
Lantana (*Lantana camara*)	Unripe fruits
Lobelia (*Lobelia* spp.)	All parts
Madagascar periwinkle (*Catharanthus roseus*)	All parts
Mountain-laurel (*Kalmia latifolia*)	All parts
Oleander (*Nerium oleander*)	All parts
Pokeweed (*Phytolacca americana*)	All mature parts
Rhododendron (*Rhododendron* spp.)	All parts

Source: Adapted with permission from Krings A: Department of Botany, North Carolina State University, Raleigh, NC.

6. Remove the patient's clothing to facilitate the examination, to look for signs of trauma, and search for pill containers.
7. Measure the temperature and, if possible, weigh the patient. A soft rectal thermometer probe measures extremes of temperature beyond the ranges of glass or digital thermometers.
8. Obtain an ABG to assess the adequacy of ventilation and the acid–base status.

Table 15-2. One pill can kill: highly toxic drugs and poisons

Drug/poison	Potentially fatal dose	Toxic dose for a 10 kg child	Toxicity
Benzocaine	20 mg/kg	2 mL of 10% gel	Methemoglobinemia, seizures
Calcium antagonists (Verapamil)	40 mg/kg	1–2 tabs	Bradycardia, hypotension, seizures, hypoglycemia
Camphor	100 mg/kg	5 mL of 20% solution	Seizures, CNS and respiratory depression
Chloroquine	30 mg/kg	1 tab	Seizures, arrhythmia, hypokalemia
Codeine	20 mg/kg	3 tabs	CNS and respiratory depression, bradycardia
Clonidine		1 tab or 1 patch	CNS and respiratory depression, bradycardia
Diphenoxylate (Lomotil)	1.2 mg/kg	2 tabs	CNS and respiratory depression
Hydrocarbons (aspiration)	One swallow		Pneumonitis, CNS depression
Lindane	6 mg/kg	2 tsp of 1% lotion	Seizures, CNS depression
Methylsalicylate (oil of wintergreen)	200 mg/kg	1/2 tsp	CNS depression, seizures, hypotension
Phenothiazines (chlorpromazine)	20 mg/kg	1 tab	CNS depression, seizures, arrhythmias
Quinidine	50 mg/kg	2 tabs	CNS depression, seizures, arrhythmias
Selenious acid (gun bluing agent)	20 mL	one swallow	CNS depression, arrhythmias, seizures
Sulfonylureas (Glyburide)	1 mg/kg	2 tabs	Hypoglycemia
Theophylline	50 mg/kg	1 tab	Seizures, arrhythmias
Tricyclic antidepressants (imipramine)	15 mg/kg	1 tab	Seizures, arrhythmias, hypotension

9. Obtain blood specimens for rapid blood glucose, CBC, liver function tests, serum electrolytes, carboxyhemoglobin (if CO poisoning cannot be ruled out by history), and methemoglobin (if cyanosis is present). Also, draw and hold tubes for type and screen and further serum tests as indicated.

10. Give 0.5 g/kg of glucose to any unresponsive patient either empirically or in response to a low bedside measured glucose.

Table 15-3. Delayed toxicity

Drug	Onset	Toxicity
Acetaminophen	24–72 h	Hepatic necrosis
Acetonitrile (acrylic nail remover)	12–24 h	Cyanide toxicity
Aspirin (enteric coated)	up to 8–12 h	Seizures, hyperthermia, acidosis, ↓ BP
Astemizole	up to 24 h	Ventricular arrhythmias
Calcium channel blockers (sustained release)	6–12 h	Cardiovascular collapse, bradycardia, ↓ BP
Diphenoxylate/atropine (Lomotil)	up to 12–24 h	Respiratory depression
Lithium	6–14 h	Seizures, bradycardia, asystole
MAO inhibitors	up to 12 h	Cardiovascular collapse
Methanol	12–24 h	Acidosis, blindness
Mushrooms		
Amanita, Glaerina	6–24 h	Hepatic necrosis
Lepiota	6–24 h	Hepatic necrosis
Gyromitra	6–12 h	Seizures, hepatic necrosis
Cortinarius	2–17 days	Renal failure
Naphthalene	1–5 days	Hemolytic anemia
Organophosphates (sulfur-containing)	days[a]	Cholinergic toxidrome, seizures, cardiac arrest
Sulfonylureas		
Chlorpropamide	up to 48 h	Hypoglycemia
Glipizide/glyburide	up to 24 h	Hypoglycemia
Thyroid hormone	6 h -11 days	Adrenergic symptoms
Tricyclic antidepressants	up to 6–24 h[b]	Seizures, arrhythmias, cardiovascular collapse

Notes: [a] Delayed toxicity with sulfur-containing organophosphates (e.g. parathion, chlorpyriphos) occurs because the compound is stored in adipose tissue and slowly released. Most patients with delayed toxicity have at least mild symptoms within the first 6 hours after ingestion.
[b] Severe arrhythmias and cardiovascular collapse may occur several days after ingestion if the patient becomes symptomatic. An asymptomatic patient with a normal heart rate at 6 hours is unlikely to develop toxicity.

In addition, delayed symptoms may occur when: medications form concretions (e.g. theophylline, aspirin, iron, meprobamate, bromides); are packaged in sustained-release formulations (calcium channel blockers, theophylline, acetaminophen, lithium); are ingested with medications that slow gastrointestinal motility (anticholinergics, opioids).

Table 15-4. Important history

Where was the patient found?
Whom has the patient visited recently?
Who has visited the patient's home recently?
Is anyone in the home taking any medications or herbals?
Is anyone else in the home suffering from headaches, seizures, fevers, or other illnesses?
Are there any pills, pill bottles, or other open containers in the house (including the garbage), or were any unusual odors noticed?
Does anyone in the house use any unusual chemicals for work or hobbies?
Was a suspect substance or pharmaceutical in the original container, or was it transferred into another one?
Was there more than one suspect substance in a container?
Was the patient given milk, clear liquids, syrup of ipecac, or food prior to arrival?
Has the patient vomited since the suspected ingestion?

11. Give naloxone 0.1 mg/kg, maximum 2.0 mg (preferably IV, but can be given IM, SC, or ET) either empirically or to correct the miosis and respiratory depression seen in opioid toxicity. If there is no response within 1–2 minutes, give a second dose. A positive response may last only 30 minutes, so repeated doses or a continuous IV infusion at 2/3 the effective dose are indicated in special situations. If habitual use is suspected in an adolescent, lower the initial dose to 0.05–0.1 mg, increasing to 0.4 mg, and then to 2.0 mg, so as to not precipitate acute withdrawal.

12. Obtain urine by catheter for dipstick examination, urine toxicology, and, in adolescent females, a pregnancy test.

13. Consider gastrointestinal decontamination as indicated if the airway is maintainable and bowel sounds are present.

In a stable or stabilized patient, attempt to ascertain the precise toxicologic diagnosis. If the ingestion was witnessed, determine the specific substance, amount, and time of the ingestion. It may be important to contact someone at the home to check information on pharmaceuticals, or to contact the pharmacy where prescriptions are typically filled. Refer to Table 15-4 for information to include in the history.

Perform a thorough physical exam (Table 15-5) including assessment of the pupils, mucosal membranes, heart, lungs, abdomen, skin, and a thorough neurologic exam (level of consciousness, pupils, motor, reflexes, and gag reflex). Certain poisons manifest consistent and unique sets of vital signs and physical exam findings, grouped into "toxidromes" (Table 15-6). Distinctive odors may also help make the diagnosis (Table 15-7).

A comatose patient with symmetric EOMs, pupillary reflexes, and motor responses probably has a toxic-metabolic basis for the coma, although hypoglycemia and toxic alcohols can cause focal motor deficits. Assume that pupillary inequality signifies a structural intracranial process. Miosis strongly suggests opioid or organophosphate toxicity. Mydriasis with reactive pupils occurs in sympathomimetic toxidromes, such as cocaine or

Table 15-5. Physical examination findings

Finding	Drugs/toxins
Vital signs	
Hyperthermia	Salicylates, amphetamines, anticholinergics, cocaine, theophylline, phencyclidine, tricyclics
Hypothermia	Barbiturates, phenothiazines, opioids, ethanol, GHB, hypotension from any cause
Tachycardia	Amphetamines, cocaine, caffeine, anticholinergics, ethanol, theophylline, hypotension from any cause, hypoglycemia, iron, phenothiazines, cannabis, ethanol or opioid withdrawal
Bradycardia	Opioids, barbiturates, digoxin, clonidine, β-blockers, hypothermia, hypoglycemia, increased intracranial pressure, calcium channel blockers, GHB
Tachypnea	Salicylates, theophylline, metabolic acidosis, amphetamines
Depressed respirations	CNS depressants (ethanol, barbiturates, opioids, sedative-hypnotics), clonidine (early), botulism
Hypotension	β-blockers, calcium channel blockers, tricyclic antidepressants, barbiturates, opioids, iron, clonidine, cardiac glycosides, ethanol
Hypertension	Sympathomimetics (amphetamines, cocaine, phencyclidine, theophylline), anticholinergics (antihistamines, atropine, phenothiazines, scopolamine, tricyclic antidepressants), clonidine, SSRIs, MAO inhibitors
Skin	
Cyanosis	Methemoglobinemia, hypoxia
Flushing	Anticholinergics, amphetamines
Diaphoresis	Amphetamines, cocaine, anticholinesterase pesticide, salicylates
Hot, dry skin	Anticholinergics
Piloerection	Opioid withdrawal
Bullae	Carbon monoxide, barbiturates
Pruritus	Vitamin A
Eyes	
Miosis	Opioids, organophosphates, clonidine, ethanol, phenothiazines, sedative-hypnotics
Mydriasis	Amphetamines, cocaine, anticholinergics, antihistamines, phenylephrine, cannabis, LSD, phencyclidine, dextromethorphan, psilocybin, hypoglycemia, ethanol, opioid withdrawal
Conjunctival injection	Direct irritants, cannabis
Nystagmus	Phenytoin, phencyclidine, carbamazepine, ketamine, alcohols
Visual disturbances	Botulism, parathion, methanol, digitalis, vitamin A

Table 15-5. (cont.)

Finding	Drugs/toxins
Neck	
Rigidity	Dystonia from phenothiazines and haloperidol, phencyclidine, strychnine
Breath sounds	
Rhonchi, wheezes	Petroleum distillate aspiration, toxic inhalants, cholinesterase-inhibitor pesticides, β-blockers
Abdomen	
Distention, ↓ bowel sounds	CNS depressants (many), anticholinergics, tricyclics
↑ bowel sounds	Amphetamines, cocaine, cholinesterase-inhibitor pesticides, drug withdrawal, food poisoning
Tenderness	Alcoholic gastritis, corrosives, salicylates, acetaminophen, iron
Distended bladder	Anticholinergics, tricyclics
Neurologic	
Ataxia	Phenytoin, benzodiazepines, sedative hypnotics, solvents, alcohols, carbon monoxide
Focal signs	Hypoglycemia, toxic alcohols, increased intracranial pressure due to a mass lesion
Tremor	Carbon monoxide, parathion, phenothiazines, mercury, ethanol, lithium, arsenic, solvents
Delirium	Sympathomimetics, anticholinergics, drugs of abuse, heavy metals, phenothiazines
Coma	Opioids, antipsychotics, anticholinergics, carbon monoxide, toxic alcohols, salicylates, organophosphates, clonidine, anticonvulsants

amphetamines, while mydriasis with poorly reactive pupils is seen in anticholinergic poisonings.

Routine testing is rarely helpful in the poisoned patient. Specific levels are available for several medications and may assist in making treatment decisions (Table 15-8). Obtain an acetaminophen level after an oral ingestion or if the patient is comatose, as it is a common co-ingestant. Urine or blood toxicology screens may be helpful in specific circumstances, but are not routinely indicated. Note that each institution's toxicology screen detects different drugs.

Acid/base status can be determined from arterial blood gas and chemistry panels. The mnemonic "MUDPILES CAT" represents the list of toxins which produce an elevated anion gap with a metabolic acidosis (Table 15-9). The anion gap is calculated by:

$$[Na^+] - ([HCO3^-] + [Cl^-])$$

The normal anion gap is typically <12, but use the upper limit of normal set by each laboratory, since this reflects differences in the methods used to calculate the electrolytes.

Table 15-6. Toxidromes

Sympathomimetic

Findings: hyperthermia, tachycardia, hypertension, mydriasis (reactive), warm/moist skin, agitated/delirium

Causes: amphetamines, cocaine, phencyclidine, theophylline, ethanol withdrawal

Anticholinergic

Findings: hyperthermia, tachycardia, hypertension, hot/red/dry skin, mydriasis (unreactive), urinary retention, absent bowel sounds, confusion/hallucinations

Causes: antihistamines, atropine, phenothiazines, scopolamine, tricyclic antidepressants

Cholinergic

Findings: SLUDGE (Salivation, Lacrimation, Urinary incontinence, Diarrhea/Diaphoresis, GI upset/hyperactive bowel sounds, Emesis), miosis, bradycardia, bronchial secretions, seizures, altered mental status, paralysis

Causes: carbamates, chemical warfare agents (VX, Soman, Sarin), organophosphates, pilocarpine eye drops

Opioid (narcotic)

Findings: miosis, respiratory depression, depressed mental status, hypothermia, bradycardia, hypotension

Causes: codeine, dextromethorphan, fentanyl, heroin, morphine, clonidine

Table 15-7. Odors

Odor	Toxin
Acetone	Aspirin, chloroform, isopropanol, ketoacidosis, methanol
Bitter almonds	Cyanide (silver polish)
Eggs (rotten)	Disulfiram, hydrogen sulfide, mercaptans
Fish or raw liver (musty)	Hepatic failure, zinc phosphide
Fruit-like	Amyl nitrite, ethanol, isopropanol, ketoacidosis
Garlic	Arsenic, dimethylsulfoxide (DMSO), organophosphates, phosphorus, selenium, thallium
Mothballs	Camphor
Peanuts	N-Pyridylmethylurea (Vacor), other rodenticides
Pear-like (acrid)	Chloral hydrate, paraldehyde
Petroleum	Petroleum distillates
Shoe polish	Chlorinated hydrocarbons, nitrobenzene
Violets (urine)	Turpentine
Wintergreen	Methylsalicylate

Table 15-8. Important drug levels

Drug	Level	Intervention
Acetaminophen	Nomogram	N-Acetylcysteine
Carbamazepine	60 mg/L	Hemoperfusion
Carboxyhemoglobin	25% (any if pregnant)	Hyperbaric oxygen
Digoxin	15 ng/mL[a]	Digoxin-specific Fab fragments
Ethanol	Low level	Necessitates search for other toxins
Ethylene glycol	20 mg/dL	Ethanol or fomepizole
	25 mg/dL	Hemodialysis
Iron	500 mcg/dL	Deferoxamine
Lithium	4 mEq/L[b] (acute)	Hemodialysis
Methanol	20 mg/dL	Ethanol or fomepizole
	25 mg/dL	Hemodialysis
Methemoglobin	20%	Methylene blue
Phenobarbital	100 mcg/mL	Hemoperfusion
Salicylate	120 mg/dL (acute)	Bicarbonate, hemodialysis
Theophylline	100 mg/L	Hemoperfusion or hemodialysis
Valproic acid	1000 mg/L	Hemodialysis

Notes: [a] Treatment with digoxin-specific Fab fragments is based on symptoms and an elevated potassium (>5.0 mEq/L). However, if the digoxin level is >10 ng/mL in an overdose, give Fab fragments, regardless of symptoms.
[b] Treatment with hemodialysis is based on symptoms (severely altered mental status, seizures, arrhythmias). However, a lithium level >4 mEq/L is indicative of severe toxicity and hemodialysis is indicated.

Table 15-9. Causes of increased anion gap metabolic acidosis (Mudpiles CAT)

Methanol or metformin	Cyanide
Uremia	Alcohol or acids (valproic)
Diabetic ketoacidosis	Toluene or theophylline
Paraldehyde or phenformin	
Iron, isoniazid, or ibuprofen	
Lactic acidosis	
Ethylene glycol	
Salicylates	

Order a serum osmolality and ethanol level in cases of suspected poisoning due to ethylene glycol, methanol, or isopropanol. Use the osmol gap to approximate serum levels and to determine therapy, such as dialysis. To calculate, subtract the calculated osmolality from the measured osmolality:

Osmol gap = measured osmolality – calculated osmolality

Calculated osmolality = $(2 \times Na^+) + (BUN/2.8) + (glucose/18) + (ethanol/4.6)$

Including ethanol in the calculated gap increases the likelihood of correctly identifying gaps attributable to methanol, ethylene glycol, or isopropanol. A normal osmol gap is $+/- 10$, while an elevated osmol gap is consistent with the presence of a toxic alcohol ingestion. However, a normal osmol gap cannot be used to exclude the diagnosis of a toxic alcohol ingestion.

Obtain an ECG for any patient who is ill or who has taken an agent known to cause cardiac disturbances. Assessment for conduction delays is important as it may precede significant rhythm disturbances. Additionally, as is the case with tricyclic antidepressant ingestions, abnormalities on the ECG may predict the development of seizures or other toxic effects.

Radiographic evaluation of the poisoned patient is generally unnecessary, however, the mnemonic CHIPES refers to the tablets that may be seen on abdominal X-ray: chloral hydrate, heavy metals (lead, iron, arsenic), iodides, phenothiazines, enteric-coated medications, and sodium and other elements (calcium, potassium, bismuth). In practice, only the heavy metals are readily visible on abdominal X-rays. "Body packers" who are intentionally transporting illicit drugs wrapped in packages in their intestines will often have visible oblong densities on X-ray. A chest X-ray, including the upper airway, is indicated if there is a possibility of aspiration or if the patient ingested a button battery or mini-magnets.

Decontamination

If the patient has dermal exposure to a toxin, remove all of the patient's clothing, using gloves, and place it in bags. Thoroughly cleanse the skin with copious amounts of water; a shower is the most effective method. Wear personal protective equipment including face mask, until the chemical is identified.

In the case of ocular exposure to chemicals, thoroughly irrigate the eyes with a minimum of one liter of saline using a Morgan lens. Check the pH of the corneal surface with pH paper prior to and after irrigation. Continue irrigation until the pH is approximately 7.0. Most ocular exposures cause an irritant conjunctivitis; however, substances which are acid or alkali may cause chemical ocular burns. These require specific therapy and ophthalmologic consultation.

Recommendations regarding the use of various modalities of gastrointestinal decontamination have changed in the last decade. Determining the indications and appropriate methods for GI decontamination requires review of the risk versus benefits of the technique as well as the toxicity of the substance ingested. The majority of pediatric ingestions are not life-threatening and therefore do not merit aggressive GI decontamination. Factors that need to be considered before administering any gastrointestinal decontamination are: the length of time since the ingestion, the likelihood the decontamination method will decrease toxin absorption, the potential adverse effects of the decontamination, the toxicity of the substance ingested, the amount of the substance ingested, and the availability of an antidote. Therefore management must be individualized.

Syrup of ipecac is no longer utilized in the emergency department. Its use is limited to the prehospital setting in the case of a life-threatening ingestion where there may be a significant delay in transport to a medical center.

Gastric lavage involves aspiration of pill fragments from the stomach using a large-bore orogastric tube size 32F–40F. Routine use is not indicated, except for an adolescent who has taken a potentially life-threatening dose of a substance without a known antidote less than 1 hour prior. Lavage can be performed only if the patient has a gag reflex and has an easily maintainable airway or if the patient is intubated. Place the patient in the left lateral decubitus position with the neck flexed 20 degrees. The appropriate tube length is the distance from the mouth to the epigastrium allowing for a curve in the pharynx. After placement, confirm the position by auscultation of air injected into the stomach. Then, instill 200 mL boluses of water or normal saline into the tube and aspirate by suction. Repeat until the effluent is clear.

Activated charcoal (AC) acts as an adsorbent to bind toxins and prevent their absorption into the systemic circulation. Activated charcoal binds to most substances except heavy metals, alcohols, caustics, hydrocarbons, and large ions such as lithium. The use of AC is limited to patients presenting within 1–2 hours of ingestion of a potentially life-threatening substance. The dose is 1 g/kg up to 50 g. Use a slurry made with a flavored beverage (cherry syrup, cola, chocolate syrup) to improve palatability. Serve the slurry in a covered opaque container to disguise the color. Do not insert a nasogastric tube solely for charcoal instillation.

Multiple doses of charcoal every 2–4 hours are useful for ingestions of delayed-release preparations or large amounts of life-threatening toxins. In addition, administer multiple doses of AC in cases of salicylate, theophylline, carbamazepine, and phenobarbital poisoning as the charcoal interrupts enterohepatic and enteroenteric circulation. Use sorbitol only with the first dose of charcoal.

Whole-bowel irrigation may be useful for an ingestion of a sustained-release or enteric-coated product, for substances which are slowly absorbed from the GI tract, and for patients in whom charcoal is not indicated. This technique involves instillation of large volumes of polyethylene glycol, which increases GI transit time, in order to decrease absorption. Instill small quantities at first (adolescent: 250 mL; toddler: 50 mL) and increase the rate to 500 mL/h in children 9 months to 6 years of age, 1 liter/h in children up to 12 years old, and 2 liter/h in older patients. Continue until the patient's effluent is clear. Periodically auscultate for active bowel sounds to ensure continued peristalsis.

Antidote

Most poisoned patients require supportive care and not specific antidote therapy (Table 15-10). However, if an antidote is available it may be indicated in certain situations in which the ingestion has the potential to cause serious toxic effects. It is important to remember that antidotes may have different pharmacokinetics than the drugs they are treating. For instance, in the case of naloxone for opioid intoxication, the antidote effects last for a shorter time than the effects of the opioid and therefore the antidote may need to be repeatedly administered.

Table 15-10. Antidotes

Poison	Antidote	Dose
Acetaminophen	N-acetylcysteine	PO: 140 mg/kg load
		IV: 150 mg/kg load over 1 h
Anticholinergic (not tricyclic)	Physostigmine	0.02 mg/kg IV (adult 2 mg)
Calcium channel blocker	Calcium gluconate	60–100 mg/kg (3 g maximum)
Cholinergic	Atropine	0.05–0.01 mg/kg (min 0.1 mg, adult 2–5 mg)
Clonidine	Naloxone	1–2 mg IV/IM
Cyanide	Cyanide antidote kit	
Digoxin	Digibind	Based on amount ingested
Ethylene glycol	Fomepizole (4-methylpyrazole)	15 mg/kg IV load, then 10 mg/kg q 12 h
	Thiamine	0.5 mg/kg (adult 100 mg)
Hypoglycemia	Dextrose	0.5–1 g/kg IV
Iron	Deferoxamine	50 mg/kg IM q 6 h
Isoniazid	Pyridoxine	Gram for gram, 70 mg/kg if amount is unknown (adult 5 g)
Methanol	Fomepizole (4-methylpyrazole)	15 mg/kg IV load, then 10 mg/kg q 12 h
	Folate	1–2 mg/kg IV q 6 h
Methemoglobinemia	Methylene blue 1%	1–2 mg/kg
Opioid	Naloxone	1–2 mg IV/IM
Oral hypoglycemic	Octreotide	1 mcg/kg q 6 h SC
Organophosphate	Pralidoxine (2-PAM)	25 mg/kg IV, adult 1–2 g
Phenothiazine	Benztropine	0.02–0.05 mg/kg
(dystonic reaction)	Diphenhydramine	1–2 mg/kg IM, IV
Sodium channel blocker	Sodium bicarbonate	1–2 mEq/kg IV
Tricyclic antidepressant	Sodium bicarbonate	1–2 mEq/kg IV
Warfarin (rat poison)	Vitamin K1	1–10 mg SC/IM/IV

Bibliography

Calello DP, Osterhoudt KC, Henretig FM: New and novel antidotes in pediatrics. *Pediatr Emerg Care* 2006;22:523–30.

Greene S, Harris C, Singer J: Gastrointestinal decontamination of the poisoned patient. *Pediatr Emerg Care* 2008;24:176–86.

White ML, Liebelt EL: Update on antidotes for pediatric poisoning. *Pediatr Emerg Care* 2006;22:740–6.

Acetaminophen

Acetaminophen is the most common oral ingestant in the United States and a common co-ingestant. It is found in many over-the-counter preparations, particularly cough, cold, and pain relief medicines. Acetaminophen overdose is a leading cause of poisoning-related deaths and it is the most common cause of acute liver failure in children in the United States.

Acetaminophen is normally metabolized in the liver by sulfonation and glucuronidation. In the overdose setting, these metabolic pathways are saturated and the excess acetaminophen is metabolized by the P450 enzymes to the toxic metabolite N-acetyl-p-benzoquinonimine (NAPQI) that causes centrilobular hepatic necrosis. Rapid diagnosis is necessary, as an antidote, N-acetylcysteine (NAC; Mucomyst), effectively prevents toxicity.

Acetaminophen usually reaches peak serum levels within 60 minutes; but this may be delayed to 2 hours if extended-release preparations are ingested. Additionally, large overdoses may result in delayed gastric emptying and a delay in peak serum levels.

Clinical presentation

In the first hours after an ingestion of acetaminophen, symptoms are generally mild and may include nausea, vomiting, and anorexia, but these are not predictive of the subsequent course. LFTs are normal during this stage. This is followed by an asymptomatic latent phase. Between 24 and 48 hours after ingestion, subclinical hepatotoxicity occurs and is evidenced by mild RUQ pain, nausea, and vomiting, with elevations of AST (SGOT), ALT (SGPT), bilirubin, and prothrombin time. Over the next several days, fulminant hepatic failure may develop with jaundice, renal failure, cerebral edema, and hypotension. Patients who survive the stage of maximum hepatotoxicity will usually recover due to hepatic regeneration.

Diagnosis

The potential for an acetaminophen ingestion to cause hepatotoxicity may be predicted by obtaining a serum level ≥4 hours after the ingestion. Plot the serum level on the acetaminophen nomogram (Figure 15-1). If the level appears above the "Possible Risk" line, then therapy with NAC is necessary. Patients whose level falls below this line do not need treatment, including those who ingested a sustained-release product.

Toxicity may be predicted less reliably by calculating whether the ingested dose is greater than 150 mg/kg. Toxicity is less common in toddlers since they generally ingest smaller quantities and have a larger relative liver size as compared with adults. In addition, young children can metabolize via the sulfonation pathway at a faster rate, limiting the production of NAPQI, and they may have greater glutathione stores. Therefore toxicity is unlikely in children <5 years of age unless >200 mg/kg was ingested.

ED management

Immediately administer 1 g/kg of activated charcoal if the ingestion was <2 hours prior to arrival. Although charcoal does adsorb some acetaminophen, it is not the treatment of choice, so do not insert a nasogastric tube simply to instill charcoal in an isolated acetaminophen ingestion.

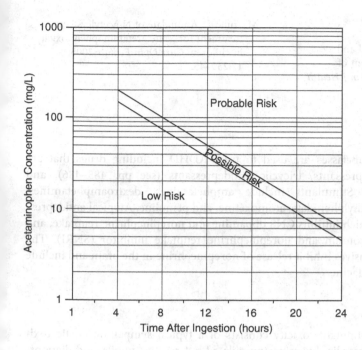

Figure 15-1. Acetaminophen nomogram.

NAC is indicated if the serum level is on or above the "Possible risk" line on the nomogram. It is 100% effective in preventing hepatotoxicity if given within 8 hours of ingestion. Both oral and intravenous routes are approved for use and are equally efficacious and available in the United States. IV administration has more side effects, including a risk of an anaphylactoid reaction, but it is preferred if the patient presents with fulminant hepatic failure or is unable to tolerate the oral formulation.

The oral loading dose is 140 mg/kg, followed by 70 mg/kg q 4 h for 17 more doses. Oral NAC is foul-smelling and often causes emesis, so dilute it 1:4 in juice to increase its palatability. In addition, give an antiemetic, such as metoclopramide (1–2 mg/kg/dose IV, IM, PO) or ondansetron (2 mg PO [8–15 kg], 4 mg PO [15–30 kg], 8 mg PO >30 kg). Giving IV NAC decreases the treatment time to 20 hours versus 72 hours for oral NAC. Give a 150 mg/kg IV load over 60 minutes, followed by 50 mg/kg over the next 4 hours, then 100 mg/kg over the final 16 hours.

If the acetaminophen level will not be available until >8 hours after ingestion give a single oral loading dose of NAC while waiting for the level. Treat a patient who arrives for care >24 hours post ingestion with a course of NAC if the level is detectable or the AST is elevated.

Obtain a CBC, electrolytes, liver function tests, PT, and PTT if the patient has a toxic level or arrives >24 hours after the ingestion.

Indications for admission

- Possible acetaminophen toxicity, based on amount ingested (>150 mg/kg) or serum levels
- Evidence of hepatotoxicity
- Suicide attempt or gesture without psychiatric clearance and appropriate follow-up arranged

Bibliography

Kanter MZ: Comparison of oral and i.v. acetylcysteine in the treatment of acetaminophen poisoning. *Am J Health Syst Pharm* 2006;63:1821–7.

Marzullo L: An update of N-acetylcysteine treatment for acute acetaminophen toxicity in children. *Curr Opin Pediatr* 2005; 17:239–45.

ADHD medications

A variety of medication subclasses are used to treat ADHD including drugs that are stimulants, atypical antidepressants, tricyclic antidepressants (see pp. 485–486), and alpha-adrenergic agonists. Stimulants include amphetamines, dextroamphetamines, methylphenidate, dexmethethylphenidate, atomoxetine, and pemoline. Atypical antidepressants include bupropion, which inhibits CNS dopamine and norepinephrine reuptake, and venlafaxine, which is a serotonin and norepinephrine reuptake inhibitor (SNRI). The centrally acting antihypertensives inhibit release of norepinephrine in the brain and include clonidine (p. 464) and guanfacine.

Clinical presentation

Amphetamine and other stimulant toxicity consists of a typical sympathomimetic toxidrome (hyperthermia, tachycardia, hypertension, dilated but reactive pupils, and diaphoresis). Clonidine toxicity resembles an opioid overdose and includes miosis, sedation, coma, hypothermia, hypotension, respiratory depression, and bradycardia. Paradoxical hypertension may develop because, early in overdose, these medications have a preponderance of peripheral alpha stimulation, prior to entry of the drug into the central nervous system. This paradoxical hypertension is then followed by hypotension. Bupropion toxicity can cause a hyperadrenergic state with agitation and seizures, although seizures can occur with normal therapeutic doses.

Diagnosis

Diagnosis is generally made by history as well as by identifying the signs and symptoms consistent with the appropriate toxidrome.

ED management

Assessment of the adequacy of the airway, breathing, circulation and vital signs are the first priority. Check the glucose level and obtain an ECG. Administer activated charcoal (1 g/kg PO) to a patient who arrives in the ED within 2 hours of ingestion. Treat agitation quickly with benzodiazepines such as midazolam (0.1–0.3 mg/kg IV, 0.2–0.4 mg/kg IM, or 0.4–0.9 mg/kg PO), as it may lead to acidosis, hyperthermia, and rhabdomyolysis. Aggressively treat severe hyperthermia (>40°C; 104°F) by covering the patient with a wet sheet and applying ice packs to the groin and axillae. The cardiovascular manifestations generally respond to benzodiazepines; also use benzodiazepines for seizures. Treat sustained tachycardia and hypertension, despite adequate sedation and cooling, with phentolamine (0.02–0.1 mg/kg IV q 10 min).

Naloxone (0.1 mg/kg IV, 2 mg maximum) is variably effective in reversing the sedation caused by clonidine toxicity. Give up to 10 mg before considering the intervention ineffective.

Indications for admission
- Abnormal vital signs or mental status
- Suicide attempt or gesture without psychiatric clearance and appropriate follow-up arranged

Bibliography

Advokat C: Update on amphetamine neurotoxicity and its relevance to the treatment of ADHD. *J Atten Disord* 2007;11:8–16.

Daviss WB, Patel NC, Robb AS, et al: Clonidine for attention-deficit/hyperactivity disorder: II. ECG changes and adverse events analysis.

J Am Acad Child Adolesc Psychiatry 2008;47:189–98.

Scharman EJ, Erdman AR, Cobaugh DJ, et al: Methylphenidate poisoning: an evidence-based consensus guideline for out-of-hospital management. *Clin Toxicol (Phila)* 2007;45:737–52.

Anticholinergics

Anticholinergic poisoning in children may be caused by ingestion of antihistamines (H_1 receptor antagonists), atropine, scopolamine, phenothiazines, antiparkinsonians, mydriatics, jimson weed (*Datura stramonium*), and tricyclic antidepressants.

Clinical presentation

The anticholinergic toxidrome must be diagnosed clinically since laboratory tests are typically not helpful. Symptoms result from peripheral blockade of acetylcholine at the muscarinic receptors and include dry mucous membranes, flushed dry skin, mydriatic and unreactive pupils, blurred vision (loss of accommodation), constipation, urinary retention, and tachycardia. Central muscarinic blockade causes temperature elevation, disorientation, hallucinations, seizures, and coma.

Symptoms have been described by the mnemonic, "Dry as a bone, mad as a hatter, red as a beet, hot as Hades, and blind as a bat."

Diagnosis

Suspect an anticholinergic ingestion in any patient with a change in mental status, hallucinations, coma, sinus tachycardia, seizures, or a wide QRS or prolonged QTc on ECG. On examination, the pupils are usually dilated and non-reactive to light and accommodation. Absent bowel sounds, dry mucous membranes, and dry flushed skin also suggest the diagnosis. Obtain blood for a CBC, electrolytes, acetaminophen level (co-ingestion in many cold preparations or attempted suicides), pregnancy test (if indicated), and fingerstick glucose determination. Also order an ECG and urine toxicology if cocaine, amphetamine, or tricyclic ingestion is a possibility.

It is important to differentiate the anticholinergic toxidrome from the sympathomimetic toxidrome, as therapy is quite different. Both the anticholinergics and sympathomimetics can cause confusion, agitation, mydriasis, and tachycardia. The pupil, skin, and abdominal examination findings may differentiate these toxidromes. Sympathomimetics cause large yet reactive pupils, with normal or increased bowel sounds, and cool, diaphoretic skin.

ED management

Initiate supportive care and cardiac monitoring. Administer activated charcoal if the ingestion is likely to have been within the previous 2 hours, as anticholinergics delay gastric emptying and increase the efficacy of activated charcoal. The treatment of coma is supportive. Treat seizures with lorazepam (0.05–0.1 mg/kg slow IV) or diazepam (0.1–0.3 mg/kg slow IV). If seizures recur give phenobarbital (loading dose 20 mg/kg IV), although propofol or general anesthesia may be necessary for intractable status epilepticus. Treat wide complex tachycardias with sodium bicarbonate (1–2 mEq/kg IV).

Physostigmine can be used in pure anticholinergic poisonings such as atropine, scopolamine, diphenhydramine, and jimson weed. Continued seizures, hemodynamic compromise, or severe agitation or hallucinations are indications for its use. Do not use physostigmine merely to arouse a comatose patient. Give a dose of 0.5 mg slowly over 5 minutes (1–2 mg for adults). This may be repeated every 10 minutes until a satisfactory endpoint is achieved. Rapid administration may cause seizures or bradycardia, and an overdose can precipitate a cholinergic crisis (salivation, lacrimation, bradycardia, hypotension, or asystole). Do not use physostigmine in patients suspected of having tricyclic antidepressant toxicity, as it may precipitate terminal cardiotoxicity, as well as in patients with gamma-hydroxybutyrate toxicity, as it may precipitate fasciculation and seizure activity. Always be prepared to give atropine (one-half the physostigmine dose) to a patient incorrectly treated with physostigmine.

Agitation may be reversed entirely with small doses of physostigmine. Although the potential side effects of physostigmine have made its use less common, it usually causes complete reversal of anticholinergic agitation. This reversal allows confirmation of the diagnosis as well as eliminating the need for further invasive diagnostic studies, i.e. CT and lumbar puncture. Repeated dosing of physostigmine at 30–60 minute intervals may be necessary. Sedation with benzodiazepines may be effective, although large doses are often necessary.

Indications for admission

- Lethargy or persistent signs of toxicity (tachycardia, confusion, sedation)
- Coma, arrhythmia, or seizures
- Suicide attempt or gesture without psychiatric clearance and appropriate follow-up arranged

Bibliography

Frascogna N: Physostigmine: is there a role for this antidote in pediatric poisonings? *Curr Opin Pediatr* 2007;19:201–5.

Henry K, Harris CR: Deadly ingestions. *Pediatr Clin North Am* 2006;53:293–315.

Spina SP, Taddei A: Teenagers with Jimson weed (Datura stramonium) poisoning. *CJEM* 2007;9:467–8.

Antidepressants

Antidepressants include the tricyclic antidepressants, monoamine oxidase (MAO) inhibitors, selective serotonin reuptake inhibitors (SSRI) and the atypical antidepressants. Tricyclic antidepressants have a unique toxicity and are discussed on pp. 485–486.

MAO inhibitors include tranylcypromine (Parnate), phenelzine (Nardil), isocarboxazid (Marplan), and selegeline (Emsam). The enzyme MAO degrades catecholamines in the CNS, liver, and intestine, as well as tyramine. Toxicity is related to enhanced catecholamine release.

SSRIs include citalopram (Celexa), escitalopram (Lexapro), fluoxetine (Prozac), sertraline (Zoloft), and paroxetine (Paxil). Receptor binding is relatively specific for the serotonin reuptake mechanism and not adrenergic receptors, and therefore SSRIs have less toxicity than their predecessors.

Atypical antidepressants include amoxapine (Ascendin), bupropion (Wellbutrin, Budeprion, Zyban), duloxetine (Cymbalta), mirtazapine (Remeron), nefazodone (Serzone), trazodone (Desyrel), and venlafaxine (Effexor). These newer medications have varying mechanisms of action, but generally block reuptake of serotonin and catecholamines.

Clinical presentation

Acute overdose of MAO inhibitors leads to a sympathomimetic toxidrome, consisting of tachycardia, tachypnea, hyperthermia, anxiety, flushing, tremor, hyperreflexia, diaphoresis, agitated delirium, and severe hypertension. The initial hyperadrenergic crisis may be followed by cardiovascular collapse and multi-system failure. These toxic effects may be delayed up to 24 hours after ingestion, so an asymptomatic patient is still at risk.

MAO inhibitors may lead to a hypertensive reaction when tyramine-rich foods (aged cheese, smoked or pickled meat, and red wine) are consumed, since MAO normally degrades tyramine in the intestine. Hypertensive reactions can also occur when additional sympathomimetic drugs are ingested. The hallmarks of such hypertensive reactions are extreme elevations in blood pressure and severe headaches.

The serotonin syndrome may develop in patients who ingest MAO inhibitors with other medications that increase serotonin in the synapse (e.g. SSRIs, meperidine, dextromethorphan). Serotonin syndrome consists of mental status changes, agitation, hyperthermia, rigidity, myoclonus, tremor, diaphoresis, and diarrhea.

SSRI overdose can cause nausea, vomiting, sedation, and very rarely seizures. Citalopram causes prolongation of the QTc interval if >600 mg is ingested.

The newer, atypical antidepressants also cause sedation and ataxia. Bupropion may cause seizures, usually within 6 hours post ingestion. Overdose also causes tachycardia, agitation, and hallucinations. Trazodone may cause priapism, as well as hypotension secondary to alpha blockade.

Diagnosis

A provisional diagnosis sufficient to initiate treatment can be made when the appropriate clinical presentation is identified.

ED management

Assessment of the adequacy of the airway, breathing, circulation and vital signs are the first priorities. Obtain an ECG. Treat severe hypertension secondary to MAO inhibitor toxicity with phentolamine (0.02–0.1 mg/kg IV bolus, repeat q 10 min) or nitroprusside (pp. 656–658).

Treat hypotension with multiple fluid boluses (20 mL/kg each), followed by a norepinephrine infusion. Begin with 0.1 mcg/kg per min and increase every 5 minutes (add a 4 mg ampule to 1 L of D_5W to make a 4 mcg/mL solution). Give activated charcoal (1 g/kg PO) to a patient who arrives within 2 hours of ingestion. Admit any patient with MAO inhibitor ingestion to a monitored setting because toxicity may occur up to 24 hours after ingestion.

Treat serotonin syndrome with aggressive cooling for hyperthermia and benzodiazepines for muscle rigidity and agitation.

Indications for admission
- Signs of severe toxicity (seizures, vital sign abnormalities)
- All ingestions of MAO inhibitors
- Serotonin syndrome
- Suicide attempt or gesture without psychiatric clearance and appropriate follow-up arranged

Bibliography

Frascogna N: Physostigmine: is there a role for this antidote in pediatric poisonings? *Curr Opin Pediatr* 2007;19:201–5.

Henry K, Harris CR: Deadly ingestions. *Pediatr Clin North Am* 2006;53:293–315.

Kokan L: Monoamine oxidase inhibitors. In Flomenbaum N, Goldfrank LR, Hoffman RS, et al. (eds), *Goldfrank's Toxicologic Emergencies*, 8th ed. New York: McGraw-Hill, 2006, pp. 1062–9.

Stork CM: Serotonin reuptake inhibitors and atypical antidepressants. In Flomenbaum N, Goldfrank LR, Hoffman RS, et al. (eds), *Goldfrank's Toxicologic Emergencies*, 8th ed. New York: McGraw-Hill, 2006, pp. 1070–82.

Antipsychotics

Antipsychotic medications are widely used for the treatment of psychosis and are now being prescribed for other conditions, such as migraine headaches, control of emesis, chemical restraint, and movement disorders. Although overdose may be common with the antipsychotics, severe toxicity is rare.

Antipsychotics are divided into typical and atypical classes. Typical antipsychotics are older medications, including chlorpromazine (Thorazine), thioridazine (Mellaril), prochlorperazine (Compazine), and haloperidol (Haldol). Their mechanism of action is via dopamine and serotonin receptor blocking in the central nervous system. In addition, they also have alpha-adrenergic blockade, anticholinergic and antimuscarinic effects, which may become more pronounced in overdose.

The newer, atypical antipsychotics include clozapine (Clozaril), olanzapine (Zyprexa), quetiapine (Seroquel), risperidone (Risperdal), and ziprasidone (Geodon). In general the atypicals are more active at serotonin receptors than dopamine receptors and therefore less likely to have adverse effects at therapeutic doses.

Clinical presentation

The most common toxicity, at both therapeutic levels and in the overdose setting, is an acute dystonic reaction which includes torticollis, opisthotonos, difficulty speaking, facial grimacing, and oculogyric crisis. Onset can be delayed up to 3 days after ingestion and spasm may wax and wane. In an overdose antipsychotics commonly cause impaired consciousness ranging from somnolence to coma. Additionally, toxicity includes postural hypotension, seizures, and an anticholinergic toxidrome (dry mouth, urinary retention, constipation, blurred vision, tachycardia). Cardiotoxicity from antipsychotics in massive overdose can be similar to tricyclic antidepressants, with widened (>10 ms) QRS complexes, terminal 40 ms right axis deviation, or a prolonged QTc.

Neuroleptic malignant syndrome is an extremely rare reaction that can be life-threatening. It is characterized by altered mental status, hyperthermia, muscular rigidity, and autonomic instability. The reaction can occur at any time following initiation of antipsychotic medications.

Diagnosis

A provisional diagnosis sufficient to initiate treatment can be made when the appropriate clinical presentation is identified. It is important to obtain a thorough history by contacting family, friends, and paramedics.

ED management

Provide supportive care as indicated, obtain an ECG, and administer activated charcoal (1 g/kg) if the ingestion has occurred within 1–2 hours. Treat a dystonic reaction with diphenhydramine (1 mg/kg IM or IV, 50 mg maximum) and/or benztropine mesylate (0.05 mg/kg IV or IM, 2 mg maximum). Prescribe a 2-day course of diphenhydramine (5 mg/kg per day div qid, 300 mg/day maximum) or benztropine mesylate (toddler: 0.5 mg bid; child or adolescent: 1.0 mg bid) to prevent a recurrence of the symptoms.

Treat seizures with lorazepam (0.05–0.1 mg/kg slow IV) or diazepam (0.1–0.3 mg/kg slow IV). Treat orthostatic hypotension with 20 mL/kg of isotonic IV fluid. The management of an anticholinergic syndrome is detailed on pp. 451–452 and the management of tricyclic cardiotoxicity is described on pp. 485–486.

Treat neuroleptic malignant syndrome with aggressive cooling, sedation with benzodiazepines, fluid resuscitation, and alkalinization of the urine if rhabdomyolysis is present.

Follow-up

- Dystonic reaction: next day

Indications for admission

- Decreased level of consciousness
- Neuroleptic malignant syndrome
- Seizures or persistent hypotension
- ECG changes
- Suicide attempt or gesture without psychiatric clearance and appropriate follow-up arranged

Bibliography

James LP, Abel K, Wilkinson J, Simpson PM, Nichols MH: Phenothiazines, butyrophenone, and other psychotropic medication poisonings in children and adolescents. J Toxicol 2000;38:615–23.

Juurlink D: Antipsychotics. In Flomenbaum N, Goldfrank LR, Hoffman RS, *et al.* (eds), *Goldfrank's Toxicologic Emergencies*, 8th ed. New York: McGraw-Hill, 2006, pp. 1039–51.

Kasantikul D, Kanchanatawan B: Neuroleptic malignant syndrome: a review and report of six cases. *J Med Assoc Thai* 2006;89:2155–60.

Beta agonists

Beta agonists such as albuterol, metaproterenol, and terbutaline are used in the treatment of bronchospasm. Overdose of these drugs rarely causes significant toxicity, although patients who ingest >0.1 mg/kg of oral albuterol are the most likely to develop symptoms.

Clinical presentation

Most patients are asymptomatic. Sinus tachycardia, tremor, agitation, nausea, vomiting, and hypokalemia may occur.

Diagnosis

The diagnosis is suggested by the history. There are no specific laboratory tests.

ED management

Typically, no treatment is required, other than reassurance.

Indication for admission

- Suicide attempt or gesture without psychiatric clearance and appropriate follow-up arranged

Bibliography

Hoffman RJ. Methylxanthines and selective β_2-adrenergic agonists. In Flomenbaum N, Goldfrank LR, Hoffman RS, *et al.* (eds), *Goldfrank's Toxicologic Emergencies*, 8th ed. New York: McGraw-Hill, 2006, pp. 989–1003.

Lang DM: The controversy over long-acting beta agonists: examining the evidence. *Cleve Clin J Med* 2006;73:973–6.

Beta blockers

Beta-adrenergic blocking drugs are widely used for the treatment of hypertension, angina, arrhythmias, migraine headaches, and various other conditions. Members of this group include propranolol, atenolol, betaxolol, bisoprolol, penbutol, carvedilol, metoprolol, nadolol, sotalol, timolol, pindolol, and acebutolol. These medications are also marketed as sustained-release preparations and also in combination with other products for the treatment of hypertension. Their main effect is through slowing the rate of SA node discharge and conduction through the atria and AV node. They also cause peripheral vasodilatation through the relaxation of vascular smooth muscle. Sotalol is a potassium channel blocker as well as a beta blocker.

Clinical presentation

Symptoms and signs occur within 6 hours of overdose unless a delayed-release preparation or sotalol has been ingested. The most common finding is bradycardia. Abnormalities on

ECG may include a widened QRS interval, increased PR interval, bundle branch block, and sinus bradycardia. Sotalol causes prolongation of the QTc, which predisposes to ventricular dysrhythmias such as torsades de pointes. Other possible ventricular arrhythmias include various escape rhythms and ventricular tachycardia.

Hypotension and cardiogenic shock can occur, but are very unlikely in younger children who have had an accidental ingestion. Patients with propranolol overdose are at particular risk for CNS manifestations, including depressed level of consciousness, delirium, coma, and seizures. Other findings may include hyperkalemia, bronchospasm in patients with asthma, and hypoglycemia in younger children.

Diagnosis

Consider β-blocker poisoning in a patient presenting with bradycardia and hypotension or seizure. Other cardiotoxic medications, such as calcium channel blockers, digitalis glycosides, and alpha agonists (clonidine) may also cause bradycardia. Serum levels are rarely necessary.

ED management

Initiate supportive care and administer a dose of activated charcoal if less than 1–2 hours has elapsed since the ingestion. Continuously monitor the ECG and blood pressure. Obtain blood for electrolytes and glucose and treat hypotension with a 20 mL/kg bolus of an isotonic fluid (normal saline or Ringer's lactate). If there is no response, consult a toxicologist and pediatric cardiologist, and arrange admission to a pediatric intensive care unit.

Glucagon is the drug of choice for severe β-blocker toxicity. The pediatric dose is 50 mcg/kg, adult dose 3–5 mg (10 mg maximum). Calcium will treat hypotension but has little effect on heart rate. Give calcium gluconate 10–20 mg/kg (0.1 mL/kg of 10% solution, 60 mL maximum) slowly IV. If calcium and glucagon are not effective, begin a norepinephrine or isoproterenol infusion. The combination of high-dose insulin and glucose has also been shown to improve cardiac function (insulin 0.5 units/kg per hr with 1 g/kg per hr glucose). Defer using other phosphodiesterase inhibitors (amrinone, milrinone) and pacing until after consultation with a toxicologist and cardiologist.

Hypoglycemia (pp. 182–186) is a particular risk in children; give supplemental glucose (1–2 mL/kg of $D_{50}W$ or 2–4 mL/kg of $D_{25}W$). Correct significant hyperkalemia (pp. 649–650). Treat seizures with lorazepam (0.05–0.1 mg/kg slow IV) or diazepam (0.1–0.3 mg/kg slow IV).

Indications for admission

- History of beta-blocker overdose, unless patient remains asymptomatic for 6 hours after ingestion and the product is not delayed-release or sotalol
- Suicide attempt or gesture without psychiatric clearance and appropriate follow-up arranged

Bibliography

Love JN, Howell JM, Klein-Schwartz W, Litovitz TL: Lack of toxicity from pediatric beta-blocker exposures. *Hum Exp Toxicol* 2006;25:341–6.

Shepherd G: Treatment of poisoning caused by beta-adrenergic and calcium-channel blockers. *Am J Health Syst Pharm* 2006;63:1828–35.

Wax PM, Erdman AR, Chyka PA, et al: Beta-blocker ingestion: an evidence-based

consensus guideline for out-of-hospital management. *Clin Toxicol (Phila)* 2005;43:131–46.

Caffeine

Caffeine is a methylxanthine which is widely available in beverages, food, over-the-counter drugs, prescription medications, and herbal and dietary supplements. It acts as an antagonist to the inhibitory function of adenosine, and as such produces CNS stimulant effects. However, at higher doses it is a cardiac, respiratory, and neuropsychiatric stimulant.

A typical cup of coffee contains approximately 100 mg of caffeine and over-the-counter supplements usually contain between 100 and 200 mg. A dose of 50–200 mg causes mild stimulation, but the lethal dose is unclear, estimated to be 150–200 mg/kg in children and adults and higher in neonates.

Clinical presentation

Most patients with caffeine ingestion will just display mild CNS stimulant effects. However, at sufficient dose, there may be headache, anxiety, agitation, insomnia, tremor and irritability, hallucinations, and seizures. Patients may also have symptoms similar to other adrenergic ingestants, including hypokalemia, and metabolic acidosis. Caffeine also has both positive inotrope and chronotropic effects. In overdose it can cause SVT, PVCs, ventricular tachycardia, and hypertension. The more serious clinical findings rarely occur without any preceding minor symptoms.

Diagnosis

Caffeine levels are not commonly available except for hospitals where neonates are routinely treated with caffeine for apnea.

ED management

Provide supportive care as needed and continuously monitor the heart rate and rhythm. Give activated charcoal (1 g/kg PO q 3 h) if there are active bowel sounds. If the patient is vomiting, give an antiemetic such as ondansetron (0.1–0.5 mg/kg per dose IV, maximum 4 mg). Treat hypotension with a pure alpha agonist such as phenylephrine (5–20 mcg/kg per dose q 10–15 min PRN) and SVT with adenosine (pp. 42–46). Give a benzodiazepine (diazepam 0.2–0.5 mg/kg per dose q 15–30 min to 5 mg <5 yr, 10 mg >5 yr) for agitation, seizures, and muscle fasciculations.

Indications for admission

- Coma, seizures, ventricular tachycardia
- Suicide attempt or gesture without psychiatric clearance and appropriate follow-up arranged

Bibliography

Hoffman RJ: Methylxanthines and selective β_2-adrenergic agonists. In Flomenbaum N, Goldfrank LR, Hoffman RS, et al. (eds), *Goldfrank's Toxicologic Emergencies*, 8th ed. New York: McGraw-Hill, 2006, pp. 989–1003.

Kerrigan S, Lindsey T: Caffeine overdose: two case reports. *Forens Sci Int* 2005;153:67–9.

Calcium channel blockers

Calcium channel blocking (CCB) drugs are widely used for the treatment of angina and hypertension. Common agents include verapamil, diltiazem, nifedipine, and amlodipine. Life-threatening poisoning can occur, especially with verapamil. In addition, several CCBs are available in sustained-release formulations (Calan SR, Covera HS, Cardizem CD, Carizem SR, Cartia XT, Adalat CC, and Procardia XL). More recently, preparations combined with angiotensin converting enzyme inhibitors (Lexxel, Lotrel, Tarka) or with angiotensin II receptor antagonists (Exforge) have been marketed. These may cause more profound hypotension. Another recent combination is with an HMG co-A reductase agent or statin (Caduet).

Clinical presentation

Toxicity reflects the distribution of calcium channels in the cardiovascular system, including the sinus and atrioventricular nodes, vascular smooth muscle, and myocardium. Overdose may cause sinus bradycardia, AV block, and hypotension. Variable degrees of CNS depression, ranging from drowsiness to coma, may occur. Metabolic effects include hyperglycemia and lactic acidosis. Adynamic ileus can manifest as hypoactive bowel sounds. Effects may be delayed 6–8 hours following ingestion of a sustained-release preparation, but have occurred as late as 12–18 hours.

Diagnosis

Consider a calcium channel blocker overdose in a patient presenting with hypotension, bradycardia, syncope, or cardiogenic shock.

ED management

Initiate supportive care and administer a dose of activated charcoal if <2 hours have elapsed since the ingestion. Gastrointestinal decontamination is paramount and orogastric lavage may alter the outcome in a life-threatening ingestion presenting within the first hour. If a sustained-release preparation was ingested, give multiple doses of activated charcoal or initiate whole-bowel irrigation. Continuously monitor the ECG and blood pressure, and obtain blood for electrolytes, glucose, CBC, ABG, and digoxin level (in an unknown toxic bradycardia).

If the patient has bradycardia or hypotension, initiate treatment immediately as these symptoms are often refractory to therapy and are an ominous sign. Consult with a toxicologist and pediatric cardiologist and arrange pediatric intensive care unit admission. Obtain large-bore IV access and give 20 mL/kg bolus of isotonic fluid and atropine (0.02 mg/kg) for bradycardia. Then administer calcium chloride (0.2–0.25 mL/kg IV) or calcium gluconate (60–100 mg/kg IV). If there is no response, start a high-dose dopamine or norepinephrine infusion. The next line of therapy includes the combination of a high-dose insulin (a myocardial inotrope) infusion (0.5–1.0 units/kg per h) with initial bolus of dextrose IV, and a glucagon (β_1 agonist) infusion (start with a 50–150 mcg/kg bolus over 1 minute, followed by an infusion of 1–5 mg/hr). Phosphodiesterase inhibitors such as milrinone may be effective in refractory cases. Clinically significant bradyarrhythmias that do not respond to the preceding management require pacing.

Indications for admission

- Symptomatic calcium channel blocker ingestion (hypotension, bradyarrhythmias, altered mental status)
- History of calcium channel blocker overdose, unless the patient remains asymptomatic for 6 hours after the ingestion
- History of sustained-release calcium channel blocker overdose
- Suicide attempt or gesture without psychiatric clearance and appropriate follow-up arranged

Bibliography

DeRoos F: Calcium channel blockers. In Flomenbaum N, Goldfrank LR, Hoffman RS, et al. (eds), Goldfrank's Toxicologic Emergencies, 8th ed. New York: McGraw-Hill, pp. 911–23.

Henry K, Harris CR: Deadly ingestions. Pediatr Clin North Am 2006;53:293–315.

Ranninger C, Roche C: Are one or two dangerous? Calcium channel blocker exposure in toddlers. J Emerg Med 2007;33:145–54.

Carbon monoxide

Carbon monoxide (CO) is a colorless, odorless, tasteless gas found in exhaust from combustion engines (automobiles, space heaters, portable generators), and in smoke from fires or tobacco products. CO competitively binds to hemoglobin 250 times more avidly than oxygen, thereby shifting the oxygen/hemoglobin dissociation curve to the left. This impairs delivery of oxygen to peripheral tissues and puts ischemic stress on the heart and CNS. In addition, carbon monoxide binds to myoglobin (potentiating myocardial ischemia), and mitochondrial cytochrome oxidase, and causes glutamate release and lipid peroxidation in the central nervous system.

Clinical presentation

Symptoms of carbon monoxide intoxication are nonspecific and often misdiagnosed. Suspect CO if multiple patients from the same environment or family are displaying symptoms. At low levels, headache, nausea, vomiting, and weakness occur. At higher CO levels, patients develop tachycardia, respiratory distress, lethargy, coma, seizures, and death. Severely CO-poisoned patients may present with cherry red colored skin (and blood) and/ or cutaneous bullae.

Diagnosis

Obtain a serum carboxyhemoglobin level from a venous blood gas (arterial puncture is not necessary). Pulse co-oximetry does not provide an accurate COHb level. If symptoms are severe, obtain serum electrolytes, CBC, urine or serum βHCG, and an ECG. Serum levels correlate poorly with symptoms, but may indicate a significant exposure and therefore guide therapy. Ascertain the interval between the end of the exposure and when the level is obtained. If the interval is long or the patient was treated with oxygen before arrival in the ED, he or she may be more severely affected than the COHb level indicates. An elevated COHb (as high as 10%) occurs in cigarette smokers.

ED management

As increasing the partial pressure of inspired oxygen significantly reduces the half-life of CO, give all patients 100% oxygen via a tight-fitting nonrebreathing mask upon arrival in the ED while awaiting the carboxyhemoglobin level. Indications for hyperbaric oxygen therapy (HBO) (pp. 207–209) include a history of unconsciousness after exposure to CO regardless of COHb level, a history of or continued mental status change or other neurologic deficit, cardiac dysfunction or ischemia, a COHb level >25% regardless of symptoms, and pregnancy with a history of CO exposure (regardless of COHb level). The only absolute contraindication to HBO is an untreated pneumothorax.

Follow-up

- Patient treated for CO poisoning: next day

Indications for admission

- Initial COHb >25%
- Any patient requiring treatment for CO poisoning who has not returned to baseline status

Bibliography

Cho CH, Chiu NC, Ho CS, Peng CC: Carbon monoxide poisoning in children. *Pediatr Neonatol* 2008;49:121–5.

Przepyszny L, Jenkins A: Prevalence of drugs in carbon monoxide related deaths. *Am J Forensic Med and Path* 2007; 28:242–8.

Tomaszewski C: Carbon monoxide. In Flomenbaum N, Goldfrank LR, Hoffman RS, et al. (eds), *Goldfrank's Toxicologic Emergencies*, 8th ed. New York: McGraw-Hill, 2006, pp. 1689–704.

Touger M, Birnbaum A, Wang J et al. Performace of the RAD-57 pulse co-oximeter compared with standard laboratory carboxyhemoglobin measurement. *Ann Emerg Med* (in press).

Caustics

Most caustic ingestions involve alkalis, such as lye, ammonia, oven or drain cleaners, Clinitest tablets, and dishwasher detergents. Non-industrial-strength household bleach (5% sodium hypochlorite) is not a strong caustic and does not cause significant injury. Some ingestions involve acids such as toilet bowl and drain cleaners, battery fluid, metal cleaners, degreasers, and industrial acids. Esophageal injury occurs in approximately 10% of cases of acid ingestion, usually in association with serious gastric damage.

Alkalis frequently cause oropharyngeal injury and serious esophageal ulcerations due to liquefaction necrosis on contact, while acids cause a coagulation necrosis, typically affecting the stomach. Consequences include esophageal perforation with mediastinitis, gastrointestinal bleeding, gastric ulceration, and strictures. Liquid products are more likely than powdered caustics to cause esophageal and stomach burns with minimal oral burns.

Clinical presentation

Oropharyngeal pain and drooling are common, and vomiting occasionally occurs. Findings may also include perioral burns, stridor, dyspnea, chest pain, or abdominal pain.

Diagnosis

The presence of oropharyngeal burns does not correlate with esophageal injury, but a serious esophageal injury (second- or third-degree burn) after an alkali ingestion is unlikely in the absence of stridor, vomiting, drooling, or other serious signs.

ED management

A patient with vomiting, drooling, or stridor is at risk for airway compromise and serious esophageal injury. For these symptomatic patients, obtain IV access, send blood for CBC, type and cross-match, and obtain a chest X-ray (mediastinal widening indicates mediastinitis). Make the patient NPO, and begin maintenance IV hydration. The following are contraindicated: inducing emesis, inserting a nasogastric tube, neutralizing the caustic, or administering activated charcoal or steroids. Consult with an endoscopist, and arrange endoscopy within 12–24 hours.

A patient with a history of possible alkali ingestion, with or without oropharyngeal burns, but without vomiting, drooling, or stridor, is at low risk of serious esophageal injury. If the chest X-ray is normal and the patient is comfortable and can drink readily, he or she can be sent home if telephone contact is possible. Arrange for immediate endoscopy if a patient who has ingested an acid is symptomatic or has oropharyngeal burns.

Indications for admission

- History of alkali ingestion and vomiting, drooling, or stridor
- History of acid ingestion with oropharyngeal burns, abdominal pain, or other symptoms
- Symptoms or signs of intestinal injury
- Suicide attempt or gesture without psychiatric clearance and appropriate follow-up arranged

Bibliography

Arevalo-Silva C, Eliashar R, Wohlgelernter J, Elidan J, Gross M: Ingestion of caustic substances: a 15 year experience. *Laryngoscope* 2006;116:1422–6.

Betalli P, Falchetti D, Giuliani S, et al: Caustic ingestion in children: is endoscopy always indicated? The results of an Italian multicenter observational study. *Gastrointest Endosc* 2008;68:434–9.

Crain EF, Gershel JG, Mezey AP: Caustic ingestions: symptoms as predictors of esophageal injury. *Am J Dis Child* 1984;138:863–5.

Fulton JA, Hoffman RS: Steroids in second degree caustic burns of the esophagus: a systematic pooled analysis of fifty years of human data: 1956–2006. *Clin Toxicol (Phila)* 2007;45:402–8.

Cholinergics

Cholinergic toxicity may be the result of a variety of agents, most notably insecticides and gases used in bioterrorism, but also products containing nicotine and plants such as hemlock. Poisoning from organophosphate insecticides and bioterror agents is life-threatening, and specific life-saving antidotal therapy is available.

Organophosphate (malathion, parathion) and carbamate (aldicarb, propoxur) insecticides block acetylcholinesterase. The subsequent elevation of acetylcholine in the CNS and peripheral nervous system is responsible for the signs and symptoms. Toxicity is usually associated with products formulated for outdoor, industrial, or bioterror settings; household "bug bombs" rarely cause significant toxicity as they contain permethrins, which do not affect cholinesterase. Plant alkaloid and nicotine excess cause symptomatology via nicotinic cholinergic receptor stimulation.

Clinical presentation and diagnosis

Carbamates and organophosphates produce a clinical state of cholinergic excess. Findings include the muscarinic symptoms of salivation, lacrimation, bronchorrhea, bronchospasm, diaphoresis, diarrhea, and miosis, and the typical pesticide odor may be apparent. Heart rate may be increased, decreased, or normal. A useful mnemonic is DUMBELS: Diarrhea, Urination, Miosis, Bronchorrhea, Bronchospasm, Bradycardia, Emesis, Lacrimation, and Salivation.

Nicotinic signs and symptoms such as muscle fasciculations, weakness, and paralysis are present, as are CNS effects such as confusion, seizures, and coma. Death is usually due to respiratory failure because of respiratory muscle paralysis, increased pulmonary secretions, and bronchoconstriction. Occasionally the patient may develop hydrocarbon aspiration pneumonitis, as some pesticides are commonly formulated in hydrocarbon suspensions.

ED management

If there was a cutaneous exposure, remove and double-bag all clothing, and thoroughly wash the patient with soap and water. The ED staff must protect themselves by wearing impervious gloves and aprons made with butyl rubber, as most hospital gloves do not prevent the penetration of these agents.

Provide supportive care, and secure a stable airway. Start an IV, administer activated charcoal if the ingestion is within 4 hours of presentation to the ED, obtain an ECG and monitor the oxygen saturation. Meticulous respiratory support is critical, and intubation and ventilation are often required.

High-dose atropine therapy is the antidote. Titrate the dose against the patient's response, which varies with the specific exposure. The endpoint is satisfactory gas exchange documented by pulse oximetry and ABGs. Start with 0.01 mg/kg (0.5 mg IV for a toddler; 2.0 mg IV for an adolescent), but be prepared to increase both the dose and the frequency. Severe cases may require a constant atropine infusion in the ICU setting.

Pralidoxime is an adjunctive antidote for organophosphate and carbamate poisonings and is indicated when more than 2.0 mg of atropine is required or for nicotinic symptoms, especially muscle weakness. Never use pralidoxime alone, especially for certain carbamates. The dose, given as a bolus, is 25–50 mg/kg IV for a child and 1.0–2.0 g for an adolescent. Pralidoxime is also available in the Mark I autoinjector kit, carried by first responders. It contains 600 mg pralidoxime and 2.0 mg atropine. The dose is one kit for children 3–7 years of age, two kits for 8–14 year-olds, and three kits for patients >15 years old.

Indications for admission

- Presence of any cholinergic clinical findings
- Suicide attempt or gesture without psychiatric clearance and appropriate follow-up arranged

Bibliography

Baydin A, Aygun D, Aydin M, Akdemir HU, Ulger F: Acute organophosphate poisoning mimicking opioid intoxication. *Eur J Emerg Med* 2008;15:245–6.

Flomenbaum N, Goldfrank LR, Hoffman RS, *et al.* eds. *Goldfrank's*

Toxicologic Emergencies, 8th ed. New York: McGraw-Hill, 2006.

Leibson T, Lifshitz M: Organophosphate and carbamate poisoning: review of the current literature and summary of clinical and laboratory experience in southern Israel. *Isr Med Assoc J* 2008; 10:767–7.

Clonidine

Clonidine is both a peripheral and a central alpha agonist. It causes central inhibition of sympathetic output and, to a lesser extent, peripheral vasoconstriction. Clonidine is often used as an antihypertensive, but it is frequently prescribed for children with significant behavior disorders including ADHD. Small children are extremely sensitive to clonidine and toxicity has been reported after ingestion of a single tablet. It is also available as transdermal patches, which present a unique danger for toddlers: a used patch when ingested can contain the equivalent of more than 50 tablets.

Clinical presentation and diagnosis

A patient may present with symptoms mimicking the classic opiate triad of coma, respiratory depression, and miosis. Onset of symptoms can occur shortly after ingestion. Occasionally, a young child is asymptomatic at presentation and suddenly develops apnea. Hypotension is usual, but transient hypertension is occasionally seen early in the course. Hypothermia and bradycardia also occur frequently. There are no specific diagnostic findings or rapidly available tests.

ED management

Institute supportive care and administer activated charcoal within 2 hours of ingestion. Treat clinically significant bradycardia with atropine (0.01 mg/kg per dose). Hypertension is usually transient and followed by hypotension, so do not give antihypertensive therapy. Treat hypotension with a fluid challenge of 20 mL/kg of isotonic crystalloid; if this fails, administer a vasopressor such as dopamine, and titrate against the patient's response. Naloxone (0.1 mg/kg) is variably effective, but it may prevent the need for endotracheal intubation in a patient with respiratory depression. Use a maximum dose of 10 mg before considering it ineffective for reversing mental status depression.

Monitor an asymptomatic patient with known or suspected clonidine ingestion for 4 hours in the ED prior to discharge.

Indications for admission

- Coma, respiratory depression, or altered vital signs
- Suicide attempt or gesture without psychiatric clearance and appropriate follow-up arranged

Bibliography

Henry K, Harris CR: Deadly ingestions. *Pediatr Clin North Am* 2006;53:293–315.

Horowitz R, Mazor SS, Aks SE, Leikin JB: Accidental clonidine patch ingestion in a child. *Am J Ther* 2005;12:272–4.

Spiller AD, Villalobos D, Johnson PB, et al. Toxic clonidine ingestion in children. *J Pediatr* 2005;146:263–6.

Cough and cold medications

Ingestion of cold preparations is common among children because the products are in most households and are available in flavored elixirs. Cold medicines may include any combination of the following: antihistamines, sympathomimetics, acetaminophen, ibuprofen, aspirin, dextromethorphan, and guaifenesin. Resultant symptoms depend on the specific contents of the ingested product. Adolescents seeking the euphoric effects of dextromethorphan and anticholinergics may knowingly ingest cold preparations.

Clinical presentation

Antihistamines such as diphenhydramine, chlorpheniramine, brompheniramine, and triprolidine produce sedation and anticholinergic effect, including tachycardia, dilated unreactive pupils, warm, dry and red skin, decreased bowel sounds, and urinary retention (see Table 15-6). In contrast, newer "non-sedating" antihistamines such as loratadine and cetirizine cause almost no toxicity.

Sympathomimetics include pseudoephedrine and phenylephrine. Phenylephrine is a selective α agonist and may cause severe hypertension. Pseudoephedrine (an isomer of ephedrine) is an α and β agonist and causes a sympathomimetic toxidrome with tachycardia, hypertension, dilated but reactive pupils, and diaphoresis (see Table 15-6). Of note, pseudoephedrine-containing products are often sought in large quantities for the illicit synthesis of methamphetamine.

Dextromethorphan is available in many OTC preparations and may be consumed in large doses by those desiring hallucinogenic effects. It is structurally similar to phencyclidine (PCP) and stimulates NMDA and opioid receptors. Depending on the dosage, there may be sedation or agitation, hypertension, and tachycardia, as well as nystagmus and mydriasis.

Diagnosis

Diagnosis is made by history. Suspect dextromethorphan ingestion in a patient with mild mental status changes and hallucinations.

ED management

Severe toxicity is rare. Administer activated charcoal to a patient arriving within 2 hours of ingestion, or longer if the preparation contains an anticholinergic agent (delays stomach emptying). While sinus tachycardia may result from either anticholinergic or sympathomimetic mechanisms, generally no therapy is needed. Treat severe hypertension associated with stimulants with phentolamine (0.02–0.1 mg/kg IV; repeat q 10 min as needed). Psychomotor agitation may be alleviated with benzodiazepines or haloperidol. See p. 452 for the use of physostigmine to reverse anticholinergic symptoms.

Always consider occult acetaminophen poisoning, as many preparations contain this drug. Obtain an acetaminophen level when the preparation is unknown or to confirm and estimate an ingestion if the timing is known.

Indications for admission

- Severe symptoms (hypotension, seizure, sedation)
- Suicide attempt or gesture without psychiatric clearance and appropriate follow-up arranged

Bibliography

Carr BC: Efficacy, abuse, and toxicity of over-the-counter cough and cold medicines in the pediatric population. *Curr Opin Pediatr* 2006;18:184–8.

Levine DA. 'Pharming': the abuse of prescription and over the counter drugs in teens. *Curr Opin Pediatr* 2007;19:270–4.

Schwartz RH: Adolescent abuse of dextromethorphan. *Clin Pediatr (Phila)* 2005;44:565–8.

Diabetic agents

Diabetic agents include the sulfonylureas (acetohexamide, chlorpropamide [diabinase], glipizide [glucotrol], glyburide [diabeta, micronase, glynase], tolazamide [tolinase], and tolbutamide [orinase]) and newer agents including the biguanides (metformin and phenformin), and the glitazones (rosiglitazone and pioglitazone).

The sulfonylureas cause hypoglycemia by stimulating pancreatic insulin release as well as enhancing peripheral insulin receptor sensitivity and inhibiting gluconeogenesis. Ingestion of a single pill may cause hypoglycemia in a small child.

Biguanides are unlikely to cause severe, persistent hypoglycemia but have been implicated in lactic acidosis. Metformin has a better safety profile than phenformin, which has been removed from the market.

The glitazones (troglitazone and pioglitazone) are also unlikely to produce hypoglycemia because they do not increase insulin release.

Clinical presentation

Signs and symptoms of hypoglycemia include pallor, diaphoresis, tachycardia, depressed level of consciousness, seizures, and coma.

Diagnosis

Consider oral hypoglycemic ingestion in all patients with hypoglycemia. The differential diagnosis of hypoglycemia is discussed on pp. 182–186.

ED management

Immediately obtain a blood sugar (bedside and venipuncture) if there is a history of possible oral hypoglycemic ingestion. Administer activated charcoal if the ingestion occurred less than 2 hours prior to arrival, and start an IV if the patient is symptomatic.

Treat hypoglycemia with 0.5 g/kg of dextrose (1 mL/kg of D_{50} for adolescents; 2 mL/kg of D_{25} for children; 5 mL/kg of D_{10} for infants and toddlers), then repeat the blood sugar.

If hypoglycemia persists give another bolus of dextrose and titrate maintenance fluids with $D_{10}W\frac{1}{2}NS$ to maintain euglycemia. Once the patient is awake, start PO feeds.

If this is unsuccessful, give octreotide to inhibit insulin secretion (25–50 mcg SC). The response is usually rapid, but a repeat dose may be required in 12–24 hours because the half-life of oral hypoglycemics is longer than that of octreotide. Glucagon has a limited effect in young children as glycogen stores are minimal and it may aggravate the emesis. Reserve the use of steroids for severe situations to create insulin resistance. Urine alkalinization to a pH of 7.0–8.0 with sodium bicarbonate (1–2 mEq/kg bolus followed by 0.5 mEq/kg per h) is effective in chlorpropamide ingestions.

Admit normoglycemic patients with a history of significant oral sulfonylurea overdose because delayed hypoglycemia occasionally occurs. Do not give prophylactic IV glucose as it complicates discharge decisions. The patient must be euglycemic without sugar supplementation. However, discharge normoglycemic patients with a history of ingestion of a biguanide or glitazone after 4 hours of observation.

Indications for admission

- Hypoglycemia
- History of oral sulfonylurea agent ingestion if close monitoring is not possible in the ED
- Suicide attempt or gesture without psychiatric clearance and appropriate follow-up arranged

Bibliography

Henry K, Harris CR: Deadly ingestions. *Pediatr Clin North Am* 2006;53:293–315.

Little GL, Boniface KS. Are one or two dangerous? Sulfonylurea exposure in toddlers. *J Emerg Med* 2005; 28:305–10.

McLaughlin SA, Crandall CS, McKinney PE: Octreotide: an antidote for sulfonylurea induced hypoglycemia. *Ann Emerg Med.* 2004;36:133–8.

Digoxin and cardiac glycosides

Ingestion of digoxin in children is uncommon and generally occurs when a patient has access to an adult relative's medications. Digoxin inhibits the function of the sodium-potassium ATPase pump, subsequently increasing calcium ion influx and binding in myocardial tissue. The minimum toxic dose is about 0.1 mg/kg. Children are more resistant to the effects of digoxin than adults, so the lethal dose may be up to 20–50 times the daily maintenance dose. Cardiac glycosides, or digoxin-like substances, are also found in several plants (rhododendron, foxglove, oleander, lily of the valley, and red squill) and licking toads (bufotoxin), but ingestion of these is very rare.

Clinical presentation

Acute ingestion almost always results in nausea and vomiting. Headache, weakness, and confusion may occur, and seizures are rare. Severe ingestions may lead to hyperkalemia, bradycardia, hypotension, and dysrhythmias. Digoxin causes an increase in automaticity and AV blockade which leads to bradycardia, and ventricular escape rhythms. Cardiac toxicity may be more profound in the setting of hypokalemia, hypercalcemia, or hypomagnesemia, or with concomitant quinidine use.

Diagnosis

Suspect digoxin overdose when either a previously well patient who lives with someone maintained on digoxin presents with an arrhythmia or a patient already taking digoxin presents with a new arrhythmia, hyperkalemia, hypotension, CNS depression, or visual disturbance.

ED management

Give activated charcoal if <2 hours have elapsed since ingestion and obtain blood for electrolytes, calcium, and magnesium. Wait until 4 hours post-ingestion to obtain a digoxin level in order to avoid overtreating a predistribution level, which may be high but nontoxic. Assess the ECG for arrhythmias or a prolonged PR interval, and attach a cardiac monitor to follow changes in the rhythm. The classic digoxin-induced dysrhythmias are paroxysmal atrial tachycardia with block or ventricular bigeminy. Other common digoxin dysrhythmias are ventricular ectopy, AV blocks, and sinus bradycardia.

Treat clinically significant bradycardia with AV or SA block with atropine, 0.01 mg/kg IV (minimum dose 0.2 mg, maximum 0.5 mg). Avoid pacemaker placement, if possible, because of an increased risk of ventricular arrhythmias. For ventricular arrhythmias give phenytoin (2 mg/kg IV slowly over 15 min), which decreases ventricular automaticity without slowing AV conduction. Lidocaine is also effective for ventricular arrhythmias (1 mg/kg IV bolus, then 20–50 mcg/kg per min continuous infusion). Avoid using any other anti-arrhythmics as they decrease AV node conduction and may worsen bradycardia. A life-threatening arrhythmia is an indication for Fab antibody fragments (Digibind).

Treat hyperkalemia (>5 mEq/L) aggressively with Fab antibody fragments as well as with conventional therapy (pp. 649–650). Potassium 5–6 mEq/L: $D_5\frac{1}{3}NS$ with 15 mEq/L of sodium bicarbonate; K^+ 6–8 mEq/L: insulin (0.1 units/kg IV), 0.5 g/kg of dextrose IV (5 ml/kg $D_{10}W$ or 2 ml/kg $D_{25}W$), and Kayexalate enemas (1 g/kg); repeat every 4 hours.

Avoid calcium products in treating hyperkalemia secondary to digoxin toxicity because of concern for a theoretical increase in cardiotoxicity.

Fab antibody fragments specific for digoxin (Digibind) are indicated for ventricular dysrhythmias, refractory bradycardia, potassium >5.0 mEq/L, and post-distribution levels >2.0 ng/mL. Be cautious treating a patient who uses digoxin therapeutically, as eliminating the therapeutic effect of the drug by treating only mild elevations of the digoxin level may not be warranted. The dose of Fab antibody fragments is:

#of vials of Fab = mg ingested × 1.6

However, if the serum level is known, the dose is:

#of vials of Fab = (digoxin level in ng/mL × weight in kg/100)

If neither the dose nor the level is known, give 10 vials empirically. If both are known, treat the level.

Indications for admission
- Ingestion of >0.10 mg/kg
- New arrhythmia, visual disturbance, headache, CNS depression, hypotension
- Suicide attempt or gesture without psychiatric clearance and appropriate follow-up arranged

Bibliography

Hack JB, Lewin NA: Cardioactive steroids . In Flomenbaum N, Goldfrank LR, Hoffman RS, et al. (eds), *Goldfrank's Toxicologic Emergencies*, 8th ed. New York: McGraw-Hill, 2006, pp. 971–82.

Hanhan UA: The poisoned child in the pediatric intensive care unit. *Pediatr Clin North Am* 2008;55:669–86.

Lapostolle F, Borron SW, Verdier C, et al: Digoxin-specific Fab fragments as single first-line therapy in digitalis poisoning. *Crit Care Med* 2008;36:3014–18.

Drugs of abuse

Adolescents frequently overdose on drugs of abuse such as cocaine, marijuana, amphetamines, and heroin. In addition, teenagers use a unique group of drugs that are quite rare in other age groups, such as MDMA ('Ecstasy'), diphenhydramine, gamma-hydroxybutyrate (GHB), ketamine, and cold medicines. Many adolescents who present with intoxication have taken multiple substances. Suicidal ideation and attempt are always a concern, so that appropriate counseling and psychiatric evaluation are necessary.

Clinical presentation
Sedative/hypnotics

Sedative/hypnotics include the benzodiazepines, barbiturates, chloral hydrate, and GHB. These agents cause CNS depression, nystagmus, ataxia, hypotension, and possible respiratory depression. Pupils are generally normal or small and vital signs often remain normal. These drugs may be used to facilitate sexual assault (ruphees).

CNS stimulants

CNS stimulants include cocaine, amphetamines, MDMA, phenylephrine, pseudoephedrine, and ephedrine. Stimulants are commonly found in weight-loss medications, cold preparations, and herbal products (Ma Huang). These produce tachycardia, hypertension, hyperthermia, dilated but reactive pupils, diaphoresis, and agitated delirium (agitation, confusion, and paranoia). Seizures, coma, arrhythmias, and myocardial infarction may occur in severe intoxications.

Cannabis

Cannabis, or marijuana, is the most commonly abused illicit drug in the United States. Most commonly smoked in "joints" or cigarettes, marijuana causes euphoria, conjunctival injection, orthostatic hypotension, xerostomia, and tachycardia. Uncommonly, patients may experience palpitations, anxiety, paranoia, and hallucinations.

Opioids

Opioids include heroine, morphine, codeine, meperidine, hydromorphone, fentanyl, oxycodone, hydrocodone, and methadone. Opioids bind to specific opiate receptors in the CNS and cause euphoria, sedation, miosis, respiratory depression, and bradycardia. Severe intoxication may lead to coma, respiratory depression, pulmonary edema, and aspiration.

Hallucinogens

Hallucinogens include lysergic acid diethylamide (LSD), phencyclidine (PCP), 3,4-methylenedioxymethamphetamine ("Ecstasy"), mescaline (peyote), and psilocybin (hallucinogenic mushrooms or "shrooms"). Several other methamphetamine derivatives exist and are commonly abused by teenagers such as "Eve," MDA, and PMA. These products bind to central serotonin and dopamine receptors and produce hallucinations and sympathomimetic effects. Patients seek medical care when unusual behavior is noted or when the patient complains of a "bad trip." PCP may cause aggressive behavior as well as seizures. MDMA causes destruction of serotoninergic neurons and may result in severe depression and memory loss for weeks or permanently. MDMA users may also develop a severe dilutional hyponatremia secondary to an intense thirst along with inappropriate ADH secretion.

Diagnosis

The diagnosis is often made through information obtained from friends, family members, and the patient. If this is not possible or not helpful, ask the paramedics whether there was drug paraphernalia at the scene (patients from a rave party or club are more likely to ingest MDMA, GHB, ketamine, or cold preparations).

A thorough physical examination will provide enough information to direct therapy and disposition (Table 15-5). The patient must be fully undressed and the clothes checked for drugs or paraphernalia. Note the presence of "track marks," or fresh needlesticks. Lethargy implies a CNS depressant or an opioid, whereas agitation suggests a CNS stimulant. Large, reactive pupils and diaphoresis imply sympathomimetic drugs. Small pupils may be seen with the sedative/hypnotics, opioids, and PCP. Paranoia and tachycardia may be seen with the hallucinogens.

ED management

The priorities in severe intoxications are of the airway, breathing and circulation, followed by treatment of grossly abnormal vital signs. Hypertension with agitation from stimulants may be initially treated with benzodiazepines such as diazepam (0.04–0.1 mg/kg per dose q 8 h), but use phentolamine (0.05–0.1 mg/kg per dose to a maximum of 5 mg) or nitroprusside (continuous IV, start with 0.3–0.5 mcg/kg per min; titrate to effect) for hypertensive urgencies. Do not use beta blockers in suspected cocaine intoxication as they may potentiate unopposed alpha-adrenergic-mediated hypertension.

Treat severe hyperthermia (>40°C, 104°F.) with aggressive cooling measures (pp. 205–206) until the core temperature is <38°C (100.4°F). Drug-related hyperthermia, in contrast to environmental hyperthermia, can continue in the hospital and must be treated immediately. Hyperthermia may lead to rhabdomyolysis, myoglobinuria, renal failure, and death.

If the patient has respiratory depression or is comatose, obtain a bedside glucose evaluation and give naloxone (up to 0.1 mg/kg, maximum 2.0 mg, preferably IV), either empirically, or to correct the miosis and respiratory depression seen in opioid toxicity. If there is no response within 1–2 minutes, give a second dose. A positive response may last only 30 minutes, so repeated doses or a continuous IV infusion at 2/3 of the dose required for the initial reversal at an hourly rate may be necessary. If habitual use is suspected in an adolescent it is suggested that the initial dose be 0.05–0.1 mg, increasing to 0.4 mg, and then to 2.0 mg, so as not to precipitate acute withdrawal.

Although flumazenil is a benzodiazepine antagonist, it is not recommended in the overdose setting because it may induce seizures in patients who co-ingest epileptogenic medications or are chronic benzodiazepine abusers. Safer therapy is careful observation and endotracheal intubation, if necessary. Infants and children are less likely to be habituated to benzodiazepines, and flumazenil may be used more safely in the setting of an established benzodiazepine overdose in this population.

Treat seizures with lorazepam (0.05–0.1 mg/kg slow IV) or diazepam (0.1–0.3 mg/kg slow IV). If necessary, sedate the agitated patient with benzodiazepines (diazepam, lorazepam, or midazolam). Haloperidol (5 mg IM) is a useful adjunct in PCP ingestions.

Treat seratonin syndrome (mydriasis, hypertension, psychomotor agitation, altered mental status) secondary to MDMA with cyproheptidine when supportive care fails (see Antidepressants, pp. 453–454).

Indications for admission

- CNS or respiratory depression
- Ventricular arrhythmia
- Serotonin syndrome
- Opiate overdose requiring naloxone treatment
- Suspected opiate or CNS depressant withdrawal
- Suicide attempt or gesture without psychiatric clearance and appropriate follow-up arranged

Bibliography

Goldstein RA, DesLauriers C, Burda AM: Cocaine: history, social implications, and toxicity–a review. *Dis Mon* 2009;55:6–38.

Reuter-Rice K: Ecstasy in the emergency department: MDMA ingestion. *J Pediatr Health Care* 2009;23:49–53.

Wood DM, Greene SL, Alldus G, et al: Improvement in the pre-hospital care of recreational drug users through the development of club specific ambulance referral guidelines. *Subst Abuse Treat Prev Polic.* 2008;3:14.

Ethanol

Ethanol is a sedative/hypnotic which works via stimulation of GABA receptors in the CNS. It is the most commonly abused drug and is the most common co-ingestant in suicide attempts. Ethanol is found in alcoholic beverages, as well as colognes, after-shave, food flavorings (vanilla extract), mouthwash, and some medicinal preparations. A standard alcoholic beverage will contain 15 g of ethanol (30 mL of 50% ethanol; 120 mL of 12% ethanol wine, 360 mL of 5% ethanol beer).

Clinical presentation

Mild intoxication, which occurs at levels of 50 mg/dL, causes euphoria, ataxia, nystagmus, nausea, and emotional lability. Moderately intoxicated patients may have aggressive behavior, vomiting, and slurred speech. With severe intoxication (serum level ≥250 mg/dL), patients may develop respiratory depression, aspiration, miosis, hypothermia, coma, seizures, and rhabdomyolysis. Young children are at high risk of hypoglycemia.

Diagnosis

The diagnosis is usually made by history. The odor of alcohol may be present on the patient's clothing and breath. Clinical signs of intoxication will be more obvious in adolescents but may be altered by co-ingestions. Infants and children with ethanol intoxication may present with hypoglycemia, repeated emesis, and altered mental status. To help estimate the risk of toxicity in an infant or toddler, note that the average volume of a swallow is approximately 0.25 mL/kg. Estimate the peak serum alcohol concentration as follows:

$$\text{peak conc (mg/dL)} = (\% \text{ alcohol}) \times (\text{volume ingested in mL})/0.6 \times (\text{weight in kg})$$

Obtain an ethanol level if alcohol toxicity is suspected. Ethanol levels may correlate with intoxication. However, experienced drinkers can tolerate higher levels of ethanol without symptoms.

An anion gap acidosis, as well as an osmolar gap, may be present. Another method for estimating the ethanol level is 4.6 times the osmolar gap.

Ethanol withdrawal may present within 6 hours of abstinence but delirium tremens (DT) rarely presents before 48–96 hours. Typical symptoms include tremors, hypertension, tachycardia, and psychomotor agitation. Progression to visual auditory and tactile hallucinations may ensue until frank psychosis, or DT, presents. Alcohol withdrawal seizures may take place during this continuum.

ED management

Management of the intoxicated patient depends on the severity of intoxication. If there is CNS depression, protect the airway (if necessary), obtain IV access, obtain a CBC, electrolytes, ethanol level, and fingerstick glucose, and give a dextrose-containing fluid. Gastric decontamination is generally ineffective. If a multiple drug ingestion is suspected and the patient has respiratory depression, give naloxone (0.1 mg/kg, 2 mg maximum).

A patient who is mildly intoxicated requires an ethanol level for confirmation, a careful physical examination to rule out organic causes of confusion (such as head injury), and observation, with frequent reassessments, until the mental status has returned to baseline. The mental status of an intoxicated patient gradually and consistently improves. However, obtain a CT scan of the head if the mental status does not improve, the ethanol level is inconsistent with the mental status, or there are signs of head trauma. An intoxicated patient is at higher risk for risky behavior and falls, so mental status changes that are attributed to alcohol may actually represent intracranial pathology. Observation may be performed at home if the parents are reliable and the patient is alert and ambulatory.

Pediatric patients rarely chronically abuse alcohol. If there is a suspicion that the patient is withdrawing from ethanol, give thiamine 100 mg, folate 1 mg, and magnesium 2 mg IV in addition to the glucose-containing IV fluid. Treat associated agitation and tachycardia with lorazepam (0.05 mg) or diazepam (0.1 mg/kg PO; 10 mg maximum). Also, arrange for psychiatric consultation.

Indications for admission

- Intoxicated preadolescent with an unstable home environment
- Persistent coma or altered mental status
- Alcohol level >250 mg/dL
- Focal neurologic findings
- Suspected ethanol withdrawal
- Suicide attempt or gesture without psychiatric clearance and appropriate follow-up arranged

Bibliography

Henry K, Harris CR: Deadly ingestions. *Pediatr Clin North Am* 2006;53:293–315.

Yip L: Ethanol. In Flomenbaum N, Goldfrank LR, Hoffman RS, *et al.* (eds), *Goldfrank's Toxicologic Emergencies*, 8th ed. New York: McGraw-Hill, 2006, pp. 1147–1161.

Foreign-body ingestion

The frequency of button battery ingestions has risen among younger children. Button batteries are used for watches, calculators, hearing aids, and some small electronic toys. While most ingestions have an uneventful course, serious complications can occur if the battery lodges in the esophagus. However, heavy metal poisoning from battery leakage is not a concern.

Recently, there have been a number of reports of morbidity from mini-magnet ingestions. While the ingestion of one magnet is usually harmless, if a child swallows multiple magnets they may attract each other, increasing the risk of GI complications. These include pressure necrosis, perforation, fistula formation, and intestinal obstruction.

Clinical presentation

Most patients will present to the ED soon after the suspected or witnessed ingestion. The majority are asymptomatic, but if the magnet or battery is lodged in the esophagus, the child may have drooling, dysphagia, or substernal pain. Patients presenting late with GI complications may have abdominal pain, vomiting, fever, hematemesis, diarrhea, and hematochezia.

Diagnosis

The diagnosis of an ingested battery or magnet is made by obtaining a single AP radiograph of the neck, chest, and abdomen. If the foreign body is seen in the esophagus or airway, a lateral radiograph is also needed.

ED management

Urgent endoscopic removal is required for any button battery lodged in the esophagus. However, spontaneous passage generally occurs if it has passed into the stomach. If the battery is <15 mm in diameter and the patient is asymptomatic, discharge the patient, who can resume normal activity. If the battery is >15 mm, there is an increased chance for lodgement in the GI tract. Repeat the radiograph in 1–2 weeks. Specific instructions are available through the Button Battery Ingestion Hotline, which is operated by the National Capital Poison Center in Washington DC, at 202-625-3333.

If a patient swallows multiple magnets, endoscopy is also required. If multiple magnets are noted on radiograph to be distal to the stomach, and the patient is asymptomatic, give GoLYTELY (p. 446) to decrease transit time. If the patient has evidence of GI obstruction or perforation, immediate surgical intervention is necessary.

Indications for admission

- Evidence of intestinal obstruction, perforation
- Multiple mini-magnet ingestion
- Lodgement in esophagus

Bibliography

Dutta S, Barzin A: Multiple magnet ingestion as a source of severe gastrointestinal complications requiring surgical intervention. *Arch Pediatr Adolesc Med* 2008;162:123–5.

Smith MT, Wong RK: Foreign bodies. *Gastrointest Endosc Clin N Am* 2007;17:361–82.

Yardeni D, Yardeni H, Coran AG, et al: Severe esophageal damage due to button battery ingestion: can it be prevented? *Pediatr Surg Int.* 2004;20:496–501.

Hydrocarbons

Hydrocarbons are organic compounds such as camphor, motor oil, gasoline, kerosene, mineral seal oil, pine oil, phenol, carbon tetrachloride, and naphthaline. The main toxicity of hydrocarbons is aspiration pneumonitis, which can occur with all products except those with very high viscosity (motor oil and petroleum jelly). The halogenated and aromatic hydrocarbons can have systemic toxicity.

Clinical presentation

Most patients who ingest hydrocarbons are asymptomatic, although asphyxiation or ventricular dysrhythmias can occur. The patient may present with acute pulmonary symptoms, including cough, tachypnea, hypoxia, and dyspnea, or the onset may be delayed for up to 4–6 hours.

Halogenated and aromatic hydrocarbons can cause coma, seizures, and arrhythmias. Pine oil may produce severe CNS depression and carbon tetrachloride may cause hepatotoxicity over several days. Benzene may cause bone marrow suppression or predispose patients to lymphoproliferative neoplasms and a large toluene ingestion may cause anion gap acidosis.

Diagnosis

Determine the type of hydrocarbon ingested. Have a family member return home and bring the container to the ED. If the chemical is unfamiliar, call the Poison Control Center or the manufacturer for assistance.

ED management

Once the specific hydrocarbon has been identified, a decision must be made whether to perform gastric decontamination. In general, gastric lavage or activated charcoal is not indicated in pediatric hydrocarbon ingestions. Do not induce emesis or perform gastric lavage if the hydrocarbon does not have significant systemic toxicity because of the serious risk of aspiration chemical pneumonitis.

The type of hydrocarbon ingested is a useful determinant in predicting toxicity. Wood-derived hydrocarbons such as pine oil are absorbed by the GI tract and may cause pulmonary edema and CNS toxicity without aspiration. In contrast, petroleum-derived hydrocarbons, such as gasoline or kerosene, must be aspirated to cause toxicity, and therefore are usually left undisturbed in the GI tract.

Observe the patient for CNS depression, seizures, and respiratory complaints for 4–6 hours. If symptoms occur, admit the patient. Obtain a chest radiograph only if the patient develops respiratory symptoms; a baseline, empiric chest radiograph is not necessary for an asymptomatic patient.

Inhalation or ingestion of hydrocarbons with systemic toxicity may lead to a sensitization of myocardial cells to catecholamines. Therefore, place all patients on a cardiac monitor and avoid catecholamines, such as epinephrine, if possible.

Indications for admission

- Ingestion of hydrocarbons with potential for significant systemic toxicity, such as heavy metals, insecticides, aniline dyes, pine oil, and camphor
- Pulmonary signs or symptoms
- Suicide attempt or gesture without psychiatric clearance and appropriate follow-up arranged

Bibliography

Gummin DD, Hryhorczuk DO: Hydrocarbons. In Flomenbaum N, Goldfrank LR, Hoffman RS, et al. (eds), *Goldfrank's Toxicologic Emergencies*, 8th ed. New York: McGraw-Hill, 2006, pp. 1429–46.

Jayashree M, Singhi S, Gupta A: Predictors of outcome in children with hydrocarbon poisoning receiving intensive care. *Indian Pediatr* 2006;43:715–9.

Lifshitz M, Sofer S, Gorodischer R: Hydrocarbon poisoning in children: a 5-year retrospective study. *Wilderness Environ Med* 2003;14:78–82.

Inhalants

Inhalation of volatile substances has increased dramatically over the last 15 years and abuse rates among adolescents are comparable to marijuana. These products are popular among adolescents because they are ubiquitous, short-acting, concealable, and inexpensive. Examples of volatile inhalants include toluene (found in model glue and spray paints), trichloroethane (found in typewriter correction fluid and spot removers), and nitrates (nitrous oxide commercially available or found in whipped cream containers).

There are a number of methods for consuming these products. These include huffing (direct inhalation of a substance adsorbed to a cloth or object held over the mouth or nose), sniffing (inhalation of vapors from an open container or heated pan), and bagging (spraying or pouring a substance into a bag which is then used to rebreathe).

Clinical presentation

Inhalation produces rapid euphoria and lightheadedness and may cause CNS depression, syncope, or hallucinations which are usually of short duration. Inhalation of volatiles can lead to sensitization of the myocardium to catecholamines, leading to ventricular dysrhythmias and "sudden sniffing death." However, this lasts for approximately 5–15 minutes after inhalation, so it is of less concern upon arrival in the ED.

Diagnosis

An inhalant abuser rarely arrives in the ED with complaints involving the inhalation. Occasionally a novice user will complain of transient lightheadedness or a patient will show evidence of abuse such as spray paint on the skin around the nose or odor of alcohol or petroleum distillates on the body or clothing. Consider inhalant abuse in an adolescent with ventricular arrhythmias or sudden arrest.

ED management
Supportive care and education is all that is necessary.

Indications for admission
- Ventricular arrhythmias
- Suicide attempt or gesture without psychiatric clearance and appropriate follow-up arranged

Bibliography
Alper AT, Akyol A, Hasdemir H, et al: Glue (toluene) abuse: increased QT dispersion and relation with unexplained syncope. *Inhal Toxicol* 2008;**20**:37–41.

Medina-Mora ME, Real T: Epidemiology of inhalant use. *Curr Opin Psychiatry* 2008;**21**:247–51.

Williams JF, Storck M; American Academy of Pediatrics Committee on Substance Abuse; American Academy of Pediatrics Committee on Native American Child Health: Inhalant abuse. *Pediatrics* 2007;**119**:1009–17.

Iron
Iron is a leading cause of fatal poisoning in younger children. It is readily available for the treatment of anemia and in prenatal and multivitamins. Most adult iron formulations contain 60–90 mg of elemental iron per tablet and children's formulations generally contain 15 mg per tablet or 10–20 mg/mL. Ferrous, gluconate is 12% elemental iron (32 mg Fe per 325 mg tablet), ferrous fumarate is 33% (100 mg Fe per 325 mg tablet), and ferrous sulfate is 20% (65 mg Fe per 325 mg tablet). Most chewable multivitamins have only 10–18 mg of elemental iron per tablet.

The minimal toxic dose is 20 mg/kg of elemental iron. Ingestion of 20–60 mg/kg is associated with mild to moderate toxicity and >60 mg/kg causes severe toxicity.

Clinical presentation
Iron toxicity results from both direct gastrointestinal injury and diffuse cellular toxicity; it presents in five stages. The initial stages are localized to the GI tract and the later stages include systemic toxicity. In the initial phase (first 6 hours), GI symptoms predominate, with vomiting, hematemesis, abdominal pain, diarrhea, and hematochezia. During the next few hours, there may be a period in which the symptoms abate (stage II). During the third stage, at 6–24 hours after ingestion, the patient develops hypotension, hepatic failure, shock, seizures, coma, metabolic acidosis, coagulopathy, and hyperglycemia. The fourth stage occurs 2–5 days post ingestion and is characterized by hepatic failure. Stage V is gastric outlet or intestinal stricture, which may occur 4–6 weeks after the ingestion.

Diagnosis
The diagnosis of iron overdose is easily overlooked if the history does not suggest the possibility of ingestion. A high index of suspicion must be maintained in young children presenting with blood in the vomit or stools or whose mother is taking prenatal vitamins.

Clinically significant iron toxicity is possible if the history suggests that more than 20 mg/kg of elemental iron was ingested or the patient is symptomatic (abdominal pain, vomiting, or diarrhea). It is extremely uncommon for a child to develop iron toxicity in the absence of vomiting. Obtain a serum iron concentration at the expected peak, 2–6 hours after ingestion. The peak iron level predicts toxicity, but the total iron-binding capacity is not a reliable marker. A level <300 mcg/dL is nontoxic, 300–500 mcg/dL correlates with localized GI symptoms and possible systemic effects, and a level >500 mcg/dL correlates with severe toxicity.

Elevation of the white blood cell count >15 000/mm^3 and glucose >150 mg/dL often occurs in patients who are iron toxic, but normal results cannot be used to rule out toxicity. Abdominal radiographs may help identify pills that are radioopaque; however, X-rays are normal in a patient who has ingested liquid or children's formulations.

ED management

Calculate the amount of elemental iron ingested. Discharge a patient who has ingested <20 mg/kg of elemental iron and is asymptomatic. For all other patients, obtain an abdominal radiograph and serum iron level.

If a significant number of tablets are seen on the radiograph, decontaminate the gut by whole-bowel irrigation (WBI) with polyethylene glycol electrolyte lavage solution (COLYTE, GoLYTELY) using a nasogastric tube. See p. 446 for the procedure for using WBI. Contraindications to WBI include an unprotected airway in a comatose patient, ileus, GI obstruction, perforation, or significant hemorrhage. Use gastric lavage only for patients with large ingestions of iron liquid. Activated charcoal does not adsorb iron significantly and is recommended only if there is a significant co-ingestant.

Provide supportive care as indicated. Start an IV, and pay special attention to perfusion and acid–base status. Large amounts of fluid and bicarbonate are frequently required.

Obtain a serum iron level 2–6 hours after ingestion; if it is >500 mcg/dL, initiate deferoxamine therapy (15 mg/kg per h IV, 6 g/day maximum; start infusion at 5 mg/kg per h to prevent hypotension). Deferoxamine chelates free iron into a water-soluble complex, which is excreted in the urine and makes the urine a vin-rosé color. Other indications for deferoxamine therapy are shock, intractable vomiting, or severe acidosis. Correct intravascular volume deficits before instituting chelation therapy because deferoxamine in the presence of decreased renal blood flow can lead to acute renal failure. Continue deferoxamine until the patient appears well, the acidosis has improved, and the urine color has returned to normal. Deferoxamine side effects include hypotension, which can be minimized by starting the infusion at a slower rate, and anaphylactoid reactions. Obtain blood for a CBC, electrolytes, coagulation profile, BUN, creatinine, liver function tests, and type and hold and a urinalysis before instituting chelation therapy.

Indications for admission

- Serum iron >500 mcg/dL
- Signs or symptoms of iron toxicity
- Suicide attempt or gesture without psychiatric clearance and appropriate follow-up arranged

Bibliography

Baranwal AK, Singhi SC: Acute iron poisoning: management guidelines. *Indian Pediatr* 2003;40:534–40.

Madiwale T, Liebelt E. Iron: not a benign therapeutic drug. *Curr Opin Pediatr* 2006;18:174–9.

Singhi SC, Baranwal AK: Acute iron poisoning: clinical picture, intensive care needs and outcome. *Indian Pediatr* 2003;40:1177–82.

Mothballs

Most mothballs in the United States contain paradichlorobenzene, which is a relatively nontoxic substance. However, older mothballs may be composed of naphthalene or, less commonly, camphor. Naphthalene can cause sedation, seizures, and methemoglobinemia, as well as severe hemolysis in G6PD-deficient patients. Camphor, which is also available as an oil in herbal preparations and ointments, also predominantly causes CNS effects such as seizures.

Clinical presentation

In most cases the patient is asymptomatic. However, the onset of hemolysis in a G6PD-deficient patient may be delayed for up to 24–48 hours. Weakness, pallor or jaundice, dark urine, and oliguria may occur. A patient who ingests naphthalene or camphor may develop lethargy, sedation, and seizures within hours of ingestion.

Diagnosis

When the chemical nature of the mothball is unknown, try dissolving a sliver in absolute ethanol: paradichlorobenzene (nontoxic) dissolves, while naphthalene does not. In addition, an X-ray of the mothball can differentiate the two: paradichlorobenzene is radioopaque whereas naphthalene is not. Another method for identifying the type of mothball is to get a large amount of salt and make a concentrated salt solution. Naphthalene mothballs float in this solution, but paradichlorobenzene does not. Mothballs containing camphor are oilier than the other two types of mothballs.

Hemolysis can be documented with serial hematocrit determinations (decreasing), the peripheral smear (fragmented red cells), and a urinalysis (dipstick positive for blood and bilirubin, but no RBCs seen). If the patient is symptomatic, a low level on a G6PD quantitative assay (not a qualitative screen) confirms that the child is at risk. In the presence of hemolysis, young RBCs, which do contain enzyme, predominate, so a qualitative screen may be falsely reassuring.

ED management

Most patients who unintentionally ingest one naphthalene or paradichlorobenzene mothball do not require medical intervention or GI decontamination. If a large number of mothballs are ingested, give activated charcoal. If the mothball contains naphthalene, determine the patient's G6PD status. For asymptomatic patients no further work-up is necessary. Instruct the family to return at once if pallor, jaundice, lethargy, or dark urine is noticed. If sedation or seizures occur, admit the patient to a monitored setting for supportive care and close observation. If camphor was ingested, observe the patient for 2–4 hours, as most seizures will occur within 1–2 hours post ingestion.

If the patient is symptomatic, obtain a CBC, type and cross-match, urinalysis, electrolytes, BUN, and creatinine. If hemoglobinuria is present, institute alkaline diuresis with $D_5\frac{1}{2}NS$ and sodium bicarbonate (1 mEq/kg q 4 h, infused over 30 min) to maintain a urine output of 3–6 mL/kg per h, using furosemide (1 mg/kg IV), if necessary. Give small transfusions (5 mL/kg) of packed red cells to maintain the hematocrit at about 80% of normal.

Treat symptomatic methemoglobinemia with IV methylene blue (1–2 mg/kg). Treat seizures with lorazepam (0.05–0.10 mg/kg slow IV) or diazepam (0.1–0.3 mg/kg slow IV).

Indications for admission

- Suspected naphthalene ingestion in a patient known to be G6PD deficient
- Significant sedation
- Seizures
- Evidence of intravascular hemolysis
- Suicide attempt or gesture without psychiatric clearance and appropriate follow-up arranged

Bibliography

Feuillet L, Mallet S, Spadari M: Twin girls with neurocutaneous symptoms caused by mothball intoxication. *N Engl J Med* 2006;355:423–4.

Kong JT, Schmiesing C: Concealed mothball abuse prior to anesthesia: mothballs, inhalants, and their management. *Acta Anaesthesiol Scand* 2005; 49:113–6.

Nonsteroidal anti-inflammatory drugs

Nonsteroidal anti-inflammatory drugs (NSAIDs) are widely used for the treatment of pain, arthritis, and dysmenorrhea. Among the many agents in this category, ibuprofen and naproxen are nonprescription, and ibuprofen is readily available as a pleasant-tasting liquid. These medications are rapidly absorbed, with peak levels occurring within 2 hours. Sustained-release preparations require 2–5 hours to reach peak level.

NSAIDs inhibit cyclooxygenase (COX), thereby decreasing prostaglandin synthesis. The most common side effects are GI, which are due to disruption of the mucosal protective effects of prostaglandin. Overdose may also cause decreased renal blood flow or CNS effects. Nonetheless, overdoses of NSAIDs rarely produce serious consequences. COX-2 inhibitors lose their selectivity for the COX-2 enzyme when ingested in overdose and display a toxicity that is similar to all other NSAIDs.

Clinical presentation

Mild GI distress, such as epigastric pain, nausea, and vomiting, is the rule, although lethargy and drowsiness sometimes occur. Very large overdoses of ibuprofen can cause metabolic acidosis. Mefenamic acid can cause seizures and muscle twitching. Apnea and cardiovascular collapse have also been reported after massive ingestions.

Diagnosis

The history suggests the diagnosis. Serum ibuprofen levels do not correlate well with outcomes. Elevation of liver transaminases, metabolic acidosis, and hypoprothrombinemia may occur in massive overdoses.

ED management

Typically, no interventions are required unless very large amounts (>400 mg/kg for ibuprofen) have been ingested. In such a case, administer activated charcoal, monitor the level of consciousness, and obtain an ABG. Treat seizures with lorazepam (0.05–0.10 mg/kg slow IV) or diazepam (0.1–0.3 mg/kg slow IV). Manage minor GI distress with magnesium hydroxide/aluminum hydroxide PO (Maalox 1 mL/kg, maximum 30 mL) and an oral or IV H_2 antagonist such as ranitidine (2–4 mg/kg per 24 hr PO div q 12 hr, 150 mg/dose maximum).

Indications for admission

*   Decreased level of consciousness or metabolic acidosis or seizures
*   Suicide attempt or gesture without psychiatric clearance and appropriate follow-up arranged

Bibliography

Belson GM and Watson WA: Nonsteroidal antiinflammatory drugs. In Flomenbaum N, Goldfrank LR, Hoffman RS, *et al.* (eds), *Goldfrank's Toxicologic Emergencies*, 8th ed. New York: McGraw-Hill, 2006, pp. 573–9.

Holubek W, Stolbach A, Nurok S, et al: A report of two deaths from massive ibuprofen ingestion. *J Med Toxicol* 2007;3:52–5.

Marciniak KE, Thomas IH, Brogan TV, et al: Massive ibuprofen overdose requiring extracorporeal membrane oxygenation for cardiovascular support. *Pediatr Crit Care Med* 2007;8:180–2.

Rat poison

The vast majority of commercial rodenticides are superwarfarins, single long-acting anti-coagulants. Included in this group are brodifacum, bromadiolone, difenacoum, valone, and dipacinone. Historically, rat poisons have been made of arsenic, thallium, strychnine, PNU, ANTU, Norbormide, and red squill. These preparations are no longer manufactured in the United States, but exposure to these and others such as tetramethylenedisulfotetramine (TETS) and aldicarb may be possible as there have been reports of these products being imported from Asia or Latin America. In view of the varied toxicity of this eclectic group of compounds, it is crucial to identify the rat poison ingested when evaluating a poisoned patient.

The superwarfarin products inhibit hepatic synthesis of the vitamin K-dependent coagulation factors (II, VII, IX, and X). Anticoagulation occurs approximately 2 days after ingestion, as new synthesis is impaired but existing functional factors remain. As the existing factors are consumed, elevation of the PT (prothrombin time) and INR (International Normalized Ratio) occur.

Clinical presentation

Most patients who ingest one of the superwarfarin products are asymptomatic on presentation and remain so. However, if the ingestion was large and occurred days prior to presentation, there may be evidence of coagulopathy, such as ecchymoses, bleeding gums, melena, hematemesis, hematuria, or intracranial hemorrhage.

Diagnosis

The diagnosis is generally made by history. Send a family member to retrieve the product, as identification of the product is absolutely necessary.

ED management

It is not necessary to routinely measure PT and INR post ingestion in a small child with accidental ingestion of a superwarfarin, unless it is known that a large quantity was consumed. The patient can be safely discharged but instruct the family to return for any bleeding problems. If a large quantity was ingested, or the ingestion was intentional, measure the PT and INR 36–48 hours post ingestion.

At time of repeat evaluation, if the INR is normal, no further management is required. If the INR is >4.0 or if the patient develops active bleeding, give vitamin K1, 10 mg/day PO div q 6–8 h, for up to 1 month. Increase the dose, as needed up to 125 mg/day, to maintain a normalized INR. Intravenous vitamin K1 can be used for severe bleeding, but it has a higher risk of anaphylactic reaction than the PO or IM routes. If the INR >9.0 or there is evidence of severe bleeding, give fresh frozen plasma (15 mg/kg). Consult with a pediatric hematologist if recombinant clotting factors might be needed to control bleeding.

Follow-up

- 36–48 hours, for coagulation studies if a large quantity was ingested

Indications for admission

- Coagulopathy
- Suicide attempt or gesture without psychiatric clearance and appropriate follow-up arranged

Bibliography

Pavlu J, Harrington DJ, Voong K, et al: Superwarfarin poisoning. *Lancet* 2005;365:628.

Spahr JE, Maul JS, Rodgers GM: Superwarfarin poisoning: a report of two cases and review of the literature. *Am J Hematol* 2007;82:656–60.

Watt BE, Proudfoot AT, Bradberry SM, et al: Anticoagulant rodenticides. *Toxicol Rev* 2005;24:259–69.

Salicylates

Salicylates are widely used because of their antipyretic, anti-inflammatory, and antiplatelet actions. Aspirin (acetylsalicylic acid) is in many nonprescription analgesics and cold preparations. Methylsalicylate is the active ingredient in some nonprescription topical creams (Icy Hot, Ben Gay, Tiger Balm; 30% methylsalicylate) and oil of wintergreen (98% methylsalicylate). One teaspoon of oil of wintergreen is equivalent to 7000 mg of aspirin.

The toxicity of salicylates is due to direct stimulation of the CNS respiratory center, which causes an initial hyperventilation and respiratory alkalosis. This is followed by an uncoupling of oxidative phosphorylation with a resultant increased anion gap metabolic acidosis.

The potentially acute toxic dose is 150 mg/kg, or about two baby aspirin per kg. Serious toxicity is possible if >300 mg/kg is ingested.

Clinical presentation

Mild poisoning causes tinnitus, abdominal pain, vomiting, and hyperpnea (respiratory alkalosis). The early signs of respiratory alkalosis are more common in adults as children tend to present with a metabolic acidosis. With larger doses, marked hyperpnea, hyperthermia, lethargy, dehydration, metabolic acidosis, and hypo- or hyperglycemia occur. Severe poisoning leads to coma, seizures, severe metabolic acidosis, oliguria, pulmonary edema, and death. An unusual presentation is acute behavior change, including confusion, agitation, hallucinations, or psychosis.

Diagnosis

Obtain serum salicylate levels at presentation and every 2 hours. In general, levels between 15 and 30 mg/dL are therapeutic, >30 mg/dL may be associated with signs of toxicity, and >100 mg/dL are very serious and may require hemodialysis. More important than the patient's serum is the patient's clinical and acid–base status. The Dome nomogram correlates poorly with serum levels and is no longer used.

An ABG and serum electrolytes will demonstrate a respiratory alkalosis early after overdose. An increased anion gap acidosis may develop at the same time or slightly later, and hypo- or hyperglycemia may occur.

Salicylate poisoning can be confused clinically with diabetic ketoacidosis (glucose usually >300 mg/dL, polyuria), influenza (myalgias, URI symptoms), pneumonia (rales, infiltrate on chest X-ray), gastroenteritis (diarrhea more common), ketotic hypoglycemia (starvation, no acid–base disturbance unless postictal), Reye's syndrome (elevated serum ammonia), or a primary neuropsychiatric disturbance See Table 15.9 for other causes of an increased anion gap are (the mnemonic Mudpiles).

ED management

Provide supportive care as needed, administer activated charcoal (<2 hours post ingestion or anytime for a symptomatic patient who may have delayed gastric emptying of the salicylate), secure an IV, and obtain blood for ABG, electrolytes, glucose, PT, and CBC. Also obtain a salicylate level at the time of presentation and every 2 hours thereafter. Consider the possibility of co-ingestion of acetaminophen, and obtain a level at 4 hours post-ingestion (pp. 448–450). Fluid losses can be significant secondary to the hypermetabolic state; treat aggressively with 20 mL/kg normal saline or Ringer's lactate boluses.

If the patient has an altered mental status, give 0.5 g/kg of dextrose IV and maintain the serum glucose level at approximately 150 mg/dL. Once there is satisfactory urine output, initiate urinary alkalization for any patient who manifests signs and symptoms of salicylate toxicity or has a serum level >40 mg/dL. Infuse D_5W with 132 mEq bicarbonate and 40 mEq/L of potassium chloride (add three 50 mL ampules of sodium bicarbonate solution to 1 liter of D_5W) at twice the maintenance rate. The goal is a urine output of 3 mL/kg per h with a pH ≥7.5. Salicylate reabsorption in the kidney tubules is inhibited at an alkaline urine pH, so the ionic form of salicylate is "trapped" in the urine. Carefully monitor the serum potassium, since it is lowered by both sodium bicarbonate administration and hyperventilation. Serum potassium in the high normal range is necessary for achieving an alkaline diuresis; otherwise hydrogen ions will acidify the urine in exchange for retaining potassium. Discontinue alkalization when the serum level is below 40 mg/dL and the patient has clinically improved and has a normal acid–base status.

Hemodialysis is indicated for an acute salicylate level >100 mg/dL, severe acidosis, oliguria or anuria, pulmonary edema, coagulopathy, intractable seizures, or progressive deterioration despite appropriate therapy regardless of the salicylate level. Hemodialysis may be indicated for chronic toxicity with a serum level >60 mg/dL in association with lethargy, mental status changes, or acidosis. Multiple doses of activated charcoal (1 g/kg q 3 h × 4) may decrease serum half-life, but are not as effective as hemodialysis. If hemodialysis is not available, exchange transfusion is an alternative.

Avoid mechanical ventilation if possible. A salicylate-toxic patient compensates for metabolic acidosis with significant tachypnea. Decreasing the respiratory rate to "normal" with mechanical ventilation may lead to severe acute acidosis, seizures, arrest, and death. If intubation is necessary, pretreat with boluses of bicarbonate and set the ventilator to a high respiratory rate.

Indications for admission

- Salicylate level >45 mg/dL 6 hours after an acute ingestion
- Signs and symptoms of salicylism in a patient taking salicylates
- Suicide attempt or gesture without psychiatric clearance and appropriate follow-up arranged

Bibliography

Davis JE: Are one or two dangerous? Methyl salicylate exposure in toddlers. *J Emerg Med* 2007;32:63–9.

Flomenbaum NE: Salicylates. In Flomenbaum N, Goldfrank LR, Hoffman RS, *et al.* (eds),

Goldfrank's Toxicologic Emergencies, 8th ed. New York: McGraw-Hill, 2006, pp. 550–64.

Henry K, Harris CR: Deadly ingestions. *Pediatr Clin North Am* 2006;53:293–315.

Toxic alcohols (ethylene glycol, methanol, and isopropanol)

The toxic alcohols include ethylene glycol, methanol, and isopropanol, as well as benzyl alcohol and propylene glycol. Ethylene glycol can be found in antifreeze (up to 95%) and is generally ingested unintentionally in children because of its sweet taste. Methanol is found in solvents, windshield-wiper fluid, and duplicating fluids. Isopropanol is the main ingredient in rubbing alcohol (70%) and is also found in solvents and disinfectants.

These alcohols may be ingested unintentionally in children or as an alcohol substitute in adolescents. All three cause intoxication similar to ethanol as well as gastritis. Isopropanol is metabolized to acetone, a CNS depressant, producing toxicity similar to ethanol in children. Methanol is metabolized to formic acid and ethylene glycol is metabolized to glycolic, glyoxylic, and oxalic acids. These "toxic metabolites" produce an anion gap metabolic acidosis and may lead to death.

Clinical presentation and diagnosis
Ethylene glycol

Ethylene glycol toxicity occurs in two distinct stages. Within the first 3–4 hours, there is inebriation, with ataxia, nystagmus, nausea, and euphoria. At this stage, the ethylene glycol level is high, the osmolar gap is elevated, but there is no acidosis. As the ethylene glycol is metabolized into toxic metabolites, the patient develops an anion gap metabolic acidosis leading to tachypnea, tachycardia, hypotension, renal failure from crystalline deposits in renal tubules, cerebral and pulmonary edema, and seizures. In this acidemic stage, the ethylene glycol levels may be lower, and the osmolar gap may be lower, but acidosis is present.

Methanol

Methanol produces a similar two-stage toxicity. The initial intoxication is not as pronounced as with ethylene glycol or ethanol. As the methanol is metabolized, an anion gap metabolic acidosis develops with tachypnea, tachycardia, visual changes, blindness, seizures, and death.

Isopropyl alcohol

Isopropyl alcohol produces inebriation that is more pronounced than ethanol. In the first few hours, euphoria, nausea, and vomiting predominate. Laboratory studies reveal an elevated osmolar gap without metabolic acidosis. Metabolism of isopropanol to acetone leads to CNS depression and a distinctive ketone odor. Because the predominant metabolite is acetone without further acidic byproducts, the hallmark of isopropanol toxicity is ketosis without acidosis.

ED management

Lethal oral doses of ethylene glycol and methanol-containing compounds are very small, approximately 1.5 mL/kg. For any potential ingestion, obtain a CBC, electrolytes, ethanol, serum osmolality and, if possible, a specific alcohol level. Calculate the osmolality and subtract it from the measured osmolality to determine the osmolar gap. Elevation of the osmolar gap may be indicative of a toxic alcohol ingestion, but it can also be secondary to ethanol, IV contrast (osmotic contrast), mannitol, acetone, ketoacidosis, or chronic renal failure (not acute). If the laboratory is unable to perform levels of the specific toxic alcohols, approximate them by multiplying the osmol gap by the following conversion factors: ethylene glycol (6.2), isopropyl alcohol (6.0), and methanol (3.2). For example, if the osmolar gap is 20, then the estimated ethylene glycol level is 124 mg/dL.

The treatment of methanol and ethylene glycol poisoning involves blocking the production and enhancing the clearance of toxic metabolites. This can be accomplished by competitively inhibiting the enzyme alcohol dehydrogenase. Hemodialysis is the mainstay of therapy, allowing both clearance of the alcohol and the acidosis. Sodium bicarbonate may be used to treat the metabolic acidosis if the pH is <7.2. Gastric decontamination is generally not beneficial because alcohols are rapidly absorbed.

Ethanol competitively inhibits alcohol dehydrogenase. Fomepizole also competitively inhibits it and is FDA-approved for the treatment of both methanol and ethylene glycol ingestions in adults. Evidence for its efficacy and safety in children has been shown in case series although no randomized controlled trials exist. The advantages over ethanol are that there are no levels to monitor and it does not cause gastritis or hypoglycemia.

Indications for ethanol or fomepizole are suspicion of methanol or ethylene glycol ingestion with one of the following: methanol >20 mg/dL, ethylene glycol >20 mg/dL, osmolar gap >10 mOsm/L, and a metabolic acidosis. Indications for hemodialysis are ethylene glycol >40 mg/dL, osmol gap >10 mOsm/L, renal failure, or metabolic acidosis. The loading dose of fomepizole is 15 mg/kg IV over 30 minutes, followed by 10 mg/kg q 12 hr for 4 doses. The dosing must be adjusted if hemodialysis is initiated to allow for clearance of fomepizole.

For ethanol, use a 10% solution and give an IV loading dose of 10 mL/kg, followed by 1–2 mL/kg per hr. An ethanol level of 100 mg/dL is sufficient to block most of the metabolite production. Serum ethanol levels and bedside glucose checks must be performed frequently. Ethanol may also be given via nasogastric tube, but this can cause a severe gastritis.

Indications for admission

- Toxic levels of ethylene glycol, methanol, or isopropanol
- CNS depression, nausea, hypoglycemia, tachycardia, or other symptoms of alcohol ingestion
- Suicide attempt or gesture without psychiatric clearance and appropriate follow-up arranged

Bibliography

Henry K, Harris CR: Deadly ingestions. *Pediatr Clin North Am* 2006;53:293–315.

Holubek WJ, Hoffman RS, Goldfarb DS, Nelson LS: Use of hemodialysis and hemoperfusion in poisoned patients. *Kidney Int* 2008;74:1327–34.

Kraut JA, Kurtz I: Toxic alcohol ingestions: clinical features, diagnosis, and management. *Clin J Am Soc Nephrol* 2008;3:208–25.

Tricyclic antidepressants

Tricyclic antidepressants (TCAs) are used for the treatment of depression, migraines, enuresis, OCD, ADD, and chronic pain. Common TCAs include amitryptyline (Elavil), amoxapine (Ascendin), clomipramine (Anafranil), desipramine (Norpramin), doxepin (Sinequan), imipramine (Tofranil), nortryptyline (Pamelor), protriptyline (Vivactil), and trimpramine (Surmontil).

Clinical toxicity results from anticholinergic effects, peripheral α-blockade, sodium channel blockade, GABA inhibition, direct myocardial (quinidine-like) depression, and acidosis. Toxic doses vary with specific drugs but all TCAs have similar side effects. The lethality of these drugs in overdose is secondary to cardiovascular and CNS effects.

Clinical presentation

The central anticholinergic effect causes hyperthermia, as well as mental status changes ranging from combativeness, delirium, and hallucinations to lethargy and coma. Peripheral anticholinergic effects include tachycardia, decreased bowel sounds, flushed skin, and urinary retention (see Anticholinergics, pp. 451–452). Transient hypertension may occur early after ingestion due to increased catecholamine release, but hypotension is more frequent and is predominantly due to the α-blockade. Sodium channel blockade slows ventricular depolarization, causing a prolonged QRS and contributing to the hypotension, and GABA inhibition leads to seizures. Ventricular arrhythmias are the primary cause of death.

Diagnosis

Suspect a tricyclic overdose in a patient presenting with an acute change of mental status, seizures, abnormal vital signs, or an arrhythmia. Attach a cardiac monitor and obtain an ECG. Toxicity can be predicted by a widened QRS >100 ms, a terminal 40 ms right axis deviation, and an R wave in AVR that generally exceeds 3 mm in amplitude. As the QRS widens and as the R wave exceeds 3 mm, there is an increasing likelihood of seizures developing.

ED management

Initiate supportive care and place the patient on a continuous ECG monitor. Perform gastric lavage if a potentially lethal dose of a TCA was taken within 1 hour of presentation; administer activated charcoal if ingestion was within 2 hours of presentation. If the QRS interval is >100 ms, give 1–2 mEq/kg of sodium bicarbonate IV over 2 minutes and repeat every 5 minutes until the QRS narrows to <100 ms. Start a bicarbonate drip and titrate the serum pH to 7.45–7.55. Sodium bicarbonate is also indicated for hypotension or a serum pH <7.1.

Do not treat hypertension, which is usually transient, since hypotension frequently follows. Treat hypotension with sodium bicarbonate (as above) and a 20 mL/kg bolus of an isotonic crystalloid (normal saline, Ringer's lactate). If fluids and bicarbonate are unsuccessful, norepinephrine (0.1–0.2 mcg/kg per min IV) is the preferred pressor and titrate the dose against the patient's response. Treat seizures with lorazepam (0.05–0.1 mg/kg IV) or diazepam (0.1–0.3 mg/kg slow IV) or phenobarbital. It is not necessary to treat supraventricular arrhythmias, but give lidocaine (1 mg/kg IV) for life-threatening ventricular arrhythmias. Electrical pacing may be needed. Do not use physostigmine, as asystole has been reported.

Consult a toxicologist and cardiologist, and admit a symptomatic patient to an ICU, where continuous cardiac monitoring and close nursing supervision can be provided, until the patient is symptom-free for 12 hours. Patients who do not develop any symptoms within 6 hours and have a normal ECG can be discharged from the ED.

Indications for admission

- Any signs or symptoms of tricyclic overdose
- History of possible tricyclic overdose, unless 6 hours has elapsed and the patient has remained asymptomatic with normal vital signs, a normal mental status, and no changes on ECG monitoring
- Suicide attempt or gesture without psychiatric clearance or appropriate follow-up arranged

Bibliography

Harrigan RA, Brady WJ: ECG abnormalities in tricyclic antidepressant ingestion. *Am J Emerg Med* 1999;17:387–93.

McFee RB, Caraccio TR, Mofenson HC: Selected tricyclic antidepressant ingestions involving children 6 years old or less. *Acad Emerg Med* 2001;8:139–44.

Rosenbaum TG, Kou M: Are one or two dangerous? Tricyclic antidepressant exposure in toddlers. *J Emerg Med* 2005;28:169–74.

Adapted with permission from Rumack BH, Matthew H: Acetaminophen poisoning and toxicity. *Pediatrics* 1975;55:871–6

Chapter 16

Neurologic emergencies

Soe Mar

Acute ataxia

Acute ataxia is usually the result of cerebellar dysfunction. However, it may also result from conditions affecting the vestibular apparatus, disorders of sensory input (from peripheral nerves, posterior roots, posterior columns), or abnormalities in the connections between the posterior columns and the parietal lobes. Although the most common causes (Table 16-1) are intoxications (alcohol, benzodiazepines, anticonvulsant medications) and parainfectious and viral infections, always consider a mass lesion (posterior fossa, brainstem, spinal cord), hydrocephalus, head trauma, meningitis, encephalitis, and a metabolic or vascular etiology.

Clinical presentation

Ataxia is manifested as an unsteady, reeling, wide-based gait or truncal instability (titubation). Dysmetria, tremor, slow, dysrhythmic "scanning" speech, and nystagmus may also be present.

Parainfectious acute cerebellar ataxia

Acute cerebellar ataxia most often occurs days to weeks after a viral infection such as varicella. Typically, a 1–3-year-old presents with a short history (hours to days) of incoordination, unsteady gait, tremor, speech abnormalities, titubation, or nystagmus. The mental status and the rest of the examination are normal. The well appearance of the child helps distinguish this syndrome from encephalitis and meningitis. The ataxia may precede or follow the appearance of an exanthem. The CSF may be normal, or there may be a mild pleocytosis or elevation of the protein. Recovery is rapid (often within days, usually within 4–6 weeks), but as many as 10–20% of patients have sequelae of variable severity.

Acute disseminated encephalomyelitis

Acute disseminated encephalomyelitis (ADEM) is an inflammatory demyelinating disease of the CNS that often presents with ataxia after a viral infection or vaccination. In contrast to acute cerebellar ataxia, patients with ADEM may have encephalopathy, a polysymptomatic presentation, and mutifocal neurological findings.

Ingestion

Accidental (toddlers) or intentional (adolescents) poisoning is a frequent cause of ataxia. The most common agents implicated are anticonvulsants, benzodiazepines, tricyclic antidepressants, phenothiazines, and alcohol. In addition, at any age, an unintentional overdose of medications, such as dilantin, carbamazepine, phenytoin, or antihistamines, including topical diphenhydramine, may produce ataxia. There may also be mental status changes.

Table 16-1. Etiologies of acute ataxia

Parainfectious acute cerebellar ataxia	*Paraneoplastic tumors*
Varicella	Posterior fossa
Mumps	Brainstem
Measles	Spinal cord
Cytomegalovirus	*Hydrocephalus*
Enteroviruses	*Sensory ataxia*
Epstein-Barr virus	Guillain-Barré syndrome
Herpes simplex	Miller-Fisher syndrome
Mycoplasma pneumoniae	*Paretic ataxia*
Acute disseminated encephalomyelitis	Frontal lobe and corticospinal lesions
Toxic-metabolic disturbances	Transverse myelitis
Drug toxicity/poisons	Spinal cord lesion compression
Ethanol	Myasthenia syndromes
Anticonvulsants	*Ischemic or vascular events*
Benzodiazepines	Cerebellar infarct or hemorrhage
Antihistamines	Vertebrobasilar dissection
Inborn errors of metabolism	Arteriovenous malformation
Hypoglycemia (*pseudoataxia*)	Sickle cell anemia
Infection	Vasculitis
Meningitis	*Trauma*
Encephalitis	Posterior fossa hematoma
Abscess	Intra-axial (cerebellar)
	Extra-axial (subdural or epidural)

Meningitis

Ataxia, with or without fever, may be the first sign of bacterial or viral meningitis (pp. 401–405). Other meningeal signs (nuchal rigidity, Kernig's and Brudzinski's signs) may be present.

Encephalitis

A viral infection affecting the brainstem can present with ataxia and cranial nerve abnormalities. There is minimal effect on the level of consciousness unless higher cortical structures are also involved. Common agents are echovirus, adenovirus, and Coxsackie virus. CSF findings are consistent with viral meningitis (pleocytosis without significant protein elevation or hypoglycorrhachia).

Posterior fossa tumor

A posterior fossa tumor usually presents with the insidious onset of headaches and vomiting, with slowly progressive ataxia. However, acute ataxia can occur as the result of obstructive hydrocephalus, hemorrhage into the lesion, or edema.

Stroke

Sickle cell disease, congenital heart disease, and hypercoagulable states can cause vertebral or basilar disease presenting with ataxia.

Transverse myelitis

Transverse myelitis is a presumed parainfectious inflammation at a specific level of the spinal cord. It may initially present with ataxia, back or neck pain, and paresthesias, followed by the rapid development of weakness at and below the level of the lesion.

Guillain-Barré syndrome

In the Miller-Fisher variant of Guillain-Barré syndrome, ataxia is accompanied by ophthalmoplegia (usually diplopia). This may be followed by areflexia, an ascending weakness and autonomic symptoms (flushing, pulse and blood pressure changes, GI symptoms). Classically, the CSF demonstrates cytoalbuminogenic dissociation (elevated protein without pleocytosis).

Migraine syndrome

Basilar migraine and hemiplegic migraines can present with ataxia. In addition, patients with migraine may have benign paroxysmal vertigo, which can be difficult to differentiate from ataxia.

Seizure disorder

Ictal or postictal phases of a seizure may present as ataxia.

Diagnosis

Attempt to ascertain the time of onset of the symptoms (chronic ataxia usually results from tumors, metabolic disorders, or hereditary ataxias) and whether there was any antecedent trauma, viral illness, rash, or toxin exposure. Inquire about the possibility of recreational drug use, ingestion, or overuse of prescription and nonprescription medications (anticonvulsants, sedatives, tranquilizers, or antihistamine preparations). Specifically inquire about over-the-counter medications, including topical diphenhydramine, which may cause intoxication if applied to a large surface area.

Pertinent physical examination findings include a typical exanthem (varicella, measles), the odor of alcohol on the breath (intoxication), or fever and meningeal signs (meningitis).

A careful neurologic exam is necessary to confirm the presence of ataxia, search for associated findings, and rule out a posterior fossa mass lesion. Note the head circumference, status of the anterior fontanel (open, bulging), and carefully examine the fundi (disk margins, presence of spontaneous venous pulsations) for evidence of intracranial hypertension. Remember that in toddlers the sutures may split before eye ground changes appear. Other evidence of a posterior fossa tumor may be neck stiffness, head tilt, cranial nerve palsies (facial weakness, ophthalmoplegia), or long-tract findings (hemiparesis, spasticity, extensor plantar responses).

Abnormal mental status suggests an ingestion, ADEM, meningitis, encephalitis, or stroke. While muscle tone and reflexes may be diminished in the ataxic patient, consider Guillain-Barré syndrome if the patient is hyporeflexic or areflexic. Check for a sensory level suggestive of a spinal cord lesion (transverse myelitis, tumor).

Acute cerebellar ataxia

In acute cerebellar ataxia, there are no meningeal signs, the sensory examination is normal, and although tone may be somewhat diminished, there is no focal weakness. In most of the disorders listed in Table 16-1, the lethargy associated with the ataxia helps to distinguish these entities from acute cerebellar ataxia.

Vertigo

It can be difficult to distinguish an unsteady gait or stance secondary to the loss of balance associated with vertigo (acute labyrinthitis, migrainous vertigo, benign positional vertigo) from similar symptoms caused by ataxia. This is particularly true in children, who may be unable to articulate a sense of motion or spinning. Nausea, vomiting, and nystagmus usually accompany vertigo, which can be provoked or worsened by changes in head position.

ED management

If the child is lethargic, immediately assess the airway, breathing, and cardiovascular functions, give oxygen, and obtain intravascular access. If there is papilledema, focal neurologic findings, bradycardia, or hypertension, begin treatment for increased intracranial pressure (pp. 516–518) and arrange for an emergency noncontrast CT scan to rule out an expanding posterior fossa lesion. Obtain a blood culture and give meningitic doses of IV antibiotics (p. 405) before obtaining the CT scan if meningitis is suspected.

After the CT scan has documented no evidence of increased intracranial pressure or mass effect, perform a lumbar puncture, including a measurement of the opening pressure. Obtain serum electrolytes for comparison of the glucose with the CSF glucose and, if intoxication is suspected, a serum osmolality (increased with ethanol). In cases of suspected ingestion or drug overdose, obtain a blood level of the drug (e.g. alcohol, phenytoin, phenobarbital, carbamazepine).

An evaluation for an inborn error of metabolism is necessary only if the patient has a past history of unexplained ataxia (recurrent episodic ataxia) and mental status changes or a family history of metabolic disorders. Obtain liver function tests, blood pH, urine organic acids, and serum levels of aminoacids, lactate, pyruvate, and ammonia. These tests are most valuable if they are obtained before IV dextrose is given.

Indication for admission

- All patients with acute ataxia until the cause has been established and the course stabilized

Bibliography

Menge T, Kieseier BC, Nessler S, et al: Acute disseminated encephalomyelitis: an acute hit against the brain. *Curr Opin Neurol* 2007;20:247–54.

Nussinovitch M, Prais D, Volovitz B, et al: Post-infectious acute cerebellar ataxia in children. *Clin Pediatr (Phila)* 2003; 42:581–4.

Ryan MM, Engle EC: Acute ataxia in childhood. *J Child Neurol* 2003;18:309–16.

Acute hemiparesis and stroke

Acute hemiparesis in children is rare. As a result, the diagnosis is often confused with other entities. The most common etiologies of acute hemiparesis are stroke, prolonged focal seizures, prolonged postictal paresis (Todd's paralysis), acute disseminated encephalomyelitis, meningitis, encephalitis, brain abscess, and mass lesions. Although bacterial meningitis was a common cause of ischemic stroke in the past, cardiac disorders, blood dyscrasias, vasculopathies, and viral infections now account for a large proportion of ischemic stroke in children. Vascular malformations and trauma are important causes of hemorrhagic stroke in children (Table 16-2).

Clinical presentation

The clinical presentation of acute ischemic stroke is related to the age of the child and size and location of the insult. In the mildest form, acute hemiparesis presents as a tendency to not use the affected arm or leg or having a hand preference in younger children. An asymmetric startle response or absent grasp reflex on the affected side might be the only finding in young infants with mild hemiparesis, while a more significant stroke typically presents with seizures, hypotonia, apnea, or decreased level of consciousness.

Older children may have visual field deficits, aphasia, dysphagia, seizures, or other neurological deficits accompanying the hemiparesis. Alteration of consciousness and seizure can occur with a large ischemic or hemorrhagic stroke, meningitis, and encephalitis. Flaccidity of the involved arm or leg is the usual presentation and the patient may adopt the decorticate posture (shoulder adduction, flexion of the elbow, wrist, and fingers; pronation of the hand; extension of the knee; and eversion and plantar flexion of the foot) after several days to weeks. Longstanding hemiparesis is usually accompanied by hyperreflexia, spasticity, and extensor plantar reflexes (corticospinal tract signs).

Arterial ischemic stroke (AIS)

AIS is defined as an acute focal neurological deficit lasting >24 hours, associated with neuroimaging evidence of cerebral infarction. The most common risk factors are congenital heart disease, RBC disorders, and genetic and acquired coagulation abnormalities, particularly sickle cell disease. Noninflammatory arteriopathies include arterial dissection, moyamoya syndrome, transient cerebral vasculopathy, and congenital hypoplastic vessel abnormalities. Implicated infections include bacterial meningitis, encephalitis, brain abscess, sepsis, and viral infections such as varicella, HIV, parvovirus B19, and influenza A.

Intracranial hemorrhage

An intracranial hemorrhage typically has a sudden onset and rapid evolution. Headache, vomiting, and obtundation are common, and there may be other signs of increased intracranial pressure, such as hypertension, bradycardia, and papilledema (pp. 516–518). Seizures may also occur early in the course.

Acute alternating hemiplegia of childhood

Acute alternating hemiplegia of childhood presents with sudden weakness and altered mental status. The motor deficit persists for minutes to days and is often followed by seizures and slowed mentation. The typical patient is <3 years of age and previously well.

Table 16-2. Etiologies of acute hemiparesis in childhood

Thrombotic events	*Congenital prothrombotic states*
Arterial thrombosis	Antithrombin III deficiency
Posttrauma/inflammation arterial occlusion	Protein S or C deficiency
Penetrating oral trauma	Plasminogen deficiency
Tonsillectomy	Factor V Leiden mutation
Posttraumatic dissection	MTHF deficiency mutation
Carotid artery	*Venous thrombosis*
Posterior circulation	Dehydration
Vertebral artery	Cyanotic heart disease with polycythemia
Hematologic disorders	Vasculitis
Sickle cell disease	Vasculopathy/vasospastic
Polycythemia	*Infections*
Leukemia or other neoplasms	Meningitis
Hemorrhage into a tumor	Mastoiditis
Acquired prothrombotic state	Encephalitis
Prothrombotic medication	Sinusitis
Lupus anticoagulant	*Collagen vascular disease*
Anticardiolipin antibodies	Systemic lupus erythematosus
Lipoprotein abnormalities	Polyarteritis nodosa
Pregnancy or puerperium	Moyamoya syndrome
	Idiopathic occlusion of intracranial carotid
	Venous angioma
Embolic events	*Mass lesion*
Congenital heart disease	Abscess
Acquired heart disease	Trauma
Subacute bacterial endocarditis	Cyanotic heart disease
Prosthetic valves	Neurofibroma
Atrial myxoma	Neoplasm
Posttraumatic (fat or air embolus)	*Other*
Intracranial hemorrhage	Mitochondrial disease
Arteriovenous malformation rupture	Fabry disease
Aneurysm (rare in prepubertal children)	
Head trauma	

Note: Hemiplegic migraine and acute infantile hemiplegia are diagnoses of exclusion.

Repeated episodes can affect one or both sides of the body, but the child is well in between and neuroimaging studies are all normal.

Diagnosis

In general, determining the cause of the hemiparesis can be deferred to the inpatient setting. However, inquire about the rate of onset of the weakness and the occurrence of seizures, fever, intraoral or head trauma, infections (URI, sinusitis, mastoiditis), or change in mental status. Ask about past or associated medical conditions (sickle cell disease, cardiac malformations, lupus, coagulopathies, neurofibromatosis, seizure disorder). Consider the possibility of non-accidental trauma, particularly in an infant or toddler.

On physical examination, check for bulging fontanel and nuchal rigidity which would suggest an infectious process (meningitis, encephalitis) or a subarachnoid hemorrhage. Examine the skin for neurofibromas and café-au-lait spots, check for cyanosis, and look for signs of head or neck trauma. Auscultate the head and neck for a bruit and the chest for a cardiac murmur.

Perform a thorough neurologic exam and assess the mental status. A limited unilateral, nonexpanding, structural hemispheric lesion does not in itself cause a change in mental status. If the patient is lethargic, consider hemorrhage, large stroke, bilateral disease, metabolic defect, infectious disease, or postictal state.

ED management

Management takes priority over etiologic diagnosis. Perform a quick survey to assess the adequacy of the airway, breathing, and cardiovascular function, and obtain a complete set of vital signs. Check the extraocular movements, the pupils for equality of size and reactivity, and the fundi for papilledema, and assess the level of consciousness. See pages 516–518 for the management of patients with evidence of increased intracranial pressure, but avoid over-aggressive treatment of the elevated blood pressure, which can worsen the cerebral hypoperfusion in children with acute stroke. Secure an IV with NS and obtain blood for a CBC, platelet count, PT and PTT, sickle prep (if patient's status is unknown), urine toxicology screen, ESR, CRP, Dextrostix, LFTs, electrolytes, ABG, Lyme titer, and culture (if the patient is febrile).

Immediately consult a pediatric neurologist or neurosurgeon, and arrange for a noncontrast CT scan. If there is no evidence of a structural lesion (tumor, acute infarct, hematoma) or increased intracranial pressure on the scan, perform a lumbar puncture (including opening pressure) and obtain specimens for cell count, protein and glucose, culture, and Gram's stain. Save an additional tube of CSF in the event that testing for varicella zoster virus, herpes simplex virus, or enterovirus is warranted (elevated CSF WBC).

In patients with AIS, thrombolytic therapy may be useful in special circumstances, but most children present too late (>24 hours) after the onset of symptoms.

If the patient has fever and altered mental status, treat with broad-spectrum antibiotics and acyclovir unless an infectious etiology can be definitively ruled out. The management of sickle cell disease (pp. 354–359), encephalitis (pp. 366–369), meningitis (pp. 401–405), and headache (pp. 405–409) is discussed elsewhere.

Indication for admission

- Acute hemiparesis or hemiplegia.

Bibliography

Bernard TJ, Goldenberg NA: Pediatric arterial ischemic stroke. *Pediatr Clin North Am.* 2008;55:323–38.

deVeber G: Arterial ischemic strokes in infants and children: an overview of current

approaches. *Semin Thromb Hemost* 2003;29:567–73.

Lynch JK, Pavlakis S, Deveber G: Treatment and prevention of cerebrovascular disorders in children. *Curr Treat Options Neurol* 2005;7:469–80.

Acute weakness

Although acute weakness is uncommon in childhood, it usually heralds a significant neurologic disorder. The possibility of rapid progression to respiratory collapse makes the onset of acute weakness a true neurologic emergency until the cause and course have been established.

Clinical presentation and diagnosis

The history is vital to defining the underlying process. Determine the time of onset, progression, pattern of weakness (unilateral, bilateral, hemi-, di-, para-, or quadriparetic, flaccid versus spastic), fluctuation of weakness with time, breathlessness (respiratory muscle involvement), difficulty in swallowing, choking, and associated systemic features. Always inquire about associated sensory changes, muscle or extremity pain, and bladder or bowel incontinence. It is also important to differentiate weakness from ataxia, which can be challenging in young children. A history of fever or a viral prodrome suggests an infectious or parainfectious origin.

Guillain-Barré syndrome

Guillain-Barré syndrome (GBS), or acute demyelinating polyneuropathy, is the most common cause of acute flaccid paralysis in healthy infants and children. It is usually a postvaccination or postinfectious phenomenon; about two-thirds of patients have a history of an antecedent respiratory tract or gastrointestinal (*Campylobacter* most frequent) infection. GBS is characterized by premonitory vague sensory symptoms or pain, ascending motor weakness, associated cranial nerve involvement (bilateral facial weakness most common), depressed or absent deep tendon reflexes, with sparing of bowel and bladder sphincters. The weakness is often asymmetric at the onset but becomes symmetrical as the disease progresses. About 10% of patients have serious respiratory, cardiac, and/or autonomic dysfunction, which may be sudden in onset and unrelated to the degree of motor weakness.

Examination of the CSF early in the course may show a mild pleocytosis, but later the classic finding is cytoalbuminogenic dissociation: striking elevation of the protein without pleocytosis.

Miller-Fisher syndrome (MFS)

Patients with this variant of GBS have external ophthalmoplegia, ataxia, and muscle weakness with areflexia. These children may also have other cranial nerve palsies. Most of these patients have cross-reacting antibodies to GQ1b ganglioside.

Myasthenia gravis

Myasthenia gravis (MG) is a rare autoimmune disorder that causes weakness by blocking the acetylcholine receptor at the neuromuscular junction. There is the subacute onset (develops over weeks or months) of weakness that most commonly presents as ptosis, diplopia, or blurry vision due to extraocular muscle weakness, with or without generalized muscle weakness. Patients with bulbar weakness may present with difficulty in chewing and swallowing, drooling, nasal voice, or poor cough. Fluctuation of the weakness and fatigability are the hallmarks of MG, as the symptoms are least prominent on awakening, and become more obvious through the day. Rarely, there may be a severe acute presentation with life-threatening weakness of the respiratory musculature (myasthenic crisis). Patients typically have normal mental status, deep tendon reflexes, pupillary reflexes, fundoscopy, sensation, and coordination. The diagnosis is confirmed by a therapeutic challenge with endrophonum (see below).

Infantile botulism

Botulism (pp. 362–363) causes a fairly rapid progression of cranial nerve dysfunction (diplopia, ptosis, pupillary dilatation, dysarthria, dysphagia) and weakness. With infantile botulism, there is a history of constipation, followed by a subacute progression of bulbar and extremity weakness, presenting as a symmetric ascending paralysis, and inability to suck and swallow, and ptosis, which may progress to generalized flaccidity and respiratory compromise.

Tick paralysis

A toxin released by dog and wood ticks prevents the release of acetylcholine at nerve endings, causing a rapidly progressive (12–48 hours), ascending, generalized paralysis. The deep tendon reflexes are depressed or absent and there may also be mild facial muscle weakness, dysarthria, dysphagia, ptosis, double vision, and respiratory compromise.

Tick paralysis must be considered in the differential diagnosis of any child presenting with acute ataxia which is then quickly followed by an acute ascending paralysis, especially during the late spring and summer seasons. In contrast to Guillain-Barré syndrome, there is no elevation of the CSF protein. A high index of suspicion is imperative as any delay of diagnosis and treatment may result in life-threatening respiratory failure.

Polio

Although poliomyelitis is very rare in the United States, it may occur in a patient with a history of incomplete or inadequate immunization. Typically, it presents with a history of a brief febrile illness, with headache, sore throat, vomiting, and fatigue, followed by a few days of recovery. The patient then has recurrent fever accompanied by weakness, lethargy, and irritability which may be associated with meningeal signs. In some patients, there is selective destruction of motor neurons, characterized by severe back, neck, and muscle pain, with the development of motor weakness. The disease tends to preferentially affect proximal muscles and the legs, and bulbar involvement may also occur, causing dysphagia, dysarthria, and difficulty handling secretions. Reflexes are decreased or absent, but the sensory examination is normal. The CSF shows a pleocytosis with protein elevation. A similar acute flaccid paralytic syndrome may be caused by other enteroviruses (echovirus, Coxsackie virus).

Diphtheria

The neurologic manifestations of diphtheria may begin during the acute illness, but most often they occur several weeks to months after the onset of the acute membranous pharyngitis. Diphtheria produces a flaccid limb paralysis, which may be accompanied by muscle tenderness and may be preceded by extraocular muscle weakness, ptosis, dysphagia, and a stocking glove sensory loss. The CSF may show an elevated protein without pleocytosis. As with polio, there may be a history of incomplete or inadequate immunization.

Spinal cord pathology

Spinal cord pathology can produce acute weakness with either paraplegia or quadriplegia. Trauma is the most likely cause. Patients with Down's syndrome or rheumatoid arthritis are particularly susceptible to C1 to C2 subluxation, which can result in quadriparesis. The presence of fever and vertebral tenderness strongly suggests a spinal epidural abscess, which is a neurosurgical emergency. Weakness can also be caused by paraspinal or spinal cord tumor with acute cord compression, spinal cord infarction (most common in the thoracic levels), or hemorrhage secondary to arteriovenous malformation.

Transverse myelitis

Transverse myelitis is defined as spinal cord dysfunction that develops over hours or days in patients in whom there is no evidence of a compressive lesion. Transverse myelitis can occur alone (known as clinically isolated syndrome) or as part of other demyelinating diseases including neuromyelitis optica, acute disseminated encephalomyelitis, or multiple sclerosis. Patients usually present with acute paraparesis, paresthesia (bilateral segmental sensory loss below the level of inflammation), sphincter dysfunction, absent deep tendon reflexes, and positive Babinski signs.

Metabolic causes

Metabolic causes (hypokalemia, hypo- and hypercalcemia, hypo- and hyperthyroidism) are rare in childhood and usually have associated systemic manifestations. Episodic paralysis, particularly during rest after exercise, suggests periodic paralysis, especially if there is a positive family history.

Other causes

Acute or subacute weakness with a rash, fever, and myalgias suggests an inflammatory process such as dermatomyositis, polymyositis, or systemic lupus erythematosus. Certain toxins, especially the anticholinesterase-inhibiting insecticides (organophosphates, carbamates), cause acute weakness.

Psychogenic causes

Consider psychogenic causes when the history and physical examination fail to suggest an organic etiology and the neurologic examination shows neurophysiologic inconsistencies. There may be a history of a stressful precipitating event or situation.

ED management

Perform a careful neurologic exam to define the extent, pattern, fluctuation, and fatigueability of the weakness, and document any associated sensory findings (particularly a sensory level). Ask about change in voice (nasal voice), dysphagia, breathlessness, bladder fullness, constipation, or incontinence of urine or stool. Percuss the lower abdomen for a distended bladder, and check the rectal tone. Examine the skin for a rash or a tick (often found hidden in hairy areas) and palpate muscles for pain. Observe the patient's respiratory efforts, and document the adequacy of ventilation with an ABG or pulse oximetry.

Obtain a urinalysis, CBC, electrolytes, and glucose and, if the patient is febrile, a blood culture and ESR. A lumbar puncture is indicated, particularly if Guillain-Barré syndrome is suspected, but it can be delayed until after consultation with a pediatric neurologist. Obtain an MRI of the spine, with contrast, if the patient has signs and symptoms suggestive of spinal cord pathology.

The management of the trauma victim is detailed on pp. 710–718. If there is any history of trauma, the patient must be maintained in neutral position. Obtain the appropriate spine films (cervical, areas of tenderness), and consult with a neurosurgeon and a pediatric neurologist.

Admit a patient with Guillain-Barré to an intensive care unit, as respiratory compromise can occur acutely. Consult a neurologist, who may recommend plasmapheresis or high-dose IV gamma-globulin. Also admit a patient with polio for close monitoring and respiratory support.

If myasthenia is suspected, perform a Tensilon (edrophonium chloride) test under the direction of a pediatric neurologist. Edrophonium is a rapid-acting cholinergic drug. Perform the test with the child on a cardiorespiratory monitor in a setting where personnel and equipment for resuscitation are readily available. Have a syringe with atropine (1 mg) available as well. Hypersensitive subjects can develop severe cholinergic reactions. The total dose of edrophonium chloride used is 0.15–0.2 mg/kg (10 mg maximum). Give one-tenth of the total dose IV, and flush the line with NS. The patient may experience a feeling of warmth or stinging sensation near the IV site, but if there are no serious autonomic effects, give the rest of the dose and assess the effect over the next 5–10 minutes. Assess the improvement of ptosis and extraocular muscle weakness, not generalized weakness, to evaluate the effectiveness of the drug. The effects of edrophonium dissipate within 10–15 minutes. Alternatively, test patients with ptosis by applying a cold pack to the lids; it will lessen the ptosis of myasthenia.

See pp. 362–363 for the treatment of botulism.

The treatment of tick paralysis is to completely remove the tick, including all mouth parts. The symptoms resolve quickly, but it is important to avoid leaving mouth parts behind in skin, as these could continue to release toxin into the host.

If a spinal epidural abscess, spinal cord compression, or transverse myelitis is suspected, obtain urgent neurology and neurosurgical consultation. Parenteral corticosteroids may be helpful in acute transverse myelitis.

Arrange for psychological counseling if the weakness is determined to be psychogenic.

Indication for admission

* Acute weakness of any origin except psychogenic

Bibliography

Agrawal S, Peake D, Whitehouse WP: Management of children with Guillain-Barré syndrome. *Arch Dis Child Educ Pract Ed* 2007;**92**:161–8.

Li Z, Turner RP: Pediatric tick paralysis: discussion of two cases and literature review. *Pediatr Neurol* 2004;**31**:304–7.

Pidcock FS, Krishnan C, Crawford TO, et al: Acute transverse myelitis in childhood: center-based analysis of 47 cases. *Neurology* 2007;**68**:1474–80.

Breathholding

Breathholding spells typically begin between 6 and 18 months of age and in 90% of cases disappear by 6 years. Most patients have no more than one attack per month, although 10% of affected children will have two or more per day. In 25% of cases, there is a positive family history of breathholding. Although the physiologic basis of breathholding is unclear, the episodes are not associated with an increased risk of epilepsy.

Clinical presentation

Breathholding spells are brief, lasting about 30 seconds. The episodes are preceded by crying, which may be due to anger, frustration, fear, or pain. After a short period of crying, the child stops breathing and loses consciousness. There may be a brief postictal period of confusion.

Breathholding spells are divided into two types, pallid and cyanotic, depending on the patient's color change. An individual child generally has only one type of spell. A cyanotic spell follows a frustrating event in which the child cries briefly, then develops apnea, cyanosis, and loss of consciousness, sometimes accompanied by rigid limbs and opisthotonos.

A pallid spell has a rapid onset after a frightening event or occipital trauma. The child starts crying, stops breathing, loses consciousness, and becomes pale and limp. Clonic jerks may be noted at the end of the episode.

Diagnosis

The diagnosis is made from the history, as the patient usually appears well and back to baseline by arrival in the ED. Breathholding spells are most often confused with seizures although before a convulsion there may be an external precipitating factor, sustained crying, or cyanosis. Also, spells may be confused with syncopal episodes. Fainting is very unusual in young children, however, and is not usually associated with rigidity or opisthotonos.

ED management

If the history of the event is typical and a thorough neurologic exam yields normal results, reassure the family about the benign nature of the episode (no risk of epilepsy). Instruct the parents to be consistent when disciplining the child and not allow him or her to derive secondary gain from the episodes (try not to pick up the child).

If the history is unusual or unclear, obtain a CBC, Dextrostix, electrolytes, glucose, and calcium, and perform an ECG and rhythm strip (see Syncope, pp. 68–71, and Cyanosis, pp. 60–61). If a seizure cannot be ruled out from the history, ask about a family history of epilepsy, examine the skin for café-au-lait or ash leaf spots, and schedule an EEG.

Follow-up

- Frequent (≥1/day) breathholding spells: pediatric neurology follow-up in 2–4 weeks

Indication for admission

- Cyanotic episode that cannot be confidently diagnosed as a breathholding spell.

Bibliography

Dewolfe CC: Apparent life-threatening event: a review. *Pediatr Clin North Am* 2005;52:1127–46.

DiMario FJ Jr: Prospective study of children with cyanotic and pallid breath-holding spells. *Pediatrics* 2001;107:265–9.

Fejerman N: Nonepileptic disorders imitating generalized idiopathic epilepsies. *Epilepsia* 2005;46 Suppl 9:80–3.

Coma

While there is no agreed-upon terminology to describe the states of arousal between normal mental status and coma, one helpful scheme uses the following definitions, in order of decreasing level of arousal.

Lethargy

Lethargy implies difficulty in maintaining the aroused state. Although the patient is able to respond appropriately when addressed, without continual stimulation he or she lapses back into a somnolent state.

Obtundation

The obtunded patient responds to verbal or tactile stimuli with cerebral alerting but does make fully appropriate responses.

Stupor

The stuporous patient responds with cerebral alerting only to painful stimuli.

Coma

Coma is a state of supreme unresponsiveness in which the patient appears as if asleep, yet does not respond to external or internal stimuli. Coma may result from medical (toxic-metabolic) causes or structural lesions. Distinguishing between metabolic causes and mass lesions is critical, as structural causes of coma may require emergency neurosurgical intervention, while metabolic coma can usually be managed medically. In addition, coma may be classified by the pathophysiology.

Toxic-metabolic

These derangements depress the cerebral hemispheres and often brainstem structures as well. They may be due to endogenous substances (uremia, liver failure, respiratory failure, DKA) or exogenous toxins (salicylates, tricyclics, sedatives, carbon monoxide, narcotics, anticonvulsants), cerebral hypoxia or hypoperfusion, hypoglycemia, or hyperammonemia. Also, subclinical seizure activity (non-convulsive status) may resemble coma.

Structural – supratentorial

Supratentorial mass lesions exert compressive forces on the cerebral hemispheres as well as brainstem structures. Large lesions of the dominant hemisphere alone can induce coma. In children, the most common mass lesion leading to coma is intracranial bleeding and swelling due to head trauma. Tumors, spontaneous hemorrhages, and ischemic strokes are rare.

Table 16-3. Toxic-metabolic causes of fixed pupils

Cause	Pupils	Diagnosis/characteristics
Anoxia	Fixed, dilated	Antecedent history of shock, cardiac or respiratory arrest, etc.
Anticholinergics (tricyclics, atropine)	Fixed, dilated	Tachycardia, QRS > 0.12 seconds Warm, dry skin
Cholinergics (organophosphates)	May be small with barely perceptible reflex	Diaphoresis, vomiting, incontinence
Opiates (heroin)	Very small with barely perceptible reflex	Needle marks, history of overdose
Hypothermia	May be fixed	History of exposure
Barbiturates, glutethimide	May be mid-sized or dilated and fixed	History of overdose

Structural – subtentorial
These destroy or compress core brainstem structures, such as the ascending reticular activating system, and may produce hydrocephalus and increased intracranial pressure.

Infection
Meningitis, encephalitis, and severe sepsis with shock may also present with coma.

Clinical presentation and diagnosis
Several elements of the physical exam help to distinguish structural from metabolic causes of coma. These include the pupillary responses, the EOMs, and the motor response to pain. Changes in the respiratory pattern may also help localize the level of the lesion, but they are more difficult to interpret.

Asymmetry of pupillary response, EOMs, or motor response to pain suggests a structural lesion. Fixed pupils are also more likely with a structural lesion. However, the earliest stage of central herniation can produce small, sluggish pupils indistinguishable from those seen in many metabolically induced coma states. Therefore, evidence of a structural origin (history or signs of trauma), other focal deficits with symmetric pupils, or signs of progressive deterioration cannot be ignored. The few medical states that can produce fixed pupils (Table 16-3) must always be considered when the pupils are non-reactive. In addition, focal neurologic findings may be seen in any metabolic encephalopathy (uremia, hypercalcemia, hepatic encephalopathy, and especially hypoglycemia), as these metabolic derangements may provoke signs and symptoms of previously subclinical lesions.

Absent EOMs or motor responses, or symmetrical posturing, may be due either to structural lesions or to profound metabolic coma. Progression from purposeful motor responses to posturing to flaccidity suggests a structural lesion.

The EOMs can be tested with the doll's-eyes maneuver or, when head or neck injury is suspected, with cold-water vestibular stimulation with the head in the midline position. Intact doll's eyes are manifested by transient conjugate deviation away from the direction of rapid head rotation. Absent EOMs on testing with the doll's-eyes maneuver may also indicate an awake patient. Intact cold caloric responses are manifested by conjugate deviation of the eyes toward the stimulated ear. Never perform cold caloric stimulation on a patient who is awake, as it causes severe vertigo, nausea, and vomiting.

The presence of asymmetric (lateralizing) findings on exam helps to make the diagnosis of a structural lesion, but the absence of asymmetry does not rule out a structural lesion, particularly in the case of midline lesions. If a metabolic cause of coma is not apparent from the history or initial exam once the patient has been stabilized, obtain a noncontrast head CT, even in the absence of lateralizing findings on the exam or a history of trauma. If there is a history or suspicion of head trauma, assume that there has been cervical spine trauma. Immobilize the neck and treat appropriately until cervical trauma has been definitively ruled out (pp. 702–704).

Nonconvulsive status is suggested by subtle findings such as eye deviation, nystagmus, or changes in tone.

ED management

The priority is stabilization of the vital signs. Initial blood tests include a CBC, electrolytes, BUN, Dextrostix and glucose, and an ABG. If the cause is unknown, also obtain a serum osmolality, PT, PTT, liver function tests, and serum levels of toxins associated with altered mental status (barbiturates, alcohol, aspirin). Save an additional red-top tube for future analysis. Administer 100% oxygen and establish IV access. Give all patients naloxone (0.1 mg/kg), and if the Dextrostix is <80 mg/dL or if it was not obtained, give IV glucose (2 mL/kg of D_{25}) for diagnostic and therapeutic purposes.

See pages pp. 509–515 for the management of head trauma.

When the cause of the coma is unknown and the vital signs are stable, treatment can be directed by the results of the coma exam as outlined above. If structural coma is suspected, management is as described for head trauma, including an emergency CT scan to identify the lesion.

The situation is generally less urgent if metabolic coma is suspected. A key exception is the patient with suspected meningitis (pp. 401–405), who requires a lumbar puncture and appropriate antibiotics immediately following the CT. If the CT is delayed, give the antibiotics prior to obtaining CSF. The general approach to medical coma requires supporting the vital signs and correcting abnormalities in acid–base and electrolyte status. A toxic ingestion may require gastrointestinal decontamination and supportive therapy (pp. 433–446).

Indication for admission

- All comatose patients

Bibliography

Halley MK, Silva PD, Foley J, Rodarte A: Loss of consciousness: when to perform computed tomography? *Pediatr Crit Care Med* 2004; 5:230–3.

Kirkham FJ, Newton CR, Whitehouse W: Paediatric coma scales. *Dev Med Child Neurol* 2008;50:267–74.

Kirkham FJ: Non-traumatic coma in children. *Arch Dis Child* 2001;85:303–12.

Facial weakness

The most common presentation of seventh cranial nerve dysfunction in children is a peripheral facial palsy. The lesion is in the facial nerve nucleus or the peripheral nerve distal to the nucleus, so both the upper and lower halves of the face are affected (including the frontalis muscle). Causes of a peripheral seventh nerve palsy include trauma, infections (Lyme disease, varicella, otitis, mastoiditis, parotitis, infectious mononucleosis), parainfectious phenomena (associated with Guillain-Barré syndrome), and neoplasms (neurofibromatosis, cerebellopontine angle tumors). A peripheral facial palsy of unknown origin is termed a Bell's palsy.

A central facial palsy affects only the lower half of the face, sparing the frontalis muscle. It is secondary to a lesion in the contralateral cerebral hemisphere, most commonly caused by stroke, demyelinating disease, or tumor.

Clinical presentation

With the exception of acute trauma, most peripheral facial palsies evolve over 24–48 hours and may be preceded or accompanied by pain around or behind the ear. The pain can be quite severe and may be the presenting complaint. The patient may note asymmetry of the face, weakness of the facial muscles, hyperacusis, excessive tearing of the ipsilateral eye, alteration of taste, or difficulty eating or drinking. Often there may also be a feeling of numbness or tingling over the affected side of the face.

A central facial palsy is not accompanied by hyperacusis or alteration of taste. In contrast to a peripheral seventh nerve palsy, wrinkling of the forehead and elevation of the eyebrow are unaffected. With a vascular origin, the onset may be acute.

Diagnosis

Acute trauma and congenital causes of facial weakness can almost always be ruled out from the history and by inspection. To determine whether the weakness is peripheral or central, note whether the patient can wrinkle the forehead.

Perform a careful neurologic exam to rule out other neurologic origins (Guillain-Barré syndrome). Test the cranial nerves, motor strength, and deep tendon reflexes. Check for an accompanying hemiparesis, particularly in infants and nonwalking children. If there is a central facial palsy, examine for aphasia, which can be manifested by mutism. This may be difficult to determine in a shy or uncooperative child.

Examine the external auditory canals and tympanic membranes for signs of infection (otitis, mastoiditis, or vesicular lesions associated with varicella or herpes simplex).

On physical examination, look for a rash (Lyme disease, varicella, herpes), café-au-lait spots (neurofibromatosis), and generalized adenopathy and splenomegaly (infectious mononucleosis).

Lyme disease

If the patient has a history of a recent tick bite or lives in an area where Lyme disease (pp. 398–401) is endemic, obtain blood for a Lyme titer. Also perform a lumbar puncture if there is a history of headache, or if other cranial nerve deficits are noted. A CSF pleocytosis is an indication for IV antibiotics. The lumbar puncture may be deferred in the absence of headache, stiff neck, and neurologic deficits other than the facial palsy.

Bell's palsy

Bell's palsy is a diagnosis of exclusion if no other cause of a peripheral seventh nerve palsy is evident.

ED management

If the patient has eye pain or discomfort, perform a fluorescein test (p. 538) to rule out a corneal abrasion. For the affected eye, give artificial tears (1–2 drops qid), Lacri-lube qhs, and an eye patch to be worn at night to prevent drying of the cornea. If the patient cannot cover the entire cornea with a blink, patch the eye and refer him or her to an ophthalmologist. Do not permit the patient to wear contact lenses. Advise the patient to report any ocular discomfort immediately (possible corneal abrasion).

If Lyme disease is suspected, obtain blood for a Lyme titer and treat for 3 weeks with either amoxicillin (<8 years old; 40 mg/kg per day div tid) or doxycycline (≥8 years old; 100 mg bid). The management of otitis media (pp. 135–138), mastoiditis (p. 146), Guillain-Barré syndrome (pp. 489–490), infectious mononucleosis (pp. 386–388), head trauma (pp. 716–717), and increased intracranial pressure (pp. 516–518) is discussed elsewhere. The presence of facial nerve weakness does not usually alter the treatment of the primary illness. If facial nerve palsy associated with an otitis media does not improve after 2 days of oral antibiotics, arrange for tympanocentesis, culture the middle-ear fluid, and admit the patient for IV antibiotics (cefuroxime, 100 mg/kg per day div q 8 h).

If the patient is seen within 48 hours of the onset of a peripheral facial weakness and the most likely diagnosis is idiopathic Bell's palsy, give a 5–7 day course of prednisone (2 mg/kg per day, maximum 60 mg). Make sure that the patient does not have other associated cranial nerve palsies or evidence of bacterial infection, as the steroids may mask a tumor or infection. Steroids have not been shown to affect the long-term prognosis for resolution of the palsy, but they may relieve associated pain. If there is no improvement noted within 3 weeks, refer the patient to a neurologist for electromyography.

If the weakness is central and is clearly of new onset, consult a pediatric neurologist and obtain a head CT scan. Neuroimaging is necessary if facial palsy is slowly progressive or associated with other cranial nerve palsies.

The prognosis of facial weakness varies with the severity of the initial palsy; approximately 80% of patients recover completely, generally within 2 months, and improvement usually begins within 1–2 weeks of diagnosis.

Follow-up

- Peripheral weakness, including Lyme disease: 2–3 days, to check the affected eye and the laboratory tests

Indications for admission

- Acute facial nerve palsy associated with progressive weakness, evidence of a mass lesion, CNS infection, intracranial hypertension, acute trauma, or other neurologic signs

Bibliography

Chen WX, Wong V: Prognosis of Bell's palsy in children–analysis of 29 cases. *Brain Dev* 2005;27:504–8.

Tiemstra JD, Khatkhate N: Bell's palsy: diagnosis and management. *Am Fam Physician* 2007;76:997–1002.

Tveitnes D, Øymar K, Natås O: Acute facial nerve palsy in children: how often is it lyme borreliosis? *Scand J Infect Dis* 2007;39:425–31.

Headache

There are many causes of headache in childhood (Table 16-4); fortunately, most are benign, such as migraine and tension-type or chronic daily headache. However, a number of life-threatening illnesses that may present with headache must be eliminated from consideration before the child is discharged from the ED.

Clinical presentation

Although the following clinical entities are discussed individually, bear in mind that many patients have headaches that do not easily fit into one particular category. Also, many patients have two or more types of headache, such as chronic tension-type headaches in a patient who also has migraines.

Common benign causes of headache

Migraine

Migraine is the most common type of headache in children of any age. In prepubertal children, the incidence of migraine is equal in boys and girls, while in adolescents and adults more females are affected. In 70–90% of cases, there is a family history of migraine in a first-degree relative. Migraine attacks may be triggered by stress, exercise, head trauma (which may be so insignificant that it is forgotten), skipping meals, particular foods, drugs, strong sunlight or odors, hormonal changes associated with the menstrual cycle and pregnancy, and possibly allergies. The frequency varies from once a year to several times a week. The duration of migraine headache is at least 2–3 hours in older adolescents, but may be as short as 30 minutes in young children. Patients with migraine are frequently treated with antibiotics for "sinus headache" before the diagnosis of migraine is finally considered.

Migraine without aura

Migraine without aura (previously called common migraine) is not preceded by any visual, olfactory, or somatosensory aura and is usually bilateral. The headache is described as pulsating or throbbing, may be paroxysmal in onset or arise in the setting of a preexisting tension-type headache, and may be accompanied by photophobia, phonophobia, nausea, vomiting, and a desire to sleep or rest in a quiet, dark room.

Migraine with aura

Migraine with aura, or classic migraine, is preceded by an aura (most commonly a visual aura of scintillating lights, scotomata, blurry vision, visual hallucinations, or, rarely, an alteration of perception of time and body image known as the Alice-in-Wonderland syndrome). The headache is usually unilateral, although it may alternate sides. If the

Table 16-4. Etiologies of headache

Common benign causes of headache	Infection-related causes of headache
Migraine	Sinusitis
Migraine without aura (common)	Dental infection
Migraine with aura (classic)	Systemic infection
Less common migraine syndromes	Group A streptococcus
Hemiplegic migraine	*Mycoplasma pneumoniae*
Ophthalmoplegic migraine	Influenza
Basilar artery migraine	Viral ("aseptic") meningitis
Cyclic vomiting	Lyme disease
Acute confusional migraine	Meningitis
Chronic tension-type headache	
Stress-related	*Headache due to increased ICP*
Visual abnormalities[a]	Brain abscess
Exo/esophoria causing convergence difficulty	Brain tumor
Posttraumatic headache	Head trauma
	Pseudotumor cerebri
	Carbon monoxide poisoning

Note: [a] Not caused by uncorrected refractive errors.

headache is always on the same side, there is more concern about the possible presence of an underlying fixed lesion.

Migraine variants

Migraine variants may present with hemiplegia, ophthalmoplegia, ptosis, an acute confusional state, or episodes of vomiting. These manifestations may or may not be accompanied by headache and are diagnoses of exclusion. The neurologic deficits are transient in most cases, but there have been reports of patients who eventually have strokes in the vascular distribution suggested by the deficit.

Chronic tension-type headache

This category of headache includes the headaches formerly known as "muscle contraction headache," "tension headache," and "psychogenic headache." The headaches are generally prolonged, may be waxing and waning in intensity, and are not preceded by an aura or accompanied by any neurologic deficits. The pain is described as dull, achy, or tight and usually begins in the occipital region; however, it may move anteriorly to the vertex or the frontal region. The headaches typically occur in the late afternoon or evening and are relieved by mild analgesics such as acetaminophen. Unlike migraines, these headaches rarely interrupt normal activities. They may be triggered by a recent emotional or traumatic event and may be associated with personality changes, as evidenced by poor school performance, sleep disturbances, aggression, lack of energy, and self-deprecatory behavior.

Heterophorias

An exo- or esophoria that forces the patient to continually exert effort to converge the eyes may cause headache. Typically, the onset is in the afternoon or evening after concentrated visual activity. Unlike heterotropia (constant misalignment of the eyes), heterophorias may be difficult to appreciate on physical exam without specific testing. Pure refractive errors such as myopia are usually not associated with headache.

Temporomandibular joint dysfunction

Disorders of temporomandibular joint function (TMJD) may present with headache. Patients with bruxism and habitual gum chewers are at increased risk. The headache of TMJD may be associated with jaw or ear pain and locking of the jaw or inability to open the mouth.

Posttraumatic headache

Early-onset posttraumatic headache is common after minor head trauma. The headache may initially be isolated to the area of impact, but often becomes generalized, and may be associated with vomiting and/or somnolence. There are no focal neurologic deficits or signs of increased intracranial pressure (ICP), but the patient may have amnesia for the events surrounding the trauma. Headache with onset minutes to days after significant head trauma may be due to an epidural or subdural hematoma. Worrisome signs are a decreasing level of consciousness, projectile vomiting, and symptoms of increased ICP (bulging fontanelle, split sutures, unequal pupils, sixth nerve palsy, hypertension with bradycardia). Head trauma (pp. 716–717) and increased ICP (pp. 576–578) are discussed elsewhere.

Occasionally, posttraumatic headache may continue for prolonged periods (weeks to years). The headache may be a migraine, triggered by head trauma in a susceptible person. Psychogenic factors or the possibility of secondary gain may be involved.

Infection-related causes of headache

Sinusitis

The headache of sinusitis (pp. 157–159) may be referred to the upper teeth, the cheek, or the frontal or retroorbital area. There may be cough, mucopurulent nasal discharge, fever, and facial pain and tenderness. Often the pain occurs in the early morning and is accentuated by leaning forward.

Dental infection

A dental infection (pp. 74–76) causes pain in the cheek or mandibular area as well as temporal headaches. The infected tooth or gum may be sensitive upon percussion or manipulation.

Systemic infection

Systemic infections, such as group A streptococcus infection, influenza, and mycoplasmal pneumonia, can cause a headache in addition to other symptoms (fever, sore throat, cough, coryza, conjunctivitis, or myalgias). Early Lyme disease (pp. 398–401) may present with headache, in addition to arthralgias, lethargy, and behavioral changes.

Meningitis

The headache of bacterial meningitis is generalized, constant, often described as "throbbing all over," and associated with fever, toxicity, nuchal rigidity (in older children), and other meningeal signs. Viral meningitis causes a similar presentation, usually during summertime epidemics. Even in older children, the absence of nuchal rigidity does not rule out meningitis, particularly early in the course of infection.

Headache caused by increased intracranial pressure

Brain abscess

A child with a brain abscess may present with a nonspecific headache, usually accompanied by fever. Vomiting, diplopia, seizures (focal, partial complex, or generalized convulsions), and altered mental status may be present. Predisposing factors are congenital heart disease with right-to-left shunting and ethmoid or frontal sinusitis that has been unresponsive to therapy.

Brain tumor

The headache of a brain tumor is intermittent initially but very quickly increases in frequency and severity. It is often present in the very early morning hours and may awaken the child from sleep, as lying supine slows the drainage of CSF, increasing intracranial pressure. There may be associated projectile vomiting in the absence of abdominal pain. Localization may be difficult, especially in the case of midline lesions. Occipital headache may indicate a posterior fossa lesion, although the pain is frequently referred to a fronto-temporal location. Thus, frontal headache may accompany either a supratentorial or a posterior fossa tumor.

Pseudotumor cerebri

Patients with pseudotumor cerebri can present with intermittent headaches, vomiting, blurred vision, papilledema, and occasionally diplopia. However, there is no alteration in the level of consciousness or intellectual functioning.

Ventriculoperitoneal shunt obstruction

See pp. 525–527.

Diagnosis

Despite the wide spectrum of causes, most childhood headaches are due to one of the common benign causes listed in Table 16-4. With the exception of children whose headaches are accompanied by severe nausea and vomiting, these patients are afebrile; appear awake, alert, and nontoxic; and have normal physical and neurologic exams.

Only a small minority of headaches in children are secondary to a serious intracranial process. However, consider one of these conditions if the patient complains of acute severe "thunderclap" headaches or sudden acute severe headaches (suggestive of subarachnoid hemorrhage), headaches that are severe, progressive and persistent for less than 6 months duration, headaches that interfere with sleep or waken the patient during the night or early morning, headaches associated with persistent vomiting, or if there is a recent history of head trauma, or change in personality or behavior. The new onset of headaches in an immunosuppressed patient is also concerning.

Obtain a complete description of the headaches, including onset, triggering factors, duration, location, quality, usual time of day they occur, what makes the pain better or worse, and whether the severity and frequency are increasing. This information may be difficult to elicit, especially if the child is less than 8–10 years old. Avoid suggesting possible descriptive terms to the preschool child, who may agree that all apply, even if they are mutually exclusive. Ask about recent emotional stress, personality changes, head trauma, warning signs (aura), family history of migraines, medications, and associated symptoms, including fever, nausea or vomiting, photophobia or visual disturbances, rash, nasal discharge or cough, and possible tick or CO exposure. CO poisoning (pp. 207–209) is rare, although it commonly causes headache, as well as fatigue and irritability, and may affect several family or group members simultaneously.

Measure the blood pressure and perform a complete physical examination, looking for fever, split sutures, bulging fontanelle, facial tenderness, gingival swelling, dental caries and tooth percussion sensitivity, otitis media, nuchal rigidity and meningeal signs, and signs of a systemic infection. A thorough neurologic exam is necessary, including ophthalmoscopy. Asymmetry of the pupils, EOMs, or motor response suggests a structural abnormality such as a brain tumor or abscess or a subdural or epidural hematoma (see Coma, pp. 499–501). Finally, check the visual acuity and visual fields, as a visual field defect may be the only neurological abnormality in a patient with a pituitary tumor or craniopharyngioma.

ED management

The priority is expeditious diagnosis and treatment of a CSF infection or increased ICP. The management of a suspected mass lesion, meningitis, head trauma, pseudotumor cerebri, sinusitis, systemic infection, and dental infection is discussed elsewhere in the appropriate sections.

Indications for CT of the head are listed in Table 16-5. However, a normal CT does not rule out subarachnoid hemorrhage or increased ICP. Perform a lumbar puncture with measurement of the opening pressure if a subarachnoid hemorrhage or increased ICP is suspected. A urinalysis, CBC, blood glucose, or carboxyhemoglobin level may be indicated, based on the clinical presentation. Obtain a shunt series, CT scan, and neurosurgical consultation for a child with a VP shunt and severe headache.

The ED treatment of chronic tension-type headaches is limited to oral analgesics (acetaminophen 15 mg/kg q 4 h, ibuprofen 10 mg/kg q 6 h) and reassurance that a serious disease process is not under way. Refer the patient to a primary care setting, where the stresses contributing to the headaches can be addressed.

Migraines

Migraines can be chronic and debilitating. For that reason, avoid treating with narcotics and other habit-forming drugs, and give only mild analgesics (as above). If ibuprofen does not help, prescribe sumatriptan nasal spray, 5–20 mg, for acute migraine in patients >12 years old. In addition, aggressive IV hydration, IV ketorolac 0.5 mg/kg (30 mg maximum), IV or PR metoclopramide (0.1 mg/kg by slow IV push, maximum 10 mg) can relieve the headache and associated vomiting. Dystonic reactions or akathisia, although rare, are possible at even minimal doses of metoclopramide. Consult a neurologist if the headache does not respond to these measures.

Table 16-5. Indications for CT in patients with headache

Focal neurologic abnormality

Papilledema

Recurrent morning headache

Persistent vomiting

Paroxysmal onset of excruciating headache

Head trauma with focal neurologic signs or lethargy

Refer children with frequent or intractable migraine to a primary care setting or a pediatric neurologist. The ED is not an appropriate site for instituting therapy with ergotamines or prophylactic agents such as propranolol, verapamil, or amitriptyline.

Ask the family or patient to keep a headache diary. For each headache, record the time of onset, duration, location, quality, exacerbating and remitting factors, and note any other associations that may help to identify the type of headache, its temporal pattern, and triggers. Have the parents of young children record any spontaneous complaints of headache, but advise them to avoid eliciting spurious complaints by asking the child whether he or she has a headache. Have the patient or family take the diary to the follow-up appointment.

Follow-up

- Migraine requiring ED treatment (other than acetaminophen or ibuprofen): 2–3 days. Otherwise, primary care follow-up in 1–2 weeks

Indications for admission

- Focal neurologic findings
- Intracranial hypertension
- Meningitis
- Acute confusional state
- Frontal sinusitis
- Severe headache after head trauma

Bibliography

Newton RW: Childhood headache. *Arch Dis Child Educ Pract Ed* 2008; 93:105–11.

Pearlman EM: Managing migraine in children and adolescents. *Prim Care* 2004;31:407–15.

Winner P: Pediatric headache. *Curr Opin Neurol* 2008;21:316–22.

Head trauma

Head trauma is very common in childhood, accounting for 76% of trauma admissions and 70% of trauma deaths. Serious head trauma most often results from falls from heights, sports injuries, and bicycle, motorcycle, and automobile accidents. Consider child abuse (shaking, whiplash injuries) in infants and young children. Always consider the possibility of associated cervical spine injury (pp. 702–704) in a patient with head trauma.

Clinical presentation

Most pediatric head trauma victims do not suffer serious injury, although soft-tissue swelling or laceration is common. The most common scenario is a toddler who runs into an object or falls. Occasionally the patient is sleepy but fully arousable; however, the neurologic examination is otherwise normal.

A less obvious presentation is the young afebrile infant with a full fontanelle who is lethargic or vomiting. The baby may be a "shaken infant," with or without other physical evidence of abuse (pp. 580–581).

Serious signs and symptoms include persistent headache, repeated episodes of vomiting, ataxia, blurred vision, altered level of consciousness, focal neurologic signs, seizures, a compound skull fracture, or evidence of increased intracranial pressure.

Contact seizures occur at the moment or within seconds of the head trauma. Although frightening to observers, contact seizures are of no clinical significance. In contrast, early posttraumatic seizures occur 1 minute to 1 week after the head trauma, whereas late posttraumatic seizures occur 1 week or more after the injury. About 25% of children with early posttraumatic seizures develop late seizures, and nearly 75% of children with late posttraumatic seizures develop epilepsy. Almost 100% of patients with penetrating head trauma eventually have epilepsy.

Specific brain injuries include the following.

Concussion

This is a brain injury that is not demonstrable by radiographic studies but may be associated with transient confusion or loss of consciousness.

Contusion

A cerebral contusion is an area of focal edema with or without hemorrhage that can be seen on CT scan. There is usually loss of consciousness, and there may be focal deficits.

Epidural hematoma

An epidural hematoma results from a tear in one of the meningeal arteries (middle meningeal is the most common site) or meningeal or diploic veins. A temporoparietal skull fracture is present in up to 75% of children. The classic presentation is a concussion followed by a lucid interval and then loss of consciousness associated with signs of increased ICP. However, this classic presentation occurs only about one-third of the time, so that in many cases there is no history of loss of consciousness or lucid interval. With a large epidural hematoma there may be ipsilateral pupillary dilatation and, less commonly, contralateral decerebrate posturing.

Subdural hematoma

With a subdural hematoma, there is tearing of the bridging veins between the cerebral cortex and the dura, with compression of the underlying brain. Subdural hematomas are often associated with more widespread shear injury to the brain, and have high morbidity and mortality rates. A subdural hematoma can present with coma or seizures, or it may develop more slowly and be associated with nonspecific signs and symptoms of increased ICP. They are most common in infancy and are suggestive of child abuse.

Diffuse axonal injury

This serious injury is produced when shearing forces generated by rapid acceleration-deceleration cause disruption of myelin and tearing of long axonal fibers. Very young children can also exhibit visible tears in the white matter. A CT scan reveals diffuse brain swelling, which develops over 24–48 hours, but no mass lesions.

Basilar skull fracture

Common fractures of the base of the skull include longitudinal or transverse fractures of the petrous portion of the temporal bone and fractures of the cribriform plate. Suspect petrous fractures when there is hemotympanum, Battle's sign, CSF otorrhea, facial palsy, or hearing loss. Hemorrhage in the nose or nasopharynx, CSF rhinorrhea, or anosmia suggests fracture through the cribriform plate. Basilar skull fractures are rarely seen on plain film. If one is suspected, noncontrast CT with thin cuts through the area of interest is necessary.

Diagnosis

The treatment of a serious head injury takes priority over obtaining the history and performing a complete physical examination. Determine the nature of the trauma, including whether the patient lost consciousness or cried immediately. Ask about vomiting, seizures, recollection of the event, activities both before and after the injury, and past medical problems (seizure disorder, neurologic handicap). Once the patient is medically stabilized, obtain a developmental history. Many victims of severe head trauma have a history of behavioral or developmental problems.

Perform a complete physical examination, including vital signs. Look for scalp lacerations and hematomas, a depressed skull fracture, and evidence of a basilar skull fracture (retroauricular or periorbital ecchymoses, hemotympanum, serous or serosanguineous rhinorrhea or otorrhea). Consider the possibility of cervical spine injury in all cases, and check for sources of bleeding and other major injuries (see multiple trauma, pp. 710–718).

Head trauma per se does not cause hypotension, except in very young infants or patients with serious scalp lacerations. Hypotension demands an immediate, thorough evaluation of the rest of the body (particularly chest, abdomen, pelvis, and thighs) for sources of blood loss. Tachycardia, particularly in association with a narrowed pulse pressure, suggests impending shock (p. 34).

Hypertension and bradycardia associated with slow or irregular respirations (Cushing's triad) indicate increased intracranial pressure, although very young children may not exhibit the full triad. Hypertension may not develop, or may be a late finding shortly before herniation. Treatment must be instituted at once (see pp. 516–518).

Perform a careful neurologic examination, paying careful attention to the signs of structural coma: asymmetry of pupillary responses, EOMs or motor response. Examine the cranial nerves, perform ophthalmoscopy (for papilledema, or loss of spontaneous venous pulsations, or retinal hemorrhage), and test the reflexes, strength, sensation, and coordination, comparing one side to the other.

Test fluid draining from the ear or nose for glucose. CSF has glucose in it; mucus does not. If the fluid is bloody, touch it with a piece of filter paper. Formation of two concentric rings suggests that CSF is mixed with the blood.

Table 16-6. Glasgow Coma Scale[a]

	Score
Eyes open	
Spontaneously	4
To speech	3
To pain	2
None	1
Best verbal response	
Oriented	5
Confused	4
Inappropriate words	3
Incomprehensible sound	2
None	1
Best motor response	
Obeys	6
Localizes	5
Withdraws	4
Abnormal flexion	3
Abnormal extension	2
None	1

Note: [a] Total GCS is the sum of the scores of the three parts.

The Glasgow Coma Scale (GCS) indicates the initial severity of the head injury and facilitates monitoring of changes in the patient's status (Table 16-6). A modified GCS has been developed for preverbal children (Table 16-7).

The neurologic exam, the nature of the injury, and the age of the patient determine the need for radiographic studies. Since CT scans provide information about the skull and, the underlying brain, skull radiographs are rarely needed. If a depressed skull fracture is suspected (trauma caused by a sharp, high-velocity object; large scalp hematoma preventing palpation of the skull below), obtain an X-ray tangential to the area in question. Skull X-rays are usually not needed to rule out a linear compound fracture in a patient with a scalp laceration, since these wounds will be explored under local anesthesia.

Risk assignment may be helpful to guide further management (Table 16-8).

ED management

The priorities are securing the airway, maintaining vital signs, stabilizing the cervical spine, and treating increased intracranial pressure. Serial examination of the patient, preferably by the same healthcare provider, is essential to the early detection of evolving injuries.

Table 16-7. Modified Glasgow Coma Scale[a]

	Score
Eyes open	
Spontaneously	4
To speech	3
To pain	2
None	1
Best verbal response	
Coos and babbles	5
Irritable cries	4
Cries to pain	3
Moans to pain	2
None	1
Best motor response	
Normal spontaneous movements	6
Withdraws to touch	5
Withdraws to pain	4
Abnormal flexion	3
Abnormal extension	2
None	1

Note: [a] Total GCS is the sum of the scores of the three parts.

First, assess the airway and adequacy of ventilation and stabilize the cervical spine with a rigid neck collar. Since a patient with a depressed level of consciousness may have inadequate ventilation despite respiratory movements, obtain an ABG, monitor oxygen saturation, and give 100% oxygen if the patient is not fully awake and alert. Intubate any patient with a GCS ≤8, using in-line stabilization of the cervical spine and the jaw thrust–chin lift maneuver. Examine the chest for the presence of bilateral breath sounds and signs of respiratory distress.

Next, measure the vital signs at least every 15 minutes, and more frequently in patients with severe head trauma or an abnormal pulse or blood pressure. Secure a large-bore IV in patients with hypotension or a GCS <15. The treatment of hypotension with 20 mL/kg boluses of isotonic crystalloid and packed red cell transfusions takes precedence over concerns about increased intracranial pressure. Once a normal BP is maintained, infuse D₅½NS at a KVO rate.

A patient with a depressed skull fracture, penetrating head trauma, focal neurologic findings, or an early posttraumatic seizure is at risk for the development of seizures. Give a loading dose of IV fosphenytoin (20 mg phenytoin equivalent/kg) slowly over 30 minutes.

Table 16-8. Risk assignment based on clinical examination

Low-risk injuries (GCS = 15)

    Asymptomatic

    Mild headache

    Dizziness

    Short-term vomiting (duration <4 hours)

    Normal neurologic examination

Moderate-risk injuries (GCS = 9–14)

    History of loss of consciousness

    Progressive headache

    Persistent vomiting (duration ≥4 hours)

    Early posttraumatic seizure

    Associated injuries (long bone fracture, contusion of internal organs)

    Altered mental status (including drug or alcohol intoxication)

    Suspected child abuse

    Basilar skull fracture

High-risk injuries (GCS <9)

    Depressed level of consciousness

    Penetrating injury to brain

    Focal neurologic examination

Give nafcillin (150 mg/kg per day div q 6 h) to a patient with a compound skull fracture before debridement, but do not give antibiotics routinely to a patient with a basilar skull fracture.

GCS <8 or GCS ≥ 8 but worsening

Immediately intubate the patient and call for neurologic and neurosurgical consultations. Hyperventilate the patient to a pCO_2 of 30–35 mmHg, keep the head in the midline, elevate the head of the bed to 30°, and restrict fluids to NS at a KVO rate. If there is pupillary asymmetry or decorticate posturing, give mannitol (0.5–1 g/kg) as an IV push. Arrange for an immediate CT scan (see Increased intracranial pressure, pp. 516–518).

GCS 9–14

Insert a large-bore IV for access, and repeat the GCS every 15 minutes. Arrange for an urgent CT scan. Admit the patient for close observation if the GCS remains <15 during the first hour in the ED.

GCS = 15

If the child has not vomited and has a normal exam, he or she may be sent home if the parents can follow instructions and return immediately for worrisonu symptoms. If there is persistent vomiting or dizziness, arrange for a CT scan or admit for observation and serial neurologic exams. Regardless of whether the CT is normal, if the parents are anxious, do not discharge a patient until he or she is back to baseline.

Admit a patient with a basilar skull fracture if a CSF leak is supected, there are associated neurologic findings, or the parents are anxious. If there is associated CSF leakage, elevate the head of the bed to 30° and consult with neurosurgery. A patient with CSF otorrhea or rhinorrhea is at risk for bacterial meningitis (10%), but prophylactic antibiotics are not indicated. Most CSF leaks resolve spontaneously within 7–10 days.

Follow-up

- GCS = 15: next day. Instruct the parents to return immediately if the patient cannot be aroused or has diplopia, unsteady gait, several episodes of vomiting, or a headache unresponsive to ibuprofen or acetaminophen

Indications for admission

- GCS <15
- Early posttraumatic seizure (not a contact seizure)
- Compound or depressed skull fracture
- Persistent vomiting, dizziness, or abnormal neurologic findings in the ED
- Basilar skull fracture with associated neurologic findings or CSF leak

Bibliography

Orliaguet GA, Meyer PG, Baugnon T: Management of critically ill children with traumatic brain injury. *Paediatr Anaesth* 2008;18:455–61.

Schnadower D, Vazquez H, Lee J, et al: Controversies in the evaluation and management of minor blunt head trauma in children. *Curr Opin Pediatr* 2007; 19:258–64.

Thiessen ML, Woolridge DP: Pediatric minor closed head injury. *Pediatr Clin North Am* 2006;53:1–26.

Implantable devices

A number of implantable devices for treatment of chronic neurologic disorders are coming into use in children and may be encountered during pediatric ED visits. These include vagus nerve stimulators (VNS) for the treatment of intractable seizures, and intrathecal baclofen pumps (IBP) for spasticity. When a patient with one of these devices presents to the ED, consult a physician experienced in the use of the device.

Vagus nerve stimulator

The VNS consists of a small pulse generator implanted under the skin, usually on the left side in the infraclavicular region. Electrodes are wrapped around the left vagus nerve, and pulses are transmitted in a retrograde fashion to the brain. The generator is programmed to emit pulses at specific intervals, with characteristics defined by the physician. A magnet, provided to the patient, can be moved once across the pulse generator to produce an extra pulse in the event of a seizure. The pulse generator can be stopped from firing by taping the magnet on top of the pulse generator and leaving it there.

A patient with the VNS may not have MRI with a body coil, although a head MRI using a transmit-and-receive head coil may be performed. Reprogram the current amplitude to 0 mA before the MRI, and reset after the procedure. Also, do not bring the patient magnet into the MRI suite. Diathermy is also absolutely contraindicated, although diagnostic ultrasound can be performed.

Problems associated with the VNS include hoarseness, cough, pain in the throat, neck, or GI tract, vomiting, and, rarely, cardiac arrhythmias or asystole. The device may also become infected, especially within the 3 months following implantation.

Intrathecal baclofen pump

The IBP consists of a medication pump and reservoir implanted under the skin, usually in the flank, with a small catheter threaded into the intrathecal space. Although the manufacturer warns that the FDA has not approved performance of MRIs on patients with the pump, MRIs have been completed successfully under the supervision of an experienced physician. Turn the pump off before the procedure and restart afterwards.

Problems with the IBP include decreased delivery of baclofen with severe spasticity (due to empty reservoir, kinking or migration of the catheter), occasional overdose of baclofen characterized by hypotonia, lethargy, and depressed respiratory drive, or infection of the pump. If the pump is empty, use oral baclofen or a benzodiazepine, although neither is as effective.

Bibliography

De Tiège X, Legros B, de Beeck MO, Goldman S, Van Bogaert P: Vagus nerve stimulation. *J Neurosurg Pediatr* 2008;2:375–7.

Motta F, Buonaguro V, Stignani C: The use of intrathecal baclofen pump implants in children and adolescents: safety and complications in 200 consecutive cases. *J Neurosurg* 2007;**107**(1 Suppl):32–5.

Increased intracranial pressure

An increase in the volume of any intracranial compartment (blood, CSF, or parenchyma) can cause an elevation in intracranial pressure (ICP) and is a true neurosurgical emergency. Head trauma is the most common cause of increased ICP in children. Although the onset of increased ICP is usually acute, onset may be delayed in patients with subdural or epidural hematomas. Other causes are brain tumor, meningitis, hemorrhage from a vascular malformation, intracerebral abscess, pseudotumor cerebri, and shunt obstruction in a patient with hydrocephalus. Intracranial hypertension is also the major life-threatening complication of Reye's syndrome.

Clinical presentation

Lethargy is an important finding in a patient with increased ICP. A patient with a GCS <9 or a falling GCS after head trauma requires an immediate evaluation for intracranial hypertension.

A patient with either a history of head injury or increased ICP on a nontraumatic basis may complain of early-morning headache and vomiting, or headaches of recent onset that have become more frequent and severe. A verbal child may complain of blurry vision, frank diplopia, or intermittent loss of vision. Altered mental status, a change in personality (constant crying or irritability in an infant), neck pain, and a head tilt are also suggestive of increased ICP. Papilledema is a highly specific but insensitive finding within the first 24-hours of acutely increased ICP.

In an infant, increased ICP causes irritability, vomiting, widening of the sutures, increasing head circumference, a full or bulging fontanelle, and possibly "sunsetting" of the eyes.

Clinical signs of imminent cerebral herniation include a deteriorating level of consciousness, unequal pupils (the dilated pupil is usually on the same side as the herniation), asymmetric EOMs, and decorticate (flexor-early) or decerebrate (extensor-late) posturing. Abnormal respirations, bradycardia, and hypertension (Cushing's triad) occur with severely increased ICP.

Diagnosis

Any patient who has suffered significant head trauma is at risk for increased ICP. Always ask about persistent vomiting or visual or behavioral changes. Check the pupillary responses, EOMs, and level of consciousness. Perform a careful ophthalmoscopic exam and a sensory and motor exam, comparing one side of the body to the other. Coma can be due to metabolic causes (see pp. 499–501), but typically the pupils are equal and reactive and there are no focal findings.

Congenital anisocoria, the use of mydriatic drops, or traumatic mydriasis or iritis can cause pupillary inequality. These are always diagnoses of exclusion in a patient with lethargy or any other signs suggesting increased ICP.

The evaluation of headaches is discussed on pp. 504–509. Morning headaches or headaches that are increasing in frequency and intensity are worrisome. However, headaches in an alert patient with no other abnormal neurologic findings are most likely to be psychogenic, tension, or migraine headaches.

ED management

If increased ICP is suspected, immediately arrange for a CT scan and notify a neurosurgeon and a neurologist to assist in further management. See pp. 509–515 for the treatment of head trauma.

If the patient has an altered level of consciousness but does not have unequal pupils, bradycardia, hypertension, or decorticate or decerebrate posturing, continuously monitor the heart rate and blood pressure and assess the adequacy of ventilation with an ABG. Secure an IV with NS for vascular access. If the patient is hypotensive, restoration of a normal BP takes priority over treatment of the increased ICP and is required in order to maintain adequate cerebral perfusion pressure. Always keep the patient's head in the midline position if there is a possible cervical spine injury and, unless he or she is in shock, elevate the head of the bed to 30°. Provide 100% oxygen, and intubate any patient who is hypoxic, hypercarbic (pCO_2 >40 mmHg), stuporous, comatose, or is leaving the ED for diagnostic procedures (and so monitoring will be difficult).

If the patient has signs of markedly increased ICP (unequal pupils, bradycardia and hypertension, abnormal posturing), employ all available modalities to lower the ICP while a neurologist and neurosurgeon are summoned. Immediately intubate and hyperventilate to a pCO_2 of 30–35 mmHg. If a mass lesion is suspected, the administer IV mannitol (0.5–1 g/kg) and dexamethasone (0.2 mg/kg, 16 mg maximum). When giving mannitol, insert a urinary bladder catheter. Limit the IV fluid rate to KVO unless the patient is in shock.

To avoid further increasing the ICP, perform intubation under controlled circumstances (see Rapid-sequence intubation, pp. 14–16). As soon as intubation has been accomplished, insert a nasogastric tube (orogastric tube if the patient has sustained head trauma), aspirate the stomach contents, and connect the tube to suction.

Order a shunt survey if there is a suspected shunt obstruction. Arrange for a neurosurgeon to tap the reservoir to obtain CSF for culture, cell count, and chemistries if a shunt infection is suspected.

Indication for admission

- Intracranial hypertension

Bibliography

Kesler A, Bassan H: Pseudotumor cerebri – idiopathic intracranial hypertension in the pediatric population. *Pediatr Endocrinol Rev* 2006;3:387–92.

Matthews YY: Drugs used in childhood idiopathic or benign intracranial hypertension. *Arch Dis Child Educ Pract Ed* 2008;93:19–25.

Mercille G, Ospina LH: Pediatric idiopathic intracranial hypertension: a review. *Pediatr Rev* 2007;28:e77–86.

Seizures

Although more than 5% of children will have at least one seizure, most seizures are either benign febrile convulsions or breakthrough seizures in a known epileptic. The priorities are to identify and treat status epilepticus appropriately and to rule out life-threatening causes such as meningitis, severe head trauma, intracranial bleeding, the long QTc syndrome (LQTS), or a metabolic derangement.

Clinical presentation and diagnosis

Some types of seizures, such as generalized convulsions, are easily recognized while other types are less familiar and subtler in appearance. Common features of seizures include rhythmic jerking movements of head or limbs, changes in tone, fixed staring with or without deviation of the eyes, myoclonic jerks, nystagmus, and unresponsiveness.

Infants, and neonates in particular, tend to have multifocal clonic seizures or more subtle types of seizure activity, including tongue thrusting and lip smacking. In infants, posturing and "funny" movements that are not accompanied by either eye deviation or alteration in vital signs are usually not seizures.

Other nonepileptic paroxysmal events, such as syncope, migraine, movement disorder, and "pseudoseizures," may be mistaken for seizures. These can usually be differentiated with a careful history. Syncope is rare in very young children and is often preceded by a stressful event, giving rise to a vasovagal reaction. Syncope may be preceded by light-headedness or nausea. Also, a syncopal episode secondary to LQTS may be mistaken for a first afebrile seizure.

Confusion or a decreased level of consciousness may accompany migraine, but headache is usually the most striking feature. Movement disorders disappear in sleep and are not associated with a decreased level of consciousness. In contrast, seizure activity frequently arises during sleep or shortly after awakening and often causes a change in level of alertness.

Pseudoseizures are also known as nonepileptic or hysterical seizures. The diagnosis may not be clear, unless the patient is known to have had previous attacks, as many patients also have true seizures. Occasionally, the differentiation of pseudoseizures from true epileptic seizures cannot be made in the ED, and extended monitoring with continuous EEG and closed-circuit television may be necessary.

For the purposes of evaluation and management in the ED, seizures are divided into status epilepticus, febrile seizures, first unprovoked seizure, and breakthrough seizures, without regard to the actual appearance of the seizure or its formal classification.

Status epilepticus

Status epilepticus is defined as either a single seizure lasting longer than 15 minutes or a series of seizures without a return to baseline mental status between each episode. If the seizure started at home and has not stopped before arrival in the ED, the patient is most likely in status. The term status epilepticus refers only to the duration of the seizure and does not imply anything about the cause, prognosis, or type of seizure activity. Generalized tonic-clonic status, partial complex status, and febrile status are the most frequent types of status.

The most common cause of status is low antiepileptic drug levels in a child with documented epilepsy. Other predisposing factors in known epileptics are fever, vomiting, and intercurrent infections. Less commonly, status is symptomatic of an acute encephalo-pathic process such as CNS infection (meningitis, encephalitis), metabolic disturbance (hypoxia, hypoglycemia, hyponatremia, hypocalcemia, hyperammonemia), intoxication or poisoning (cocaine, theophylline, tricyclic antidepressants, amphetamines, camphor), mass lesion, or head trauma.

Children generally tolerate status epilepticus well, although there may be hypoxia and hypercarbia with metabolic and respiratory acidosis significant enough to require intub-ation and mechanical ventilation. Increased cerebral oxygen consumption and cerebral blood flow occur and may cause intracranial hypertension. This can lead to exacerbation of brain damage, if the seizure is due to trauma or spontaneous intracranial hemorrhage. Physical injury and vomiting with aspiration are additional hazards. Therefore, treat status epilepticus as quickly as possible, but avoid the overuse of sedating antiepileptic drugs, which may exacerbate respiratory depression or alteration of mental status.

Febrile seizure

A febrile seizure occurs in 2–5% of otherwise normal children between 6 months and 6 years of age. By definition, the seizure occurs during the course of a febrile illness that does not involve the CNS. The characteristics of febrile seizures are noted in Table 16-9.

Meningitis or encephalitis must be ruled out. This is often possible during the history and physical examination of older children. However, young children can have meningitis without the typical signs (stiff neck, headache, Kernig's and Brudzinski's signs). Therefore, a lumbar puncture (LP) is indicated for any febrile patient <12 months of age unless he or she has an identified source of fever, appears well, and is functioning in a normal baseline fashion. Be particularly cautious with infants who are too young to sit, as clinical assessment

Table 16-9. Characteristics of febrile seizures

Family history in 10%	
No prior CNS dysfunction or neurological disorder	
Simple	*Complex*
Brief (<15 minutes)	Prolonged duration
Generalized	Focal (before, during, after)
Single event	Multiple occurrences within 24 hours
	Febrile status epilepticus

may be difficult. For patients >12 months of age, indications for an LP include lethargy, irritability, toxic appearance, and febrile status epilepticus, regardless of whether a possible source of infection is identified on clinical exam (e.g. otitis media). Have a low threshold for lumbar puncture in children who are pretreated with oral antibiotics. In addition, neuro-imaging (MRI preferred) is required if the child has focal neurological signs.

About two-thirds of patients have only one febrile seizure episode. Of patients who have a second episode, about one-half to two-thirds will have three or more febrile seizures. Recurrences are more likely in children <18 months old at the time of the first seizure and those who have febrile seizures with temperatures <40°C (104°F). Simple febrile seizures do not indicate an increased risk of epilepsy, although the risk is slightly higher than the general population for children with complex febrile seizures. Some children who are eventually diagnosed with epilepsy do present initially with seizures in the setting of a febrile illness.

First unprovoked seizure

An unprovoked seizure is one that is not associated with fever, infection, trauma, ingestion, metabolic abnormality, or any other identifiable cause. The first such episode can some-times be the initial presentation of epilepsy, although the majority of patients never have another seizure.

Breakthrough seizure

A breakthrough seizure occurs in a patient taking chronic antiepileptic drugs. The most common cause is low antiepileptic drug level secondary to noncompliance (particularly common in teenagers), inability to obtain the medication(s), having outgrown the drug dose(s), or change in the patient's metabolism of the drug(s). Antibiotics, birth control pills, and other drugs metabolized through the hepatic P450 system may reduce antiepileptic drug levels. In contrast, erythromycin may lead to an increased carbamazepine (Tegretol) level, and any new medication that is protein-bound may displace phenytoin (Dilantin) from protein-binding sites and lead to transient toxicity. Adding a second antiepileptic agent can also change other drug levels. Finally, a febrile illness or any other type of stress can lower the child's seizure threshold.

ED management

The priorities are evaluation and stabilization of the patient's airway and vital signs, termination of ongoing seizure activity, prevention of recurrent seizures, diagnosis of CNS infection, and determination of the cause of the seizure. If the patient has seizure activity in the ED, document the features of the seizure, including any focal movements, gaze deviation, presence and direction of nystagmus, and alteration in autonomic function.

Obtain a complete history, including an accurate description of the seizure and how and where it started; any "aura" at the onset of the seizure, the time of day and the patient's activity at the time of the seizure (particularly whether the seizure had onset in sleep or early morning), and the postictal state. Inquire about medications taken, family history of epilepsy or other neurologic or neurocutaneous disorder, developmental history, and past medical history. On physical exam, check the skin for neurocutaneous stigmata, perform a thorough general exam and neurologic exam, including a complete mental status exam appropriate to the patient's age, and assess the patient's developmental status.

Once it is clear that the patient did have a seizure and is not in status epilepticus, the ED work-up and management are directed by the answers to the following questions:

1. Is this a first seizure, or is there a history of seizures? If there have been previous seizures, is this seizure similar with regard to type of activity, duration, and frequency?
2. Is the patient taking antiepileptic drugs? Has the child "outgrown" the dose, or has there been a problem with adherence to the drug regimen?
3. Is the patient febrile? Is this a febrile seizure in an otherwise normal child with a fever and an infection that does not involve the CNS? Is this a child with an underlying neurologic disorder who has seizures when febrile?
4. Is there evidence of meningitis?
5. Could the seizure have been provoked by something other than fever, such as hypoxia, hypoglycemia, ingestion of cocaine or another drug, electrolyte abnormality, or head trauma? Has the patient had previous syncopal episodes, raising the possibility of LQTS?

Status epilepticus

Assess the airway, breathing, and circulation before proceeding with treatment. Suction the oral cavity, apply a face mask with 100% oxygen over the nose and mouth, and monitor the vital signs and oxygen saturation. Secure an IV with D_5NS (at KVO if the vital signs are stable), and obtain blood for laboratory tests as indicated by the history. These may include blood for antiepileptic drug levels, serum toxicology screen, CBC, electrolytes, glucose, calcium, and magnesium. If acute exposure to lead is a possibility, also obtain a lead level. Always obtain a rapid Dextrostix estimate of the serum glucose and an extra red-top tube. If the child is febrile and appears toxic, obtain a blood culture. If the cause of the seizure is not clear, obtain a urine sample drug screen, including cocaine metabolites.

Protocol for treatment of status epilepticus

While monitoring the blood pressure, ECG, and respiratory status, give:

1. Lorazepam, 0.05–0.1 mg/kg, 2–4 mg maximum, slow IV over 2 minutes (preferred), IO, PR, or intrabuccally. Alternatives include diazepam 0.1–0.3 mg/kg given slow IV over 2 minutes (5–10 mg maximum), IO, or PR and midazolam 0.05–0.2 mg/kg slow IV over 2 minutes, IO, or IM (5 mg maximum). Respiratory depression and hypotension may

occur. Do not give lorazepam or diazepam IM, because of erratic absorption. Repeat the dose if the seizure does not stop within 5 minutes.

2. Fosphenytoin, 20 mg/kg phenytoin equivalents IV (preferred) or IO given by slow push over 10–15 minutes. Alternatively, give phenytoin, 20 mg/kg IV given by slow push over 20–30 minutes. If the seizure does not stop within 5 minutes after the dose is complete, proceed to step 3, and contact a pediatric neurologist. Fosphenytoin has significant advantages over phenytoin, since it can be given quickly with much less risk of cardiac arrhythmia or asystole. As the pH is 8 (as opposed to 13 for phenytoin), it is much less likely to cause extensive tissue necrosis in the case of extravasation. Fosphenytoin can be diluted in NS or dextrose-containing fluids to concentrations from 1:2 to 1:25 as convenient, while phenytoin is only compatible with NS. However, do not give fosphenytoin IM for status epilepticus, due to its slow absorption.

3. Phenobarbital, 20 mg/kg IV. Phenobarbital can cause respiratory depression and hypotension, especially if given in combination with benzodiazepines. If there is any sign of respiratory depression or if the patient does not have good airway protection reflexes (gag and cough), prophylactic intubation prior to administration of phenobarbital is recommended. If the seizure does not stop, consider steps 4 and 5, and contact a pediatric intensivist or anesthesiologist.

4. Pentobarbital coma, in an intensive care unit.

5. General anesthesia, in an intensive care unit.

If the seizure activity is stopped by lorazepam, the patient usually needs no further antiepileptic medication. This includes a patient with febrile status, breakthrough seizures due to low antiepileptic drug levels that can be adjusted once the patient returns to baseline, or metabolic derangements, which are easily correctable. However, if a patient is unconsciousness, intubated, or has received paralytic agents, it is necessary to treat with IV fosphenytoin or phenobarbital as seizures may not be detectable clinically.

For the rare patient who does not have a history of epilepsy and does not respond to lorazepam or diazepam, check the electrolytes and obtain an ABG. A patient with a metabolic or hypoxic basis for the status needs correction of the underlying problem and usually does not require treatment with anticonvulsants. Treat hyponatremic seizures with water restriction and normal saline (see Hyponatremia, pp. 186–189). If needed, give hypertonic (3%) saline (2–4 mL/kg IV push). Correction of the sodium to 125 mEq/L is generally sufficient to stop seizures, but avoid a rapid correction to a "normal" sodium. Treat hypertensive seizures with IV labetalol (0.25 mg/kg over 10 minutes) or IV diazoxide miniboluses (1 mg/kg), which can be repeated up to five times at 10–15 minute intervals (see Hypertension, pp. 656–658).

Fever, irritability, or lethargy are indications for a blood culture and a lumbar puncture, once the seizure has been terminated. It is essential that the child's respiratory status be stable before a lumbar puncture is attempted. If there is apnea, hypoventilation, or signs of increased ICP such as papilledema or posturing, give antibiotics and delay the procedure. If the Dextrostix reading is low (<70 mg/dL), give an IV push of 0.5 g/kg glucose (2 mL/kg of D_{25}) after obtaining blood for glucose and insulin levels. Obtain urine to check for ketones, if the patient is hypoglycemic.

A patient with evidence of focality (except for known stable neurological deficits without new findings) or increased ICP on neurologic exam must undergo immediate CT scanning (see Increased intracranial pressure, pp. 516–518). However, a patient with generalized seizures with no residual defects does not require radiographic imaging in the ED. An EEG is indicated for a patient with new-onset status epilepticus with focal features, focal neurological deficits, or if the onset of seizure activity was unwitnessed, but it is more useful if deferred until after the immediate postictal period. An EEG is indicated in the ED when there is reason to suspect subclinical status epilepticus (subtle seizure activity that continues after convulsive status epilepticus has been treated).

Febrile seizures

A patient with a febrile seizure lasting more than 15 minutes has status epilepticus; treat as described above. For most children with febrile seizures, vigorous antipyresis with acetaminophen (15 mg/kg q 4 h) and/or ibuprofen (10 mg/kg q 6 h) is commonly used to prevent recurrences, although there is no evidence that these measures are effective. Consult a neurologist to consider treatment with antiepileptic drugs or rectal diazepam for a patient whose seizures are unusually severe, frequent, or accompanied by aspiration or a need for intubation.

A patient with a febrile seizure without focality may be discharged from the ED when all infectious disease issues have been resolved, his or her condition has returned to baseline status, and the family has an adequate supply of antipyretics, with instructions for their use.

First unprovoked seizure

Long-term antiepileptic drug treatment for a first-time unprovoked seizure in an otherwise normal child may be postponed until the child has a second or third seizure. Defer these decisions to the primary medical provider or pediatric neurologist. Metabolic derangements are rare, although the likelihood increases in younger children and infants. For an older child who appears well and has returned to a normal neurological baseline following a seizure, routine electrolytes, calcium, and magnesium determinations are seldom helpful. However, if the patient has a history of syncopal episodes or a family history of arrhythmia, syncope, sudden death, or deafness, obtain an ECG and rhythm strip to rule out LQTS (see Syncope, pp. 68–71).

A patient with a new-onset unprovoked seizure without focality may be discharged from the ED when his or her condition has returned to baseline status, arrangements for appropriate follow-up have been made, and the immediate concerns of the child and family have been addressed.

Breakthrough seizure

If the patient is known to have had a recent therapeutic anticonvulsant level, give an extra dose of that medication rather than a full loading dose. For example, give 5 mg/kg of either fosphenytoin, phenytoin, or phenobarbital IV over 15–20 minutes. Do not give either drug IM. If there are subsequent seizures, treat as for status epilepticus, as described above. Valproic acid, but not carbamazepine, is now available in IV form. Use the same dose as for oral administration, over 1 hour.

A patient with a history of epilepsy and breakthrough seizures may be discharged from the ED when his or her condition has returned to baseline status, there is a therapeutic antiepileptic drug level, and the patient has an adequate supply of all necessary anticonvulsants.

Follow-up
- Febrile or first unprovoked seizure: next day
- Breakthrough seizure: 2–3 days, to check anticonvulsant levels

Indications for admission
- Status epilepticus
- Increasing number of breakthrough seizures or new types of seizures in a known epileptic
- Focality or evidence of increased intracranial pressure
- CNS infection
- Structural lesion (trauma, tumor, hemorrhage)
- Child who does not return to baseline mental status within 1–2 h of the seizure

Bibliography

Haut SR, Shinnar S: Considerations in the treatment of a first unprovoked seizure. *Semin Neurol* 2008;28:289–96.

Jones T, Jacobsen SJ: Childhood febrile seizures: overview and implications. *Int J Med Sci* 2007;4:110–4.

Riviello JJ Jr, Ashwal S, Hirtz D, et al: Practice parameter: diagnostic assessment of the child with status epilepticus (an evidence-based review): report of the Quality Standards Subcommittee of the American Academy of Neurology and the Practice Committee of the Child Neurology Society. *Neurology* 2006;67:1542–50.

Walker DM, Teach SJ: Update on the acute management of status epilepticus in children. *Curr Opin Pediatr* 2006;18:239–44.

Sleep disorders

Nightmares, night terrors, and sleepwalking can occur with enough frequency to bring a patient to the ED.

Clinical presentation and diagnosis

Nightmares

Nightmares are frightening dreams that occur during rapid eye movement (REM) sleep. The child is easily arousable or awakens spontaneously, and typically has a good recall of the dream. Nightmares are fairly common in children beginning at about age 3, but it is important to obtain a careful medication history, since withdrawal from minor tranquilizers, anticonvulsants, and sedative-hypnotics can be associated with nightmares.

Night terrors

Night terrors occur within 2 hours of falling asleep, most often in children 3–8 years old. The child will be frightened and crying inconsolably. In contrast to a nightmare, it is very difficult to arouse the patient. Signs of autonomic arousal are common, including increased heart rate, pupillary dilatation, sweating, and even combativeness. After a few minutes, the child will return to sleep and will have little, if any, recall of the episode. A patient with night terrors frequently also has somnambulism (see below). Night terrors are easy to confuse with nightmares or nocturnal seizures. A thorough history is of primary importance in making the diagnosis.

Somnambulism

Somnambulism, or sleepwalking, occurs in 1–6% of the population (particularly boys), and there is often a positive family history. The child will be out of bed, often performing some sort of purposeful behavior, and may even respond somewhat to verbal commands, although there is usually no recall for the event when the patient is fully awake. Somnambulism can be confused with psychomotor seizures, which do not occur exclusively at night.

Take a careful history of the event, and review the patient's general health status and medication history. Ask about recent stresses in the child's life.

ED management

Nightmares

Occasional nightmares are of little concern. Recurrent episodes, especially if a particular dream occurs frequently, may be indicative of stress or emotional upset that requires further attention.

Night terrors

Generally, a patient "outgrows" night terrors, so that reassurance is all that is needed. However, frequent recurrences suggest underlying stress. If nocturnal seizures cannot be ruled out (episodes also occur during the day or more than 2–3 hours after falling asleep), order a sleep-deprived EEG.

Somnambulism

Sleepwalking is difficult to prevent and, once it begins, it may continue into adulthood. Advise the parents to secure the child's area to prevent injury during sleepwalking (protect stairways, doors, windows).

Follow-up

- Primary care follow-up in 2–4 weeks

Bibliography

Heussler HS: 9. Common causes of sleep disruption and daytime sleepiness: childhood sleep disorders II. *Med J Aust* 2005;182:484–9.

Moore M, Meltzer LJ, Mindell JA: Bedtime problems and night wakings in children. *Prim Care* 2008;35:569–81.

Morgenthaler TI, Owens J, Alessi C, et al: Practice parameters for behavioral treatment of bedtime problems and night wakings in infants and young children. *Sleep* 2006; 29:1277–81.

Ventriculoperitoneal shunts

The survival of premature infants has led to a significant increase in the number of patients with ventriculoperitoneal (VP) shunts. A VP shunt places a patient at risk for malfunction, leading to increased ICP, infection, and in some cases, low-pressure headache due to over-draining of the CSF.

Clinical presentation

While the presentation may be dramatic, with signs of increased ICP or CNS infection, the parent may note only that the child "looked just like this the last time he or she had a shunt problem." Although most parents will mention that the patient has a shunt, occasionally this part of the patient's history may be forgotten, particularly if the shunt has been functioning well for a long time or if the presenting complaints are primarily referable to the abdomen.

Shunt malfunction

Proximal (intracranial) obstruction can be caused by CSF protein, choroid plexus, or embedding of the tube in the brain parenchyma. Distal obstruction to CSF flow may result from the formation of an abdominal pseudocyst around the end of the shunt. Malfunction may also result from disconnection or kinking of elements of the shunt leading to symptoms of shunt obstruction. Proximal obstruction causes headache, vomiting, neck pain, lethargy, sixth nerve palsy, persistent downward gaze ("sunsetting" eyes), and feeding intolerance (see Increased intracranial pressure, pp. 516–518). If the obstruction is distal, the patient may also have nausea, abdominal pain, and a distended abdomen.

Shunt infection

Meningitis and ventriculitis present with fever, irritability or lethargy, meningismus, and signs of increased ICP. Infection is most likely to occur in the first 3 months after placement of the shunt, secondary to contamination at the time of the procedure. A late infection is due to hematogenous spread. Occasionally, a patient may develop peritonitis, followed by an ascending infection of the shunt.

Low-pressure headache

While newer shunts have anti-syphoning devices and may have programmable valves to allow for adjustment of the opening pressure, an older patient may have a shunt without these devices. The shunt may intermittently overdrain with subsequent tension on the dura and other pain-sensitive structures, causing nausea and severe headache. On CT scan, the ventricles appear slit-like. This syndrome is annoying but not life-threatening; consult with the neurosurgeon.

Diagnosis

Perform a thorough evaluation for shunt problems if a patient with a VP shunt has headache, lethargy, vomiting, or abdominal pain. Inspect the overlying skin along the entire course of the shunt for erythema, erosions, or induration, which may suggest a source of infection. Evaluate for possible obstruction by depressing the subcutaneous reservoir. Inability to depress the reservoir suggests distal obstruction, while if the reservoir is depressible but does not refill within 10 seconds, there may be obstruction proximal to or within the one-way valve at the cranial end of the reservoir. If an obstruction is suspected, obtain a noncontrast CT of the brain and compare with previous studies to determine whether there has been an increase in the size of the ventricular system. However, an unchanged CT does not rule out obstruction, particularly in cases where the patient has been shunted for a long time and the ventricles are no longer compliant. Also obtain a shunt series (a series of plain films that show the full extent of the shunt) to rule out malfunction due to disconnection or kinking of the elements of the shunt.

If a distal obstruction is suspected, obtain an abdominal ultrasound to look for a pseudocyst or fluid collection.

If infection is suspected, consult a neurosurgeon to obtain a specimen of CSF for cell count and culture. Although a lumbar puncture can be attempted in any patient except those with meningomyelocele (in which case the location of spinal cord elements is unclear), the procedure is often unsuccessful because of alterations in CSF flow due to the presence of the shunt. Most shunts can be tapped directly by inserting a butterfly needle through the skin into the reservoir under sterile conditions.

ED management

Assess the airway, breathing, and cardiovascular status, give oxygen, and obtain IV access, if necessary. Consult a neurosurgeon to assess shunt function and tap or externalize the shunt, if necessary. If there is papilledema, focal neurologic findings, bradycardia, or hypertension, begin treatment for increased ICP (pp. 516–518) while arranging for radiologic assessment of the shunt.

If the patient has Cushing's triad or asymmetry of the pupils suggesting that herniation is imminent, summon a neurosurgeon to insert a spinal needle through the bony defect along the track of the intracranial portion of the shunt catheter into the ventricle and allow CSF to drain out. Follow the neurologic exam carefully before and during this procedure. If a shunt infection is suspected, obtain appropriate blood and urine cultures and begin antibiotic treatment (vancomycin 60 mg/kg per day div q 6h) only if the patient is unstable or the shunt cannot be tapped within a reasonable amount of time. *Staphylococcus epidermidis* and *Staphylococcus aureus* are the most common organisms.

Indication for admission

- All patients in whom there is evidence or strong clinical suspicion of shunt infection or malfunction

Bibliography

Browd SR, Gottfried ON, Ragel BT, Kestle JR: Failure of cerebrospinal fluid shunts: part II: overdrainage, loculation, and abdominal complications. *Pediatr Neurol* 2006; 34:171–6.

Browd SR, Ragel BT, Gottfried ON, Kestle JR: Failure of cerebrospinal fluid shunts: part I:

Obstruction and mechanical failure. *Pediatr Neurol* 2006;34:83–92.

Desai KR, Babb JS, Amodio JB: The utility of the plain radiograph "shunt series" in the evaluation of suspected ventriculoperitoneal shunt failure in pediatric patients. *Pediatr Radiol* 2007;37:452–6.

Ophthalmologic emergencies

Carolyn Lederman and Martin Lederman

Anatomy

Knowledge of anatomy is required in order to adequately evaluate the eye and related structures (refer to Figure 17-1).

The eye is protected by the lids and surrounding orbital bones. The most anterior part of the eye is the tear film layer covering the cornea (clear front portion of the eye). The corneal margin, where the cornea meets the sclera, is referred to as the limbus. The conjunctiva is a thin membrane covering both the white sclera (where it is called the "bulbar conjunctiva"), and the inside of the lids (where it is referred to as the "palpebral conjunctiva"). Because the bulbar and palpebral conjunctivae join in the superior and inferior fornix (the area where they join is known also as a "cul-de-sac"), objects such as foreign bodies and contact lenses cannot slip behind the eye and be lost.

Behind the cornea is the anterior chamber, which is approximately 1–2 mm in depth and is filled with clear fluid, known as aqueous humor. The aqueous circulation begins in the ciliary body located behind the iris and flows through the pupil and out through the trabecular meshwork located in the angle between the iris and the peripheral cornea.

The iris contains a circular constrictor muscle and radial dilator muscles, each controlling the circular pupil.

Behind the iris plane is the crystalline lens, which functions as the focusing mechanism of the eye. It is kept in place and controlled by fine suspensory ligaments (zonules) that form an attachment from the lens to the ciliary body.

The inner volume of the eye is filled with a clear gel, the vitreous body. Lining the inner sclera is the retina, a fine network of blood vessels and photosensitive nerve cells which are the first receptors of the visual pathway.

The bony orbit surrounds, supports, and protects the globe. In addition to the globe, the contents of the orbit include connective tissue, blood vessels, fat, and the six extraocular muscles that control eye movement.

Evaluation

Except for chemical injury, when immediate flushing is indicated, an adequate examination of the eye must include an evaluation and recording of its sensory function, i.e. visual acuity. While parts of the following eye examination can be omitted when appropriate, always assess visual acuity.

The standard Snellen chart at 20 feet is best, but other distances may be used as long as that distance is noted. The numerator of the Snellen Fraction denotes the distance from the chart and the denominator is an arbitrary number given to each line. A smaller denominator refers to a smaller letter (optotype), i.e. a letter on the "20" line is half the size of a letter on

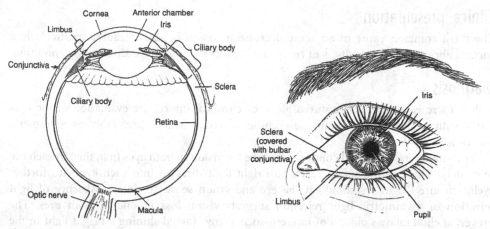

Figure 17-1. Anatomy of the eye.

the "40" line, and ten times smaller than a letter on the "200" line. Thus, 20/200 means that a letter on the "200" line was correctly identified at 20 feet and 4/40 (its equivalent) means that the "40" line letter (5 times smaller) was correctly identified at 4 feet (5 times closer).

Charts using other symbols have been constructed for preliterate children but other methods can be used if a chart is not available, such as counting fingers at a specified distance, hand motions at a specified distance, observed eye closure when a light is directed in the eye (light rejection), or reading a newspaper headline at some distance. It is important to check each eye separately. Use a sterile gauze pad to occlude the non-tested eye without pressing on the globe, then check both eyes together. For children who wear corrective glasses, test visual acuity with and without the glasses. Test the "good" eye first in order to reduce anxiety. For infants and preverbal children, test visual acuity by assessing whether the child can fix on and follow an object.

Assuming that there are no other life-threatening or organ-threatening injuries, evaluate the eyes in a systematic manner, starting from the most anterior aspect of the eye to the most posterior. Look first at the lids and surrounding structures, palpate the bony orbital rim, assess the tears, look at the anterior aspect of the eye including the conjunctiva, cornea and sclera, and assess ocular mobility by having the patient follow a finger (not a bright light, which may cause photophobia) moving in all positions of gaze (up, down, left, right, and oblique). Note the depth and clarity of the anterior chamber, and observe pupillary motility and quality. In a semi-darkened room, at a distance of 1–2 feet, dial the ophthalmoscope to sharply define iris markings (usually black or plus 1 or 2) and assess the clarity and symmetrical color of the pupils. Use the ophthalmoscope to evaluate the retina, noting the sharpness and color of the optic nerve, vascular pattern, foveal reflex and retinal contour. Finally, palpate the globes if a ruptured globe is not suspected.

Decreased vision

Decreased vision can be caused by life-threatening intraocular or intracranial tumors, eye-threatening diseases (trauma, iridocyclitis, pseudotumor cerebri, glaucoma, retinal detachment), or minor conditions (corneal foreign body, conjunctivitis, tearing). In addition, decreased vision may be a functional complaint.

Clinical presentation

The most common cause of an acute decrease in vision is ocular trauma, particularly a corneal abrasion. The priority is to rule out a life-threatening or eye-threatening condition.

Diagnosis

Unless there is an obvious ruptured globe or chemical injury, the evaluation of the eyes starts with a determination and description of visual acuity, preferably as a numeric function.

For infants and preverbal children, describe the vision in both eyes first, then in each eye separately. The sleeping infant reacts to bright light directed into each eye with further eyelid closure ("light rejection") if the eye and vision sense are intact. Absence of light rejection or asymmetric light rejection suggests vision loss in one or both eyes. The preverbal child follows objects of interest, such as toys (avoid shining a bright light in the awake child's eyes), by fixing centrally on the object and following it. Test each eye separately, using the examiner's or parent's thumb as an occluder. For an older child, a Snellen chart that has been calibrated at 20 feet is most accurate, especially if the light is constant and reproducible, and the examining area is quiet. Testing can be done at a distance of 5 to 10 feet, although using shorter testing distances may miss subtle differences between the eyes. In the absence of a Snellen chart, ask the patient to count fingers held a few feet away or check the ability to read a newspaper headline at a set distance. The testing distance must be noted.

ED management

Treat the chief complaint or primary illness. Indications for immediate ophthalmologic evaluation include a sleeping infant who does not reject light, an awake infant who does not follow with either or both eyes, and asymmetry in the vision testing results, particularly if there has been ocular trauma.

Bibliography

Committee on Practice and Ambulatory Medicine, Section on Ophthalmology. American Association of Certified Orthoptists; American Association for Pediatric Ophthalmology and Strabismus; American Academy of Ophthalmology. Eye examination in infants, children, and young adults by pediatricians. *Pediatrics* 2003;111(4 Pt 1):902–7.

Curnyn KM, Kaufman LM: The eye examination in the pediatrician's office. *Pediatr Clin North Am* 2003; 50:25–40.

Tingley DH: Vision screening essentials: screening today for eye disorders in the pediatric patient. *Pediatr Rev* 2007;28:54–61.

Excessive tearing

Tears are produced immediately after birth, but the volume increases after the sixth week. Excess tearing is very common and is secondary to either excess production or insufficient drainage. Excess production is usually due to irritation, infection, foreign body, trauma, iritis, or glaucoma. Insufficient drainage is caused by a stenotic or blocked lacrimal system, usually at the level of the nasolacrimal duct, which conducts tears from the lacrimal sac into the nose.

Clinical presentation

Excess production

Tearing due to excess production is often accompanied by conjunctival injection in older children, but injection is usually absent in the newborn. Lid swelling and nasal discharge are common.

Congenital glaucoma (elevated intraocular pressure)

Congenital glaucoma is accompanied by excess growth of the eye (buphthalmos), photophobia, loss of vision, and tearing, with discharge at the nares. The clarity of the cornea may be reduced with obscuration of the iris markings. It may be unilateral or bilateral, and there may be a positive family history.

Iritis

Iritis is accompanied by photophobia, ciliary flush (circumcorneal conjunctival injection), a small pupil with diminished response, and decreased visual acuity. It is uncommon in infancy, except after eye trauma.

Insufficient drainage

Dacryostenosis (nasolacrimal duct obstruction)

Dacryostenosis is the most common ophthalmologic cause of excess tearing in infancy, usually presenting in the first 3 months of life. A persistent mucoid or mucopurulent discharge is usually present, in addition to recurrent conjunctivitis. Nasolacrimal duct obstruction may be accompanied by dermatitis of the lids due to the chronic tearing, but there is no nasal discharge or photophobia (to distinguish dacryostenosis from congenital glaucoma).

Hydrops (amniotocele)

Hydrops of the lacrimal sac is usually present at or shortly after birth and is secondary to blockage of the proximal and distal portions of the lacrimal sac. It presents as a bluish discoloration at the location of the lacrimal sac and can be confused with a meningocele. Secondary infection is common.

Dacryocystitis

Acute dacryocystitis is a suppurative infection of the lacrimal sac. It presents with tenderness and swelling of the lacrimal sac, with erythema and swelling of the overlying skin. There is usually a history of nasolacrimal duct obstruction.

Diagnosis

The priority is to rule out excessive tear production as the cause before diagnosing nasolacrimal duct obstruction. Photophobia, eyelid closure (blepharospasm), ciliary flush, pain, and nasal discharge suggest excessive production. See Table 17-1 for the differential diagnosis of excessive tearing.

Consider a foreign body or corneal abrasion if the tearing started suddenly, especially if it is accompanied by pain and blepharospasm. The diagnosis of glaucoma is confirmed by evaluation of the intraocular pressure. Consider iritis after trauma.

Table 17-1. Differential diagnosis of excessive tearing

Diagnosis	Differentiating features
Congenital glaucoma	Photophobia, nasal discharge
	Corneal clouding, buphthalmos
Iritis	Photophobia, miosis, ciliary flush
	May have a history of trauma
Nasolacrimal duct obstruction	Onset in 2nd or 3rd month of life
	Discharge, recurrent conjunctivitis, dermatitis of lids
Corneal foreign body or abrasion	Sudden onset of tearing
	Pain, blepharospasm

The diagnosis of nasolacrimal duct obstruction is suggested by constant tearing beginning in the second or third month of life, associated with concurrent eye discharge and conjunctivitis. There may be swelling of the lacrimal sac with reflux of material from the punctum when digital pressure is applied to the side of the nose overlying the lacrimal sac. Dacryocystitis is likely if there is erythematous swelling of the lacrimal sac. Discharge from the punctum is rarely present.

ED management

The management of excessive tearing secondary to a foreign body (pp. 535–541) or conjunctivitis (pp. 541–545) is detailed elsewhere. Glaucoma and iritis require immediate ophthalmologic consultation.

Dacryostenosis

In most cases, dacryostenosis clears spontaneously by 6–12 months of age. Treatment consists of massage of the lacrimal sac three times a day to express the contents. Using the pad of a clean finger, direct the massage from the area of the medial canthal ligament down the side of the nose to the level of the nostril. Prescribe a topical ophthalmic antibiotic (erythromycin ointment, bacitracin ointment, sulfacetamide or polymyxin-trimethoprim drops) tid to suppress infection. Refer the patient to an ophthalmologist for evaluation if the condition does not clear by the sixth month, especially if there have been frequent infections.

Hydrops

Refer immediately to an ophthalmologist.

Dacryocystitis

After obtaining a culture of any material in the palpebral fissure, treat acute dacryocystitis with oral antibiotics. Use amoxicillin-clavulanate (875/125 formulation; 45 mg/kg per day div bid) or cephalexin (25–50 mg/kg per day div tid). Topical ophthalmic antibiotics (bacitracin, erythromycin, or moxifloxacin) qid and warm compresses qid are useful adjunctive therapies. Urgent referral to an ophthalmologist is indicated. Probing of the nasolacrimal duct may eventually be necessary in order to avoid recurrence.

Follow-up

- Dacryocystitis: return in 2–3 days if there is no improvement.

Indications for admission

- Congenital glaucoma
- Dacryocystitis, if close outpatient follow-up is not ensured

Bibliography

Forbes BJ, Khazaeni LM: Evaluation and
management of an infant with tearing
and eye discharge. *Pediatr Case Rev*
2003;3:40–3.

MacEwen CJ: Congenital nasolacrimal duct
obstruction. *Compr Ophthalmol Update*
2006;7:79–87.

Eyelid inflammation

The eyelids can be affected by dermatologic conditions that also involve other areas of the skin. However, the unique structures of the eyelids make them prone to particular and characteristic diseases. The protective function of the eyelids, their constant movement, and their prominent location make abnormalities particularly noticeable and troubling.

Clinical presentation and diagnosis

Hordeolum

A hordeolum, or stye, is an infection (*Staphylococcus* most common) of a sebaceous gland of the lid (gland of Zeis). It usually presents as a localized erythematous swelling of the lid margin, although the entire lid may be affected. The area is tender, and the abscess may point at the base of a lash. Several styes may be present simultaneously.

Chalazion

A chalazion is a granulomatous swelling of the other sebaceous gland of the lid (Meibomian gland). It begins as a firm, painless, circular swelling within the lid itself. There may be multiple chalazia. Secondary infection leads to increased swelling and pain, with the abscess pointing onto the skin surface or the conjunctival side of the lid.

Blepharitis

Blepharitis is inflammation of the margin of the lid, usually secondary to *Staphylococcus aureus* infection. Blepharitis is often chronic and may lead to the development of hordeola and chalazia. Typically, the lid margins are erythematous, crusted, and swollen, and there may be an associated conjunctivitis. Pruritus, burning, a foreign-body sensation, tearing, blurry vision, and loss of lashes are common complaints.

Seborrheic dermatitis

Seborrheic dermatitis is an erythematous, scaly, or crusting eruption with overlying yellowish greasy scale. The eyelids can be affected, in addition to the scalp, postauricular areas, ears, and neck. Conjunctivitis is uncommon in the absence of blepharitis.

Herpes simplex

Eyelid involvement may be the sole finding or may be part of a more generalized herpetic infection. It presents with grouped vesicles on an erythematous base. The surrounding skin and lips may also be affected, and there may be associated conjunctivitis, keratitis, iritis, and preauricular lymphadenopathy. Recurrences are common.

Varicella

The characteristic papular, vesicular, and crusting rash of varicella may affect the eyelids and surrounding skin. Conjunctivitis can be present, particularly if the lid margin is affected. Photophobia, iritis, pupillary abnormalities (irregular or sluggishly reacting), and loss of vision are worrisome, but rare findings. Zoster causes pain in the affected area, followed by swelling of the eyelids. Several days later, the characteristic vesicles develop.

Molluscum contagiosum

Molluscum appear as 1–5 mm flesh-colored umbilicated papules, usually associated with similar lesions on the periorbital skin. Patients are usually asymptomatic, although involvement of the lid margins can produce a concomitant conjunctivitis.

Parasitic infestation

The crab louse (*Phthirus pubis*) can infest the eyelids. The infestation is pruritic, and lice and ova or "nits" (tiny white dots) can be seen attached to the lashes and eyebrows. Severe conjunctivitis can result.

ED management

Hordeolum and chalazion

Treat hordeola and infected chalazia with warm (not hot) compresses for 3 to 5 min three times a day. Apply about 2–3 mm of an ophthalmic antibiotic ointment (e.g. erythromycin, bacitracin) tid after the compress. Treat an associated blepharitis (see below) to prevent recurrence. Usually a hordeolum disappears within a week. Refer the patient to an ophthalmologist if improvement does not occur within 2 or 3 days. A chronic chalazion may remain for weeks to months and does not require excision as long as vision is unaffected.

Blepharitis

Blepharitis is a chronic disorder, and treatment is directed toward keeping the disease under control. Use warm-water compresses to loosen the scales at the base of the lashes. The scales can then be removed with an applicator stick moistened with diluted baby shampoo. Apply erythromycin or bacitracin ophthalmic ointment tid to reduce bacterial overgrowth.

Seborrhea

Treat seborrhea with gentle cleansing with diluted baby shampoo to remove the crusts. Shampoo the scalp every other day with a keratolytic shampoo (Sebulex, Selsun). Ophthalmologic referral is needed before treatment with topical corticosteroids.

Herpes simplex

If conjunctivitis is present or keratitis is suspected, refer the patient immediately to an ophthalmologist for antiviral therapy.

Varicella and zoster

Varicella and zoster eyelid infections do not require treatment unless intraocular or corneal involvement is suspected. If the patient demonstrates ciliary flush, photophobia, pupillary abnormalities or visual loss, refer to an ophthalmologist immediately.

Molluscum contagiosum

Molluscum is usually a self-limited disease, so no treatment is necessary unless the lesions are cosmetically unacceptable, increase in number, or occur at the lid margin and are associated with conjunctivitis. Refer to an ophthalmologist for incision and curettage.

Lice

Treat pediculosis with bid applications of a bland ophthalmic ointment (Lacri-Lube or erythromycin) to the base and length of the lashes. Repeat at weekly intervals to kill the emerging lice. Defer forceps removal of lice and nits to an ophthalmologist. Check for and treat pubic lice, and thoroughly wash clothing and bedding. Investigate the child's sleeping arrangements and the possibility of infestation in other household members and consider the possibility of abuse.

Follow-up

- Chalazion, blepharitis, seborrhea, and lice: primary care follow-up in 1–2 weeks.

Bibliography

Jackson WB: Blepharitis: current strategies
for diagnosis and management. *Can
J Ophthalmol* 2008;43:170–9.

Lederman C, Miller M: Hordeola and chalazia.
Pediatr Rev 1999;20:283–4.

Ocular trauma

Consider ocular trauma in cases of sudden reduction of vision, blepharospasm (uncontrollable closure of one or both eyes), facial trauma, and high-velocity projectile injury. In the setting of multiple trauma, delay the search for and treatment of ocular injuries only until more serious priorities have been addressed. If trauma to the eye is suspected, however, apply a protective shield until it can be adequately evaluated. Eye trauma may also be the presentation of abuse.

Clinical presentation

Lid lacerations

Lid lacerations, particularly if vertical, are easily seen. However, a search for lid lacerations is required in all cases of facial trauma. There may also be an associated injury to the underlying globe. Vertical lacerations through the lid margin result in wide gaping of the wound because of the circular nature of the orbicularis oculi muscle. Lacerations through the medial one-sixth of the lid margin may be associated with a severed canaliculus.

Ruptured globe

Always suspect a ruptured or lacerated globe in cases of blunt facial trauma or when there is an eyelid laceration. The findings may be subtle and can include reduction of vision, subconjunctival hemorrhage, swelling of the conjunctiva, deformity or obvious laceration of the cornea or sclera, shallowing or absence of the anterior chamber, deformity of the iris, cataract, softness of the globe, and extrusion of intraorbital contents. Iris tissue may plug the perforation, so the only finding may be a distorted pupil (peaked, pointed, pulled to one side, or flattened on one side). Staining the tears with fluorescein can help diagnose a subtle perforation of the cornea because the clear aqueous stream leaking from the perforation will be more obvious in the fluorescein (Seidel test). Do not use an open solution of fluorescein because of possible bacterial contamination, particularly with *Pseudomonas aeruginosa*.

Hyphema

A hyphema is caused by bleeding of vessels of the anterior uvea with leakage of blood into the anterior chamber. It is usually associated with blunt trauma, but a spontaneous hyphema can occur with iris neovascularization or intraocular tumors (malignant and benign). The findings can be subtle, particularly in the supine patient, if small amounts of blood are mixed with the aqueous. Look for obscuration of the iris markings. Larger quantities of blood are more obvious and cast a reddish glow on the iris. In the upright patient, the blood settles because of gravity, and a blood-aqueous level can usually be seen. The vision is usually reduced, the conjunctiva hyperemic, and the pupil is often irregular and pointed. Pain is almost always present.

A dangerous rise in intraocular pressure may result, especially in patients with sickle cell disease or trait. Persistent hyphemas may cause opacification (blood staining) of the cornea with vision loss. Rebleeding can occur, usually within the first 5 days after the injury. It is associated with the sudden onset of pain, increased intraocular pressure, and eventual opacification of the cornea.

Corneal and conjunctival abrasions

Superficial abrasions of the conjunctiva and cornea present with pain that can be severe, photophobia, conjunctival hyperemia, and tearing. The vision is variably affected. An abrasion can often be seen as an irregularity of the normally smooth surface of the globe or as a shadow cast on the iris when a light is directed into the eye.

Fluorescein dye instilled into the cul-de-sac will stain areas of epithelial cell loss and glow bright yellow-green under cobalt blue or Wood's lamp. A subtle perforation of the cornea can be diagnosed when fluorescein staining reveals clear aqueous leaking from the perforation site (Seidel test). Do not use an open solution of fluorescein because of possible bacterial contamination, particularly with *Pseudomonas aeruginosa*.

Foreign bodies

Superficial foreign bodies present with poorly localized discomfort. Vision is variably affected, but tearing, photophobia, and blepharospasm are common. Lid eversion may be required for the object to be seen, and magnification may be needed if the object is small or transparent. A foreign body can adhere to the conjunctiva of the upper lid at the edge of the tarsal ridge and cause a vertical linear abrasion of the superior cornea. There may be one or more foreign bodies.

Intraocular foreign bodies may present with variable signs of ocular irritation. The expected findings of visual reduction, irritation, pain, and signs of penetration may be absent. A high index of suspicion is required, particularly if the patient experienced pain or a foreign-body sensation while hammering nails or other metal objects. The history is very important in establishing the diagnosis.

Orbital fracture

An orbital fracture is caused by blunt trauma to the bony walls of the orbit. A ruptured globe may occur as well. Edema and ecchymosis of the lids and surrounding tissues are usually present; swelling and tenderness of periorbital tissues can limit the examination. Fracture of the floor or walls of the orbit can injure the extraocular muscles or surrounding tissues and result in decreased ocular mobility and diplopia (double vision). Enophthalmos can result from orbital contents prolapsing into a sinus. Fracture of the floor of the orbit can result in injury to the infraorbital nerve, with resultant hypesthesia in the lower lid and cheek. Air may be introduced subcutaneously from the affected sinus, causing crepitus (orbital emphysema). Injury to the ciliary ganglion causes dilatation of the pupil and loss of accommodation (ability to focus) so that near vision is more affected than distance vision.

Burns

Thermal and chemical burns can cause both immediate and delayed damage. Burns due to acids coagulate and denature surface proteins but generally do not penetrate the eye, whereas alkali burns penetrate and damage internal ocular structures. In addition to the globe, the skin of the face and lids may be affected. Presentation depends on the extent of the injury but may include blepharospasm, tearing, photophobia, decreased vision, conjunctival swelling, hyperemia or ischemia, loss of corneal clarity, and variable pain.

Iris tear

A tear of the iris occurs after blunt or penetrating injuries to the eye. The muscles of the iris are circular and radial, and a tear in the iris causes deformity in the size, shape, and motility of the iris. Despite the highly vascular content of the iris, hyphema after an iris tear may not occur.

Retrobulbar hemorrhage

A retrobulbar hemorrhage causes acute proptosis, chemosis, variable subconjunctival hemorrhage, reduction of vision, pain, reduced corneal clarity, glaucoma, and limitation of ocular motion. It can occur after blunt or penetrating injury and may lead to loss of vision because of central retinal vessel occlusion.

Traumatic iritis

Traumatic iritis is due to exudation of protein and inflammatory cells into the aqueous humor and can occur after any injury to the eye. It is characterized by reduction of vision, photophobia, conjunctival hyperemia, ciliary flush, and miosis (pupillary constriction).

Child abuse

Child abuse victims may present with injury to the face and eyelids, subconjunctival hemorrhage, hyphema, pupillary abnormalities, eye movement abnormalities, papilledema, and retinal hemorrhages.

Diagnosis

A thorough history and determination of visual acuity in each eye with and without glasses are the first steps in the evaluation of all cases of possible ocular injury. The exception is for cases of chemical (especially alkali) burns to the eye, which require immediate lavage. For all other injuries, ascertain the precipitating event, the nature of the implicated vehicle or substance, the time of the injury, visual loss or disturbance in one or both eyes, onset of pain and injection, presence of light intolerance, and any previous trauma or other ocular abnormality.

Check vision with a standard Snellen chart (see pp. 528–529). Test the uninjured eye first in order to reduce anxiety. Unless there is a suspected ruptured globe, place one drop of an anesthetic in the eye (e.g. proparacaine 0.5%) to reduce the pain and aid in the evaluation. Make a note about the eye tested (it is customary to test the right eye first), the vision test used, the distance from the object of regard to the examined eye, and the result.

Examine the face, lids, lashes, and brows. Look for ptosis and deformity of the lid and the surrounding orbit. Observe the extraocular movements, look for strabismus, and note any complaint of diplopia, limitation of movement, or pain caused by movement. Examine the palpebral and bulbar conjunctivae, and look for evidence of laceration, localized injection, or foreign body.

To evert the upper lid, hold an applicator stick horizontally at the midportion of the lid. Grasp the lid lashes with the thumb and forefinger of the other hand and evert, using the applicator stick to help form a hinge. Look for foreign bodies at the ridge formed by the top of the tarsal plate or lodged deep in the upper or lower fornix (junction of bulbar and palpebral conjunctivae).

Check the clarity of the cornea, and look for lacerations, particularly at the corneoscleral junction. Suspect a ruptured globe if the anterior chamber is shallower or deeper than that of the other eye or if the pupil is distorted.

A hyphema can be as obvious as a definite aqueous-blood level in the anterior chamber or as subtle as a faint red tinge to the iris. It may be visible only on magnification with a biomicroscope (slit lamp). Pupillary distortion and pain often accompany a hyphema.

An abrasion can be delineated with fluorescein dye instilled in the cul-de-sac, which will adhere to areas of epithelial cell loss and fluoresce bright yellow-green under cobalt blue or Wood's lamp.

The red reflex of light from the direct ophthalmoscope illuminating the pupil can be used to estimate and compare the clarity of the ocular media. In a darkened room, set the dial of the ophthalmoscope to zero, stand 1 foot away from the patient's eyes, and direct the light beam so that the two pupils are equally illuminated and can be viewed through the aperture of the instrument (you may have to change the dial setting of the ophthalmoscope to focus on the iris). A shadow of a corneal abrasion or cataract may be illuminated in the red pupillary reflex, and there can be a difference in the color and brightness of the reflex. Use the ophthalmoscope to examine the optic nerve head for papilledema and the retina for hemorrhage, tears, or detachment.

The diagnosis of a foreign body may require ultrasound, radiography, or computed tomography (CT) scanning, but avoid magnetic resonance imaging (MRI) if a magnetic foreign body is suspected.

To evaluate a possible orbital fracture and compare the position of the eyes, stand above and behind the patient and sight down the forehead. With the patient's eyes open, compare the position of the most forward point of each cornea. With the patient's eyes closed, compare the most anterior point of the upper lid. Palpate the orbital rim for any irregularity.

ED management

For eye injuries in which the integrity of the eye is not ensured, avoid increasing intraocular pressure. Do not manipulate the eyes. Have the patient rest in a supine position with the head of the bed elevated to 30° and avoid excessive movement. Tape a protective shield from forehead to cheekbone over the injured eye until a definitive diagnosis can be made. Avoid a bulky pad under the shield to prevent placing pressure on the globe. Topical cycloplegics are not necessary in the initial evaluation of the patient, but topical anesthesia can be very helpful with chemical burns, abrasions, and foreign bodies.

Lid lacerations

Refer the patient to an ophthalmologist if the laceration is vertical through the lid margin, extends through the full thickness of the lid, or affects the nasal one-sixth of the lid and may therefore damage the tear excretory apparatus. Always check for injuries to the underlying globe.

Ruptured globe

Immediately refer the patient to an ophthalmologist. Delay radiographs to search for foreign bodies until after the evaluation. Avoid topical agents and do not remove pigmented material from the surface of the globe, as it may represent intraocular contents. Use a protective shield without a pad, and place the patient supine with the head of the bed elevated to 30°. Assume surgical intervention will be required and keep the patient NPO.

Hyphema

Refer immediately to an ophthalmologist. Put the patient at rest in a quiet area with the head of the bed elevated to 30°, place a protective shield, and avoid excessive manipulation. Do not give aspirin or NSAIDs, which may prolong bleeding time. Test for sickle hemoglobinopathy, when appropriate.

Corneal abrasion

Treat with a topical ophthalmic antibiotic (e.g. polysporin-trimethoprim, erythromycin, bacitracin) tid. Do not use an occlusive dressing unless close supervision can be ensured, as they have not been shown to shorten healing time or decrease pain, and can be associated with infection. Avoid using occlusive dressings in young children, because they may open the eye under the dressing. If an occlusive dressing is used in an older child, instill 2 drops of a topical anesthetic, followed by a topical antibiotic. Avoid repeated instillation of topical anesthetics because they interfere with healing and can cause keratitis. Refer the patient to an ophthalmologist the next day if the abrasion is large, pain or photophobia are still present, vision is affected, or the eye remains red. Small corneal abrasions often heal within a day. If pain seems out of proportion to the size of the abrasion or if there is corneal haze around the abrasion, consider a corneal ulcer and refer immediately to an ophthalmologist.

Foreign bodies

Superficial corneal and conjunctival foreign bodies may be irrigated off the anesthetized eye with a forceful stream of sterile saline or other ocular irrigating solution (Dacriose). A swab can be used to remove or loosen a foreign body and the remainder irrigated off the eye.

Check for multiple foreign bodies. Treat any remaining corneal or conjunctival abrasion as above. Refer the patient immediately if the foreign body cannot be easily removed or there is a retained rust deposit.

Intraocular and intraorbital foreign bodies require an immediate ophthalmologic consultation. Apply a protective shield.

Orbital fracture

Refer any patient with an orbital fracture to an ophthalmologist, particularly if there is enophthalmos, limitation of extraocular motion, diplopia, pupillary inequality, or hypesthesia in the region of the infraorbital nerve. A CT scan is not routinely indicated unless one or more of the above signs is noted. Antibiotics are not necessary, but advise the patient to use a nasal decongestant and avoid blowing the nose. Refer the patient to an ophthalmologist within 5 days so that surgical repair, if necessary, can be performed in a timely fashion.

Burns

Chemical burns require immediate lavage with 1–2 liters of sterile saline. Tap water may be used if sterile saline is not available. Use a topical anesthetic and lid retractors. A Morgan lens (a clear plastic scleral shell with cannula attached) will deliver irrigation to the eye more thoroughly. Sweep the fornices with applicator sticks to remove foreign bodies, and check the pH of the tears with litmus paper 30 minutes after irrigation is complete to ensure that neutralization has occurred. Normally, tears are approximately neutral (pH 7). Do not use an irrigant of opposite pH, as more damage will occur. Consult an ophthalmologist immediately.

Thermal burns are rarely isolated to the lids or globe except in cases of cigarette burns, which are treated as a simple abrasion with antibiotic ointment. More extensive burns of the face also require an ophthalmologic evaluation of the eye and lid function.

Traumatic iritis

Refer immediately to an ophthalmologist for evaluation of the globe and for treatment with topical cycloplegics.

Retrobulbar hemorrhage

Immediate ophthalmologic evaluation is necessary for treatment with pressure-lowering drugs (intravenous mannitol), surgery (lateral canthotomy), and intravenous steroids.

Follow-up
- Corneal abrasion: return the next day.
- Hyphema: daily ophthalmology visits.

Indications for admission
- Ruptured globe
- Hyphema, if compliance with follow-up visits and bed rest cannot be ensdured
- Lid laceration requiring surgical repair in operating room

- Intraocular foreign body
- Orbital fracture, if compliance with follow-up care cannot be ensured
- Retrobulbar hemorrhage

Bibliography

Garcia TA, McGetrick BA, Janik JS: Ocular injuries in children after major trauma. *J Pediatr Ophthalmol Strabismus* 2005;42:349–54.

Kuhn F, Maisiak R, Mann L, et al: The Ocular Trauma Score (OTS). *Ophthalmol Clin North Am* 2002;15:163–5.

Levine LM: Pediatric ocular trauma and shaken infant syndrome. *Pediatr Clin North Am* 2003;50:137–48.

Salvin JH: Systematic approach to pediatric ocular trauma. *Curr Opin Ophthalmol* 2007;18:366–72.

The red eye

The conjunctiva is normally transparent. When it is inflamed, the numerous fine blood vessels become engorged; hence the term "pink eye." Inflammation is most often secondary to infection. Organisms include bacteria (*Staphylococcus aureus, Streptococcus viridans, Streptococcus pneumoniae, Haemophilus influenzae, enterococci, Neisseria gonorrhoeae*), viruses (herpes simplex, adenovirus, enterovirus, molluscum contagiosum), and *Chlamydia trachomatis* (trachoma).

Conjunctival hyperemia can be secondary to keratitis (superficial corneal inflammation) or uveitis. Keratitis is most often caused by ocular trauma or infection (adenovirus, herpes, *Chlamydia, Staphylococcus, Streptococcus*). The anterior uvea (iris and ciliary body) can be inflamed by trauma, infection (Lyme disease, tuberculosis, varicella, herpes simplex), or a corneal foreign body.

Other causes of a red eye include allergy and reaction to dust, smoke, foreign bodies, chemicals, and other irritants. Finally, conjunctival hyperemia can accompany serious acute conditions such as preseptal and orbital cellulitis, erythema multiforme, or Kawasaki disease.

Clinical presentation and diagnosis
Preseptal and orbital cellulitis

The orbital septum connects to both the periosteum of the orbital bones and the tarsal plates of the lid, and separates the lid structures from the orbital contents. Infections can spread from contiguous structures or be blood-borne from distant sites. The organisms most frequently implicated are *S. aureus, S. pyogenes,* and *S. pneumoniae*.

Both preseptal (or periorbital) and orbital cellulitis present with lid swelling, erythema, and pain. Preseptal cellulitis can arise from a break in the skin (insect bite, laceration), trauma, dacryocystitis, chalazia, hordeola, or sinusitis. The vision is usually normal.

Orbital cellulitis is characterized by the diagnostic triad of proptosis, limitation of extraocular movement, and pain with extraocular movement. Vision may be decreased, and an afferent pupillary defect (APD) may be present.

To assess for an APD, shine a bright light into one pupil for a few seconds, and note the pupillary response. Swing the light quickly to the other eye ("swinging light test") and observe the pupillary response. Repeat this process several times until the pupillary response is clear. Normally there is a consensual response, with both pupils constricting when one eye is illuminated. With an APD, both pupils gradually dilate when the affected eye is illuminated.

The patient with orbital cellulitis frequently appears toxic, with fever and lethargy. Most often, there is a history of recent upper respiratory symptoms, and the sinuses are involved. A CT scan is indicated to determine the extent of sinus and/or bony involvement, or if the differentiation between preseptal and orbital cellulitis is in doubt.

Conjunctivitis

Inflammation of the bulbar and palpebral conjunctival mucous membranes produces vascular engorgement, appearing as diffusely distributed discrete red vessels. Although itching or a "sandy" sensation is frequently noted, there is no ocular pain, and photophobia, if present, is mild. Visual acuity is normal. On examination, a discharge ranging from mucous and crusting to frank pus may be present, along with lid edema and erythema.

A viral cause is suggested by a watery or mucoid discharge during a URI, especially if there is preauricular adenopathy or an associated pharyngitis (typical of adenovirus, which may be called pharyngoconjunctival fever). With an enteroviral infection there may be associated subconjunctival hemorrhage. Herpes simplex can be diagnosed from viral culture or with immunofluorescence. A bacterial cause is more likely if there is a purulent eye discharge with or without otitis media. Allergy is suggested by a seasonal pattern (spring or autumn), watery or mucoid discharge, edema, pruritus, and multiple creases and discoloration of the lower lid. In general, the quality of the eye discharge is not diagnostic of the etiology of the conjunctivitis, and there is some overlap in the clinical picture among causes.

Neonatal conjunctivitis was more frequent in the past when silver nitrate prophylaxis was routinely used in the delivery room. Currently, a purulent discharge in the first week of life suggests a gonococcal or chlamydial infection, but a definite diagnosis cannot be made without confirmatory tests. Gram-negative intracellular diplococci and PMNs are found on Gram's-stained smears of eye discharge caused by N. *Gonorrhea*, and the organism can be grown on nonselective chocolate agar with incubation in 5% to 10% carbon dioxide, or on specialized culture media. *Chlamydia trachomatis* is diagnosed by cell culture or direct fluorescent antibody staining of conjunctival scrapings.

Obtain the specimen by rolling a saline-moistened sterile swab along the lower palpebral conjunctiva. A sample of the exudate is not adequate, as it often yields a false-negative result. Do not use a topical anesthetic when obtaining the culture of the discharge, because the preservatives in the anesthetic can interfere with growth.

Corneal disease (keratitis)

Corneal involvement is generally accompanied by conjunctival hyperemia. Pain, photophobia, and visual reduction are common. A disruption of the corneal epithelium can be diagnosed by fluorescein staining of the cornea, followed by illumination with a cobalt blue or Wood's light. Areas of epithelial disturbance or loss will fluoresce a bright yellow-green in the midst of the yellow fluorescein. Do not use an open solution of fluorescein because of the frequency of bacterial contamination, particularly with *Pseudomonas aeruginosa*.

Uveitis

Inflammation of the interior pigmented vascular structures of the eye can be associated with conjunctival hyperemia. The presentation is variable and may include photophobia, reduced vision, pain on reading, conjunctival hyperemia, ciliary flush (a pink halo of dilated episcleral vessels that surround the cornea), and pupillary miosis.

Erythema multiforme

Erythema multiforme major (Stevens-Johnson syndrome, pp. 107–108) is a bullous eruption with skin and mucous membrane involvement. Bullae form on the conjunctiva, which can result in symblepharon (adhesions between the bulbar and palpebral conjunctivae) with shrinkage of the fornices, loss of tear production, and resultant dry eye symptoms. There may be purulent conjunctival discharge, conjunctivitis, keratitis with corneal ulceration, or uveitis. Long-term sequelae include entropion and trichiasis.

Kawasaki disease

Kawasaki disease (pp. 395–396) is characterized by a constellation of symptoms including prolonged fever, cervical lymphadenopathy, stomatitis, erythematous polymorphous rash, edema of the peripheral extremities, and transient conjunctivitis without discharge. Ocular signs can be a presenting feature of the disease; these include bilateral, painless, nonexudative bulbar conjunctival injection, bilateral anterior uveitis, and, less commonly, superficial punctate keratitis, vitreous opacities, and papilledema.

ED management

The determination of visual acuity is of paramount importance; any acute reduction is an indication for immediate ophthalmologic referral. Evidence of intraocular involvement includes severe photophobia or ocular pain, vascular engorgement at the limbus, and pupillary abnormalities. Always inquire about a history of ocular trauma.

Preseptal and orbital cellulitis

Mild preseptal cellulitis can be treated on an outpatient basis with oral amoxicillin-clavulanate (875/125 formulation; 90 mg/kg per day div bid). However, if orbital cellulitis cannot be ruled out, obtain a CT scan of the orbits. If orbital involvement is confirmed, admit the patient and treat with IV antibiotics (nafcillin or oxacillin 200 mg/kg per day div q 6 h and either cefotaxime 150–200 mg/kg per day div q 8 h or ceftriaxone 80–100 mg/kg per day div q 12 h; if methicillin-resistant *S. aureus* is a concern, use vancomycin 40–60 mg/kg per day div q 6 h instead of nafcillin or oxacillin). Consult an ophthalmologist. Obtain blood cultures prior to giving IV antibiotics, and perform a lumbar puncture if meningeal or cerebral signs are present. Consult an otolaryngologist if sinus involvement extends beyond the ethmoid sinuses.

Conjunctivitis

In general, bacterial cultures are not needed. Treat with a topical ophthalmic antibiotic, either tid application of a solution (ciprofloxacin, ofloxacin, polymyxin B/trimethoprim, tobramycin) or an ointment (bacitracin, erythromycin, polymyxin B/bacitracin, tobramycin). The antibiotics will rapidly treat most uncomplicated bacterial cases and retard secondary bacterial infection, if the origin is viral. Do not prescribe steroid preparations without ophthalmologic consultation. Continue treatment for 5 days, or for 2 days after clinical resolution. Instruct the patient or parent of a younger child to gently wipe away any crust with a warm, damp gauze pad or cottonball before instilling the drops. Meticulous hygiene (no shared towels or washcloths) and frequent handwashing are also necessary, and advise the patient to discard any eye makeup. Refer the patient to an ophthalmologist if there is persistent infection, severe photophobia or pain, or visual complaints.

Table 17-2. Topical ophthalmic antiallergics

Medication	Brand name	Dosing
Ketorolac	Acular	qid
Cromolyn	Crolom	qid
Lodoxamide	Alomide	qid
Naphazoline/pheniramine	Naphcon-A	qid
Naphazoline/antazoline	Vasocon-A	qid
Azelastine	Optivar	bid
Epinastine	Elestat	bid
Ketotifen	Zaditor	bid
Nedocromil	Alocril	bid
Olopatiaine	Patanol, Pataday	bid or q day

Neonatal conjunctivitis

The presence of Gram-negative diplococci in PMNs on a Gram's stain is diagnostic of gonococcal conjunctivitis until cultures are available. Admit the infant and treat with one dose of ceftriaxone (25–50 mg/kg, 125 mg maximum) IM or IV. Isolate the infant for 24 hours, and remove any discharge with frequent sterile saline irrigations, taking care to avoid splashing the pus into the caregiver's eyes.

If the Gram's stain in an infant 1–12 weeks of age with a purulent discharge reveals PMNs but few organisms, and antigen detection or culture for *Chlamydia* are not available, treat for presumed *Chlamydia* conjunctivitis with oral erythromycin (50 mg/kg per day div q 6 h) for 2 weeks to avoid systemic complications such as pneumonitis. Topical ophthalmic antibiotics are optional; use erythromycin ointment qid for 3 days.

Allergic conjunctivitis

Treat with 1 drop qid of a topical antihistamine (levocabastine, naphazoline/antazoline, naphazoline/pheniramine) and mast cell stabilizer (lodoxamide, cromolyn) beginning 2 weeks before the start of the allergy season. Alternatively, use a topical nonsteroidal anti-inflammatory (ketorolac) alone. Topical combination drugs (mast cell stabilizer, H_1-antagonist NSAID) are convenient with bid dosing (see Table 17-2). Do not give topical steroids. If there is no improvement in 7 days or the symptoms worsen, refer the patient to an ophthalmologist.

Immediately refer all cases of keratitis and uveitis to an ophthalmologist.

The treatment of erythema multiforme major (pp. xx–yy) requires an ophthalmologist and includes topical antibiotics, steroids, and lubricants. Surgery, including lysis of synechiae, is sometimes necessary. If Kawasaki disease is suspected, refer the patient to an ophthalmologist.

Follow-up

- Preseptal cellulitis: 1 day
- Conjunctivitis: 5 days, if no improvement

Indications for admission

- Orbital cellulitis
- Preseptal cellulitis if compliance not ensured
- Stevens-Johnson syndrome
- Gonococcal conjunctivitis

Bibliography

Greenberg MF, Pollard ZF: The red eye in childhood. *Pediatr Clin North Am* 2003;50:105–24.

Patel H, Goldstein D: Pediatric uveitis. *Pediatr Clin North Am* 2003;50:125–36.

Wald ER: Periorbital and orbital infections. *Pediatr Rev* 2004;25:312–20.

Wagner RS, Aquino M: Pediatric ocular inflammation. *Immunol Allergy Clin North Am* 2008;28:169–88.

The white pupil (leukocoria)

Light entering the eye is absorbed by the pigmented interior and does not leave in sufficient quantity to illuminate the pupil. If an opacity exists in the normally clear optical media, light will reflect off the opacity and be seen in the pupil as a white reflection (leukocoria).

The most common causes of leukocoria are cataracts, infections (syphilis, toxocara, toxoplasmosis, tuberculosis), intraocular hemorrhage, retinopathy of prematurity, detached retina, retinoblastoma, coloboma, and persistent hyperplastic primary vitreous. Therefore, opacities can represent static conditions that interfere with vision (cataracts), active diseases that can lead to visual difficulties (early retinal detachment), or life-threatening illnesses (retinoblastoma).

Clinical presentation and diagnosis

Examine both pupils, using a direct ophthalmoscope set at zero at a distance of 12 to 18 inches from the eye. Normally, the red reflex is symmetrical and the pupil size equal. If there is an opacity in the media, all or part of the pupil will appear dark or off-white instead of red. Depending on the extent of the abnormality, the eyes and/or pupils may be asymmetric in size. There may be no pupillary light response, or it may be slower than in the opposite eye.

Leukocoria can be unilateral or bilateral. If a unilateral problem is suspected, covering the "good" eye will cause upset in a small child, while covering the affected eye will not change the child's behavior.

ED management

Consult an ophthalmologist immediately whenever leukocoria is suspected.

Indication for admission

- Any case of leukocoria, if adequate outpatient follow-up cannot be ensured

Bibliography

Abramson DH, Beaverson K, Sangani P, et al: Screening for retinoblastoma: presenting signs as prognosticators of patient and ocular survival. *Pediatrics* 2003;112(6 Pt 1):1248–55.

Haider S, Qureshi W, Ali A: Leukocoria in children. *J Pediatr Ophthalmol Strabismus* 2008;45:179–80.

Lee YC, Kim HS: Clinical symptoms and visual outcome in patients with presumed congenital cataract. *J Pediatr Ophthalmol Strabismus* 2000;37:219–24.

Chapter 18

Orthopedic emergencies

Sergey Kunkov and James Meltzer

Contributing author
Katherine J. Chou: Splinting

Back pain

In contrast to adults, back pain is a relatively uncommon complaint in children. Back pain in a prepubertal child is particularly concerning and may indicate significant underlying pathology.

Etiologies of pediatric back pain can be classified as mechanical (musculoskeletal/ orthopedic), medical (infection, masses, systemic disease), and miscellaneous (reflex sympathetic dystrophy, fibromyalgia). Of note, idiopathic scoliosis is not a cause of pediatric back pain.

Clinical presentation

Mechanical conditions

Spondylolysis and spondylolisthesis

Spondylolysis and spondylolisthesis are the most common causes of back pain in children >10 years of age. Spondylolysis is a defect in the pars interarticularis, a bony process on the posterior spine, usually caused by repetitive stress. This defect may take the form of a fracture, stress fracture, or sclerotic change, and is most common at L5. The incidence is higher in children who participate in activities involving hyperextension of the spine, such as dance, figure skating, gymnastics, football, tennis, and weight training.

A patient with spondylolysis generally complains of low back pain worsened by activity, often associated with tight hamstrings and buttock pain. Spondylolysis may become complicated by spondylolisthesis, which is a forward slippage of one vertebra upon another (usually L5 on S1). The physical examination may be normal, although there may be a palpable step-off in the lower lumbar region and tight hamstrings with limited forward flexion.

Scheuermann's kyphosis

Excessive kyphosis in either the thoracic or lumbar regions is a frequent cause of back pain in adolescents. The patient has poor posture and complains of dull pain over the deformity, which is worsened by activity. On examination, the kyphosis is obvious, accentuated by bending forward, and persists despite the patient's conscious efforts to stand erect. X-rays will show anterior wedging of several vertebrae.

Disk injury

The intervertebral disk is a gelatinous substance that provides shock absorption to the spine and allows for a smooth range of motion. A disk may be injured (bulging) or herniated; the most common sites are L4–L5 and L5–S1. Affected patients are usually older than 10 years and complain of back pain with or without sciatica (pain down the back of the thigh). Physical examination findings include decreased lumbar lordosis, limited forward flexion, paraspinal muscle spasm, and a positive straight leg-raising test (see below).

Lumbar sacral sprain

This is an injury or tearing of the ligaments and/or muscle fibers (interspinous or paraspinal) that connect one vertebra to another or support a vertebra. A common mechanism for the sprain is a sudden twisting motion; a patient who is inflexible and overweight is more likely to suffer from this type of injury. This variety of injury can occur in children who carry heavy backpacks.

Trauma

Often when a child presents with back pain secondary to trauma, the parent or child will be able to describe some preceding event as the cause. Most often the trauma is benign and without sequelae. The practitioner must be cautious, however, when the child's injury or degree of pain appears disproportionate to the event described. A more thorough investigation is then necessary.

Fractures of the spine are uncommon and usually are associated with a significant amount of force. Occasionally trauma to the back can lead to an epidural hematoma that can compress the spinal cord as it expands. This is most relevant in patients with hemophilia or other clotting disorders.

Medical etiologies

Infection

Orthopedic infections including diskitis, osteomyelitis (pp. 571–573), and spinal epidural abscess can cause back pain.

Diskitis

Diskitis usually occurs in younger children (average 3 years old), and may present with fever, malaise, low back pain, refusal to walk or crawl, and associated hip or abdominal pain. On physical examination, there may be tenderness over the involved disk, decreased back motion, and pain with hip flexion. While the ESR and CRP are usually elevated in diskitis, the WBC is generally normal. The blood culture is usually negative but sometimes yields an organism, most often *S. aureus*.

Vertebral osteomyelitis

Vertebral osteomyelitis presents similarly to diskitis, but is more common in the older child (average 7 years old). Unlike diskitis, the blood culture is positive in about 50% of cases (usually *S. aureus*). Uncommon entities, such as *B. henselae*, salmonella, and tuberculosis, can also cause vertebral osteomyelitis but generally are associated with recognized risk factors (cat scratch, sickle cell anemia, risks for TB).

Epidural abscess

An epidural abscess most often results from hematogenous spread of bacteria into the epidural space, but it can also occur secondary to direct extension from an underlying osteomyelitis or superinfection of a traumatic hematoma. Organisms responsible for epidural abscesses are similar to those for vertebral osteomyelitis. Because not all children with vertebral infections will present with fever and back pain, some go undiagnosed until they present with neurologic symptoms. Children with infections (i.e. abscess or pyomyositis) involving the paraspinal or pelvic muscles often complain of back pain. In addition, various nonorthopedic infections, such as pyelonephritis, pneumonia, and pancreatitis, can occasionally present with back pain.

Rheumatologic diseases
Ankylosing spondylitis
Ankylosing spondylitis is a spondyloarthropathy involving the sacroiliac joints and lumbar spine. It is most common in adolescent boys, and the majority of affected patients are HLA-B27 positive. The patient may experience transient arthritis of large joints, followed by back involvement later in the disease course. Pain in the lower back, hips, and thighs is associated with morning stiffness that is relieved by movement. There may also be an acute iridocyclitis and/or aortitis. The spinal involvement begins in the sacroiliac joints and ascends progressively to involve the rest of the spine, including the cervical vertebrae. In contrast, JRA affects the cervical spine, but spares the lumbar spine.

A patient with inflammatory bowel disease may have associated spondylitis similar to ankylosing spondylitis. The patient may present with low back pain prior to the onset of gastrointestinal symptoms.

Neoplasm
Spinal tumor
A spinal tumor is a rare but concerning cause of back pain in children. The majority are benign, including osteoid osteomas, eosinophilic granulomas, and unicameral bone cysts. However, possible malignancies include Ewing sarcoma, osteosarcoma, and metastatic lesions (neuroblastoma, etc.). A history of nighttime pain, pain not associated with activity, or a painful scoliosis raises the concern of a tumor. Leukemia may present as persistent back pain secondary to infiltration of the bone marrow.

Sickle cell crisis
Back pain is a common complaint in children with sickle cell disease. Most patients will be identified early in life on the newborn screen, unless they come from a country that does not routinely screen newborns for hemoglobinopathies.

Miscellaneous conditions
Reflex sympathetic dystrophy (RSD)
The hallmark of this syndrome is severe pain associated with autonomic dysfunction (swelling, edema, skin color changes, mottling). RSD may occur in the back after trauma. The initial injury may be a sprain or a disk injury, with ongoing pain out of proportion to what is expected for the original injury (allodynia, dysthesias).

Fibromyalgia
This condition is defined as chronic musculoskeletal pain (>6 months duration) associated with trigger points and nonspecific symptoms (sleep disturbance, headache, irritable bowel, weakness, swelling or stiffness in the morning). A child may present with severe lower and upper back pain.

Diagnosis

A thorough history is essential in determining whether the patient's back pain requires urgent or immediate intervention. Ascertain the onset of the pain, its timing, severity, and radiation, as well as factors that alleviate or trigger it. Inquire about sports participation, including the intensity of the involvement and the initiation of any new sports. Ask specifically about trauma. Determine the child's activity level since the onset of symptoms; back pain that forces the child to refrain from usual activities requires a thorough evaluation.

Determine whether the pain is related to sleep or resting in bed. Specific difficulty in moving from side to side in bed may suggest a disk problem or lumbar sprain. Importantly, any patient awakened and kept awake by back pain must be thoroughly evaluated for a tumor, infection, or inflammatory condition. In contrast, back pain from overuse syndromes, muscle pain, Scheuermann's disease, or spondylolysis (with or without spondylolisthesis) usually improves with rest.

In addition, always check for the presence of systemic symptoms, such as fever, malaise, irritability, or weight loss. In these children, ask about pets (i.e. kittens) and risk factors for tuberculosis such as travel to or immigration from endemic areas. A positive history for ankle or foot weakness, changes in bowel or bladder function, and/or an altered gait is suggestive of neurologic impairment. Ask about medications or therapies already tried, including chiropractic manipulation and acupuncture. Note any chronic medications that cause osteoporosis (i.e. steroids) because these increase the risk for fracture.

Physical examination

Have the patient undress down to his or her underwear and observe the gait and posture. Note any muscle asymmetry and signs of splinting; assess the back for a midline defect or lesion such as a tuft of hair or hemangioma. Check carefully for tenderness by palpating over the vertebra, spinous processes, vertebral spaces, and interspinal ligaments, as well as the shoulders and paraspinal muscles.

For the lumbar spine, check forward flexion, lateral rotation, lateral bending, and extension. The forward bend test helps reveal any deformities of the spine; low back pain increased by hyperextension suggests spondylolysis and/or spondylolisthesis.

Perform a complete neurological examination, paying particular attention to symmetry and DTRs (knee jerk and ankle jerk). Look for quadriceps and hamstring asymmetry, which can result from a low back problem. Check the strength of each lower extremity, isolating each joint and comparing it to the other: hip (flexion, extension, abduction, and adduction), knee (flexion and extension), and ankle/foot (plantar flexion/dorsiflexion, inversion, eversion). Lower limb weakness may be a sign of spinal cord compression and is a particularly ominous finding requiring immediate attention. Also check for signs of meningeal irritation (Kernig's and Brudzinski's signs).

A straight leg-raising test will frequently be positive in patients with disk herniation. For the straight leg-raising test have the patient lie supine, grasp the ankle, and, with the knee held in extension, bring the leg upward to assess range of flexion of the hip joint. Note the angle and location of any elicited pain. Then repeat the maneuver and dorsiflex the foot as the painful angle is approached; this should aggravate the pain. Back pain radiating down the back of the leg indicates sciatic nerve irritation and a herniated disk.

Table 18-1. Clinical features of back pain requiring immediate evaluation

Age <4 years

Pain for >1 month

Systemic symptoms: fever, lethargy, irritability

Point tenderness over spine or intervertebral space

Pain triggered by usual activities

Pain awakens patient from sleep

Neurologic abnormalities: foot or ankle weakness, changes in bowel or bladder function, altered gait, abnormal DTRs or Babinski, asymmetric strength, meningeal signs

Radiologic studies

Children with abnormal physical findings, pain that has lasted 3 months or more despite conservative treatment, nighttime or constant pain, or pain due to significant trauma require radiologic evaluation. Obtain anteroposterior and lateral radiographs of the spine; oblique lumbar spine views are also needed if spondylolysis is suspected. Obtain a technetium-99 bone scan if a febrile patient has an examination that is consistent with diskitis or osteomyelitis, but the plain films are normal. A CT scan can further define spinal pathology located by bone scan, and a fine cut CT scan (1–3 mm cuts) is useful in diagnosing and evaluating spondylolysis. Obtain an MRI for any abnormal neurologic findings. The MRI is a valuable tool in evaluating spinal cord tumors, tethered cords, disk herniations, diskitis, and other spinal pathology, but clinically insignificant disk herniations or degenerative disk disease may be over-read. A concern about spinal cord compression is one of the few indications for an emergent MRI.

Laboratory studies

If a medical cause is suspected, order a CBC, serum electrolytes, CRP, ESR, urinalysis, and a blood culture. If a rheumatologic cause is suspected, also obtain an ANA, rheumatoid factor, and HLA-B27.

ED management

The priority is to identify conditions requiring immediate treatment, including mass lesions, diskitis, or osteomyelitis. If the patent has any of the clinical features outlined in Table 18-1, arrange for immediate radiologic evaluation (see above) and consultation with a neurologist and/or orthopedist. Immediately consult a neurosurgeon if the patient has any signs of spinal cord compression.

If an older child with back pain for less than one month appears well, has a normal neurologic examination, and does not have point tenderness, nighttime pain, or restriction of daily activities, refer him or her to a primary care provider, orthopedist, or sports medicine specialist for follow-up within 1 week. In general, appropriate management for these patients includes referral to a physical therapist, avoidance of the offending activity (usually hyperextension), and occasionally, a back brace. Bed rest has virtually no role in the management of back pain. Encourage the patient to walk and go to school as soon as possible. Reserve ibuprofen (10 mg/kg q 6 h) for acute pain (sprains, fractures, disk injuries).

Follow-up

- Within 1 week; patient to return immediately for worsening pain, especially at night, neurologic symptoms, or systemic symptoms

Indications for admission

- Diskitis, osteomyelitis, or spinal epidural abscess
- Suspected neoplasm

Bibliography

Baker RJ, Patel D: Lower back pain in the athlete: common conditions and treatment. *Prim Care* 2005;32:201–29.

Bernstein RM, Cozen H: Evaluation of back pain in children and adolescents. *Am Fam Physician* 2007; 1669–76.

Curtis C, d'Hemecourt P: Diagnosis and management of back pain in adolescents. *Adolesc Med State Art Rev* 2007;18: 140–64.

Fractures, dislocations, and sprains

Skeletal injuries account for 10–15% of all injuries in children and 15% of these involve the physis or growth plate. Always consider the possibility of child abuse in young children.

Clinical presentation and diagnosis

Obtain a complete history, including the mechanism of the injury; location of maximal pain; previous orthopedic or rheumatologic problems (fractures, dislocations, joint pain, or swelling); chronic medical problems (rickets, renal failure, liver disease, malignancy); and drug use (phenytoin can produce a rickets-like picture). For open fractures, ascertain the patient's tetanus status and whether the trauma occurred in a dirty environment (farm and field injuries are at risk for clostridial infections).

On physical examination, focus on the area(s) of pain and tenderness, as well as the joints above and below the suspected injury. However, perform a complete examination, looking for associated and/or additional traumatic injuries.

Begin the examination with assessment of the neurovascular status of the affected extremity. Palpate the pulses; check the warmth, capillary filling, and active motion of the fingers or toes; and evaluate sensation, using the uninjured limb for comparison. The presence of any of the "six Ps" distal to the fracture site suggests neurovascular compromise: pain, pulselessness, pallor, paralysis, paresthesias, and painful passive motion. The presence of a pulse does not ensure adequate circulation; however, assume that absence of a pulse means compromise.

Inspect the extremity and compare it to the uninjured side, looking for asymmetry, swelling, abrasions, ecchymoses, and deformity. Significantly displaced fractures and dislocations may cause an obvious deformity. Swelling and ecchymosis may be present or may develop over several hours. Check for point tenderness, which is often, but not always, associated with a fracture. In some cases, the pain may not be well localized, but is usually present in the affected bone.

Next, evaluate the joints. Have the patient attempt an active range of motion of the injured joint, using the other side for comparison. If the child is unable to complete a full range of motion, gently perform a passive examination of joint mobility.

An orthopedic injury is obvious if there is a history of significant trauma (fall from height, pedestrian struck, etc.) or if the patient complains of pain after an injury. However, the cause may have been unwitnessed or not noticed, so that an injury is not suspected until significant swelling is apparent. Toddlers and young children may take an unwitnessed fall and present with crying or unwillingness to bear weight on the affected leg. Paradoxical irritability (more crying when picked up by a caregiver) can be a sign of rib fractures. In addition, children can self-splint injuries, particularly buckle fractures of the distal forearm.

Fracture

A fracture is a break in the continuity or architecture of a bone. It is described by the skin integrity (open or closed) overlying the site of the injury; the name of the bone; the location within the bone (intra-articular, distal, proximal, or midshaft); the character of the fracture (comminuted, spiral, greenstick, transverse, oblique); and the direction of displacement (displaced, nondisplaced, dorsally angulated, etc.). The clavicle, radius, and ulna are the most frequently fractured bones in children.

A fracture usually presents with point tenderness, ecchymosis, and swelling after an episode of trauma. An infant or toddler, however, may merely refuse to use the affected limb, which is neither swollen nor markedly tender. (e.g., the patient may suddenly refuse to walk). Significant blood loss, leading to shock, can occur with a fracture of the femur or pelvis.

Open fracture

An open or compound fracture communicates with the outside environment by means of a puncture or laceration through the skin.

Pathologic fracture

A pathologic fracture can occur in areas of bone weakness. Causes include rickets, bone cysts, osteogenesis imperfecta, and malignancies.

Buckle fracture

A buckle or torus fracture is caused by compression of the metaphysis in a young child's bone. There is disruption of at least one side of the cortex, without a visible fracture line.

Greenstick fracture

A greenstick fracture, which usually involves the diaphysis, occurs when an angulated force breaks one, not both, sides of the cortex.

Complete fracture

A complete fracture is a break of the cortex through and through (displaced or nondisplaced).

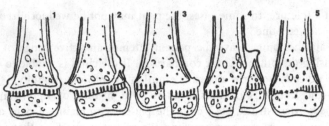

Figure 18-1. Salter-Harris classification of growth plate injuries. Adapted with permission from Salter RB, Harris WR: Injuries involving the epiphyseal plate. *J Bone Joint Surg* 1963;45A:587.

Plastic deformation (traumatic bowing)

This is bowing of a bone without obvious radiographic fracture.

Epiphyseal injury

Determining whether a growth plate is injured is critical. Although many growth plate injuries do not result in growth arrest, serious deformity and disability can result despite optimal medical care. The Salter classification scheme of epiphyseal injury (Figure. 18-1) is useful for describing the fracture. This system correlates well with the degree of injury and is useful in treatment and prognosis.

Dislocation

A dislocation is a complete disruption of the normal articular relationships of a joint. The most common sites are the shoulder (anterior), metacarpophalangeal and interphalangeal finger joints (pp. 557–561), and patella. Posterior elbow and knee dislocations are rare, but they are significant because of the risk of vascular compromise.

Subluxation

A subluxation is an incomplete dislocation. The most common bone subluxed is the radial head of a toddler (nursemaid's elbow).

Sprain

A sprain is disruption of a ligament. Young children are more likely to have physeal fractures than sprains because of the relative weakness of the physis compared to the surrounding ligaments. Joint injuries, dislocations, and ligamentous injuries are therefore less common in the young child. Sprains occur more frequently in the adolescent with closed or closing growth plates. Sprains of the knees and ankles are the most common sports-related injuries.

Sprains present as joint swelling, with ecchymosis and tenderness over the affected ligament. Usually there is a clear history of trauma. There may be pain on palpation over the ligament without any instability (grade I), increased joint laxity upon stress (grade II), or total joint instability (grade III).

Strain

In contrast to a sprain, a strain is an injury to the musculotendinous unit.

Dislocation

A dislocated joint appears deformed, with a limited, painful range of motion. A subluxed joint may appear normal, as with a nursemaid's elbow.

Radiographs

Confirm a fracture or dislocation with radiographs, including standard anteroposterior (AP) and lateral views to assess the presence and nature of a fracture. Although CT, MRI, and bone scan are helpful in making a detailed assessment of a fracture or dislocation, these are not the primary means of making the diagnosis.

AP and lateral X-rays are indicated if there is an obvious deformity, point tenderness, or marked swelling or ecchymosis. Splint the extremity first, and obtain views that include the joints above and below the site of injury. If the radiologist or orthopedist is experienced in interpreting pediatric films, comparison views of the uninjured extremity are not routinely indicated (with the exception of the elbow). Obtain oblique views if a "toddler's fracture" is suspected.

For patients with an ankle injury, use the Ottawa ankle rules and obtain ankle films for patients with any of the following: tenderness over the distal 6 cm of the fibula or tibia, medial or lateral malleolus tenderness, navicular or fifth metatarsal tenderness, or inability to bear weight both immediately and in the emergency department (four steps). In the case of a knee injury, obtain knee films if there is isolated tenderness to the patella, tenderness at the fibular head, and/or inability to bear weight both immediately and in the emergency department (four steps).

When viewing the radiographs, carefully follow the cortex, looking for any discontinuity, which is diagnostic of a fracture. Evaluate the growth plates and joints for displacement, disruption, or widening.

The differentiation between sprains and Salter I epiphyseal injuries can be difficult, as both can present with minimal swelling over the growth plate and normal radiographs. However, growth plate injuries are more common in young children, while sprains are more likely in adolescents. With a sprain the ligament is tender and the joint may be lax, while Salter I injuries cause tenderness over the growth plate. Do not stress the ankle when there is tenderness over the lateral malleolus; a nondisplaced Salter I fracture may be counverted into a more serious injury.

A number of fractures are suspicious for child abuse: metaphyseal (bucket-handle), rib (especially posterior), scapular, spinous process, and sternal fractures and long bone fractures in young non-ambulating children. Other injuries that are associated with inflicted trauma include epiphyseal separations, vertebral body fractures and subluxations, digital fractures, complex skull fractures, and multiple fractures, especially if bilateral or in various stages of healing. Common fractures that have a low specificity for abuse include subperiosteal new bone formation, clavicular fractures, long bone shaft fractures in older children, and linear skull fractures.

ED management

Time is critical with neurovascular compromise, open fractures, and joint sepsis. These orthopedic emergencies demand prompt intervention to avoid complications and possible loss of limb.

After stabilization of vital signs and assessment of nonorthopedic injuries, the priority is assessment of the neurovascular status of the injured extremity. As discussed above, the presence of any of the "six Ps" suggests neurovascular compromise and is an indication for immediate orthopedic consultation. If orthopedic consultation is not immediately available, place the extremity in longitudinal traction and align any gross deformities.

If there is an open fracture, priorities before obtaining radiographs are to: obtain a culture of any exposed bone or soft tissues; cover the wound with sterile dressings; start an IV; give the first dose of antibiotics (nafcillin 40 mg/kg; cephalothin 25 mg/kg; clindamycin 10 mg/kg if penicillin-allergic); and give tetanus toxoid unless there is documentation of adequate immunization.

Pain relief is the next priority. Splint the extremity in a comfortable position, and elevate and apply ice to minimize swelling. Splints can be made from any firm material and tape. Give acetaminophen (15 mg/kg PO), ibuprofen (10 mg/kg PO), or codeine (0.5 mg/kg PO). For patients with severe pain, give morphine, 0.1 mg/kg IV or IM.

Obtain radiographs after the initial assessment is conducted. Splint all deformities in physiologic position (pp. 573–579), apply ice, and elevate while awaiting radiographs and/ or orthopedic consultation.

Fractures

Definitive treatment ranges from a simple sling to complex surgical reconstruction. In general, most nondisplaced extremity fractures can be treated with *in situ* immobilization with a cast or splint. Refer all displaced fractures and growth plate fractures to an orthopedist. These usually require reduction to an anatomic position, followed by immobilization. If the patient must travel to see an orthopedist, splint the extremity in a physiologic position to avoid further displacement of the fracture.

Dislocations

Reduce a finger dislocation promptly, with axial traction, after finger block anesthesia. See below for the reduction of a glenohumeral dislocation. Elbow, hip, and knee dislocations are at risk of neurovascular compromise and therefore require orthopedic consultation.

Contusions and first-degree sprains

Treat with RICE therapy: Rest, Ice (for 24–48 hours), Compression (with an elastic bandage), and Elevation (to reduce swelling). Advise that activities can be resumed as tolerated. Most minor injuries will resolve over 5–7 days. Instruct the patient to follow up if there is no improvement.

Severe sprains

A second- or third-degree sprain requires splinting for several weeks. In the ED, apply any of the commercially available splints or a Jones dressing. Give crutches if the patient has a severe sprain of a lower extremity.

Cast care

After casting, follow-up must be arranged by the orthopedist. Instruct the patient to keep the extremity elevated, move the fingers or toes, keep the cast dry, and avoid putting any objects into the cast. Advise the family to check for pain out of proportion to the injury, color change of the distal extremity, and numbness or tingling. These signs suggest excessive cast tightness or neurovascular compromise and require an immediate return to the ED.

Bibliography

Jadhav SP, Swischuk LE: Commonly missed subtle skeletal injuries in children: a pictorial review. *Emerg Radiol* 2008;15:391–8.

Myers A, Canty K, Nelson T: Are the Ottawa ankle rules helpful in ruling out the need for

x ray examination in children? *Arch Dis Child* 2005;90:1309–11.

Young SJ, Barnett PL, Oakley EA: 11. Fractures and minor head injuries: minor injuries in children II. *Med J Aust* 2005;182:644–8.

Common orthopedic injuries
Upper extremity
Clavicle

Clavicular fractures are particularly common in newborns (5 per 1000 births). They are associated with a breech or difficult delivery but may not be noticed until about 1 week of age, when a grossly obvious callus is found in the area of the fracture. In older children, they are caused by a fall on an outstretched hand or by a direct blow, and present with crepitus, swelling, and tenderness. It is important to tell parents to expect a large, possibly tender, swelling (callus) 7–10 days after the injury. Most clavicle fractures heal with minimal supportive treatment. Either immobilize the arm with a sling or apply a figure-of-8 clavicle splint. A full return of function requires 3–4 weeks.

True sternoclavicular and acromioclavicular (AC) joint dislocations are relatively uncommon in children and more often actually represent physeal fractures. However, the treatment is usually the same, outpatient management with a sling. Rarely, the clavicle may be severely displaced and require reduction. Medial clavicular injuries require particular attention when displaced posteriorly because they may compress the trachea, great vessels, and brachial plexus. An emergency CT scan and orthopedic consultation are required if this injury is suspected.

Shoulder

Shoulder dislocations are rare in childhood, as the proximal humeral epiphysis is weaker than the shoulder joint capsule. As the growth plate closes, shoulder dislocations can occur with a fall on an outstretched hand, forced abduction of an externally rotated arm, or a posterior blow to an elevated, abducted arm. Anterior dislocation is the most common, presenting with the arm held slightly abducted and in external rotation, with a squared-off appearance to the shoulder. There may be numbness and tingling of the arm. The recurrence rate approaches 90% after an initial dislocation in a teenager.

Test for neurovascular compromise before and after any attempt at shoulder reduction by comparing bilateral brachial pulses and examining sensation over the deltoid muscle. Reduce an anterior shoulder dislocation with the Stimpson method. After providing adequate sedation (pp. 682–691), have the patient lie prone on a stretcher, with the affected arm hanging down. Application of a 5–10 lb weight to the arm will cause gradual reduction over 15–30 minutes. During the reduction rotate the inferior edge of the scapula medially with gentle pressure. Place the arm in a sling and obtain post-reduction radiographs to evaluate for an associated fracture.

Proximal humerus

Injuries to the proximal humerus usually involve the growth plate, occurring with a fall onto an outstretched arm. Neurovascular compromise is rare. This area has tremendous remodeling potential, so growth disturbances are uncommon. Angulations up to 30° and displacement of up to 50% may not require reduction. Treat with a sling and immobilization. More significantly displaced fractures require reduction.

Overhand sports (baseball pitching, swimming, etc.) can place stress and injure the proximal humeral physis by the same mechanism that causes a rotator cuff injury in older athletes. Typically, the pain has a gradual onset over months and is most severe when performing the overhand activity. Patients often present with tenderness over the proximal humerus, but many are asymptomatic at rest. Radiographs of the humerus may be normal or show widening of the physis, fragmentation, demineralization, or sclerosis. Treat with rest, ice, and analgesia.

Humeral shaft

These fractures are less common than proximal and distal humeral fractures. They can be associated with a unicameral bone cyst of the humerus. Carefully assess the radial nerve (wrist dorsiflexion), which may be injured as it passes close to the bone in the distal half of the shaft. Treat with closed reduction and neurovascular checks before and after reduction.

Elbow injuries

If a fracture is suspected, splint the extremity and obtain true AP and lateral radiographs. If there is an obvious deformity, do not test passive range of motion, because of the risk of displacing a fracture. Apply ice and elevate the extremity above the level of the heart to reduce swelling.

Since a child's elbow is a maze of growth centers, surrogate markers for fracture are often helpful when a fracture line is not obvious. On the lateral radiograph, the anterior humeral line normally intersects the middle third of the capitellum on a true lateral; if it does not, suspect a fracture. Similarly, the radius typically aligns with the capitellum; if it does not, suspect a dislocation. A normal elbow will have a visible thin anterior fat pad that is flush up against the humerus. The posterior fat pad normally lies deep in the olecranon fossa and is not visible when the elbow is flexed. When the joint capsule is distended by blood or an effusion, however, the anterior fat pad is lifted away from the humerus (sail sign) and the posterior fat pad will be visible as it is pushed posteriorly out of the olecranon fossa.

CRITOE is a helpful mnemonic (Table 18-2) that represents the order in which the growth centers of the elbow ossify (appear as bone on radiograph). When a bony fragment appears out of this order, be suspicious for an occult fracture. Comparison views of the contralateral uninjured elbow may be helpful.

Supracondylar fractures

These account for about two-thirds of elbow fractures and typically occur in children <10 years of age who fall on an outstretched arm with a hyperextended elbow. Fractures of the distal end of the humerus pose a high risk (12%) of neurovascular compromise, most often involving the median and radial nerves. Supracondylar fractures may present with ischemic pain in the forearm from a compartment syndrome or injury to the brachial artery. An attempt to extend the fingers may cause considerable pain. This is a more reliable sign of ischemia than the presence or absence of the radial pulse. Prompt orthopedic intervention is required to prevent a Volkmann's contracture. If compartment syndrome is suspected, compartment pressure of the forearm must be measured.

Table 18-2. Ossification of growth centers of the elbow (CRITOE)

Growth center	Age of ossification (years)
Capitellum	1
Radial head	3
Internal or medial epicondyle	5
Trochlea	7
Olecranon	9
External or lateral epicondyle	11

Treat nondisplaced fractures with *in situ* immobilization; these heal well. Displaced fractures require accurate anatomic reduction and immobilization, often necessitating pin fixation. Admit patients with displaced supracondylar fractures and/or marked swelling for repeated neurovascular checks.

Fractures of the lateral and medial condyles and epicondyles

These represent Salter IV fractures involving both the growth plate and the elbow joint. Lateral epicondyle fractures are one of the few types of pediatric fractures that may proceed to nonunion. Radiographs may not reveal the true extent of the displacement; an arthrogram may be required. Suspect a fracture if there is instability on valgus and varus stress. Treat nondisplaced fractures with immobilization, but displaced fractures require surgery for precise anatomic reduction.

Little League elbow is a common overuse injury that results in an apophysitis about the medial epicondyle. The act of throwing places excessive valgus stress on the medial epicondyle. Typically, the pain worsens during throwing and improves with rest. Examination may be normal or demonstrate point tenderness over the medial epicondyle. Radiographs may be normal or show a widened physis, fragmentation, or hypertrophy about the medial epicondyle. If the radiographs are normal, treatment consists of rest, ice, and analgesia. Otherwise, orthopedic consultation is indicated.

Fractures of the proximal radius

These can also occur from a fall onto an outstretched hand. Characteristic findings are pain over the radial head and decreased forearm pronation and supination. Neurovascular compromise is unusual. Other parts of the elbow are frequently injured (50%), so obtain a dedicated ipsilateral elbow radiograph if only a forearm X-ray was taken. Normally, a line drawn through the shaft of the radius always intersects the capitellum, no matter what the position of the arm. In the absence of any angulation or displacement, treat symptomatically with either a sling or a splint. Otherwise, consult an orthopedist for evaluation and possible reduction because of the increased risk of avascular necrosis and subsequent loss of function.

Nursemaid's elbow (radial head subluxation)

This is a common problem that may be recurrent, but it can be managed without radiographs or orthopedic consultation. Classically, it occurs when a young child's

(1–3 years) arm is suddenly pulled while the elbow is extended and the arm pronated. It is not uncommon for children to suffer a nursemaid's elbow after a minor fall. The toddler with a nursemaid's elbow is comfortable but refuses to actively flex the elbow, preferring an extended, internally rotated position. There is no swelling and minimal tenderness around the elbow or wrist, unless passive flexion of the elbow is attempted.

To reduce a nursemaid's elbow, cup the elbow in one hand and the wrist in the other. Rapidly supinate the forearm while simultaneously flexing the elbow. Usually a click is felt, and within 10–15 minutes (sometimes longer) the child actively flexes the elbow. If the success of the reduction is in question, obtain radiographs of the elbow to evaluate for an occult fracture before attempting to reduce again. Hyperpronation of the forearm is another technique useful for reduction.

Elbow dislocations

Posterior dislocations of the elbow are the most common type and are associated with significant neurovascular compromise. Contact orthopedics for reduction. Afterward, obtain post-reduction radiographs to look for associated fractures and admit the patient for observation for compartment syndrome.

Forearm fractures

These are the most common fractures of childhood (45% of the total) and are usually caused by falls. About 75% occur in the distal third of the forearm and most others in the middle third. Over half are greenstick fractures presenting with pain and swelling without significant deformity. If only one forearm bone is fractured, image the elbow and wrist to evaluate for concurrent dislocation of the other bone. A Monteggia fracture consists of a fracture of the ulna with angulation and dislocation of the radial head, and a Galeazzi fracture is a fracture of the radius with shortening and dislocation of the distal ulna.

Treat a nondisplaced fracture with splinting or casting. A displaced or angulated fracture requires closed reduction and casting under sedation. Use a long arm cast for a midshaft fracture, but a short arm cast will suffice for a distal fracture. In patients <10 years of age, the forearm and wrist will remodel with no lasting deformity, if proper reduction is achieved.

Wrist and hand fractures

Carpal fractures are unusual in children; the scaphoid (navicular) is the most commonly fractured carpal bone. They are caused by a fall on an outstretched hand. Carpal fractures present with pain in the wrist but little deformity or swelling. These fractures may occur without definite radiologic abnormalities. Point tenderness in the anatomic snuff box suggests a scaphoid fracture as does pain in the snuffbox with axial loading of the thumb. Obtain a wrist radiograph with dedicated scaphoid views. Treat nondisplaced scaphoid fractures with a thumb spica cast. Displacement is a sign of wrist instability and requires open reduction and internal fixation. Radiographs may not detect subtle scaphoid fractures so place all patients with snuffbox tenderness and negative X-rays in a thumb spica splint.

Metacarpal fractures are usually the result of fighting. The neck of the fifth metacarpal is most often affected (boxer's fracture). The patient may present 1–2 days after the injury with swelling of the dorsum of the hand and decreased range of motion. In the absence of significant angulation or displacement, treat with a hand and wrist splint. Consult orthopedics for multiple metacarpal fractures or metacarpal fractures with rotational deformity causing finger overlap.

Finger fractures and injuries

Most finger fractures are simple, nondisplaced distal phalangeal shaft injuries. They are commonly seen in toddlers who get a finger caught in a door. A subungual hematoma is often associated with the fracture. Reduction is indicated if there is a displaced phalangeal fracture with >20° of volar angulation. Use a dorsal splint to immobilize a fractured digit, maintaining the MCP joints at 35–40° of flexion, ensuring that the rotational alignment of the digits is preserved. Injuries to the base of the thumb may require a thumb spica cast, and significantly unstable fractures may require pin fixation.

Finger dislocations are easily recognized from the deformity of the digit. The most frequently dislocated metacarpophalangeal joint is the second. Anesthetize the finger using a digital nerve block and reduce the finger dislocation with simple traction. Afterward, splint for 7–10 days.

Lower extremity

Pelvic fractures

Fractures of the pelvis are rarely isolated, occurring most often in a multiple trauma victim who has pain with movement or palpation of the pelvis. There may be associated injuries to the viscera and bladder or a vaginal or rectal laceration. There may be a large hematoma superficially beneath the inguinal ligament or in the scrotum (Destot's sign), a bony prominence or a large hematoma as well as tenderness on rectal examination (Earle's sign), or a decreased distance from the greater trochanter to the pubic spine on the affected side with a lateral compression fracture (Roux's sign). If there is any suspicion of a pelvic injury, obtain pelvic X-rays. Most pelvic fractures are stable, so treatment is directed toward fluid resuscitation and hemodynamic stabilization.

Do not insert a urinary catheter in any patient with blood at the urethral meatus or a male with a high-riding prostate or scrotal hematoma because of the risk of converting a partial urethral tear into a complete one. Consult urology for an emergency urethrogram.

Pelvic apophyseal avulsion injuries are fairly common and usually isolated injuries in children. They occur after a strong contraction of the attached muscle. The patient most often is an athlete with localized pain. The anterior superior and inferior iliac spines, the iliac crest, and the ischeal tuberosity are the sites most often involved. Pelvic radiograph findings vary from a widening of the physis (apophysitis) to complete avulsion. Treat simple apophysitis symptomatically with analgesia and rest. Consult an orthopedist for complete avulsion fractures.

Hip injuries

Hip fractures are rare, occurring with significant high-energy trauma. In 30% of cases, there are associated injuries. Observe how the patient holds the leg while lying supine. The affected leg is shortened and externally rotated, while the hip may be flexed. Compare the skinfolds of young patients; asymmetry can occur with dislocation or fracture. Obtain AP and lateral (frog-leg) radiographs. Prompt surgical reduction is required to prevent avascular necrosis, especially with femoral neck fractures and hip dislocation. A delay in treatment can cause permanent deformity.

A traumatic hip dislocation is rare, most often posterior, and usually secondary to low-energy trauma. It is, however, associated with significant morbidity if not relocated within 6 hours.

Femoral shaft fractures

Typically, femur fractures are easily identified, presenting with swelling, deformity, and tenderness in the thigh. Occasionally, they may be detected while evaluating a crying child who refuses to bear weight on the affected leg. Look for other injuries, such as ipsilateral hip dislocation, femoral neck fracture, epiphyseal injury, tibial fracture, and fracture of the contralateral femur. While a femoral shaft fracture can occur with falls and play, suspect child abuse in non-ambulatory children or those with other signs of inflicted trauma (pp. 580–581). Treatment varies with the patient's age. In general, children <6 years of age require a spica cast. Older children and adolescents are treated with either internal fixation or delayed casting after traction. If there are no concerns about abuse, young children in spica casts can be discharged with outpatient follow-up.

Knee injuries

The knee is a common site of sports injuries, especially in football players and skiers. The history of the mechanism of injury, including the position of the knee and foot at the time and whether there was any contact, helps suggest the most likely diagnosis. The patient may complain of pain or swelling or may be limping or unable to bear weight. A sensation of "tightness" behind the knee suggests a small effusion.

Obtain AP and lateral radiographs of the knee to rule out fracture in patients who have any bony tenderness, are unable to bear weight, or cannot flex their knee to 90°. Order an additional patellar skyline view if a patellar fracture is suspected and a tunnel view if a tibial plateau injury is a possibility. It is quite common for an acutely injured knee to be so swollen and painful that an examination is impossible. In this situation, provide analgesia (see p. 556) and aspirate the joint to relieve some of the pain. Use the RICE protocol with a knee immobilizer, and refer the patient to an orthopedist for definitive diagnosis and treatment. If a fracture is present, immediate consultation is required.

Knee sprains

Knee sprains are rare in young children; they occur more frequently in adolescents with closed or closing growth plates. The medial collateral ligament (MCL) is the most common site of sprain, caused by a lateral blow to the knee. Injuries to the anterior cruciate ligament (ACL) can occur without contact by abrupt deceleration maneuvers, jumping, missed landing, or "cutting" maneuvers such as those seen in basketball, football, or tennis. Lateral collateral ligament (LCL) and posterior cruciate injuries are less common.

After the initial evaluation of the injured extremity, the integrity of the knee ligaments must be checked. For each ligament, assess the range of motion and whether there is a definite endpoint, using the other side as a reference. With the patient supine, the hip extended, and the knee at 0° (fully extended), place one hand above the ankle and the other on the lateral aspect of the distal femur. Abducting the lower leg then causes valgus knee stress, testing the medial collateral ligament. Place the upper hand on the medial aspect of the distal femur, and adduct the lower leg (varus stress, lateral collateral). If there is instability, stop the examination; if the knee is not unstable, repeat the exam at 30° flexion.

Medial collateral ligament sprains cause medial pain; lateral collateral injuries result in pain on the lateral side of the knee.

Next, test the cruciate ligaments by performing a Lachman test. With the knee flexed 20°, stabilize the femur with one hand and draw the tibia downward with the other. A sharp endpoint indicates anterior cruciate integrity. Then flex the hip to 45° and the knee to 90° with the foot flat on the table. Sit on the patient's toes, place four fingers of both hands on either side of the patient's calf and your thumbs on the femoral condyles, and pull the tibia forward (anterior draw, anterior cruciate), feeling for a definite endpoint. Then push it backward (posterior draw, posterior cruciate).

With anterior cruciate ligament tears the patient or bystanders may report having heard a "pop" or "snap," the patient refuses to bear weight, and swelling begins almost immediately. Treat knee sprains with a knee immobilizer and crutches. Radiographs may demonstrate an avulsion fracture of the superior lateral tibia (Segond fracture).

Meninscal injuries

Meniscal injuries occur on weightbearing with the foot externally rotated, pushing off, often during squatting and twisting (baseball catchers); lateral meniscus injuries are uncommon. Meniscal injuries present with painful ambulation and inability to fully extend the knee. To evaluate the menisci, perform McMurray's test. While the knee is hyperflexed, rotate it internally and externally by applying torque at the ankle. Palpitate over the medial and lateral joint lines; clicking or grinding reflects a positive test.

Patellar dislocation

A lateral patellar dislocation is most common in adolescent girls. It can be caused without contact by an acute strong contraction of the quadriceps muscles or by a direct blow to the knee. A ripping sound is often reported by the patient, and the knee is held semiflexed, appears deformed, and cannot be straightened. Patellar dislocation is obvious when the patella is lateral to the joint, and the anterior aspect of the knee appears concave and empty. Reduction can usually be achieved by manipulating the patella medially when the quadriceps muscle is at its shortest, with the knee fully extended and the hip flexed. Many patients often present after self-relocation, complaining of knee pain with no obvious deformity. The patellar apprehension test is useful if relocation has occurred. Slightly flex the knee and prepare to push the patella laterally. The patient will become anxious and stop the procedure. Apply a knee immobilizer and give the patient crutches. Consult an orthopedist if reduction is unsuccessful or if there is an associated fracture on X-ray.

Knee fractures

Intraarticular fractures of the knee are uncommon with sports injuries. However, pain, deformity, decreased range of motion, and fluid in the knee joint suggest the possibility. The distal femoral growth plate (which can be displaced and lead to growth disturbance), tibial tubercle, and proximal tibial metaphysis are the most common areas fractured. Movements that would normally cause an ACL tear in an adult will cause a fracture of the tibial spine in a child. Fractures of the patella are uncommon, resulting from a forceful blow directly to the knee.

Perform a careful neurovascular examination to ensure that the popliteal vessels are intact. If there is neurovascular compromise, apply gentle longitudinal traction in line with the extremity. Comparison X-rays are helpful in assessing the degree of displacement of the tibial tubercle and tibial spine. Treatment of tibial fractures usually consists of closed reduction, but fractures of the distal femoral epiphysis usually require surgical reduction and fixation.

Osgood-Schlatter disease

Osgood-Schlatter disease (pp. 568–571) is an apophysitis of the tibial tuberosity. It typically presents in physically active athletes who complain of anterior knee pain and swelling that is at its worse during exercise. The patient will have point tenderness over the tibial tubercle. Radiographs are not needed to confirm the diagnosis but demonstrate thickening of the patellar tendon and, often, fragmentation of the tibial tubercle. The disease is self-limited and improves with rest, ice, and NSAIDs.

Tibia and fibula fractures

These are most frequently caused by motor vehicle accidents and falls from height. Many are greenstick-type fractures. Spiral fractures of the tibia, caused by rotational force on a foot that is fixed, are a common sports injury. Pain and swelling occur with nondisplaced tibial fractures but may not be seen in isolated fibula fractures. Beware of any signs of compartment syndrome. Treat tibia fractures with long leg casting.

A toddler's fracture is a nondisplaced fracture of the distal diaphysis of the tibia or fibula. It most commonly occurs between 9 months and 3 years of age, sometimes without a history of significant trauma. The child presents with a limp, and the initial radiograph may show a faint line in the tibial shaft. A callus can be seen on repeat films 1 week later. If a toddler's fracture is missed, however, it will heal without sequelae.

Isolated fibula fractures are rare; careful examination and radiographs are necessary to rule out any displacement. An isolated nondisplaced fibula fracture requires supportive specific therapy only.

Ankle injuries

Ankle injuries are among the most common in all age groups. Patients most often present after twisting or "rolling" their ankle with localized pain, swelling, and decreased range of motion. While older teenagers are more likely to sprain their ankle, younger children are more likely to have a fracture. Carefully examine the ankle for tenderness over the medial and lateral malleoli. Always examine the ipsilateral foot and knee for associated injuries.

If the radiograph does not demonstrate a fracture and the patient has closed physes, treat the patient for an ankle sprain with RICE therapy. Crutches may be used until the patient is able to bear weight on the affected ankle.

If the radiograph does not demonstrate a fracture and the patient has open physes, immobilize the ankle. Skeletally immature patients (i.e. with open physes) may have a Salter 1 fracture although the radiograph appears normal. A later radiograph will demonstrate callous formation as evidence of fracture. Immobilize patients with medial malleolar (tibial) tenderness in a short leg cast or a posterior splint; give them crutches and keep them non-weightbearing. Patients with lateral malleolar tenderness can be placed in an air-cast or splinted and allowed to walk because the fibula is a non-weightbearing bone.

Consult orthopedics for physeal fractures seen radiographically. Some ankle fractures may need additional "stress view" radiographs to determine whether there is any ankle joint instability. Tillaux and triplane fractures can occur during adolescence when the tibial physes are beginning to close. Operative treatment may be required and subsequent growth arrest can be significant. Displacement of ankle fractures usually requires operative management.

Tarsal and metatarsal injuries

These most commonly occur secondary to a direct blow to the foot. Ninety percent of foot fractures occur in the metatarsals, presenting with pain and swelling. Treat with a padded support dressing and protected weightbearing with crutches. A common error is confusing the growth center of the first metatarsal (located proximally) as a fracture; the growth centers of the other metatarsals are located distally.

Avulsion fractures of the base of the fifth metatarsal are common injuries, but they can be confused with secondary ossification centers. These fractures most commonly occur with an inversion injury and present with point tenderness and mild swelling. Treat them like most other metatarsal fractures with a short-leg walking cast.

A true "Jones fracture" occurs at the proximal diaphysis of the fifth metatarsal, is perpendicular to the long axis of the bone, and extends into joint between the fourth and fifth metatarsals. Treat these patients with a short-leg cast or posterior splint, give them crutches, and keep them non-weightbearing because of the risk of nonunion.

Metatarsal stress fractures

These occur in patients who have recently become physically active, such as adolescents beginning participation in sports. The usual complaint is pain on weightbearing, with less discomfort at rest. Swelling is minimal, but localized tenderness is marked. Anterior, lateral, and oblique X-rays are normal early, but after 2–3 weeks callus formation can be seen. Treat with rest and avoidance of the offending activity.

Tarsometatarsal dislocation

A dislocation of the tarsometatarsal joint can occur when violent plantar flexion of the forefoot occurs if the foot is in the "tiptoe" position (foot used to break a fall from a bicycle or motorcycle). These dislocations are generally accompanied by metatarsal shaft or neck fractures. The patient presents with swelling of the dorsum of the foot overlying the tarsometatarsal joints, with marked pain and tenderness and inability to bear weight. Often, a deformity is not present because of the high rate of spontaneous reduction. Reduction, with immobilization or pinning, is required.

Fractures of the phalanges of the foot

These are rare in young children but more common in adolescents. They are caused by direct trauma secondary to a falling object or kicking a hard object. The patient presents with pain, swelling, and, occasionally, deformity. Treat with alignment and buddy taping.

Indications to consult an orthopedist

• Compound, complete, open, or pathologic fracture
• Displaced fracture requiring reduction
• Growth plate injury other than Salter I
• Suspected neurovascular compromise
• Specific fractures: supracondylar, pelvis, hip, femur
• Specific dislocations: elbow, patella, tarsometatarsal

Follow-up

- Fracture treated with casting: immediately for pain out of proportion to the injury, color change of the distal extremity, and numbness or tingling; otherwise as per orthopedist
- Injury treated with sling, splint, or immobilizer: immediately for unremitting pain; otherwise 1–2 weeks
- Nursemaid's elbow: 24 hours, if the child is not moving the arm in a normal fashion

Bibliography

Carson S, Woolridge DP, Colletti J, Kilgore K: Pediatric upper extremity injuries. *Pediatr Clin N Am* 2006;53:41–67.

Cassas KJ, Cassettari-Wayhs A: Childhood and adolescent sports-related overuse injuries. *Am Fam Physician* 2006;73:1014–22.

LaBella CR: Common acute sports-related lower extremity injuries in children and adolescents. *Clin Pediatr Emerg Med* 2007;8;31–42.

Quick TJ, Eastwood DM. Pediatric fractures and dislocations of the hip and pelvis. *Clin Orthop Relat Res* 2005;432:87–96.

Limp

Limp in children is most often secondary to trauma. Other causes are infections, connective tissue disorders, malignancies, and sickle cell disease (Table 18-3). In addition, if the pain can be localized to either the hip or knee joint, there are specific age-related disorders to consider.

Clinical presentation

Trauma

The etiology may be a minor trauma, such as a sore from an ill-fitting shoe or a foreign body in the sole of the foot. However, there may be a more serious injury, such as fracture, sprain, or dislocation, with ecchymosis, swelling, localized tenderness, decreased range of motion, ligamentous laxity, or obvious deformity. A history that is inconsistent with the traumatic injury raises the concern for possible child abuse.

Infections

Osteomyelitis

Osteomyelitis (pp. 571–573) causes fever and limp or unwillingness to use the extremity. Point tenderness is typical, with or without overlying cellulitis.

Septic arthritis

Septic arthritis presents with the sudden onset of fever and limp or complete unwillingness to move the leg. There is erythema, increased warmth, and tenderness over the affected joint, and the patient resists passive range of movement. When the hip is affected, it is maintained in flexion, external rotation, and abduction. Classically, children with septic arthritis will be unable to bear weight on the affected limb, have fever ($>38.9°C$; $102°F$), an elevated ESR (>60 mm/h), CRP (>2.0 mg/dL) and an elevated WBC ($>10,000/mm^3$).

Table 18-3. Etiologies of limp trauma

Trauma	Hip diseases
Dislocation	Developmental dysplasia (DDH)
Foreign body	Legg-Calvé-Perthes disease
Fracture	Slipped capital femoral epiphysis
Soft-tissue injury (bruise)	Transient synovitis
Sprain	Knee diseases
Infections	Chondromalacia patellae
Intervertebral diskitis	Osgood-Schlatter disease
Lyme disease	Osteochondritis dissecans
Osteomyelitis	Arthritis
Septic arthritis	Acute rheumatic fever
Viral infections	Henoch-Schönlein purpura
Other	Inflammatory bowel disease
Abdominal or pelvic pathology Neoplasm	Juvenile rheumatoid arthritis
Sickle cell disease	Serum sickness
	Systemic lupus erythematosus

Lyme disease

In the first stage of Lyme disease (pp. 398–401), there may be arthralgias and the patient may favor an extremity. Fever, lethargy, and headache may occur along with the pathognomonic rash, erythema migrans. Frank arthritis (especially of the knee) is a manifestation of the early disseminated stage. Typically, the joint is swollen and tender but not warm or erythematous.

Intervertebral diskitis

Intervertebral diskitis is an infectious or inflammatory disease occurring primarily in 2–7-year-olds. The patient may present with limp, back pain, refusal to sit or walk, irritability, and low-grade fever. Physical examination findings include localized tenderness directly over the spine, paravertebral muscle spasm, and limited straight leg raising.

Viral infections

Many viral infections can present with arthritis or arthralgias usually during the viral prodrome. Possible etiologies include herpesviruses (HSV, varicella, EBV, CMV), parvovirus, hepatitis, rubella, HIV, mumps, adenovirus, Coxsackie, and echovirus. Children may also experience arthralgia or arthritis after receiving the MMR or rubella vaccine. The arthritis is usually symmetric.

Hip diseases

With hip diseases, the pain may be in the groin or anterior thigh, or it may be referred to the anteromedial aspect of the knee.

Transient synovitis

Transient synovitis is a benign, self-limited, inflammatory hip disease that occurs predominantly in 3–8-year-olds. There is an acute or gradual onset of limp and either hip or referred knee pain. Fever is variable and the child does not appear toxic, but there may be a URI. The hip is held in mild flexion, external rotation, and abduction, but there is no erythema or increased warmth. Abduction and internal rotation are limited by pain only at the extremes of motion. WBC, ESR, and CRP are generally normal or slightly elevated. X-rays and sonography may show a hip effusion. Transient synovitis is a diagnosis of exclusion and must be distinguished from an early septic arthritis of the hip.

Legg-Calvé-Perthes disease

Legg-Calvé-Perthes disease, or osteochondrosis of the femoral head, usually occurs in 4–9-year-old boys. There is a gradual onset of limp and pain in the hip, groin, or medial knee. Abduction and internal rotation of the hip are limited. The radiographic findings may be confused with avascular necrosis associated with corticosteroid use, sickle cell disease, or Gaucher's disease.

Slipped capital femoral epiphysis

A slipped capital femoral epiphysis (SCFE) is a displacement of the normal relationship between the femoral head and neck. Ten to 20% of cases are bilateral; some, especially in patients with short stature, are associated with hypothyroidism. The typical patient is an obese adolescent who presents with a limp and subacute or chronic groin pain, which may be referred to the anterior thigh or knee. The hip is held in flexion and external rotation. Passive hip flexion may accentuate the external rotation deformity, while internal rotation and abduction may be limited. Long-term morbidity (i.e. arthritis) is directly linked to the degree of displacement on presentation.

Developmental dysplasia of the hip (DDH)

DDH occurs most often in girls who underwent a breech delivery. Those not detected in the newborn period will develop a limp once they begin walking. Unlike many other causes of limp, these children are often pain-free.

Knee diseases

Although there are a number of specific disorders that affect the knee, remember that the obturator nerve can cause hip diseases to present with knee pain. Therefore, examine the hips carefully in all patients with knee pain.

Osgood-Schlatter disease

Osgood-Schlatter disease, or apophysitis of the tibial tuberosity, is a self-limited "overuse" disorder that usually occurs in physically active adolescents. Patients present with a gradual onset of limp, especially after exercise. On examination, there is unilateral or bilateral tenderness and swelling over the tibial tuberosity, but the knee joint is otherwise normal.

Chondromalacia patellae

Also known as "runner's knee" or "painful patella syndrome," this overuse injury is thought to be due to misalignment of the patella in the femoral groove, which leads to erosion of the cartilage. Typical findings of chondromalacia patellae include patellar pain after activity (especially stair climbing), episodes of buckling (but not locking), and crepitance and tenderness on palpation of the patellar articular surface. The "patella grind test" will be painful in patients with this condition. The test is performed while the patient is supine and the knee is extended. The practitioner then gently pushes the patella inferiorly while the patient contracts the quadriceps muscle. A joint effusion is uncommon and suggests other diagnoses.

Osteochondritis dissecans

With osteochondritis dissecans, an area of bone, usually on the lateral aspect of the medial femoral condyle, develops ischemic necrosis and subsequent fracture. A piece of bone and cartilage may then break loose into the joint. This causes intermittently painful limp after exercise, buckling, locking, and a tender medial femoral condyle. The cause is unknown but is most common in adolescent boys involved in organized sports.

Other causes
Arthritis

Arthritis (nonseptic) presents with swelling, erythema, tenderness, decreased range of motion, and increased warmth of single or multiple joints (pp. 671–675). Associated findings may include fever, rash, heart murmur, generalized adenopathy, and hepatosplenomegaly.

Sickle cell disease

Sickle cell bone infarcts (p. 356) can cause diffuse bone pain with tenderness and limp. Associated findings may include fever, jaundice, abdominal pain, and, in younger children, swelling of the dorsum of the hands and feet (dactylitis).

Neoplasms

Rare causes of limp include both benign (osteoid osteoma, osteochondroma) and malignant (osteosarcoma, Ewing's sarcoma) bone tumors. Metastatic bone cancer (i.e. neuroblastoma) and leukemia and can also present as bone pain and limp.

Abdominal or pelvic pathology

Diseases that irritate the psoas or obturator muscles, such as PID or appendicitis, can cause hip or thigh pain which then manifests as limping.

Diagnosis

The priority is the prompt diagnosis of a septic arthritis, osteomyelitis, or SCFE. Inquire about trauma, rate of onset (acute versus chronic), similar previous episodes, past medical history, fever, weight loss, malaise, easy bruising, and location and radiation of the pain. Perform a full physical examination, looking for a source for the limp, paying particular attention to the abdomen, back, and genitals. Observe the patient's gait, if able, while barefoot, attempting to locate the area of concern. Next, thoroughly evaluate the affected extremity(ies), looking for erythema, warmth, and tenderness. Put all joints through complete active and passive ranges of motion, then evaluate the neurovascular status of the extremity.

Thoroughly examine the hip of any child with a complaint of knee pain. Flex and extend the hip from 0° to maximal flexion. While the hip is flexed, check internal and external rotation. Pain on rotation may be the first sign of hip disorders.

Unless it is clear that the cause of the limp is minor trauma, obtain standard AP and lateral X-rays of the suspicious area(s). If the limp is associated with decreased hip range of motion, obtain AP pelvis and frog-leg lateral radiographs of both hips. Possible findings include fractures, SCFE (on the frog-leg view), joint space widening (septic arthritis, transient synovitis, Legg-Calvé-Perthes disease), increased density of the femoral epiphysis (Legg-Calvé-Perthes disease), or subchondral bone fragmentation (osteochondritis dissecans). An MRI is needed to diagnose early Legg-Calvé-Perthes disease. X-rays of the knee are not necessary when Osgood-Schlatter disease is suspected, and radiographs are normal in chondromalacia patellae.

If the limp is associated with back pain, consider diskitis or osteomyelitis, particularly if the patient is febrile. Obtain plain X-rays and arrange for an MRI scan.

Obtain a CBC, ESR, CRP, and Lyme titer (in endemic areas) when there are fever and/or constitutional symptoms and no definite history of trauma. Leukocytosis, a shift to the left, and a markedly increased ESR (>60 mm/h) and CRP (>2.0 mg/dL) may occur in inflammatory conditions such as septic arthritis, osteomyelitis, and diskitis. With transient synovitis, the ESR is elevated, but usually <60 mm/h and the CRP is <2.0 mg/dL.

ED management

It may be impossible to make a specific diagnosis of the cause of a limp. If the fever is not high, the WBC, ESR, and CRP are normal, and the radiographs are unremarkable, the patient may be discharged with close follow-up. Many such children have a soft tissue injury without fracture or transient synovitis. Instruct the patient to return at once if there is high fever or an inability to ambulate or bear weight.

Infection

If septic arthritis or osteomyelitis is suspected, refer the patient immediately to an orthopedist for aspiration of joint fluid or subperiosteal pus. Intravenous antibiotics are then indicated. The treatment of Lyme disease (pp. 398–401) is detailed elsewhere. Since diskitis is difficult to distinguish from osteomyelitis, admit the patient for bed rest and IV antibiotics. Use nafcillin (150 mg/kg per day div q 6 h) or, if MRSA is a concern, vancomycin (40 mg/kg per day div q 6 h).

Hip diseases
Transient synovitis

Patients who are well appearing, with a normal WBC and an ESR <60 mm/h, CRP (>2.0 mg/dL) may be treated at home with bed rest and acetaminophen (15 mg/kg q 4 h) or ibuprofen (10 mg/kg q 6 h) until the symptoms have resolved. For a patient with more severe symptoms, consult an orthopedist and admit for bed rest and skin traction, until the range of motion is normal.

SCFE

Immediately obtain orthopedic consultation, as minor trauma can cause complete displacement of the femoral epiphysis. Weightbearing must be discontinued and the patient placed at rest. Long-term morbidity (i.e. arthritis) is directly linked to the degree of displacement on presentation. If the patient has short stature, obtain thyroid function tests in addition to any labs needed prior to an operation.

Legg-Calvé-Perthes

Although no emergency treatment is required, refer these patients to an orthopedist so that a comprehensive plan of treatment can be arranged.

Knee diseases

Osgood-Schlatter disease

Treat with ibuprofen (as above) and limitation of activity until the acute symptoms resolve (2–6 weeks). Then, increase the activity level slowly.

Painful patella syndrome

The treatment is the same as for Osgood-Schlatter disease. In addition, recommend quadriceps strengthening exercises (straight leg lifting).

Osteochondritis dissecans

Refer patients with suspected osteochondritis dissecans to an orthopedist, since treatment usually requires immobilization or possible surgery.

Follow-up

- Transient synovitis: 2–3 days, if symptoms have not resolved
- Legg-Calvé-Perthes, osteochondritis dissicans: orthopedist in 1–2 weeks
- Osgood-Schlatter, painful patella syndrome: primary care follow-up in 2–4 weeks

Indications for admission

- Slipped capital femoral epiphysis
- Possible septic arthritis, osteomyelitis, diskitis, rheumatic fever, or neoplasm
- Transient synovitis with fever, leukocytosis, ESR >60 mm/h, CRP (>2.0 mg/dL), or markedly decreased range of motion

Bibliography

Abbassian A: The limping child: a clinical approach to diagnosis. *Br J Hosp Med (Lond)* 2007;**68**:246–50.

Caird MS, Flynn JM, Leung YL, et al: Factors distinguishing septic arthritis from transient synovitis of the hip in children. A prospective study. *J Bone Joint Surg Am* 2006;**88**:1251–7.

Leung AK, Lemay JF: The limping child. *J Pediatr Health Care* 2004;**18**:219–23.

Osteomyelitis

Osteomyelitis is a bacterial bone infection, caused by organisms introduced either hematogenously or by direct spread from a contiguous local focus. The usual site is the metaphysis; the distal femur and proximal and distal tibia are the most commonly involved bones. In the newborn, the proximal humerus is a frequent location.

Staphylococcus aureus causes the majority of infections. Other etiologies include group A *Streptococcus, S. pneumoniae* and *Kingella* in young children and toddlers, and group B *Streptococcus* and enteric bacteria in neonates. Children with hemoglobinopathies (sickle cell disease) are at risk for infection with *Salmonella. Pseudomonas* can infect the bones of the foot after a puncture wound through the sole of a shoe. *H. influenzae* type B is no longer a concern due to the success of widespread vaccination.

Clinical presentation

The usual presentation in a child or adolescent is pain and point tenderness at a long-bone site, with decreased range of motion in the adjacent joints. Swelling, erythema, and warmth are generally not seen unless purulent material ruptures through the cortex and spreads to the subcutaneous tissues. The patient may be febrile and often refuses to use or bear weight on the limb, holding it as motionless as possible. With vertebral osteomyelitis, there is chronic back pain or torticollis with spasms of the paraspinal muscles.

An infant may occasionally have nonspecific signs, such as fever, irritability, vomiting, and decreased mobility of an extremity, but more often there is swelling and tenderness of the affected area. In infants, because of the relatively thin cortex and loose periosteum, osteomyelitis spreads to contiguous structures in muscle and joints more often than in an older patient. Seventy percent of neonates have an associated septic arthritis.

Diagnosis

The diagnosis of osteomyelitis is clinical. The typical combination of fever, point tenderness, and unwillingness to use an extremity is not invariably seen, but when present is highly suggestive of osteomyelitis. The CRP and ESR are almost always elevated, whereas elevation of the WBC count is typical but less predictable. Aspiration of the pus from the bone and positive blood cultures confirm the diagnosis.

Plain films may show soft-tissue changes and swelling as early as 3 days after onset of symptoms; however, routine X-rays do not show bone changes until 10–20 days after the onset of the infection. In contrast, a 99mTc phosphate bone scan can detect bone changes earlier than plain films, and prior aspiration of the bone does not affect results. MRI has emerged as the most sensitive tool for detecting osteomyelitis and gauging the extent of the disease. However, bone scan is less expensive, usually does not require sedation in young children, and can detect multiple foci of infection.

Osteomyelitis is an unusual entity and can mimic many common diagnoses. Trauma can cause pain, swelling, and limitation of movement. Usually there is a history of an injury or radiographic evidence of a fracture, and the ESR and CBC are normal. Cellulitis of a distal extremity can be mistaken for a manifestation of osteomyelitis, although there is no point tenderness over the bone.

Sickle cell disease (pp. 354–359) can cause pain secondary to infection or vasoocclusive crisis. Distinguishing between the two may be difficult, although the pain of a crisis tends to recur in the same sites, can be in several locations at once, and often resolves with IV hydration. Pain in a single bone that has not been affected in the past is suspicious for osteomyelitis.

Other considerations include bone tumor, Caffey's disease (infantile cortical hyperostosis), and Langerhans' cell histiocytosis. All of these can be excluded by X-ray.

ED management

When osteomyelitis is suspected, obtain a blood culture, CBC with differential, ESR, CRP, and X-rays of the extremity. If available, order a 99mTc phosphate bone scan or MRI to confirm the diagnosis. Consult with an orthopedist to perform needle aspiration to drain the pus and provide specimens for culture and Gram's stain. If no pus is obtained, send bone marrow for culture and Gram's stain. Needle aspiration can also exclude a sickle cell vasoocclusive crisis when the clinical picture is unclear.

Admit a patient with osteomyelitis and treat with an IV penicillinase-resistant antistaphylococcal drug. For a patient >5 years of age use nafcillin (150 mg/kg per day div q 6 h). Add vancomycin (40 mg/kg per day div q 6 h) if MRSA is a concern. Add *Salmonella* coverage (ceftriaxone 100 mg/kg per day div q 12 h) for a patient with a hemoglobinopathy such as sickle cell disease and *Pseudomonas* coverage (piperacillin/tazobactam 250 mg/kg per day IV div q 6 h or ceftazidime 100 mg/kg per day div q 8 h) for osteomyelitis of the foot secondary to a puncture through a shoe. For patients 2 months to 5 years of age, use ceftriaxone and either nafcillin or vancomycin (doses above). Treat a neonate with cefotaxime (150 mg/kg per day div q 8 h) and either nafcillin or vancomycin. The doses may need to be adjusted for patients in the first week of life.

Indication for admission

- Osteomyelitis

Bibliography

Gutierrez K: Bone and joint infections in children. *Pediatr Clin North Am* 2005;52:779–94.

Kaplan SL: Osteomyelitis in children. *Infect Dis Clin North Am.* 2005;19:787–97.

Shetty AK, Kumar A: Osteomyelitis in adolescents. *Adolesc Med State Art Rev* 2007;18:79–94.

Splinting

Many simple, nondisplaced fractures can be managed with splinting alone. Splinting is also useful in the treatment of ligamentous injuries, soft-tissue injuries and infections, and joint infections.

Equipment

1. Cotton padding (Webril) between the fingers or toes to prevent maceration, and against the skin to be covered by plaster or fiberglass.
2. Plaster of Paris, fiberglass rolls, or Ortho-Glass.
3. Elastic bandages.

Splint application

Wrap cotton padding around the affected limb; be sure to separate the fingers or toes. Measure the appropriate length of the splint needed and cut the plaster or fiberglass to that size. For elbows and ankles, cut a notch where the splint bends to allow for a smooth corner about the joint. Dip the plaster or fiberglass into a basin of room-temperature water until

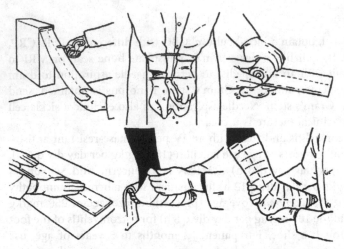

Figure 18-2. Splint application. Adapted from Roberts JR, Hedges JR: *Clinical Procedures in Emergency Medicine*, 3rd ed. Philadelphia: Saunders, 1997, with permission.

no bubbles are seen; then roll or "squeegie" the slab until excess water is removed. Smooth the plaster to avoid wrinkles, and apply it to the affected limb in the position desired. Roll a layer of Webril, followed by an elastic bandage, over the splint. Smooth and mold the splint with the palms of both hands, taking care to avoid using fingertips or excessive force (Figure 18-2).

In many institutions, the traditional plaster or fiberglass rolls have been replaced by Ortho-Glass, which consists of a roll of fiberglass with a cotton covering. Measure the appropriate length of material and then cut that amount from the larger roll. Wet the Ortho-Glass under the faucet and then pat it dry using a towel. Make certain that the edges of the fiberglass are covered because when dry they will become sharp and may hurt the patient. Apply the splint and cover it with an elastic bandage. Smooth and mold the splint into the desired position.

As a splint hardens, heat will be generated and the splint will shrink slightly. Before the patient is discharged, after the splint hardens, perform a careful neurovascular examination of the fingers or toes. Instruct the patient and family about rest, ice, and elevation in the first 24 hours, and arrange appropriate follow-up to check the injury and remove the splint at the appropriate time.

Suggested lengths of immobilization

Contusions or abrasions 1–3 days
Mild sprains 5–7 days
Soft-tissue lacerations 5–7 days
Fractures as per orthopedist
Tendon lacerations as per orthopedist or plastic surgeon

Commonly used splints

See Table 18-4 for the indications for various splints.

Table 18-4. Common splinting indications

Splint	Indications
Volar wrist	Wrist sprain, contusion, soft-tissue injury
Sugar tong forearm	Simple and buckle distal forearm fractures
Radial gutter	2nd or 3rd metacarpal or proximal phalange fracture
Ulnar gutter	4th or 5th metacarpal or proximal phalange fracture
Thumb spica	Scaphoid fracture
	Ulnar collateral ligament injury (gamekeeper's thumb) Nonangulated, nonrotated, thumb or first metacarpal fracture
Long arm posterior	Reduced elbow dislocation
	Supracondylar fractures
	Nondisplaced radial head or midshaft forearm fracture
Short posterior leg	Ankle sprain
	Fracture of the foot, ankle, or distal fibula
Long posterior leg	Knee injuries
Buddy tape/dorsal finger	Simple phalangeal fracture
	Reduced interphalangeal dislocation

Volar splint

This splint (Figure 18-3) extends from the distal aspect of the metacarpals to the proximal aspect of the forearm, leaving the phalanges and elbow free. Apply the splint along the volar surface of the arm with the wrist in a neutral or slightly hyperextended (10–20°) position.

Sugar tong forearm splint

This type of splint (Figure 18-4) will immobilize the elbow, preventing pronation and supination. Apply Webril from above the elbow to the distal edge of the palm. With the elbow in 90° of flexion, apply the plaster or fiberglass in a U-shape starting at the distal edge of the palm, wrapping around the elbow, and ending just proximally to the knuckles. Place the wrist in a neutral to slightly extended (10–20°) position and allow the thumb to move freely.

Gutter splint

Separate the fingers with gauze or Webril, apply the plaster along either the radial or ulnar aspect of the forearm, and wrap it around the two fingers to be immobilized (Figure 18-5). Flex the metacarpophalangeal joints to 90° and the interphalangeal joints to 10–20°; place the wrist in the neutral position or hyperextend it slightly (10–20°). Note for the radial gutter you will have to cut a hole to allow for the thumb to move freely.

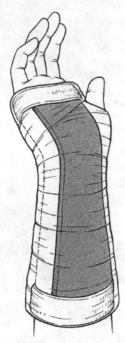

Figure 18-3. Volar forearm splint. Adapted from Roberts JR, Hedges JR: *Clinical Procedures in Emergency Medicine*, 3rd ed. Philadelphia: Saunders, 1997, with permission.

Figure 18-4. Sugar tong splint. Adapted from Roberts JR, Hedges JR: *Clinical Procedures in Emergency Medicine*, 3rd ed. Philadelphia: Saunders, 1997, with permission.

Figure 18-5. Gutter splint. Adapted from Roberts JR, Hedges JR: *Clinical Procedures in Emergency Medicine*, 3rd ed. Philadelphia: Saunders, 1997, with permission.

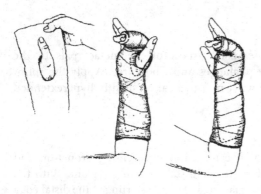

Thumb spica

Apply the splint (Figure 18-6) along the radial aspect of the forearm and wrap it around the thumb, extending to the thumbnail. Keep the wrist in a neutral or slightly extended position (10–20°) and the thumb abducted and slightly flexed (10–20°).

Posterior arm splint

Apply the plaster to the posterior aspect of the upper arm and forearm, extending to the midpalmar area (Figure 18-7). Flex the elbow to 90°, and place the wrist in a neutral or

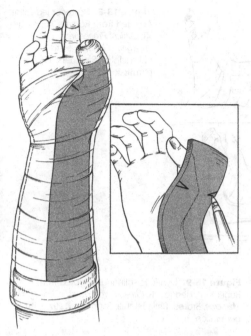

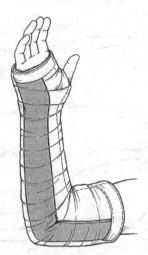

Figure 18-7. Posterior arm splint. Adapted from Roberts JR, Hedges JR: *Clinical Procedures in Emergency Medicine*, 3rd ed. Philadelphia: Saunders, 1997, with permission.

Figure 18-6. Thumb spica splint. Adapted from Roberts JR, Hedges JR: *Clinical Procedures in Emergency Medicine*, 3rd ed. Philadelphia: Saunders, 1997, with permission.

slightly extended (10–20°) position. Put the arm in a sling after the splint is applied. While these splints are useful in managing many types of fractures, consult an orthopedist for more complicated fractures (e.g. supracondylar).

Posterior leg splint

Apply a short leg splint from the head of the metatarsals to the midcalf, with the ankle in as close to a neutral position (90°) as possible. For a long leg posterior splint, extend the plaster to the mid-thigh and keep the knee in slight flexion (Figure 18-8).

Finger splints

Perform a careful examination of the injured finger and review the radiographs to determine the presence of a rotational or unacceptably angulated deformity, growth plate injury, or collateral ligament injury, all of which require orthopedic consultation.

A simple phalangeal fracture or a reduced interphalangeal dislocation may be managed with splinting alone. A soft-tissue injury or laceration will also benefit from finger splinting. Dynamic splinting, or "buddy taping" (Figure 18-9), permits movement at the MP joint and slight movement at the IP joints. Splint the injured finger to the adjacent finger, or "buddy," to provide support.

An alternative splint is the foam-backed aluminum splint (Figure 18-10), which may be cut and bent to fit. It is preferably applied to the dorsal surface of the finger, which preserves dexterity more effectively than splints applied to the volar surface. The splint should

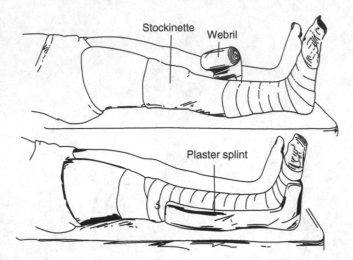

Stockinette   Webril

Plaster splint

Figure 18-8. Posterior leg splint. Adapted from Roberts JR, Hedges JR: *Clinical Procedures in Emergency Medicine*, 3rd ed. Philadelphia: Saunders, 1997, with permission.

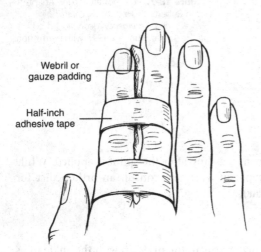

Webril or gauze padding

Half-inch adhesive tape

Figure 18-9. Dynamic splinting. Adapted from Roberts JR, Hedges JR: *Clinical Procedures in Emergency Medicine*, 3rd ed. Philadelphia: Saunders, 1997, with permission.

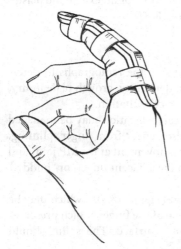

Figure 18-10. Foam splint. Adapted from Roberts JR, Hedges JR: *Clinical Procedures in Emergency Medicine*, 3rd ed. Philadelphia: Saunders, 1997, with permission.

immobilize as few joints as possible; measure it to include only one joint above and one joint below the injury. Place the finger in the position of function or slightly flexed (10–20°) at the IP joints. Two-finger injuries require specific splinting techniques other than buddy taping or dorsal splinting.

Mallet finger

The mallet finger is caused by a rupture of the extensor tendon at the DIP joint. Splint the finger only over the dorsal aspect of the DIP in full extension or slight hyperextension. The splint must remain for at least 8 weeks, and the finger must not be flexed at any time during that period.

Boutonnière deformity

The boutonnière deformity is a rupture of the central slip of the extensor digitorum communis tendon, resulting in the PIP "buttonholing" through the torn extensor hood. Splint the finger only over the dorsal aspect of the PIP in full extension or slight hyperextension. Keep the splint in place for at least 4 weeks; the finger must not be flexed during that time.

Bibliography

Abraham A, Handoll HH, Khan T: Interventions for treating wrist fractures in children. *Cochrane Database Syst Rev* 2008;(2): CD004576.

Boyd AS, Benjamin HJ, Asplund C: Principles of casting and splinting. *Am Fam Physician* 2009;79:16–22.

Halanski M, Noonan KJ: Cast and splint immobilization: complications. *J Am Acad Orthop Surg* 2008;16:30–40.

Plint AC, Perry JJ, Correll R, Gaboury I, Lawton L: A randomized, controlled trial of removable splinting versus casting for wrist buckle fractures in children. *Pediatrics* 2006;117:691–7.

Physical and sexual abuse

Stephen Ludwig, Mary Mehlman and Scott Miller

Contributing author
Olga Jimenez: Chart documentation in child abuse and *Medical testimony and court preparation*

Physical abuse

Physical abuse is defined as nonaccidental physical injury to a child by the actions or omissions of a parent or caregiver. There has been an alarming increase in reported cases of child abuse throughout the United States in the past three decades. In all states, health professionals are now legally required to report their suspicions of abuse to their state child protection services (CPS) or police.

Clinical presentation and diagnosis

Determination of suspected abuse is based on compilation from five data sources: (1) history, (2) physical examination, (3) laboratory and radiographic information, (4) observation of the child/caregiver interaction, and (5) a detailed family social history.

When examining any child with an injury, be suspicious of abuse if the history reveals an unusual delay in seeking medical care, the parents' explanation of the injury is not compatible with the physical findings, the cause of the injury is unknown or "magical," or there is a history of similar episodes. Parents may be reluctant to give information, or their reaction may be inappropriate to the severity of the injuries. Other worrisome signs are a lack of primary care (no immunizations, no source of healthcare), a history of parental mental illness or substance abuse, and high levels of family stress.

While examining the child, maintain a high index of suspicion for abuse or neglect if the child's weight is below the third percentile for age and there is poor personal hygiene, lack of adequate clothing, behavioral disturbance (especially undue compliance with the examiner), or an abnormal interaction between the parent and child (unwarranted roughness or extreme aloofness).

Remove all of the child's clothing and examine the skin carefully for contusions, abrasions, burns, and lacerations in various stages of resolution. Any bruise on a child who is not yet independently mobile is unusual. Certain skin lesions are typical for specific types of abuse, such as circular cigarette burns, human bite marks, J-shaped curvilinear or loop-shaped marks from a wire, cord, or belt, circumferential rope burns, "grid" marks from an electric heater, and symmetrical scald burns on the buttocks or extremities. Other dermatologic manifestations are cutaneous signs of malnutrition (decreased subcutaneous fat, increased creases), scalp hematomas, and signs of trauma to the genital area.

Fractures are suggested by refusal to bear weight or move an extremity, gross deformity, or soft-tissue swelling and point tenderness over an extremity. However, most metaphyseal chip fractures are not associated with deformity. Neurologic manifestations may include retinal hemorrhages, unexplainable irritability, coma, or convulsions. Finally, an acute abdomen, poisoning, or any traumatic injury that cannot be explained may in fact represent forms of child abuse.

The differential diagnosis of the abused child includes conditions with skeletal involvement: accidental trauma, osteogenesis imperfecta, Caffey's disease, scurvy, rickets, birth trauma, and congenital infection. Diseases with dermatologic manifestations include bleeding disorders (idiopathic thrombocytopenic purpura, leukemia, hemophilia, von Willebrand's disease), recurrent pyodermas, and scalded skin syndrome. Sudden infant death syndrome and accidental poisonings may be mistaken for child abuse. The most common clinical problem is the differentiation between accidental and nonaccidental trauma.

ED management

If there is any fracture or other suggestion of abuse in a child <2 years of age, obtain a complete skeletal survey for trauma. For older patients, if the physical exam suggests a fracture, obtain specific X-rays. Order other radiologic studies, such as a head CT or MRI scan, as indicated by the nature of the injuries.

If the parents deny any knowledge of the cause of skin bruises, obtain a CBC with differential, platelet count, PT, PTT, and a bleeding time. The differential diagnosis and other possible laboratory studies are shown in Table 19-1.

Physicians and other health-care workers are required to report the suspicion of abuse. Use the information gathered in the assessment phase to determine the level of concern. Notify the CPS or police by telephone if abuse or neglect is suspected. Generally, the CPS is required to initiate action in all cases reported and may not refuse a referral made in good faith by a competent reporter. Usually, a physician, nurse, or social worker must complete a report within 48 hours. However, do not delay reporting if there are other children at home, as up to 20% will have also been abused.

The CPS worker must evaluate the case and decide whether the child can safely return home or must go to a temporary shelter or foster care setting. Hospitalize the child if medical care is needed or if the inpatient setting is the only option to ensure safety. Arrange appropriate follow-up for patients who do not require hospitalization. Notify the parents about your intention to report and/or hospitalize the child. If the parents refuse to allow hospitalization, it may be necessary to have law enforcement officials intervene. In most states, hospital personnel may place a child under temporary protective custody without either parental consent or a family court order, although it is the responsibility of the CPS worker to decide whether the child can be placed in the custody of a relative or guardian.

Working with the families of abused children can be a difficult experience. Avoid an accusatory attitude, as most of these parents love their children and deserve a supportive approach. Keep the parents informed and involved, and emphasize that the goal of all concerned is to keep the child safe and, when possible, the family together. Explain the role of the social worker and supportive services, and assure confidentially. Careful documentation is critical (see pp. 587–591); the record will be needed for legal reference.

Follow-up

- Patient discharged home or to a shelter: primary care follow-up in 1 week

Indications for admission

- Medical care required
- Extent of injury uncertain
- Need for protection unavailable through community resources

Table 19-1. Differential diagnosis and abnormal laboratory studies to support nonabuse diagnosis

Findings	Differential diagnosis	Distinguishing features and tests
Bruising (extensive or deep)	Trauma	Physical examination
	ITP	↓ platelets
	Hemophilia	↑ PT and PTT
	Von Willebrand's disease	↑ bleeding time
	Henoch-Schönlein purpura	Rash on lower extremities
		Rule-out sepsis; normal platelet count
	Purpura fulminans	Clinical appearance (findings of sepsis)
		↓ platelet count
	Ehlers-Danlos syndrome	Joint hyperextensibility
Dehydration	Renal or prerenal	↑ BUN, creatinine, and urine specific gravity
		Prerenal: BUN/creatinine >20:1
Failure to thrive	Organic or nonorganic	History, physical examination
		Abnormal studies based on symptoms
Abdominal pain	Trauma	Hematuria; increased liver enzymes
	Tumor	↑ amylase; abdominal ultrasound; abnormal urinalysis
	Infection	↑ WBC, ESR, CRP; abdominal ultrasound
Fractures (multiple or in various stages of healing)	Trauma	Location, may be multiple
	Osteogenesis imperfecta	Blue sclerae; X-ray: ↓ bone density
	Rickets	Increased calcium; ↓ phosphorus, ↑ alkaline phosphatase
		X-ray: cupping at ends of long bones, widened metaphysis
	Hypophosphatasia	Decreased calcium, alkaline phosphatase; increased phosphorus
	Leukemia	Abnormal peripheral smear, bone marrow, biopsy
	Previous osteomyelitis or septic arthritis	↑ WBC, ESR, CRP; positive culture
	Neurogenic sensory deficit	Detailed neurologic examination

Table 19-1. (cont.)

Findings	Differential diagnosis	Distinguishing features and tests
Metaphyseal/epiphyseal lesions	Trauma	X-rays; consistent mechanism of injury
	Scurvy	X-rays: periosteal elevation; nutritional history
	Rickets	(See above)
	Menkes' syndrome	Decreased copper, ceruloplasmin; hair analysis
	Syphilis	Abnormal serology (VDRL)
	Little League elbow	History of use
	Birth trauma	Neonatal history
Subperiosteal ossification	Trauma	History
	Osteogenic malignancy	X-ray; biopsy
	Syphilis	(See above)
	Infantile cortical hyperostosis	No metaphyseal changes
	Osteoid osteoma	Dramatic clinical response to aspirin
	Scurvy	(See above)
CNS injury	Trauma	CT and/or MRI scan
	Aneurysm	CT and/or MRI scan
	Tumor	MRI scan

Bibliography

Chiesa A, Duhaime AC: Abusive head trauma. *Pediatr Clin North Am* 2009;56:317–31.

Hudson M, Kaplan R: Clinical response to child abuse. *Pediatr Clin N Am* 2006;53:27–39.

Kellogg ND: American Academy of Pediatrics Committee on Child Abuse and Neglect: Evaluation of suspected child physical abuse. *Pediatrics* 2007;119:1232–41.

Mudd SS, Findlay JS: The cutaneous manifestations and common mimickers of physical child abuse. *J Pediatr Health Care* 2004;18:123–9.

Pierce MC, Bertocci G: Fractures resulting from inflicted trauma: assessing injury and history compatibility. *Clin Pediatr Emerg Med* 2006;7:143–8.

Sexual abuse

Sexual abuse is the exposure of a child to sexual stimulation inappropriate for his or her age, cognitive development, or position in the relationship. The legal definition is nonconsensual sexual contact. Incest is legally defined as marriage or intercourse (oral, anal, genital) with a person known to be related as an ancestor, descendant, brother, sister, uncle, aunt, nephew, or niece. Rape is legally defined as nonconsensual sexual intercourse. The typical perpetrator in sexual abuse incidents is a person who has legitimate access to the child.

Clinical presentation

A number of signs, symptoms, and behavioral changes may signal the possibility of sexual abuse, including difficulties in school, sudden changes in behavior, fears, unwillingness to go to certain places, enuresis and encopresis, sleep disturbances, running away, and attempted suicide. Sexual abuse victims may exhibit seductive or regressive behavior. More specific complaints include difficulty walking or sitting and genital trauma, discharge, pain, or itching. A sexually transmitted disease (STD) in a child <12 years of age is sexual abuse until proven otherwise. Consider sexual abuse in girls who become pregnant.

Diagnosis

Maintain a high index of suspicion in order to identify sexual abuse promptly. Ensure privacy for the patient and whoever accompanies the child, and keep the number of staff members involved to a minimum. Because sexual abuse usually evokes intense feelings, maintaining objectivity may require effort on the part of the healthcare provider.

The key to establishing the diagnosis in sexual abuse cases is a careful history. Use language that is appropriate for the child's age and ask specifically about all types of sexual contact. It may be useful to use anatomically correct dolls or pictures to encourage the child to describe the sexual contact in as much detail as possible. Try to ascertain when the last sexual activity occurred and what the child has done since the assault (changed clothes, bathed, urinated, defecated). Assure the child that he or she was right to reveal information about the sexual abuse.

Consent for physical examination is often an issue. However, consent from the minor (regardless of age) is all that is required, since the examination also serves to rule out STDs. Do not force the patient if the examination is refused.

If the abuse has occurred within the past 72 hours, be aggressive in terms of evidence collection; most emergency departments have sexual assault evidence collecting kits for this purpose. If the patient has not changed clothes since the sexual activity, have him or her undress on a sheet and save all clothing for legal evidence. If the child has changed but not bathed, collect only the underwear. If the child has pubic hair, comb it onto a paper towel and seal the towel, combings, one plucked pubic hair, and the comb in a labeled envelope. These samples may be used for DNA evidence. Perform a complete and careful physical examination looking for marks, bruises, or other signs of physical injury or illness, and note the child's Tanner stage of pubertal development.

In most cases, the revelation of sexual abuse occurs long after the actual contact. If sexual contact has not occurred within 72 hours and there are no physical complaints (e.g. bleeding), refer the patient to a specialized sexual abuse center.

With either prompt or delayed revelation, a careful genital examination is necessary. Perform a perineal-genital examination in young children in the frog-leg, supine, or knee-chest prone position. Using a saline-moistened cotton q-tip, swab any areas of possible seminal fluid deposition and place it on a labeled slide to air-dry. In girls, spread the labia with two fingers to examine the hymenal ring, the introitus, and the area between the labia majora and minora. In the prepubertal girl, if there are no acute signs of pelvic injury, a speculum exam is not necessary. If there are obvious signs of physical injury (bleeding, lacerations), consult with a pediatric gynecologist or pediatric surgeon on the need for pelvic examination under anesthesia.

In boys, examine the penis and scrotum for bruises, swelling, teeth marks, erythema, or other signs of trauma. In both boys and girls, spread the buttocks with both hands to

Table 19-2. Possible laboratory studies in sexual abuse

Neisseria gonorrhoeae cultures: oropharynx, vagina/urethra, rectum

Chlamydia trachomatis cultures: vagina/urethra, rectum

Clothing, hair, fingernail scrapings, and other physical evidence

Serum pregnancy test (if appropriate)

HIV testing (depending on the locale and nature of the abuse)

Stool hematest (in cases of anal penetration)

If contact occurred within 96 hours:

 Detection of sperm: obtain specimens from the mouth/vagina/rectum, place the swaps in saline, then dry mount on slide

 Determination of blood group: saliva

examine the anus and perineal area. If there are obvious signs of physical injury or severe pain, anoscopy or sigmoidoscopy is indicated, under anesthesia if necessary.

Table 19-2 lists the specific laboratory evaluation of a sexually abused child. Obtain gonorrhea and chlamydial cultures from the cervix (postmenarchal), vagina (premenarchal), urethra, rectum, and pharynx if the symptoms of an STD are present. Examine vaginal specimens for the presence of *Trichomonas*. Obtain wet preps from all affected areas to look for sperm: mouth up to 6 hours after assault, rectum and vagina up to 96 hours. If a speculum exam is performed, obtain a Pap smear and ask the hospital laboratory to specifically note the presence of sperm. Immotile sperm are present up to 2½ weeks after intercourse. Obtain a pregnancy test on all pubertal females, but do not obtain a VDRL; a positive result can be used as damaging evidence during subsequent court proceedings. Encourage HIV testing (at 1 month, 6 months, and 1 year after contact), especially in areas of high incidence or if the perpetrator has any risk factors for HIV infection.

ED management

If the alleged perpetrator is a family member or someone with family-like contact with the child, report the suspected sexual abuse to the CPS. It is not the responsibility of the ED staff to determine whether or not the abuse actually occurred. In many jurisdictions, child sexual abuse is also reported to the police. Make careful documentation, in writing, of all findings on the physical exam; diagrams and drawings are very useful. Take photographs of any bruises or other evidence of physical injury. Label all specimens taken for evidence, and place them in evidence envelopes to be logged and secured by the security department of the hospital or given directly to the police. Ensure that the chain of legal evidence is unbroken.

Give treatment for gonorrhea and chlamydial infections as outlined in Table 12-4 (Sexually transmitted diseases, pp. 320–325) if there is a high suspicion of infection or if the patient is not likely to return (emancipated minor).

Offer a postcoital contraceptive to the postmenarchal adolescent girl who is seen within 72–120 hours. Plan B (levonorgestrel) and Preven (ethinyl estradiol and levonorgestrel) are two FDA-approved emergency contraceptives that are given in two doses, 12 hours apart. Alternatively, "off-label" formulations of typical oral contraceptives may also be used as emergency contraceptives, as shown in Table 19-3.

Table 19-3. FDA-approved and oral contraceptives for use as emergency contraception

Brand	Pills per dose[a]
Plan B (FDA-approved)	1 white pill
Preven (FDA-approved)	2 blue pills
Alesse	5 pink pills
Aviane	5 orange pills
Levlen	4 light orange pills
Levlite	5 pink pills
Levora	4 white pills
Low-Ogestrel	4 white pills
Lo/Ovral	4 white pills
Nordette	4 light orange pills
Ogestrel	2 white pills
Ovral	2 white pills
Ovrette	20 yellow pills
Tri-Levlen	4 yellow pills
Triphasil	4 yellow pills
Trivora	4 pink pills

Note: [a]Emergency contraception treatment consists of 2 doses taken 12 hours apart. Give the first dose within 72–120 hours of the sexual assault/abuse.

Reassure the child that his or her body is not harmed, that he or she was not responsible for the sexual assault, and that you believe the patient and will do everything to protect him or her from further assault. Some victims and parents may need reassurance that the encounter will not alter the child's sexual preference in the future.

Follow-up

- Within 1–2 days, with a skilled psychotherapist or child abuse specialist
- With a physician in 2 weeks (for repeat cultures) and in 6 weeks (to obtain a VDRL)

Indications for admission

- Sexual abuse that occurred very near the home or when the patient's family is unable to provide the necessary support
- Active vaginal or rectal bleeding

Bibliography

Adams JA, Kaplan RA, Starling SP, et al: Guidelines for medical care of children who may have been sexually abused. *J Pediatr Adolesc Gynecol* 2007;20:163–72.

American Academy of Pediatrics Committee
on Adolescence: Emergency contraception.
Pediatrics 2005;116:1026–35.

Kellogg N: American Academy of
Pediatrics Committee on Child Abuse
and Neglect: The evaluation of sexual

abuse in children. *Pediatrics* 2005;
116:506–12.

Watkeys JM, Price LD, Upton PM, Maddocks A:
The timing of medical examination
following an allegation of sexual abuse:
is this an emergency? *Arch Dis Child*
2008t;93:851–6.

Chart documentation in child abuse

Medical professionals conducting evaluations of children suspected of being abused must assume that the medical record will be subpoenaed and be subjected to close scrutiny. Thus, all documentation needs to be legible, thorough, and objective. This includes a clear and careful recording of the detailed medical history, interview, physical findings, impression, and plan.

Verbal evidence

The principal diagnostic component of the child abuse assessment lies in the history obtained from the parent, primary caretaker, and the child suspected of being abused. Always document the time and place of the interview and who was present. If a translator was involved, document his or her name and the language spoken.

When interviewing a child, use appropriate interviewing techniques, allow free narrative, ask nonleading and nonsuggestive questions, and use language suitable for the child's developmental level. Basic nonleading questions usually begin with "who," "how," "what," "when," "where" or "why"; these types of questions allow the patient the freedom to describe details of what happened without jeopardizing the integrity of the interview. For example, if the patient discloses that her stepfather touched her inappropriately, a leading follow-up question might be "Did he touch you on your vagina?" In contrast, a nonleading question might be phrased "Where did he touch you?" Record the patient's statements verbatim; do not correct grammatical errors or paraphrase the child. Use quotations as often as possible.

Statements made by a child are often considered "hearsay," a statement made out of court offered into evidence in order to establish the truth of the matter asserted in the statement. In other words, the child's words are offered in court to prove that what the child said is actually the truth. Generally, hearsay statements are not admissible in court, although exceptions to this rule exist. The two pertinent exceptions to the hearsay rule are the *Excited Utterance* exception and the *Medical Diagnosis or Treatment* exception. Documentation of the features that allow a statement to qualify as a hearsay exception increases the chances the child's words will be admissible in court.

Excited utterance

The excited utterance exception is a hearsay statement that relates to a stressful event. Three requirements are necessary for a statement to fall under this exception: the child must have experienced a stressful event, the child's statement must be associated with the event, and the child must still be experiencing the emotions caused by the event. Document in the chart the type of stressful event, the amount of time that passed between the event and when the child first made the statement, the child's speech, spontaneity and emotions, what questions led to the disclosure, and what was the first secure opportunity the child had to disclose.

Medical diagnosis or treatment exception

This relates to the belief that people are honest with medical professionals and therefore the information provided is trustworthy. Under this exception the information obtained in the medical history, including chief complaint, review of systems, past medical history, and the child's description of the cause of injury, are admissible in court.

It is also important to document the characteristics of the patient's statements that enhance their reliability, including the child's advanced knowledge of anatomy, description of distinctive sensory/visual details of sexual acts, and emotions displayed when the statement was made.

Documentation of the medical history

The medical record is a summary of the child abuse evaluation and is an essential part of this assessment. The information is most useful if it is obtained from the parents and the child separately. Include the following components in the medical record:

1. Birth history: include complications during delivery, traumatic birth, prematurity, etc.
2. Developmental history: if parents report that the child's injury was self-inflicted, try to corroborate the child's developmental capabilities (i.e. rolling over, climbing, etc.) that led to the injury. Note whether the examiner or another objective observer was able to substantiate the information provided.
3. Current medical conditions: note whether the child suffers from preexisting conditions that may be pertinent when conducting the abuse evaluation (e.g. lichen sclerosis).
4. Hospitalizations/injuries: note any hospitalizations, motor vehicle accidents, fractures, burns, or other serious injuries.
5. Surgeries: it is important to include anogenital surgeries or procedures that may have left residual findings.
6. Note the name of the child's primary care medical provider. Also obtain the patient's immunization record, as children who are abused may not be up to date with their vaccinations or have a regular healthcare provider.
7. Chief complaint:
   a. Interview with the parents. Clearly document the mechanism, time and place, and witnesses of the injury.
   b. Interview with the child. Ensure that the patient understands the importance of providing accurate information and that the purpose of the interview and examination is to provide diagnosis and treatment. In sexual abuse cases, the history from the child remains the single most important diagnostic feature in coming to the conclusion that a child has, in fact, been sexually abused (see verbal evidence above).
8. Review of systems: when evaluating a child for sexual abuse, pay particular attention to the genitourinary and gastrointestinal systems. Note the presence of specific symptoms and the time of presentation in relationship to the sexual contact. Ask about a history of vaginal pain, bleeding, discharge, vaginal foreign bodies, surgery, use of tampons, self-stimulation, history of genital trauma, dysuria, frequency, urgency, enuresis, and a history of urinary tract infections. Dysuria, pain and bleeding have been highly associated with genital-to-genital contact. Regarding the GI system, document any history of constipation, anal pain, bleeding, itching, hemorrhoids, encopresis, or infections.

9. Family history: include any condition that may be confused with abuse, such as osteogenesis imperfecta, bleeding disorders, etc.

10. Social history: document the names of the child's caretakers, other people residing in the home, and the alleged offender, as well as his/her relationship to the patient. This information will help determine whether it is safe for the patient to go home.

Documentation of the physical examination

A thorough and complete physical examination is indicated for all children and adolescents suspected of being abused or neglected. Include the following in the medical record:

1. Growth parameters: these are especially important when evaluating a child for failure to thrive and possible neglect. Chart current values on a growth curve and compare them with previous measurements.

2. Describe the pattern, shape, location, size and color of any marks, bruises, burns, bites, scars, and/or other lesions suggestive for abuse. Areas of the body frequently unnoticed during the physical examination are the frenulum of the tongue and lips, pinna, scalp, and medial aspects of arms and legs.

3. Include all positive and pertinent negative findings (e.g. no retinal hemorrhages noted in a child with suspected inflicted head trauma).

Emergency medical providers may need to perform examinations on children suspected of being sexually abused when a child abuse expert is not immediately available. In order to properly document genital findings, refer to the American Professional Society on the Abuse of Children published guidelines for standardized language to describe normal, and variants of normal and abnormal genital findings. Use the clock face to describe the location of the injury. The 12 o'clock position is anterior (urethra being 12 o'clock). The anal examination can be performed in the lateral decubitus, supine, or knee-chest position. Document the following about the anogenital examination:

1. Position in which the patient was examined (e.g. supine, knee-chest).

2. Tanner stage.

3. Any use of magnification (colposcope or other magnifying instrument).

4. Whether the exam was photographed or videotaped (see below, under "photographic documentation").

5. Each anatomical structure (labia, clitoris, vestibule, hymen, fossa navicularis, posterior fourchette, vagina). Mention the presence or absence of lesions, bruises, petechiae, etc. (for example, "hymen with a tear at 6 o'clock, the tear extends to the fossa navicularis").

6. The shape of the hymen (crescentic, annular, redundant, etc.). Make note of the presence of warts, bruises, tears, petechiae, and/or ecchymoses (e.g. "hymen crescentic-shaped with an acute complete transection at 6 o'clock, few petechiae noted at 3 and 5 o'clock"). Avoid terms like "virginal" or "intact."

7. Utilize body and/or genital diagrams demonstrating the site and type of injury.

8. Any anal tags, fissures, bruises, lacerations, scars, rashes, discharge, bleeding, and/or other lesions. Note the normal variants of the anal examination so that these are not confused with abnormal findings.

9. For the male genitalia, a description of the penis and scrotum, noting the presence of circumcision and any hematomas, lacerations, scars, ecchymoses, rashes, discharge, erythema, and/or other lesions.

Photographic documentation

Documentation of medical findings with photographs is an essential element of the child abuse evaluation. Photographs give clinicians an opportunity for later review of the medical findings; in some cases additional information initially overlooked may be found. If a second opinion is sought, the photos can be reviewed instead of having the child endure repeated examinations. In court, photographs provide a visual impact that may surpass the best-written chart. In addition, photographs can be used to compare examinations over time.

It is the role of the medical personnel caring for the child to photograph the injuries found. Before taking a picture, explain to the child in simple language what is going to happen, who will see the pictures, and why pictures are being taken. Label the photographs, including the date, patient's name, identification number, date of birth, the area being photographed, and the name of the photographer. Take an identifying picture of the child's face and as many pictures as needed of each injury, including an anatomic landmark. The inclusion of a knee, elbow or other body part identifies the location of the injury. When the child presents with burns, it is particularly important to take pictures before a dressing is applied. For bite marks, take the photograph such that the angle of the camera lens is directly over and perpendicular to the plane of the bite to avoid distortion. Include in the picture a measuring device. The ABFO No. 2 reference scale was developed specifically for this purpose as well as for documenting patterned injuries. Photo- or video-colposcopy is helpful for documenting the genital exam. However, photographs are not a substitute for body diagrams and a detailed description of the injury. Although digital photography is now widely utilized for legal reasons, one must not change the images in any way. Each institution must have a policy for photographing, storing, releasing, and handling pictures.

Documentation of laboratory and radiologic tests

Document the results of all laboratory tests performed. If cultures for sexually transmitted infections (STIs) are taken, document the type of culture and the site from which it was obtained (e.g. vagina, rectum). At the present time, cultures are still the gold standard for evaluating STIs in children suspected of being sexually abused. Follow the Centers for Disease Control/American Academy of Pediatrics recommendations for testing children and adolescents in the context of sexual abuse. Include in the medical record the interpretations of radiographs, MRIs, and CT scans performed. Order a skeletal survey, looking for occult fractures acute or chronic, for any child under the age of two with evidence or strong suspicion of abuse.

Impression and plan

1. Clearly document the disclosure of abuse and findings of the physical examination. Avoid using terms such as "alleged sexual assault" or "rule out abuse." It is important to note that a normal genital or anal examination does not exclude sexual abuse and that most sexually abused children do not have medical findings.
2. List any medications prescribed, including indications, length of treatment, and potential side effects.
3. If a report to child protective services was made, state the name of the child protective worker and any detectives or police officers involved.

4. In acute sexual abuse/assault cases in which forensic evidence was collected, the name and badge number of the police officer receiving the forensic evidence must be documented. It is of utmost importance to maintain the "chain of custody" at all times.

5. Increasing rates of adolescent sexual assault has been associated with the availability of drugs used to incapacitate the victim. If "rape drugs" are suspected, collect a drug-facilitated sexual assault kit with the adolescent's signed consent. Maintaining the chain of custody is vital.

6. In those cases when collected evidence is not immediately handed to the police, follow hospital policy for storing, discarding, and releasing the evidence.

7. If other providers were consulted, state their recommendations clearly.

8. Arrange an appointment for medical follow-up to discuss results of the tests performed, repeat certain tests, or repeat a physical examination, if necessary.

9. Document whether a referral was made to a specialized program for a sexual or physical abuse evaluation. In most cases of sexual abuse, a comprehensive evaluation including a detailed genital examination can be deferred until a later date in a more appropriate setting. Consult the hospital's Child Protection Team or affiliated Child Advocacy Center.

10. Offer a follow-up mental health appointment to all abused children and their families.

11. Collaborate with child protective and law enforcement agents to establish the safest environment for the child. A representative for child protective services will determine whether the child may stay at home or should be placed in foster care temporarily.

Bibliography

Adams JA: Guidelines for medical care of children evaluated for suspected sexual abuse: an update for 2008. *Curr Opin Obstet Gynecol* Oct 2008;20:435–41.

DeLago C, Deblinger E, Schroeder C, Finkel MA: Girls who disclose sexual abuse: urogenital symptoms and signs after genital contact. *Pediatrics* 2008;122:e281–6.

Finkel MA: Sexual abuse: the medical evaluation. In Giardino AG, Alexander R (eds), *Child Maltreatment: A Clinical Guide and Reference*, 3rd ed. St Louis, MO: GW Medical Publishing, 2005, pp. 253–88.

Waller EM, Daniel AE: Purpose and utility of child custody evaluations: the attorney's perspective. *J Am Acad Psychiatry Law* 2005;33:199–207.

Medical testimony and court preparation

The testimony of a medical provider can be one of the most critical pieces of evidence supplied to the court in cases of child abuse and maltreatment. Typically, abuse cases, and child sexual abuse cases in particular, are difficult to prove. Attorneys rarely have the luxury of providing the court with eyewitness accounts of the incident in question. Cases may not be heard by the court for months or even years, while children may be reluctant to speak about the abuse until much later in their lives. Many times, even where abuse has occurred, there may be no medical findings as anticipated or expected by the jury or judge. The medical provider's observations and documentation of observations, at the time of care, are of critical importance to the adjudication of these matters. Therefore, the testimony of the medical provider who cared for the child may be pivotal in the final determination of the matter before the court.

Medical providers are mandated reporters of suspected child abuse and maltreatment. As such, they have both an ethical and legal responsibility to participate in and cooperate with any investigatory and/or court process. Medical providers may be subpoenaed to testify in two distinct venues. One such venue is Family Court (for civil cases), where the focus will be on determining the safe placement of the child; alternatively, the case may be tried as a criminal matter, in Criminal Court, where the court will make a factual determination and decide upon a verdict of guilty or not guilty. In either case, the role of the medical provider remains essentially the same.

Expert qualification

A medical provider may testify at trial as an expert in the field of child abuse only after the court qualifies her or him to do so. The expert brings his or her experience and knowledge to the case, and as such plays an important role in helping the court reach a proper verdict. There is a foundational threshold that must be met in court in order for the medical provider to be deemed an expert. To accomplish this, the court must be shown that the individual has knowledge and experience beyond the realm of the average layperson. Having been qualified at previous trials does not automatically ensure one's qualification at future court proceedings.

The subpoenaing attorney will prepare the provider for this portion of the proceeding. Advance preparation is essential to ensure that the qualification process is completed without incident. The qualification process assumes a series of questions posed by both attorneys and court. This portion of the proceeding is called a *voir dire*. The provider must provide his or her current curriculum vitae, which will serve as a vital source of information for both the attorneys and the court. The medical provider should also review all questions that he or she will be asked by the subpoenaing attorney as well as any hypothetical questions that may arise, and be prepared to explain any technical terminology that may be used in the trial. In addition, the potential expert must be able to discuss his or her practical experience in the field and all authored publications, including why and how they differ from other respected publications and treatises.

Proper preparation is crucial also in readying the provider for the qualification process or *voir dire*. Both attorneys will question the provider as to his or her qualifications. The subpoenaing attorney will ask direct questions. Once completed, the opposing counsel is provided an opportunity to cross-examine the provider on the topic of their qualifications as an expert. At this juncture, cross-examination will be limited to questions about the medical provider's experience and knowledge in the field. The ultimate purpose of *voir dire* is to either confirm or prevent qualification of the provider as an expert in the field. At the end of this portion of the proceeding, the court will be asked to deem the provider expert.

Factual witness

In addition to providing general expertise, medical testimony serves a second function of eliciting factual evidence, including details of patient interviews and/or medical procedures performed by the provider. Not uncommonly, the only witness to the alleged incident is the victim; in such cases, the medical provider's testimony can substantially influence the outcome of the case. In some instances, the provider is the first person to whom the child disclosed the abuse. A detailed record of the patient interview is therefore crucial.

The provider must show documentation not only of the patient's exact statements, but also of the circumstances surrounding the disclosure. Include all observations made, both medical and nonmedical in nature, during the course of patient treatment and care. More credibility and weight may be given to the medical provider's testimony if he or she is able to provide extensive details of the interview (see Child abuse, pp. 587–589).

Any cross-examination will attempt to discredit the testimony by showing that the patient's statements were, in fact, misunderstood, fabricated, or otherwise tainted through inappropriate or misguided interviews. The fewer details documented by the provider, the more likely that opposing counsel will be able to weaken the case by injecting doubt into the minds of the court or jury. Cross-examination is distinctly different in nature from a direct examination, in which a witness is allowed relative freedom to explain any findings and observations. During cross-examination, opposing counsel may attempt to discredit and/or confuse the witness with a barrage of questions. In a criminal matter, opposing counsel is under no legal obligation to affirmatively put forth a case. As a result, cross-examination is often the venue by which opposing counsel presents their version of events or theory of the case to the judge or jury. Proper preparation and thorough review of all medical documentation by the provider will ease a witness's tension and anxiety.

The provider's only objective during testimony is to answer questions posed by either attorney in a clear and direct manner. If, during the course of testimony, the provider does not understand a question, she or he may ask the examining attorney to repeat or rephrase the question. The role of the provider during trial is simply to state the facts as they are known while preserving the integrity of the testimony. Regardless of his or her personal feelings, the provider must remain as unbiased and unprejudiced as possible. It is the role of the attorney, not the provider, to object when there is an evidentiary or legal problem with the testimony; the judge will then determine whether to sustain or overrule the objection.

Impact of documentation upon court proceedings

Opposing counsel may call into question the notes and observations of a medical provider during a court proceeding. Therefore, it is crucial that medical providers always document patient interviews so as to preserve details for future court testimony. Medical providers must be especially careful when interviewing children and ask only open-ended and nonleading questions (see p. 587).

In addition to documenting details of the actual disclosure, medical providers' records must include the circumstances in which the patient first presented to medical care, how and when the disclosure was made, who was present at the time of the disclosure, where the disclosure was made, the physical state of the patient (i.e. nervous, calm, shifting in seat, eyes downcast, etc.), and observations of any family members present with the child. Information that may not seem pertinent at the time of the initial interview with the patient may be precisely the detail sought at trial. In addition, there may be a long delay before a trial starts and without proper documentation the provider may be unable to recall clearly the details of the interview and circumstances during trial.

It is equally important to document all aspects of medical procedures performed on the child. For instance, if the child discloses sexual abuse and a "Rape Trauma Kit" is collected, it is crucial to include not only the details of the interview and examination, but also to whom the kit was given, so that the attorney(s) can trace the "chain of custody" of the evidence at trial. Documentation of the proper handling of physical evidence will support the premise that there has been no tampering with the evidence.

While medical providers are accustomed to speaking and writing in medical shorthand, the average layperson is not accustomed to such language. The testimony of a medical witness/expert can be difficult for the jury to understand. If the medical provider must use technical language, he or she should always define and explain the terms. If the testimony is complicated and/or confusing, ask the attorney to provide visual aids, which facilitate the jury's understanding and focus them on the topic at hand.

Bibliography

Evans AD, Lee K, Lyon TD: Complex questions asked by defense lawyers but not prosecutors predicts convictions in child abuse trials. *Law Hum Behav* 2009; 33: 258–64.

Holcomb MJ, Jacquin KM: Juror perceptions of child eyewitness testimony in a sexual abuse trial. *J Child Sex Abus* 2007;16:79–95.

Palusci VJ, Hicks RA, Vandervort FE: "You are hereby commanded to appear": pediatrician subpoena and court appearance in child maltreatment. *Pediatrics* 2001;107:1427–30.

Abandonment and physical neglect

Abandonment of infants and small children is the most extreme form of parental neglect. Abandoned children may suffer physical and psychological harm unless there is immediate and appropriate intervention. Other forms of neglect may be less pervasive as parents fail to meet a child's need for food, clothing, shelter, medical care, education, or supervision. The long-term effects of neglect may be more injurious than those of abuse, since the indolent nature of neglect causes it to be underreported and uncorrected.

Clinical presentation and diagnosis

Every abandoned child must undergo a thorough physical examination, with particular attention to a general assessment of the state of hydration, nutrition, body temperature, and hygiene. Undress and examine the child thoroughly for physical stigmata of abuse or neglect.

ED management

The first priority is to try to locate the parent or another family member known to the child. Then perform the physical examination and obtain appropriate laboratory studies to document any harm resulting from abandonment and to find any treatable conditions. The next step is to report this form of child neglect to the local CPS and/or police, depending on local child abuse reporting laws and protocols.

Disposition options in the management of an abandoned child include transfer to the custody of a relative who is judged suitable by the CPS worker or placement in temporary shelter or foster care. However, if medical care is necessary, or if community-based resources do not exist, admit the child to the hospital. In most states, abandoned children who are referred to the local CPS may be legally placed, on a temporary basis, in another home without a court order. Proper court proceedings must follow to justify the continuation of this emergency placement.

In the ED, parents who have abandoned their child may be extremely defensive and at times hostile to the ED staff. Do not induce further hostility by raising the levels of parental guilt or fear. Instead, focus on the mutual concern for the child.

For children with neglect short of abandonment, meticulously document the aspects and findings of neglect and refer the family to their primary care provider.

Indications for admission
- Abandoned child who requires medical care
- Abandoned child when community placement resources do not exist

Bibliography

Dubowitz H, Bennett S: Physical abuse and neglect of children. *Lancet* 2007;369:1891–9.

Dubowitz H: Tackling child neglect: a role for pediatricians. *Pediatr Clin North Am* 2009;56:363–78.

Legano L, McHugh MT, Palusci VJ: Child abuse and neglect. *Curr Probl Pediatr Adolesc Health Care* 2009;39:31.e1–26.

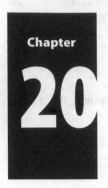

Psychological and social emergencies

Stephen Ludwig, Mary Mehlman, and Scott Miller

Contributing author
Daniel Mason: Psychiatric emergencies and *Suicide*

Death in the emergency department

The loss of a child has a devastating effect on a family, particularly when it is unexpected or without any readily identifiable cause. These families do not have the opportunity for "preparatory grief." Proper ED management is critical to the family's long-term adjustment.

Clinical presentation and diagnosis

When the ED is notified of the transport of a child in extremis, assign a resuscitation team member to work with the parents. Take the parents to a quiet area not far from the resuscitation scene, and have that team member act as a liaison to keep the family informed. In some centers, parents may be allowed in the resuscitation room, but a staff member who can interpret the events must accompany them.

At the time of the child's death, notify the parents privately, clearly, and directly. Specify the word "dead" to avoid any confusion. Avoid using euphemisms such as "He has passed." Once the death has been announced, the management phase begins.

ED management

Family members may display many emotional reactions, from hysterical screaming to anger to silence. All responses are normal. Once the immediate reaction has had time to occur, be available to answer any questions. There is no need for excuses, although parents may appreciate expressions of personal emotion and concern. Respond to parental expressions of guilt with a realistic appraisal of the circumstances. Gain history that may be helpful in establishing a diagnosis. If abuse is suspected, it will be confirmed at autopsy; there is no need to confront the grieving family.

Provide the family with assistance: phone, coffee, tissues. Do not assume that they want a particular relative or clergyman unless they so request.

Encourage parents to see the child's body once it has been prepared for their viewing (removal of medical equipment, soiled linen, etc.). Allow parents to hold the child's body and say their farewells. A prayer said over the body is a good way to bring closure after a brief period of contact with the child.

Inform the family of any requirements concerning an autopsy. In most states an autopsy is not mandated if the child had a chronic condition in which death was expected. If there are no requirements, encourage autopsy in order to answer any questions pertaining to the cause of death. Instruct a trusted family member or friend about hospital policy on claiming the body and other necessary arrangements.

Give the parents your name and phone number for follow-up questions and concerns, and document the chart and death certificate appropriately. Afterward, a brief staff meeting may pull staff members together and allow them to express their feelings.

Bibliography

Knapp. J, Mulligan-Smith D: Committee on Pediatric Emergency Medicine: Death of a child in the emergency department. *Pediatrics* 2005;115:1432–7.

Knazik SR, Gausche-Hill M, Dietrich AM, et al: The death of a child in the emergency department. *Ann Emerg Med* 2003t;42:519–29.

Parker-Raley J, Jones BL, Maxson RT: Communicating the death of a child in the emergency department: managing dialectical tensions. *J Healthc Qual* 2008;30:20–31.

Psychiatric emergencies

Although minor behavioral problems are common in pediatrics, true psychiatric emergencies are rare. However, with the relative lack of mental health services for children, the ED is often the portal of entry into the mental health system. The priorities in the ED are assessment of whether the patient is dangerous to him- or herself or others, and whether the family can adequately care for the child at home.

Clinical presentation

Depression

The depressed patient may present with recurrent somatic complaints (stomachaches, headaches, myalgias) for which no organic cause can be found. Sometimes depression can present with acting-out behavior, running away, stealing, fire-setting, or being accident-prone. Occasionally, the parent is concerned about a loss of appetite, poor school performance, or a change in the sleep pattern.

Psychosis

The psychotic patient, who cannot distinguish reality from fantasy, may present with a history of hallucinations, extreme variations in mood, and, occasionally, violent behavior. The adolescent with schizophrenia has delusions, auditory hallucinations, and inappropriate affect, although memory and orientation may remain intact.

Conduct disorders

The child with a conduct disorder acts out or behaves in an antisocial way. There are many psychodynamic factors in conduct disorder, and often the child will be brought to the ED by police or by parents unable to provide supervision. Although the use of drugs or alcohol may exacerbate conduct disorders, deviant or disruptive behavior usually occurs without such intoxicants.

Diagnosis and ED management

Depression

Somatic complaints with no identifiable organic basis, or changes in the patient's normal behavior or mood, suggest depression. Ask the patient how he or she is sleeping, whether or not he or she enjoys school, and what he or she does for fun. Ask about a family history of depression and suicide. Have the patient name his or her best friend and tell you when he or she last saw that person. Ask about future plans, hopes, and aspirations. If the patient appears to be depressed (loss of interest in school, friends, usual hobbies, sports), ask whether he or she has ever thought of committing suicide. Far from putting thoughts in the patient's mind, these types of questions may actually help the patient feel better, since he or she can now discuss something troubling. A patient who has considered suicide must be seen immediately by a psychiatrist or psychologist. If the suicidal ideation has reached the point of actual planning, hospitalization is indicated. Consider whether an organic disorder (hypothyroidism, anemia, diabetes, AIDS, CMV, EBV, Lyme disease, Addison's disease) may be making the patient depressed.

Psychosis

The first step is to rule out an organic origin for the psychosis. The most common organic cause is drug ingestion (LSD, PCP, Ecstasy, amphetamines, cocaine, anticholinergics, over-the-counter cough remedies). Teenagers who are "thrill seeking" will often experiment with polypharmacy, making their presentation and medical management complicated. Other causes of psychosis are hypoglycemia, increased intracranial pressure (tumor, brain abscess, arteriovenous malformation), temporal lobe seizures, encephalitis, porphyria, uremia, and Wilson's disease.

Ask about possible drug ingestion, and have the family bring in all medications in the home and from the homes of friends or relatives the patient has visited recently. Stimulants commonly used to treat ADHD have been known to trigger psychotic episodes, even at pharmacologic doses. Therefore, determine whether the patient has recently started taking a new medication. Inquire about a family history of schizophrenia, and try to determine when the symptoms were first noticed. With an organic psychosis, the onset is acute and the hallucinations are often visual, olfactory, tactile, or gustatory, rather than auditory. With schizophrenia and other functional psychoses, the hallucinations are typically auditory and the onset is more insidious.

On physical examination, there may be fever (anticholinergic or amphetamine ingestion, brain abscess, encephalitis), tachycardia (sepsis or anticholinergic, hallucinogen, or amphetamine ingestion), and hypertension (anticholinergic, amphetamines, cocaine, LSD, or PCP ingestion). The vital signs may be normal in patients with psychosis of functional origin. Note the pupillary size and reactivity; there may be inequality (mass lesion, brain abscess), mydriasis (hypoglycemia or LSD, amphetamine, cocaine, or anticholinergic ingestion), or miosis (cholinergic, opiate, or PCP ingestion).

Immediately order a CT scan for patients with any focal neurologic abnormalities, signs of increased intracranial pressure, or fever. Febrile patients require a lumbar puncture after the CT (if it is normal). Also obtain a CBC, electrolytes, serum glucose and Dextrostix, liver function tests, and urinalysis.

Unless an organic cause for the psychosis can be definitely ruled out in the ED, admit the patient to a pediatric service to continue the evaluation after consultation with a psychiatrist. Do not initiate antipsychotic medications in the ED unless a psychiatrist, who can provide the necessary close follow-up, has examined the patient. If sedation is required for agitation or uncontrolled acting out, use an agent listed in Table 20-1.

Table 20-1. Medications for restraint of uncontrolled patients

Drug	Dose
Haloperidol (Haldol)	1–10 mg IM q 30 min[a]
Risperidone	1–2 mg PO[a]
Quetiapine (Seroquel)	100–200 mg PO[a]
Ativan	0.5–1.0 mg IM/PO[b]

Note: [a]Up to three doses may be given, as needed.
[b] Give in combination with risperidone, quetiapine, or haloperidol.

Conduct disorder

In managing children with conduct disorder, the goals are to (1) ensure the safety of the child, family, and staff; (2) rule out medical conditions; and (3) gather information for appropriate disposition.

When the child is aggressive, the behavior must be controlled. If a medical condition or an intoxicant may be inducing the behavior, acute hospitalization is indicated. This is especially true of males with conduct disorder who are also abusing substances, as their suicide risk is increased. If the aforementioned conditions have been ruled out, psychiatric hospitalization is indicated to promote healthier ways of functioning.

Indications for admission

- Suicide attempt or gesture
- Depression with concrete suicidal plan (relative)
- Depression with inability to function
- Psychotic episode thought to be organic
- Conduct that will harm self or others
- Complications of substance abuse

Bibliography

American Academy of Pediatrics, Committee on Pediatric Emergency Medicine; American College of Emergency Physicians and Pediatric Emergency Medicine Committee, Dolan MA, Mace SE: Pediatric mental health emergencies in the emergency medical services system. *Pediatrics* 2006;118:1764–7.

Baren JM, Mace SE, Hendry PL, et al: Children's mental health emergencies–part 2: emergency department evaluation and treatment of children with mental health disorders. *Pediatr Emerg Care* 2008;24:485–98.

Elliott GR, Smiga S: Depression in the child and adolescent. *Pediatr Clin N Am* 2003;50:1093–106.

Sudden infant death syndrome

Sudden infant death syndrome (SIDS) is defined as "the sudden death of an infant or young child, unexpected by history, in which a thorough postmortem examination and death scene investigation fail to demonstrate an adequate cause for death." SIDS is the leading cause of death among infants 1 month to 1 year old.

Clinical presentation

The peak incidence is at 2–4 months, although there have been autopsy-proven occurrences up to 12 months of age. The incidence is higher in males, premature infants, and if the mother is a smoker, drug addict, or of lower socioeconomic status. Most cases occur between midnight and 9 a.m. during the cold-weather months. Typically, a previously healthy baby either does not awaken for a morning feed or is found cold and lifeless in the crib.

On occasion, the infant is found pale or cyanotic, apneic, or limp, and resuscitation is initiated at home or en route to the ED. It is not clear whether these near-miss episodes are part of the SIDS spectrum.

There have been many theories that attempt to explain the cause of SIDS. Prone positioning of infants during sleep has been most strongly implicated, and the incidence of SIDS in the USA has dramatically decreased since the advent of the "Back to Sleep" campaign. However, no single theory has been able to account for all cases of SIDS. In addition to "back to sleep," the American Academy of Pediatrics recommends use of a firm sleep surface, removal of soft objects and loose bedding from the crib, no co-sleeping, cessation of maternal smoking during and after pregnancy, offering a pacifier at sleep time, and avoidance of overheating. They also discourage sleep positioning devices and home monitors.

Diagnosis

SIDS is a diagnosis of exclusion and cannot be confirmed until an autopsy and other postmortem studies have ruled out other possible causes of sudden death in infancy, including adrenal insufficiency, overwhelming pneumonitis, bacterial sepsis (especially in sickle cell disease), child abuse, and poisoning. Near-miss episodes may also result from prolonged sleep apnea, gastroesophageal reflux-induced apnea, cardiac dysrhythmias, metabolic disorders, and seizures.

ED management

The management of the SIDS victim requires a detailed history of the circumstances surrounding the infant's death. An autopsy must be performed by the medical examiner. The management of a bereaved family is discussed on pp. 596–597.

If the resuscitation of a near-miss victim is successful, admit the infant to an ICU for continuous cardiopulmonary monitoring and further evaluation (see The critically ill infant, pp. 747–753). Obtain an ECG with rhythm strip, chest X-ray, and blood for a CBC with differential, electrolytes, glucose, and culture. Perform a lumbar puncture for cytology, chemistries, and culture, and obtain a urinalysis and urine culture.

Indication for admission

- Near-miss episode

Bibliography

American Academy of Pediatrics Task Force on Sudden Infant Death Syndrome: The changing concept of sudden infant death syndrome: diagnostic coding shifts, controversies regarding the sleeping environment, and new variables to consider in reducing risk. *Pediatrics* 2005;116:1245–55.

American Academy of Pediatrics, Hymel KP,
  Committee on Child Abuse and Neglect,
  National Association of Medical Examiners:
  Distinguishing sudden infant death

syndrome from child abuse fatalities.
Pediatrics 2006;118:421–7.

Moon RY, Horne RS, Hauck FR: Sudden infant
death syndrome. *Lancet* 2007;370:1578–87.

Suicide

Suicide is the third leading cause of death among teenagers, although it also occurs in younger children. Reported rates have steadily increased since the 1960s. Suicide gestures, which are seen more frequently in girls, are perhaps 100 times more common than successful suicides, which occur more often in boys. Girls are more likely to employ nonviolent methods (ingestion), whereas boys more often use violence (firearms, blades). Many suicides go undiagnosed and are attributed to accidental trauma.

Clinical presentation and diagnosis

Suicide usually occurs in a depressed patient. The attempt is usually triggered by a "crisis" situation, such as the death or departure of a loved one, a fight with a boyfriend or girlfriend, or an argument with a parent. There are a number of danger signals that may signify that a patient is potentially suicidal (Table 20-2).

In the ED, these patients may present as trauma or overdose victims, or in a coma of unknown origin. Every child older than 5 years who takes a medication overdose or ingests a household product (caustics, hydrocarbons, insecticides) is making a suicide attempt until proven otherwise.

Table 20-2. Findings suggesting a high risk of suicide

Recent previous suicide attempt
Multiple ED visits for trauma
Suicidal threat made
"Accidental" ingestion in child over 5 years old
Signs of depression
Medical concerns accompanied by depression
Recent withdrawal behavior
Exposure to violence
Underlying psychiatric condition:
Psychosis
Conduct disorder
Attention deficit disorder
Substance abuse
Mental retardation
Family history of suicide
Recent cluster of suicides in the community

ED management

The patient's clinical condition and the method of attempted suicide determine the priorities of ED management. However, most patients are well enough to be interviewed when first seen, although a suicidal patient requires continuous one-to-one observation. Assess the seriousness of the attempt. Greater "lethality" of intent is suggested by a previous suicide attempt, a plan to commit suicide, no communication of intent to others, no request for help after the attempt (discovered accidentally), and taking action that is clearly lethal (jumping from a rooftop). Differentiating between a suicide "attempt" and "gesture" is critical as the latter focuses on inflicting pain, but not death. Patients who perform suicide gestures use physical actions (cutting, scratching) to treat emotional distress and may not require hospitalization if they can be discharged into a safe environment with appropriate psychiatric follow-up.

Once medically stable, a child psychiatrist must evaluate all patients making suicidal gestures or attempts. Hospitalize those with medical complications in a pediatric unit. Admit patients who are medically stable to a psychiatric unit unless they have been cleared by a psychiatrist to be discharged home.

Follow-up

- Primary care follow-up in 1 week
- Psychiatric follow-up within 1 week

Indications for admission

- Suicide attempt that requires medical care
- All patients unless cleared for family-based care by a child psychiatrist

Bibliography

Baren JM, Mace SE, Hendry PL, et al: Children's mental health emergencies–part 2: emergency department evaluation and treatment of children with mental health disorders. *Pediatr Emerg Care* 2008;24:485–98.

Bridge JA, Goldstein TR, Brent DA: Adolescent suicide and suicidal behavior. *J Child Psychol Psychiatry* 2006;47:372–94.

Shain BN, Committee on Adolescence: Suicide and suicide attempts in adolescents. *Pediatrics* 2007;120:669–76.

Munchausen syndrome by proxy

Munchausen syndrome (MS) was first described in adults who subject themselves to diagnostic tests and therapeutic procedures in order to gain the safety and security of being hospitalized. Munchausen syndrome by proxy (MSBP) is a subset of the child abuse syndrome in which signs or symptoms of medical illnesses are either feigned by the parent or produced in the child, so that the parent and child can be hospitalized. It is therefore an extension of MS in adults. Similar psychopathology occurs in both; the difference is that in MSBP, the child is used by the parent as the focus of medical attention.

Clinical presentation

MSBP has many varied presenting signs and symptoms, including apnea, near-miss SIDS episodes, hematuria, hematochezia, hematemesis, fever, seizures, frequent infections, failure to thrive, hypoglycemia, and poisonings. Virtually any complaint can be feigned or artificially produced in MSBP. In some series, MSBP has a 10% mortality rate.

Diagnosis

A high index of suspicion is required to diagnose MSBP. Suspect it in any clinical situation that has baffled physicians at other centers or has a "one of a kind" dimension. The identified parental characteristics include a parent (the mother in 90% of cases) who has some medical background, is often by the bedside, appears very devoted, and is invested in the illness. MSBP parents are usually very intelligent, verbal, and appealing to the medical staff. Generally, it is the parent who notes the episodic nature of the signs and symptoms. In addition, the parent is usually distant from her spouse, and she may have a history of being a patient herself.

ED management

MSBP is rarely diagnosed in the ED, as careful observation over time is required. The ED staff should be alert to parents who seem to be frequent, inappropriate ED users or who seem to exaggerate their children's symptoms. If the diagnosis is suspected in the ED, admit the child and notify the child abuse team. Depending on the nature of the MSBP, there are many strategies for proving the diagnosis, including laboratory tests (blood type, insulin level, etc.), blood cultures, covert videotaping of the parent, monitoring devices, and limitation of parental visitation. If the ED staff can make the diagnosis of MSBP by direct observation, report the case to the child protection services and place the child in a protected environment.

Indication for admission

• Suspected victim of MSBP

Bibliography

Shaw RJ, Dayal S, Hartman JK, DeMaso DR: Factitious disorder by proxy: pediatric condition falsification. *Harv Rev Psychiatry* 2008;16:215–24.

Stirling J Jr and the Committee on Child Abuse and Neglect: Beyond Munchausen syndrome by proxy: identification and treatment of child abuse in a medical setting. *Pediatrics* 2007;120:1026–30.

Interpersonal violence

Interpersonal violence is an altercation between two or more non-caretaker individuals in which at least one of the participants intended to harm the other. These altercations frequently occur in the school, schoolyard, or street. However, it is not useful to apply the terms "victim" and "perpetrator," as the "victim" that presents to the ED may have instigated the fight that he or she subsequently "lost." It has recently been reported that as many as 25% of all adolescents seen in a pediatric ED were treated for injuries resulting from interpersonal violence.

In contrast, family violence, such as child abuse and domestic violence, is characterized by one individual having significant power over another within the relationship. While most healthcare systems have protocols for the management of family violence, there is no mandated reporting system for interpersonal violence.

Clinical presentation and diagnosis

Violently injured patients present with a wide range of injuries and injury severity. Prior to the interview, assure the patient that all responses are confidential, with the exception of

Table 20-3. Priorities in the evaluation of the violently injured patient

Circumstances	Safety issues
What caused the event	Retaliation plans by patient, family, friends[a]
Relationship to the other participants	Suicidal ideation[b]
Use or appearance of weapons at the scene	Access to weapons
Police involvement	Depression: long-term plans, presence of family and close friends

Note: [a] Requires immediate referral to police.
[b] Requires immediate referral to psychiatry and social work.

suicidal or homicidal statements and the disclosure of child abuse. Let the patient tell the story in his or her own words, in private, and listen nonjudgmentally. After the interview, ask the youth's permission to involve the family in the discussion. Enlisting the help of the family can often facilitate follow-up and ongoing support for the patient.

The responses to a few suitable questions can determine the need for immediate referral to social work, mental health, or law enforcement (Table 20-3). Clearly document these responses in the medical record. The legality of access to the medical record by law enforcement agencies varies among communities. Contact the hospital's legal counsel regarding local statutes and recommendations pertaining to documentation.

A thorough evaluation of the violently injured patient includes an understanding of what caused the violent event, the location and time of the event, the relationship of the patient to others involved in the incident, and the use or appearance of weapons at the scene. Explore issues related to the patient's safety. Ask specific questions regarding any intention to hurt themselves or others. Also inquire if a family member or friend plans to retaliate. Although open-ended questions such as, "Once you leave here, what are you going to do?" can clue a physician into potentially dangerous plans, ask directly about retaliation and suicidal thoughts. Similarly, ask the patient about drug selling, access to weapons, and possible gang affiliation. When present, these risk factors may predict the lethality of future actions. Inquire about the patient's friends and acquaintances when asking about substance use and abuse, in order to ascertain exposure to this lifestyle. If the youth admits to using marijuana or other drugs, ask why. Patient responses to these questions may expose the adolescent who is self-medicating his or her stress, anger, or depression.

Assess the patient's present emotional state and reaction to the trauma. Since there is a strong correlation between depression and the risk of violent injury, ask about the patient's long-term plans for the future and the presence or absence of close friends or family members as confidants and allies.

ED management

The primary goals of ED care of a violently injured youth are to stabilize the patient, ensure the immediate safety of the patient and other participants, and to assess the patient's risk for further injury. If the patient reveals suicidal or homicidal intent, contact a psychiatrist immediately. Also, the medical staff is obligated to contact the police if there are legitimate concerns about retaliation.

It is also important to assess and address the psychosocial comorbidities, including depression, substance abuse, school failure, and family violence. Refer a depressed or hopeless patient to a psychiatrist urgently. However, provide psychosocial support to all violently injured patients, regardless of the situation that caused the injury. Consult a social worker, who can help provide access to available community resources. Give contact information for appropriate crisis hotlines, community support groups, and available local shelters. Information about these resources is often also available from municipal social service agencies.

If the patient is being admitted, communicate any safety concerns to the inpatient medical and nursing staff, security officers, and social workers. One-to-one observation is necessary for suicidal or homicidal patients.

Follow-up
• Primary care follow-up in 1 week

Indication for admission
• Active suicidal or homicidal ideation

Bibliography

Cheng TL, Schwarz D, Brenner RA, et al: Adolescent assault injury: risk and protective factors and locations of contact for intervention. *Pediatrics* 2003;112:931–8.

Lin AJ, Raymond M, Catallozzi M, Ryan O, Rickert VI: Relationship violence in adolescence. *Adolesc Med State Art Rev* 2007;18:530–43.

Ozer EJ, Tschann JM, Pasch LA, Flores E: Violence perpetration across peer and partner relationships: co-occurrence and longitudinal patterns among adolescents. *J Adolesc Health* 2004;34:64–71.

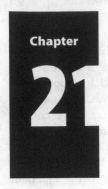

Pulmonary emergencies

Ellen F. Crain and Sergey Kunkov

Contributing author
Sandra J. Cunningham: Pulse oximetry

Asthma

Asthma is characterized by reversible hyperresponsiveness, obstruction, and inflammation of the lower airways. More than 10% of children are affected and, despite recent therapeutic advances, morbidity continues to be substantial, especially among inner-city residents.

Inflammation contributes to airway edema, abnormal mucociliary clearance, and mucous plugging. Following exposure to a triggering event, an acute asthma exacerbation has an early allergen response (EAR) phase, accompanied by the release of leukotrienes, and, in up to 50% of the cases, a late allergen response (LAR) phase, induced by T_h2 helper cells. Common triggers include irritants (cigarette smoke, gases), viral infections, weather changes, allergens (dust, animals), exercise, cold air, and emotional stress. Children with a history of bronchopulmonary dysplasia (BPD) or other acute lung injury (smoke inhalation, hydrocarbon ingestion, near-drowning) are at increased risk for hyperactive airways or asthma. The greatest risk of mortality is in children who have a history of respiratory failure or hypoxic seizures, are under-treated (at home or after a medical visit), or delay seeking medical attention.

Clinical presentation

Acute asthma presents with dyspnea, cough and expiratory and, to a lesser extent, inspiratory, wheezing. Children with cough-variant asthma have recurrent episodes of dry or productive cough and little or no wheezing. Airway obstruction can lead to retractions and decreased air entry, with little or no audible wheezing. Tachycardia, tachypnea, and, in severe attacks, cyanosis may be present; altered mental status (agitation, lethargy) occurs with impending ventilatory failure. Findings of a URI are also often present.

Complications

Atelectasis is common. Other respiratory complications are pneumomediastinum, which requires no specific treatment, and, rarely, pneumothorax, which may be under tension and require immediate evacuation. Respiratory failure may occur suddenly from large-airway collapse or exhaustion.

Diagnosis

Immediately evaluate a patient with a reported asthma exacerbation or wheezing. After the initial brief assessment, institute treatment promptly. While the first bronchodilator treatment is given, perform a focused history and physical examination related to the acute exacerbation. A more detailed history and physical examination can be delayed until after the initial therapy is given.

A trial of an inhaled β_2 agonist may simultaneously confirm the diagnosis and provide clinical improvement. Relief of airway obstruction occurs in <15 minutes (often <5 minutes), and peak flow typically improves by >20% from baseline. Less improvement may occur with severe or prolonged episodes associated with more inflammation, leaving the diagnosis uncertain unless the patient has a history of previous wheezing episodes. Laboratory studies do not help in establishing the diagnosis of asthma, and chest X-rays are not necessary for most first episodes of wheezing. A chest X-ray occasionally may be indicated in the setting of localized posttreatment findings in association with significant tachypnea (rate >60/min in infants, >40/min in older children) or persistent tachycardia (rate >160/min) 20–30 minutes after the completion of a β_2 agonist treatment in an afebrile child.

Inquire about a history of prematurity, mechanical ventilation, BPD, previous wheezing episodes, or heart disease. Check for a family history of asthma, recurrent bronchitis, eczema, allergic rhinitis, or other allergies.

Consider the possibility of complicating factors or a diagnosis other than asthma if a child or infant has protracted (>3 days), recurrent, or persistent localized wheezing in the face of adequate therapy for asthma. See Table 21-1 for the differential diagnosis and Table 21-2 for selected risk factors for death from asthma.

ED management
Acute treatment
Rapidly assess the airway and breathing, measure the peak expiratory flow rate (PEFR) in all children >5–6 years of age, and determine whether the patient has mild, moderate, or severe asthma (Table 21-3). To facilitate evaluation of the PEFR and changes following therapy, always record the PEFR as a percent of the child's predicted normal PEFR from a table of standards by height or best value (if known), rather than an absolute number. Provide supplemental oxygen (40% by mask) to a patient with moderate wheezing; use 100% oxygen if the attack is severe. The supplemental oxygen is important for treating hypoxemia; some patients may have an initial drop in pO_2 during β_2 agonist therapy due to ventilation-perfusion (V/Q) mismatch, particularly if the aerosol is administered with room air rather than oxygen. Monitor a severely ill patient with pulse oximetry, provide continuous albuterol nebulization, IV access for steroids and magnesium sulfate if the breath sounds are barely audible and do not improve within 5–10 minutes following the initial therapy.

Inhaled β_2 agonists
Give 0.15 mg/kg (2.5 mg minimum; 5 mg maximum) of albuterol every 20 minutes for 3 doses then, 0.15–0.3 mg/kg every 1–4 hours as needed for mild to moderate exacerbations. Substitute 4–8 puffs of an albuterol MDI (90 mcg/puff) with a spacer every 20 minutes for nebulized albuterol if the patient is cooperative. For severe exacerbations, give 0.5 mg/kg/hr by continuous administration. Levalbuterol does not appear to provide superior therapeutic effect or diminish adverse effects (tachycardia, tremulousness, etc.); use it only for patients with a history of extreme tachycardia following albuterol administration. The efficacy of albuterol is comparable to that of epinephrine, but with fewer side effects and no painful injection. Onset of action is within 5 minutes and the duration is 4–6 hours. Repeat doses are given every 20–30 minutes until no further improvement is noted in peak flow, oxygen saturation, or respiratory rate.

Table 21-1. Differential diagnosis of asthma

Diagnosis	History	Physical examination	Radiography/laboratory
Upper-airway obstruction			
Croup	Cough	Barking cough	"Steeple" sign
	Fever	Inspiratory stridor	Radiographs usually unnecessary
Foreign-body aspiration	Choking episode	Upper: inspiratory stridor	Radioopaque object
		Lower: localized wheezing	Expiration: contralateral mediastinal shift
Laryngotracheomalacia	May be present from birth	Degree of stridor depends on body positioning	Laryngo- or bronchoscopy usually diagnostic
Retropharyngeal abscess	Fever	Drooling	Lateral neck: wide retropharyngeal space
		Inspiratory stridor	
Vascular rings/ laryngeal webs		Localized wheeze	Bronchoscopy usually diagnostic
Vocal cord dysfunction	Adolescents	Monophasic wheeze that is loudest over glottis	
	May have psych history	Can mimic severe asthma attack	
Lower-airway obstruction			
Atypical pneumonia (*Mycoplasma, Chlamydia*)	Cough	Bilateral wheezing	Patchy bilateral infiltrates
	Fever		40–50% with (+) cold agglutinins
Cardiac asthma		Tachycardia, heart murmur	Cardiomegaly
		Hepatomegaly	Pulmonary overperfusion
		Pedal edema	
Cystic fibrosis	Malabsorption		
	Failure to thrive		↑Sweat chloride
	Excessive salt loss		
Gastroesophageal reflux	Nighttime cough	Bilateral wheezing, poorly responsive to bronchodilators	

Table 21-2. Selected risk factors for death from asthma

Previous severe asthma exacerbation necessitating ICU care or intubation

Two or more hospitalizations in the past year

Hospitalization or ED visit for asthma during past month

Difficulty in perceiving asthma symptoms

Low socioeconomic status or inner-city residence

Psychological/psychiatric problems

Table 21-3. Clinical severity classification of acute asthma

	Symptoms	Peak expiratory flow rate
Mild	Dyspnea only during activity	≥70% predicted or personal best
Moderate	Dyspnea interferes with usual activity	40–69% predicted or personal best
Severe	Dyspnea at rest	<40% predicted or personal best
	Interferes with speech	
Life-threatening	Too dyspneic to speak	<25% predicted or personal best

Source: Adopted from *Guidelines for the Diagnosis and Management of Asthma*, National Heart, Lung, and Blood Institute, 2007.

Subcutaneous epinephrine and terbutaline

A dose of subcutaneous epinephrine or terbutaline may be given for severe attacks (peak flow <15% predicted or nearly absent breath sounds) when aerosolized medication may not reach the target small airways. For epinephrine the dose is 0.01 mL/kg to 0.3 mL maximum of the 1:1,000 preparation; for terbutaline, use 0.01 mL/kg up to 0.25 mL maximum. It is no longer recommended to give up to three repeated injections. Common side effects of epinephrine injection include nausea, palpitations, tachycardia, agitation, tremor, and, less frequently, hypertension and ventricular dysrhythmias. Terbutaline may cause less nausea and vomiting. Simultaneously begin nebulized β_2 agonist treatments.

Corticosteroids

Promptly give an oral dose of a corticosteroid if the patient meets any of the following criteria:

- requires two or more β_2 agonist aerosol treatments to meet criteria for discharge
- oxygen saturation is <93% on any assessment
- >2 days of coughing or awakening from sleep due to asthma in the past week
- chronically uses (every day or every other day) oral corticosteroids
- ED visit within the past 2 weeks, has had a past ICU admission
- hospitalized (for asthma) within the past 2 weeks
- three or more hospitalizations during the past year.

Use prednisone or prednisolone, 1–2 mg/kg (40 mg maximum) or dexamethasone 0.6 mg/kg (10 mg maximum). If the patient cannot tolerate oral medication, give IM dexamethasone (same dose as above). For a patient with impending respiratory failure, give a bolus of IV methylprednisolone (2 mg/kg, 125 mg maximum, followed by 1 mg/kg q 6 h).

Ipratropium bromide

Ipratropium bromide is a quaternary ammonium congener of atropine. Anticholinergic agents produce bronchodilatation by antagonizing the activity of acetylcholine at the level of its receptors, particularly those found on airway smooth muscle. Compared to inhaled β agonists, the effect on airway obstruction is modest and generally results in approximately a 10% improvement in FEV_1. Some asthmatics with severe airway obstruction may respond better to a combination of inhaled albuterol and ipratropium than to albuterol alone. Dilute albuterol (0.03 mL/kg) in a vial of ipratropium (250 mcg < 12 years of age or 500 mcg >12 years of age). Give three consecutive ipratropium-albuterol inhalations to a patient whose asthma score or PEFR fails to improve after the initial albuterol treatment. The onset of action of ipratropium is relatively slow (20 minutes), and the peak effect occurs in about 60 minutes.

Ipratropium, unlike atropine, is poorly absorbed across mucous membranes and has little toxicity at the stated dose. In particular, it does not inhibit mucociliary clearance. However, there are infrequent reports of paradoxical bronchoconstriction with the administration of anticholinergic agents to some asthmatics. Monitor the patient carefully, and stop the nebulization if there are any signs or symptoms of worsening asthma.

Magnesium sulfate

The IV administration of magnesium sulfate may be useful for a patient whose condition worsens or fails to improve significantly (peak flow increases <50% from presentation and is <60% of predicted, intercostal retractions persist, or oxygen saturation <93%) after administration of β agonists and systemic corticosteroids. Mechanisms of action include inhibition of calcium channels in airway smooth muscle, blockade of calcium-mediated muscle contraction, reduction in acetylcholine release from neuromuscular end plates, parasympathetic-induced airway smooth-muscle constriction, and inhibition of histamine-induced bronchospasm.

The dose is 40 mg/kg (3 g maximum) in 50 mL of normal saline administered IV over 30 minutes. Side effects include hypotension, mild sedation, and cutaneous flushing; do not use the drug in patients with significant hypotension or renal failure. Monitor the blood pressure every 10 minutes during the infusion and every 30 minutes thereafter for 4 hours, but do not stop the infusion for mild reductions in blood pressure in the absence of hypotensive symptoms.

Hydration

Encourage oral fluids; provide IV hydration if the patient is seriously ill. However, limit IV hydration to maintenance plus replacement of ongoing losses. Assess the hydration status, obtain blood for electrolytes when placing the IV line, and monitor for the syndrome of inappropriate ADH excess (pp. 186–189) if a patient with severe asthma (absent or minimal breath sounds, PEFR <15% of expected) has been vomiting or drinking poorly.

Intravenous terbutaline

Although IV administration of β agonists may not offer any significant advantage over continuously administered aerosols, consider IV terbutaline for a patient with impending respiratory failure as manifested by continued poor air exchange, CNS depression, or rising pCO_2 (>50 mmHg with pH <7.3). A terbutaline infusion requires frequent ABGs as well as either continuous intraarterial or noninvasive blood pressure measurement. Start with 0.4 mcg/ kg per min, and increase by 0.1–0.2 mcg/kg every 15 minutes until a clinical response is achieved (improved air entry or 10% reduction in pCO_2) or a serious complication ensues (hypotension).

Heliox

Heliox (a mixture of helium and oxygen) can be used as a nebulizing agent for albuterol when there has been a poor response to conventional therapy. Heliox provides a low-density gas mixture which can decrease turbulence in air flow through constricted airways and improve gas exchange and albuterol delivery. Request heliox (70% helium/30% oxygen) in a premixed tank from the respiratory therapy department, then administer a continuous nebulization of albuterol via nonrebreathing mask at 10 L/min. Discontinue heliox if the oxygen saturation is <93% and initiate treatment with 100% oxygen.

Mechanical ventilation

If the above-described therapy fails to achieve adequate oxygenation, endotracheal intubation and mechanical ventilation are necessary. Use ketamine (1–2 mg/kg) to provide sedation and bronchodilatation. In general, use smaller tidal volumes than average (6–8 mL/kg instead of the standard 10 mL/kg) on a volume-preset ventilator, with normal-to-somewhat-lower respiratory rates for age, and long expiratory times. The required inspiratory pressures can exceed 50–60 cm. Assess breath sounds and obtain an ABG. Permissive hypercapnia may lessen the risk of barotrauma; limit the goal of mechanical ventilation to incomplete correction of the respiratory acidosis (pCO_2 >50–60 mmHg). An intubated asthmatic will usually require a sedative (midazolam 0.1–0.3 mg/kg IV q 1–2 h, 5 mg maximum) and a neuromuscular relaxant (vecuronium 0.05–0.1 mg/kg IV q 1–2 h, 10 mg maximum) to minimize barotrauma.

Aminophylline

Aminophylline (85% theophylline) is a potent bronchodilator, but it adds little to the effects of inhaled β_2 agonists during an acute episode. IV aminophylline is therefore not indicated in the ED treatment of status asthmaticus.

Discharge management

A patient with acute asthma can be discharged home when the peak flow is >60–70% predicted for height, the oxygen saturation is >92% in room air, wheezing is minimal, and there are no signs of significant obstruction (retractions, tachypnea, decreased air entry). Ensure that the parent can give the medications confidently, knows how to use a spacer device with an MDI, can monitor the child frequently, and is able to return to the ED if necessary. Ongoing bronchodilator therapy is usually necessary for 2 weeks. Review all medications for home use with the parent and child and have the patient demonstrate proper use of the MDI (if one was prescribed). Be sure that the family has a written action plan for worsening symptoms and a follow-up appointment within a week or two of the ED visit.

β₂ agonist

Inhaled β_2 agonists are preferred for all patients with documented asthma and are first-line therapy, sometimes as single drug therapy, but more commonly in combination with steroids. An older child (>3 years) can use an MDI or an inhaler with a spacer (Aerochamber, InspirEase); an infant or younger child can use an MDI attached to a spacer with a face mask. For an inhaler (with or without spacer), use 2 puffs q 6–8 h of albuterol. For a nebulizer, use albuterol 0.5% (0.5–1.0 mL) or levalbuterol (0.63 mg <10 kg or 1.25 mg >10 kg) in 3 mL of normal saline given over 5–10 minutes.

Corticosteroids

Give a dose of oral steroids if the patient required two or more acute albuterol treatments. In addition, prescribe steroids for a patient who has required acute therapy twice (or more) within 24 hours or three times in the past week. Avoid steroids in a child who has been exposed to viruses in the herpes family (especially varicella). Give oral prednisone or methylprednisolone (1 mg/kg per day, 40 mg maximum q day or div bid, half-life 12–36 hours) for 4 days. For children who cannot tolerate prednisone because of vomiting, a single dose of oral dexamethasone (0.6 mg/kg q day, 10 mg maximum, half-life 36–72 hours) is an alternative.

Prescribe inhaled steroids to patients whose risk (likelihood of exacerbations) and impairment (frequency and intensity of symptoms and functional limitations) characteristics classify them as having persistent asthma. Use fluticasone (44 mcg/puff 4–11 years; 110 mcg/puff ≥12 years) 1 puff bid. Prescribe budesonide inhalation suspension for nebulization (0.25–0.5 mg) for children 0–4 years of age whose asthma medications are nebulized.

Follow-up

- Mild to moderate first wheezing episode >1 year of age, new or altered medications or steroids prescribed: primary care follow-up in 1–2 weeks

Indications for admission

- Status asthmaticus: continued moderate or severe wheezing or other evidence of significant airway obstruction after therapy with nebulized β_2 agonists, ipratropium, corticosteroids, or subcutaneous epinephrine, or any wheezing after IV magnesium sulfate
- Repeated emergency visits over several days when therapy is maximal or compliance uncertain
- Persistent tachypnea, inability to tolerate fluids or medications, altered mental status
- Hypercapnia: pCO_2 >40 mmHg
- Hypoxemia: pO_2 <60 mmHg or oxygen saturation < 93% in room air despite aggressive therapy
- Pneumothorax, pneumomediastinum, or significant atelectasis

Bibliography

Chou KJ, Cunningham SJ, Crain EF: Metered-dose inhalers with spacers vs. nebulizers for pediatric asthma. *Arch Pediatr Adolesc Med* 1995;149:201–5.

Kim I, Phrampus E, Venkataraman S, et al: Helium/oxygen-driven albuterol nebulization in the treatment of children with moderate to severe asthma exacerbations: a randomized, controlled trial. *Pediatrics* 2005;116;1127–33.

Mannix R, Bachur R: Status asthmaticus in children. *Curr Opin Pediatr* 2007;19:281–7.

National Heart, Lung and Blood Institute: *Expert Panel Report 3: Guidelines for the Diagnosis and Management of Asthma.* United States Department of Health and Human Services National Institutes for Health, Bethesda, MD, 2007 (NIH publication no. 08–4051).

Bacterial tracheitis

Bacterial tracheitis (BT) is the most common life-threatening bacterial infection of the airway, including the larynx, trachea, and bronchi. The pathology involves copious purulent secretions and pseudomembranes within the trachea. *Staphylococcus aureus* is most frequently implicated, followed by *Streptococcus pyogenes, Moraxella catarrhalis*, and *Streptococcus pneumoniae. Influenza* type A is often detected as well, suggesting a primary viral process followed by bacterial superinfection.

Clinical presentation

Patients of any age can be affected, although the mean is about 4 years of age. Following a brief prodrome of cough, rhinorrhea, and low-grade fever, the initial presentation resembles moderate to severe viral croup, with hoarseness, sore throat, barking cough, and stridor. However, instead of improving after several days, the patient develops high fever with significant respiratory distress. Drooling is uncommon.

Diagnosis

Suspect BT in a febrile child with stridor that does not respond to racemic epinephrine administration or that gets worse after a number of days (when croup is usually resolving), particularly if the cough seems productive. In a stable patient, a portable lateral neck radiograph obtained in the ED may reveal an irregular tracheal margin characteristic of BT. Viral croup (pp. 620–622), epiglottitis (pp. 622–624), retropharyngeal abscess (pp. 156–157), and foreign-body aspiration (pp. 624–626) are major differential diagnostic considerations.

ED management

If BT is suspected, allow the patient to assume a position of comfort on the parent's lap. Provide supplemental oxygen in an unobtrusive manner, but defer completing a physical examination or inserting an IV. Immediately notify an anesthesiologist and otolaryngologist to prepare for laryngoscopy and possible orotracheal intubation in the operating suite. If the patient's respiratory status suddenly deteriorates (usually due to movement of a pseudomembrane within the airway) perform bag-mask ventilation.

Definitive treatment includes airway stabilization, most frequently with tracheal intubation in the operating suite and meticulous pulmonary toilet and suctioning of secretions. Give broad-spectrum antibiotics, such as nafcillin (100 mg/kg per day div q 6 h) or cefotaxime (150 mg/kg per day IV div q 6 h), but add vancomycin (40 mg/kg per day div q 6 h) if MRSA is a concern.

Indication for admission

- Suspected bacterial tracheitis

Bibliography

Hopkins A, Lahiri T, Salerno R, Heath B:
Changing epidemiology of life-threatening
upper airway infections: the reemergence of
bacterial tracheitis. *Pediatrics*
2006;118;1418–21.

Loftis L: Acute infectious upper airway
obstructions in children. *Semin Pediatr Infect
Dis* 2005;17:5–10.

Rafei K, Lichenstein R: Airway infectious disease
emergencies. *Pediatr Clin North Am*
2006;53:215–42.

Bronchiolitis

Bronchiolitis is the most common wheezing-associated respiratory illness in children <2 years of age. Epidemics in the winter (December through early February) are most frequently caused by respiratory syncitial virus (RSV). Human metapneumovirus (hMPV) causes bronchiolitis in somewhat older children (median age 11 months) typically in the spring (March through April). Less common causes of bronchiolitis include parainfluenza, influenza, and adenovirus, *Mycoplasma*, pertussis, *Chlamydia*, and *Ureaplasma*.

Clinical presentation

Typically, there is a prodromal URI with rhinorrhea and coryza, followed by cough, audible wheezing, and varying degrees of respiratory distress. An infant with severe disease has tachypnea (>50/min), subcostal and intercostal retractions, poor feeding, nasal flaring, and grunting. In all cases, symptoms are likely to be most prominent at night. An associated otitis media is present in >50% of cases, but fever is variable and usually low grade. Although wheezing is the typical auscultatory finding, rhonchi and coarse rales may also be heard. In most patients, the condition worsens for 3–4 days and then rapidly resolves, although some patients may have a persistent cough for weeks afterward. Neonates and young infants may present with apnea and a sepsis-like picture.

Diagnosis

Acute wheezing, cough, and respiratory distress in a young infant are most often secondary to bronchiolitis. Other diagnoses are as follows.

Asthma

Asthma (reactive airway disease) can cause a clinical picture with wheezing that is indistinguishable from bronchiolitis. Some infants with a first RSV exposure may already manifest hyperreactive airways. Consider asthma if the patient has had previous episodes of wheezing that were responsive to bronchodilators, a history of bronchopulmonary dysplasia, eczema, or a family history of asthma or atopic disease.

Foreign-body aspiration

An aspirated foreign body may present with wheezing after a coughing or choking episode in an infant typically >6 months of age. There is no URI prodrome. Unless there is acute infection distal to the foreign body, there is usually no fever. Auscultatory findings are often localized. An esophageal foreign body can impinge on the trachea and also cause respiratory distress.

Congenital malformations

These conditions can cause airway obstruction and wheezing, which are exacerbated by a URI. Consider congenital lobar emphysema and intrapulmonary cysts (bronchogenic or cystadenomatoid malformation) when the wheezing is unilateral or localized. The chest X-ray is often diagnostic. With tracheomalacia, stridor from inspiratory collapse of a floppy trachea predominates over expiratory wheezing. Wheezing from a vascular ring is typically loudest over the trachea and midlung fields.

Cardiac disease

Mitral stenosis or obstruction (cor triatriatum) or myocardial dysfunction from other causes can occasionally present with pulmonary edema, which can mimic bronchiolitis. Usually there is significant tachycardia and a gallop, and cardiomegaly is seen on chest X-ray.

Gastroesophageal reflux

GER presents with nighttime cough and wheeze typically unresponsive to bronchodilator therapy. There may be associated gagging with feeding or dysphagia, and, in some infants, intermittent or frequent episodes of apnea.

ED management

Inquire about a history of wheezing, prematurity, or mechanical ventilation (BPD), and check for a family history of asthma or allergies. Perform the examination with the infant undressed from the waist up and sitting on the parent's lap. Obtain an accurate respiratory rate, note any signs of respiratory distress (flaring, grunting, retractions, cyanosis) or heart disease (murmur, hepatosplenomegaly), and assess the activity level and ability to drink.

Respiratory rate >60/min or signs of respiratory distress

Check the oxygen saturation in room air by pulse oximetry, and give supplemental oxygen. Suction the nares if necessary. Give a trial dose of nebulized epinephrine (1:1,000, 0.5 mL/kg, 2.5 mL maximum, in 3 mL NS) or albuterol (0.5%, 0.50 mL in 3 mL NS) over 5–10 minutes. Occasional side effects in young infants include tachycardia and irritability. Assess the effectiveness of therapy by reevaluating the respiratory rate, signs of respiratory distress, and oxygen saturation. If there is no substantial improvement, admit the patient. If the respiratory rate slows to 40–60/min and there is no respiratory distress, discharge the patient with a trial of a β_2 agonist (see below), provided oral intake is adequate and daily follow-up can be arranged. Oral corticosteroids are unlikely to be helpful except in patients with a past history of wheezing.

Respiratory rate 40–60/min

Supportive therapy (fluids, acetaminophen as necessary) is all that is needed if the infant is alert, is tolerating fluids well, and has no signs of distress. Close follow-up is warranted. Do not use bronchodilators routinely. However, a trial of inhaled albuterol, via MDI and a spacer with a face mask (2 puffs q 4–6 h), may be useful if the patient required mechanical ventilation as a newborn, has BPD, there is a family history of asthma or allergies, or the child improved following acute bronchodilator therapy in the ED. Do not use oral theophylline.

Provide supplemental oxygen (usually 30–40% by oxyhood or nasal prongs) to hypoxic patients to maintain an oxygen saturation >95% or a pO_2 >85 mmHg. Start an IV and give maintenance fluids with $D_5\frac{1}{2}NS$ unless the patient is dehydrated (see pp. 18–19). If the patient responded to nebulized albuterol, continue the nebulizations q 4–6 h, although albuterol can be administered as often as every hour if there is documented improvement and the patient is carefully monitored. Clinical deterioration, with persistent hypoxemia, elevation of pCO_2, or the development of acidosis may portend exhaustion and respiratory failure requiring mechanical ventilation.

Chest radiographs are not routinely indicated in patients with bronchiolitis. In general, obtain a chest X-ray if the infant has known underlying pulmonary or heart disease or does not respond to aggressive inpatient management.

Follow-up
- Persistent tachypnea (> 60/min), difficulty feeding: return at once
- All infants in 24 hours for reevaluation of feeding, respiratory effort, weight

Indications for admission
- Respiratory rate >70/min after maximal ED therapy, regardless of clinical appearance
- Respiratory rate 60–70/min with lethargy or poor oral intake
- Infant <3 months of age with a respiratory rate 60–70/min after maximal ED therapy
- Respiratory distress, oxygen saturation <93% or pO_2 <65 mmHg in room air, or normal-to-elevated pCO_2 (>40 mmHg)
- Infant with congenital heart disease, chronic lung disease, or immunodeficiency (at risk for complications of RSV infection) in the progressive stage (first day or two) of the illness
- Parents uncomfortable with the severity of illness or with limited resources at home (especially if the infant is <3 months of age)

Bibliography

American Academy of Pediatrics, Subcommittee on Diagnosis and Management of Bronchiolitis: Diagnosis and management of bronchiolitis. *Pediatrics* 2006;118; 1774–93.

Gadomski AM, Bhasale AL: Bronchodilators for bronchiolitis. *Cochrane Database Syst Rev* 2006;3:CD001266.

Yanney M, Vyas H: The treatment of bronchiolitis. *Arch Dis Child* 2008;93;793–8.

Cough
Cough is a very common symptom that is most often caused by a minor URI. However, a cough may also signal a more serious problem, such as pneumonia, asthma, or congestive heart failure. A thorough clinical evaluation is necessary before assuming that the patient just has a "cold."

Clinical presentation and diagnosis
The clinical presentation varies, depending on the etiology (Table 21-4). Usually these can be differentiated with a careful history and physical exam, with only the occasional need for laboratory tests. Three features of a cough that help determine the cause are its quality, timing, and whether it is productive of sputum.

Table 21-4. Differential diagnosis of cough

Anatomic site	Emergency/potentially emergency	Common/other
Upper airway	Croup (severe)	URI
	Foreign-body aspiration	Pharyngitis
	Pertussis	Sinusitis
	Aspiration	Noxious fumes
	Congenital anomalies, such as TE fistula, etc.	Tracheal compression
	Laryngeal edema	GERD
Lower airway	Asthma	Foreign-body aspiration
	Bronchiolitis	Cystic fibrosis
	Pneumonia	Pulmonary hemosiderosis
	Anaphylaxis	
	Congestive heart failure	
Nonrespiratory	Impaired gag reflex	Aural foreign body
		Psychogenic cough
		Diaphragmatic irritation
		Phrenic or vagus nerve irritation

Quality

Quality refers to both the sound and pattern of the coughing episodes; it is best ascertained from hearing the cough, rather than relying on the history. Coughs are often described as "wet" or "dry"; however, these descriptions may not be useful. A barking cough suggests croup, and a loud, honking cough is often associated with a psychogenic cough. Paroxysmal episodes (a series of coughs with no breathing between them), especially when followed by apnea, cyanosis, or a whoop, are consistent with a pertussis syndrome. A staccato cough (a series of coughs with short breaths between them) suggests an "afebrile pneumonia" (*Chlamydia, Mycoplasma*).

Timing

Cough that is related to feeds and includes either choking or emesis suggests aspiration. The possible causes include gastroesophageal reflux (cough may be the only symptom), mechanical abnormalities (tracheoesophageal fistula), and neurologic abnormalities. Night cough is consistent with asthma, sinusitis, postnasal drip, gastroesophageal reflux (GERD) and croup; an early-morning cough suggests a suppurative process. Seasonal cough, exercise-related cough, and cold-air-related cough occur with reactive airway disease. Finally, "school-day-only cough" suggests a psychogenic origin.

The patient's age suggests different causes. During infancy, consider congenital anomalies, pertussis, bronchiolitis, *Chlamydia*, and pulmonary edema (usually cardiogenic). Cough during the first 2 months of life is more probably related to serious pathology than at any other age. Consider foreign-body aspiration in toddlers and older children. Among adolescents, consider smoking and mediastinal masses.

Sputum production

Productivity is difficult to judge, as children tend to swallow sputum. Green sputum reflects leukocyte breakdown and not necessarily a bacterial process. Blood-streaked sputum suggests pneumococcal pneumonia. Hemoptysis may reflect foreign-body aspiration, a chronic suppurative process (cystic fibrosis), tuberculosis, and more rarely, pulmonary hemosiderosis.

Physical findings help localize the origin to a specific part of the respiratory tract. Pharyngitis, otitis media, rhinorrhea, swollen turbinates, sinus tenderness, snoring, and stridor are consistent with upper-airway disease. Wheezing, rales, rhonchi, and decreased breath sounds occur with lower respiratory tract pathology. Also look for signs of congestive heart failure (gallop, hepatomegaly, jugular vein distention) and diaphragmatic irritation (right or left upper-quadrant tenderness).

ED management

The priority is prompt recognition and treatment of respiratory distress and emergency conditions. Assess oxygenation and perfusion, and initiate appropriate resuscitation, if necessary. Look for signs of upper-airway obstruction, assess the patient's preferred position of breathing, and listen carefully for stridor (place the stethoscope on the side of the neck). If there are any signs of obstruction, maintain the patient in the position of maximal airway opening (see pp. 622–624). If oxygenation and perfusion are not compromised, consider the potentially urgent and most common causes for each age group (Table 21-4). If the history and physical exam are not conclusive, obtain a chest X-ray and room air pulse oximetry to screen for serious pathology.

Infants <2 months

Rule out serious pathology as this age group is at relatively high risk for apnea. Serious causes include pneumonia, bronchiolitis, and pulmonary edema (cardiogenic and noncardiogenic). Potential emergencies include pertussis, *Chlamydia* and other afebrile pneumonias (*Ureaplasma* and *Mycoplasma*), bronchiolitis, aspiration, and congenital mechanical obstruction. Measure the oxygen saturation, and obtain a chest X-ray and CBC looking for lymphocytosis (pertussis) or eosinophilia (*Chlamydia*).

URIs and GERD are common nonemergency causes. Treat a URI with normal saline nose drops, but avoid neosynephrine nose drops, which may cause dysrhythmias (SVT) and severe rebound congestion. For reflux, if there is associated apnea, consult with a gastroenterologist or pulmonologist to determine whether an immediate upper GI series is needed. Otherwise, further work-up can be deferred to the outpatient setting.

Older infants and children

Emergent etiologies include pneumonia, reactive airway disease (bronchiolitis/asthma), and pulmonary edema. Upper-airway obstruction in this age group is usually related to foreign-body aspiration or laryngeal edema (croup).

Common causes in this age group include asthma, sinusitis, postnasal drip, and GERD. Asthma may have no corroborating physical findings, and the peak flow may be normal. If the history is suggestive (night cough, family history of atopy, other atopic symptoms, exercise-induced cough), a diagnostic/therapeutic trial of bronchodilators is warranted (pp. 607–609). If the history and physical exam suggest sinusitis (worsening rhinorrhea for >7 consecutive days, periorbital swelling, halitosis, swollen turbinates), treat with a 14-day course of antibiotics (pp. 137–138). Finally, postnasal drip may cause a persistent cough. If sleep is disturbed, recommend a trial of an oral antihistamine such as chlorpheniramine (2–6 years: 1 mg/dose q 4–6 h, 4 mg/day maximum; 6–12 years: 2 mg/dose q 4–6 h, 12 mg/day maximum). Do not use sustained-release products in children <6 years of age.

GERD can cause persistent cough, despite the absence of GI symptoms, and should be suspected when systematic investigation for other common causes of cough are negative. Although a 24-hour esophageal pH monitoring study can confirm the diagnosis, first assess the response to an empiric trial of anti-reflux medication (ranitidine, 4–5 mg/kg per day div bid).

Older children and adolescents

ED management is similar to the approach outlined above. Emergency resuscitation and upper-airway clearance are the priorities. Common causes are similar to those in younger children. If a patient presents with persistent symptoms, obtain a chest X-ray (mediastinal mass) and check for a history of exposure to TB.

Finally, treat the cause of the cough and not the cough itself. Consider cough suppression only when the cause is known and the cough severely impairs the patient's daily life (sleep deprivation, not permitted in school). In such cases, try a cough suppressant with 100% dextromethorphan or codeine (0.5 mg/kg q h, 30 mg maximum).

Follow-up

- Refer a patient with chronic cough (> 2 weeks) to a primary care provider

Indications for admission

- Respiratory distress or patient requires oxygen
- Pertussis (infant <6 months old)
- Bronchiolitis or *Chlamydia* pneumonia (infant <2 months, because of risk of apnea)
- Interstitial pneumonia (infant <2 months)
- Lobar pneumonia (infant <6 months)
- Pulmonary edema
- Foreign-body aspiration
- Persistent upper-airway obstruction from any cause
- Laryngeal edema
- Croup with significant upper-airway obstruction and stridor at rest

Bibliography

Carr BC: Efficacy, abuse, and toxicity of over-the-counter cough and cold medicines in the pediatric population. *Curr Opin Pediatr* 2006;18:184–8.

Chang AB: Cough. *Pediatr Clin North Am* 2009;56:19–32.

Smith SM, Schroeder K, Fahey T: Over-the-counter medications for acute cough in children and adults in ambulatory setting. *Cochrane Database Syst Rev* 2008;1: CD001831.

Croup

Laryngotracheobronchitis, or croup, is an acute subglottic inflammatory process generally caused by parainfluenza virus, types 1 and 3, during the late fall and early winter months. Other causes are influenza viruses A and B, measles, *Mycoplasma pneumoniae*, human metapneumovirus and respiratory syncitial virus. Croup primarily occurs between 6 months and 3 years of age, but morbidity is greatest in the first year of life, when the subglottic airway is relatively narrow. Although exhaustion may lead to obstruction of the airway by mucus, death is infrequent.

Spasmodic croup is probably an allergic disease that occurs mainly in patients with personal or family histories of asthma and allergies.

Clinical presentation

Croup causes varying degrees of acute upper airway obstruction. Clinically, this presents with inspiratory stridor, suprasternal retractions, tachypnea, and tachycardia. Croup usually begins with low-grade fever and rhinorrhea, followed by hoarseness and a barking, "seal-like" cough. The amount of stridor is highly variable, but with increasing obstruction there are suprasternal and intercostal retractions, decreased air entry, and increased work of breathing. The illness lasts 3–5 days, with the second or third day being the peak of clinical symptoms. High fever, dysphagia, and drooling are usually absent. Exhaustion and respiratory failure ensue in a small number of cases (<2%). Patients with preexisting upper-airway problems (congenital or acquired subglottic stenosis, webs, tracheomalacia, choanal narrowing, micrognathia, macroglossia) are at particular risk.

Spasmodic croup presents in the middle of the night with the sudden onset of loud stridor and croupy cough which resolves quickly and often improves with cool mist. There is little or no viral prodrome, and dysphagia, drooling, high fever, and toxicity are notably absent. The croup may recur on successive nights, and recurrent episodes are common. Some children have recurrent croup-like illnesses induced by infection or allergens that may have associated reversible lower-airway obstruction suggestive of asthma.

Diagnosis

Croup is a clinical diagnosis based on history and physical findings. When epiglottitis cannot be ruled out clinically, or when other entities are being considered, radiographs are helpful. A lateral neck film can exclude entities such as epiglottitis or a retropharyngeal abscess. With croup, on a PA view of the chest, the upper airway is narrowed to appear like a "steeple," and the infraglottic region is hazy.

Epiglottitis

The onset of epiglottitis (pp. 622–624) is sudden, sometimes suggestive of spasmodic croup. However, a patient with epiglottitis is toxic, with high fever, dysphagia, and drooling. The barking cough is absent, and there is a tendency to adopt a characteristic "sniffing" position, sitting up with the neck extended. On lateral neck X-ray there is classic "thumb"-shaped epiglottis and swelling of the aryepiglottic folds, the normal cervical lordosis is lost, and the hypopharynx is distended with air.

Foreign body

An upper-airway foreign body (pp. 624–626) can present with the sudden onset of stridor. The object may be seen only on radiograph or by direct visualization. However, hoarseness and the "barking" cough are not usually present.

Bacterial tracheitis

Bacterial tracheitis is a form of acute subglottic obstruction usually caused by *S. aureus*. It generally occurs in patients who have had croup for several days, and resembles epiglottitis, with the sudden onset of high fever, toxicity, and severe respiratory distress.

Laryngomalacia and subglottic stenosis

These are common causes of mild stridor in infants. The stridor is accentuated during respiratory infections and is not associated with hoarseness, and the child's activity is usually normal.

Retropharyngeal abscess

Fever is accompanied by drooling and dysphagia. Respiratory distress is variable but may be pronounced, and meningismus or torticollis may also be present (pp. 156–157). Examination of the oropharynx reveals bulging tissue in the rear of the mouth.

ED management

Mild-to-moderate croup

Make a rapid assessment of color, perfusion, work of breathing, retractions, and air entry. If the patient is in mild-to-moderate distress, administer humidified oxygen, 4 L/min by face mask. Some infectious croup episodes and almost all spasmodic croup attacks will respond to mist with diminished stridor and lessened respiratory distress. Give a dose of oral or IM dexamethasone (0.3–0.6 mg/kg, 10 mg maximum) to a patient with a barking cough or cough with hoarseness or rhonchi.

Most often, the condition of a patient with spasmodic croup is markedly improved by the time of ED arrival; however, caution the parents that the illness may recur the following night.

Severe croup

Administer humidified oxygen, 4 L/min by face mask; use 100% O_2 delivered by a nonrebreather mask for a patient with severe distress, and continuously monitor with a pulse oximeter. Treat with either nebulized racemic epinephrine (Vaponephrine, 0.05 mL/kg [0.5 mL maximum] in 3 mL NS) or L-epinephrine (1:1,000, 0.5 mL/kg in 3 mL NS; ≤ 4 years 2.5 mL maximum, >4 years 5 mL maximum) over 5–10 minutes. Also treat a patient with stridor at rest with nebulized epinephrine. Epinephrine acts as a local vasoconstrictor that shrinks airway swelling; its effects last approximately 2 hours unless steroids are given. Therefore, to prevent a rebound in the airway swelling, give dexamethasone to any patient who receives nebulized epinephrine treatment and observe for at least 2 hours prior to discharge from the ED. Maintain the humidified oxygen after the treatment.

Discharge the patient who clearly has croup if there is no significant stridor at rest, for at least 2 hours, after treatment with epinephrine and dexamethasone. Arrange for follow-up in the next 24–48 hours.

A patient whose severe respiratory distress persists despite racemic epinephrine or L-epinephrine and dexamethasone requires intubation. Use a tube 0.5 mm smaller than usual to prevent pressure necrosis of the airway lumen. Start an IV if the patient is not drinking adequately and administer a 20 mL/kg bolus of isotonic crystalloid if the patient appears dehydrated. Obtain an ABG after epinephrine treatment if the child is agitated or has increased work of breathing, as carbon dioxide retention can occur in a young infant with moderate-to-severe croup. In addition, obtain radiographs of the chest and lateral neck if the patient is in moderate-to-severe distress or the diagnosis is unclear.

Follow-up

- Immediately if stridor at rest develops at home, otherwise daily for the first 2–3 days

Indications for admission

- Stridor at rest that fails to resolve with epinephrine and dexamethasone
- Rebound during a 2-hour observation period following epinephrine and dexamethasone treatment for stridor at rest
- Inadequate fluid intake
- Impending respiratory failure (pCO_2 >40 mmHg; O_2 saturation <93% in room air)

Bibliography

Bjornson CL, Johnson DW: Croup. *Lancet* 2008;371:329–39.

Cherry JD: Clinical practice. Croup. *N Engl J Med* 2008;358:384–91.

Everard ML: Acute bronchitis and croup. *Pediatr Clin North Am* 2009;56:119–34.

Epiglottitis

Epiglottitis (supraglottitis) is a life-threatening bacterial infection of the upper airway almost always caused by *Haemophilus influenza* type b (HIB). The incidence has declined dramatically as a result of the HIB vaccine. Other causes of supraglottic inflammation are *S. aureus*, herpesvirus, and *Candida albicans* infections and thermal injury from hot liquid aspiration. Immediate, aggressive management of the airway in a child with suspected epiglottitis is the first priority to ensure survival without morbidity from the complications of sudden upper-airway obstruction.

Clinical presentation

Most patients with epiglottitis are 3–8 years of age, although it occurs in young infants as well as adults. Typically there is a sudden onset of fever, lethargy, and respiratory distress with stridor. Drooling occurs in about 50% of patients, and the barking cough of croup is notably absent. Occasionally a patient (usually older child or teenager) presents in a more indolent fashion with mild stridor and a severe sore throat.

Most patients with epiglottitis will place themselves in the position of comfort, the "sniffing" position, sitting up with the neck extended. Physical findings include respiratory distress, tachypnea, stridor, and, often, retractions (suprasternal). Inspiratory breath sounds are prolonged but diminished throughout all lung fields. Adventitious breath sounds are uncommon in uncomplicated epiglottitis. If the obstruction is more severe, the child may have signs of respiratory failure, including obtundation, cyanosis, absent breath sounds, or apnea.

Diagnosis

The clinical picture is usually so characteristic that the diagnosis is suspected immediately. Epiglottitis is most safely and efficiently confirmed by direct visualization of the inflamed upper airway in an operating room. If a cooperative older child can open his or her mouth wide, direct visualization of the cherry-red epiglottis may be possible in the ED. However, do not use a tongue depressor; there is the potential danger of causing acute airway obstruction. When epiglottitis is not the primary suspected diagnosis, using a tongue depressor to visualize the oropharynx is generally safe. Be careful when evaluating a patient with an upper-airway problem, especially when there may be secretions or a foreign body in the posterior pharynx.

If epiglottitis is unlikely (prolonged course, low-grade fever) but has not been ruled out clinically, order a lateral neck radiograph of the soft tissues. Obtain a portable film in the ED, with the emergency staff and airway equipment at the child's bedside. Allow the patient to remain in the sitting position for the X-ray, with the parent at the bedside. Radiographic findings reveal a distended hypopharynx, an obliterated vallecula, a large and indistinct epiglottis (thumbprint), thickened aryepiglottic folds, and loss of the normal cervical lordosis. The subglottic region appears normal.

Croup (pp. 620–622) is most common in infants from 6 months to 3 years of age, although it does occur in older children. The onset is more indolent, with low-grade fever, hoarseness, a "barking" cough, and varying degrees of stridor. Often a normal supraglottic region can be seen during a careful examination of the oropharynx. If obtained, the lateral neck radiograph is normal in the supraglottic region, and there may be some subglottic haziness.

A retropharyngeal or parapharyngeal abscess most commonly occurs in a young child <3–4 years of age. Fever is usually accompanied by excessive drooling and dysphagia. Respiratory distress is variable but may be pronounced, and meningismus or torticollis may also be present. Examination of the oropharynx reveals bulging tissue in the rear of the mouth. The lateral neck radiograph shows a swollen prevertebral soft-tissue space (much more than half the width of the vertebral bodies).

Foreign-body aspiration (pp. 624–626) with upper-airway obstruction is generally of very acute onset, with cough and varying degrees of stridor. Aspiration is most common in children 6 months to 5 years of age. Fever is unusual, and the chest radiographs may be normal or a radioopaque density may be seen in the upper airway.

Bacterial tracheitis (pp. 613–614) is an acute bacterial infection of the trachea associated with a membranous obstruction. It is usually caused by *S. aureus*, and it most often affects children 2–10 years of age. Most characteristic is the severe stridor. Diagnosis is usually made by direct visualization of the normal supraglottic region and intubation of the airway with suctioning of thick inspissated secretions.

ED management

The management varies according to the clinical presentation.

Epiglottitis likely, airway stable

Place the patient in a position of comfort, with the parents, in a room with immediate access to airway equipment. Give supplemental oxygen if possible, but do not agitate the child. Pulse oximetry is advisable if it does not upset the patient. Immediately notify the operating room staff, and assemble the physician team best able to handle airway intubation (usually an attending anesthesiologist and otolaryngologist). Delay IV placement and laboratory studies until after the child is taken to the operating suite. The airway can be secured best under light general anesthesia without neuromuscular relaxation.

Epiglottitis likely, patient in extremis with an unstable airway

Place the child supine, and open the airway with a chin lift. Perform bag-valve-mask ventilation with a tight seal and 4–5 cmH$_2$O pressure to maximize air entry past the obstructing epiglottis. Occasionally this will not be sufficient, and intubation will be necessary. Rarely, needle cricothyrotomy is required to provide a temporary airway until a team can assemble in the ED to manage the airway.

Mild suspicion of epiglottitis, airway stable

Obtain a lateral neck radiograph to differentiate among the other potential problems. If there is significant stridor or respiratory distress, perform the radiograph in the ED with the physician at the bedside. If epiglottitis is confirmed, proceed with operating room management.

Indications for admission

- Suspected or confirmed epiglottitis
- Undiagnosed upper-airway obstruction with stridor at rest

Bibliography

Loftis L: Acute infectious upper airway obstructions in children. *Semin Pediatr Infect Dis* 2005;17:5–10.

Rafei K, Lichenstein R: Airway infectious disease emergencies. *Pediatr Clin North Am* 2006;53:215–42.

Sobol SE, Zapata S: Epiglottitis and croup. *Otolaryngol Clin North Am* 2008;41:551–66.

Foreign body in the airway

Aspirated foreign bodies cause more deaths in the United States than croup and epiglottitis combined. Determining the presence of a foreign body requires an accurate history, a high degree of clinical suspicion, and often a direct look down the airway. The peak incidence coincides with the period of oral behavior, between 6 months and the early school years.

Clinical presentation

Aspiration of a foreign body classically presents with an immediate episode of coughing, gagging, choking, or cyanosis. In infants and small children, a foreign body lodged in the esophagus can impinge on the trachea and cause respiratory embarrassment. Some foreign bodies will be promptly vomited or swallowed, eliminating the immediate risk of hypoxemia and the complications of the foreign body lodging in the pulmonary tree.

Extrathoracic (laryngeal or tracheal)

The patient presents with stridor, a croupy cough, varying degrees of dyspnea, or acute hypoxemia and cyanosis. The symptoms may vary with the degree of obstruction of the airway. The sound elicited by air moving over the object varies with the size of the airway and degree of inflammation induced.

Intrathoracic (lower trachea and bronchial)

A lower-airway foreign body presents with an initial choking episode and varying periods of quiescence, followed by persistent and often progressive symptoms. Commonly, there is cough, wheezing, and dyspnea. With inflammation or secondary atelectasis, fever and signs of pneumonia may predominate, leading to a misdiagnosis of asthma or recurrent pneumonia. A focal foreign body may produce unilateral hyperinflation with widening of intercostal spaces. On auscultation, localized or diffuse wheezing, rales, or decreased air entry may be appreciated.

Diagnosis

The clinical symptoms of a foreign-body aspiration may be subtle. Suspect an aspiration if an afebrile patient presents with the sudden onset of significant respiratory distress, an "asthmatic" has localized wheezing or decreased breath sounds, or a patient has recurrent pneumonias on the same side. The only certain method for verifying the diagnosis is with bronchoscopy. However, if foreign-body aspiration is suspected and the patient is not in extreme respiratory distress, obtain radiographs, which can assist in the diagnosis.

Extrathoracic

Radiographs of the lateral neck and chest are generally normal, as only a small number of aspirated foreign bodies are radioopaque. There may be signs of upper-airway obstruction, such as ballooning of the hypopharynx, gastric distention, or diminished lung volumes. Esophageal foreign bodies can occasionally compress the trachea from behind; these tend to be larger objects that are more likely to be radioopaque. Orientation of a radioopaque foreign body in the sagittal plane on the PA film of the chest (slit-like image) confirms its presence in the trachea or larynx.

The differential diagnosis of an extrathoracic foreign body includes epiglottitis, croup, bacterial tracheitis, tracheomalacia, retropharyngeal abscess, and congenital anomalies of the airway. The abrupt onset suggests aspiration, but in cases with moderate symptoms, bronchoscopy is required to confirm the diagnosis.

Intrathoracic

Most are radiolucent, but there is a high incidence of abnormal chest radiographs (80%). Hyperinflation, atelectasis, and pneumonia are the most common abnormalities. In rare instances, a pneumothorax may be present. In the older child, inspiratory and expiratory chest films may reveal persistent hyperinflation of the ipsilateral side during expiration. Unilateral hyperinflation on the inspiratory film may be seen, but it is less common. For a toddler, when cooperation for an inspiratory film is unlikely, obtain bilateral decubitus films, which may reveal increased lucency on the affected side when that side is dependent. Fluoroscopy may sometimes be useful to distinguish small areas of air trapping or mediastinal shifting.

An intrathoracic foreign body is often confused with asthma, pneumonia, congenital lobar emphysema, or other syndromes associated with hyperinflation or atelectasis. History, clinical response to therapy (i.e. bronchodilators in asthma), and chronicity may help distinguish these entities.

ED management

Assess the patency of the airway and breathing. Complete obstruction demands immediate BLS maneuvers: five back blows followed by five chest compressions in a patient <12 months of age and 6–10 subdiaphragmatic abdominal thrusts (Heimlich maneuver, pp. xx–yy) for an older child. If there is an incomplete obstruction, place the child in the sniffing position (maximal airway opening), provide supplemental oxygen, and permit the child's own ventilation through a partly occluded airway to be maintained. Maneuvers that dislodge the foreign body may move the object to the central airways, causing complete obstruction. Continuously monitor the patient with pulse oximetry while awaiting an anesthesiologist and bronchoscopist (pediatric surgeon or otolaryngologist) to perform rigid bronchoscopy.

Lower-airway foreign bodies generally present with less severe signs of obstruction. Chest physiotherapy, may cause occlusion of a major airway and hypoxemia, and is therefore contraindicated. Provide supplemental oxygen, and arrange for semi-elective removal by rigid bronchoscopy under general anesthesia.

Indications for admission

- Clinical suspicion of an airway foreign body
- Respiratory symptoms after expulsion of an airway foreign body

Bibliography

Daines CL, Wood RE, Boesch RP: Foreign body aspiration: an important etiology of respiratory symptoms in children. *J Allergy Clin Immunol* 2008;121:1297–8.

Gregori D, Salerni L, Scarinzi C, et al: Foreign bodies in the upper airways causing complications and requiring hospitalization in children aged 0–14 years: results from the ESFBI study. *Eur Arch Otorhinolaryngol* 2008;265:971–8.

Kadmon G, Stern Y, Bron-Harlev E, et al: Computerized scoring system for the diagnosis of foreign body aspiration in children. *Ann Otol Rhinol Laryngol* 2008;117:839–43.

Hemoptysis

Hemoptysis is the expectoration of blood from the lower respiratory tract. Hemoptysis is uncommon in childhood; most suspected cases are the result of vomiting blood swallowed from the esophagus, nasopharynx, or oropharynx. The cause of true hemoptysis is usually a pulmonary infection or other pulmonary disease (Table 21-5).

Clinical presentation

Hemoptysis usually presents with signs and symptoms of the underlying disease, an acute exacerbation of that process, or a pulmonary infection. For example, pneumonia presents with fever, cough, tachypnea, and rales or decreased breath sounds. A patient with cystic fibrosis may have chronic diarrhea and failure to thrive.

Bronchiectasis

Bronchiectasis can occur with cystic fibrosis, tuberculosis, fungal infections (e.g. coccidioidomycosis). Airway erosion leads to acute hemorrhage that is frightening but usually self-limiting, although the bleeding may be life-threatening if a major vessel is affected. The usual presentation is fever, cough, and expectoration of blood.

Table 21-5. Etiologies of hemoptysis

Infectious causes (bronchiectasis, airway erosion)

Bacterial infections

Bronchopulmonary dysplasia

Coccidioidomycosis

Cystic fibrosis

Measles

Tuberculosis

Noninfectious causes

Foreign-body aspiration

Airway compression: carcinoid, bronchogenic cyst, cystadenomatoid malformation, mediastinal tumor

Arteriovenous malformation

Bleeding diathesis

Pulmonary embolus

Pulmonary hemosiderosis

Pulmonary sequestration

Rib fracture with pulmonary contusion

Wegener's granulomatosis

Foreign body

An airway foreign body generally presents with cough, localized wheezing, and varying degrees of respiratory distress. A chronic foreign body may cause erosion of a bronchus or distal bronchiectasis.

Trauma

Trauma to the chest and airways is often associated with rib fractures and pulmonary contusion. In most instances there is point tenderness over the rib, pleuritic chest pain, and dyspnea in addition to the hemoptysis.

Mass

A patient with an intrinsic pulmonary or endobronchial mass may be relatively asymptomatic, or they may have cough or wheezing. Weight loss or fatigue can also occur.

Bleeding diathesis

The patient will have other manifestations of bleeding (petechiae, ecchymoses, hematemesis, epistaxis, hematochezia).

Diagnosis

Initially, confirm that the blood is truly pulmonary in origin and exclude the oral cavity, nasopharynx, or GI tract as the site of the bleeding. If necessary, pass a nasogastric tube to exclude an upper GI bleed.

Inquire about a history of possible aspiration of a foreign body, trauma, acute infection, or exposure to fungus or TB. Check for an underlying history of bronchopulmonary dysplasia, cystic fibrosis, or bleeding dyscrasia.

Perform a careful physical examination of the chest, including observation of abnormality in chest excursion, palpation for external tenderness, and auscultation for air entry and adventitious sounds (rales or wheezes). The area of pulmonary hemorrhage may not alter the breath sounds heard over the chest wall.

Radiographs of the chest may be unchanged from previous films or may demonstrate an infiltrate, evidence of a foreign body (hyperinflation of the affected side, radioopaque foreign body, or infiltrate distal to the foreign body), or a mass or density. With pulmonary hemosiderosis there may be fluffy infiltrates that change location with each episode.

ED management

Admit a patient with true hemoptysis (>60 mL) and consult with a pulmonologist or thoracic surgeon. Obtain a chest radiograph, CBC, platelet count, PT, PTT, and type and cross-match. If the patient has tachypnea or respiratory distress, measure the oxygen saturation with either pulse oximetry or an ABG. Insert a large-bore IV and transfuse packed RBCs for volume depletion or evidence of significant ongoing blood loss. Place a 5TU PPD (0.1 mL) if the patient is not known to have a positive skin test.

Hemoptysis with blood-streaked mucus can be treated on an outpatient basis if the patient is not in respiratory distress. The ED management of pneumonia (pp. 629–633), foreign-body aspiration (pp. 624–626), and a bleeding diathesis (pp. 337–339) are discussed elsewhere.

Follow-up

- Pulmonology or primary care follow-up within 1 week

Indications for admission

- Hemoptysis >60 mL
- Hematocrit <30% or signs of acute severe blood loss
- Underlying chronic disease requiring parenteral antibiotics or inpatient therapy
- Mediastinal mass or peripheral lung density
- Suspected foreign-body aspiration, pulmonary embolus, TB

Bibliography

Bidwell JL, Pachner RW: Hemoptysis: diagnosis and management. *Am Fam Physician* 2005;72:1253–60.

Dine AP, Werner SL: Pediatric hemoptysis with pulmonary hemorrhage and respiratory

failure. *Am J Emerg Med* 2008;26: 639.e3–4.

Godfrey S: Pulmonary hemorrhage/hemoptysis in children. *Pediatr Pulmonol* 2004;37:476–84.

Table 21-6. Etiologies of pneumonia

Age	Agent
Less than 2 weeks	Group B streptococcus
	Coliform bacteria
	Respiratory syncitial virus (RSV)
	Staphylococcus aureus
2 weeks – 3 months	*Chlamydia trachomatis*
	RSV
	Parainfluenza virus
	Streptococcus pneumoniae
	Haemophilus influenzae type b (very rare if immunized)
	S. aureus
3 months – 5 years	Viral (especially RSV, influenza)
	S. pneumoniae
	H. influenzae type b (very rare)
Over 5 years	Viral
	Mycoplasma pneumoniae
	S. pneumoniae
	Chlamydia pneumoniae
Other agents to consider	*Mycobacterium tuberculosis*
	Pertussis (<1 year old)
	Pneumocystis carinii (HIV positive)
	Legionella sp.

Pneumonia

Pneumonia is a common disease with an incidence of 1–4.5 cases per 100 children per year. Pathogens can reach the lung parenchyma via either microaspiration or hematogenous spread. While just 20–30% of pneumonias are bacterial in origin, these are responsible for the majority of severe complications.

Streptococcus pneumoniae remains the most common bacterial pathogen. Although universal immunization has decreased the frequency of pneumococcal infections, certain virulent subtypes, such as 19A, are now more common and are causing severe disease. In addition, many organisms have become penicillin-resistant.

RSV is the most frequent viral cause and *Pneumocystis carinii* is the most likely opportunistic infection in HIV-positive infants. Methicillin-resistant *Staphylococcus aureus* (MRSA) has emerged as an important pathogen, especially in very ill-appearing children with pleural effusions. Table 21-6 lists the most likely etiologies in each age group.

Clinical presentation

Cough, tachypnea, and fever are the common symptoms of childhood pneumonia, while pallor, fatigue, and other constitutional symptoms are variable. Posttussive vomiting can be a common complaint in young children. A neonate or young infant may present with tachypnea, decreased activity, and poor feeding. With progression of the pneumonia, there may be signs of respiratory distress, including nasal flaring, intercostal or substernal retractions, dyspnea, cyanosis, or apnea. On auscultation, inspiratory rales may be heard or the breath sounds may be locally decreased or tubular, although adventitious sounds are harder to appreciate in a young child. Dullness and diminished breath sounds may indicate an effusion. Abdominal pain can occur with lower-lobe pneumonia and meningismus with upper-lobe infection.

Chlamydia trachomatis is the most common non-viral cause of pneumonia in infants between 2 weeks and 3 months of age. The classic presentation is a staccato cough in an afebrile, tachypneic infant with nasal congestion and fine rales. There may be a history of or concurrent conjunctivitis in approximately 50% of cases, as well as wheezing, bilateral patchy infiltrates on chest X-ray, and eosinophilia ($>300/mm^3$).

Mycoplasma pneumoniae and *Chlamydia pneumoniae* present with the gradual onset of a nonproductive hacking cough in a school-age child. The patient does not appear very sick, wheezing is more common than rales, headache and myalgias may also occur, and other family members may have had a similar illness.

Infection with *Bordatella pertussis* (pp. 414–416) may also lead to a secondary lobar or diffuse pneumonia. Typically there is a URI with rhinorrhea (catarrhal stage), which progresses to a harsh, episodic cough (paroxysmal stage), followed by the resolution of the cough over weeks to months (convalescent stage).

Staphylococcus aureus infection can be present in a very ill child with clinical signs of pneumonia. Pneumatoceles may be noted on the chest X-ray. Consider MRSA in a patient with concurrent soft-tissue or bone/joint infection and in any patient with suspected empyema.

Diagnosis

Pneumonia can be diagnosed clinically when fever, cough, and rales are present; a radiograph does not often alter the patient's management. Obtain a chest X-ray (PA and lateral) when the patient is in respiratory distress, the diagnosis is uncertain, there is concern about a pleural effusion, or an infant <2 months of age has respiratory signs (including cough). Also obtain a chest radiograph if a patient is not responding to appropriate therapy. Various patterns on the radiograph may help with the differential diagnosis (Table 21-7). Generally, pyogenic bacterial infections appear as bronchopneumonia or lobar infiltrates, sometimes with pleural effusion. Viral infections often present with diffuse airway involvement and hyperinflation.

The abdominal pain sometimes associated with pneumonia can suggest gastroenteritis or early appendicitis. However, a history of cough as an early symptom and a higher temperature suggest a primary respiratory disease.

Asthma

Asthma, which may be difficult to distinguish from pneumonia, can predispose to pneumonia, and accompanying atelectasis can lead to localized decreased breath sounds. Asthma

Table 21-7. Chest X-ray pattern as a guide to etiology

Diffuse pattern

   Viral (90%) of cases

   Chlamydia trachomatis (afebrile infants, eosinophilia common)

   Mycoplasma pneumoniae and *Chlamydia pneumoniae* (school-age children)

   Haemophilus influenzae type b (rare)

   Mycobacteria (uncommon)

   Fungi (uncommon)

   Rickettsia (uncommon)

   Pneumocystis carinii (usually central pattern, elevated LDH, hypoxia)

Lobar pattern

   Streptococcus pneumoniae (90%)

   Staphylococcus aureus

   H. influenzae type b (rare)

   Other bacteria (uncommon)

Pneumonia with effusion

   S. pneumoniae (commonest effusion)

   H. influenzae type b (empyema common)

   Group A *streptococcus*

   Staphylococcus aureus (often cavitation and/or empyema)

   Mycoplasma pneumoniae (effusions uncommon)

   Mycobacteria (unilateral effusion can occur without pneumonia)

   Adenovirus (small effusion)

is suggested by the presence of diffuse wheezing, coarse rales and rhonchi, and a response to bronchodilators.

Congestive heart failure

Congestive heart failure can present with tachycardia, tachypnea, rales, a gallop, and evidence of the primary cause (muffled heart sounds in myocardial disease, a murmur in volume overload shunts, poor perfusion or diminished pulses with left ventricular obstruction). Hepatosplenomegaly may be noted, and cardiomegaly and congestion can be seen on the chest radiograph.

Foreign-body aspiration

A foreign body can cause decreased breath sounds or predispose to pneumonia. The history and radiographs may be suggestive; bronchoscopy is often required for a definitive diagnosis.

Inhalation injury

Inhalation injury or any pulmonary toxic agent may induce findings consistent with intrapulmonary inflammation, mimicking pneumonia.

Recurrent pneumonia

Recurrent pneumonia is usually associated with asthma but may be caused by immunologic dysfunction, cystic fibrosis, foreign-body aspiration, or external airway compression (tumor, node).

ED management

Most children have infections with viral agents and require supportive care (fever control, fluids) only. Nonetheless, it is critical to immediately assess the adequacy of breathing. If the patient is dyspneic or in respiratory distress, assess the oxygen saturation with pulse oximetry. Consider an ABG if the patient has poor breath sounds and is lethargic, and administer supplemental oxygen if the patient is in distress or has decreased oxygenation (oxygen saturation <95%; pO_2 <80 mmHg). The goal is an oxygen saturation >95% or pO_2 >80 mmHg. Obtain a chest radiograph, if indicated (see above). Perform a lumbar puncture to exclude meningitis if there is fever and irritability, obtundation, lethargy, or meningismus. If the patient is febrile, give antipyretics to decrease the temperature and its effects on work of breathing (acetaminophen 15 mg/kg; ibuprofen 10 mg/kg). Place a PPD (0.1 mL, 5 TU) intradermally on the forearm unless the child is known to be positive for TB. If the patient is discharged from the ED, arrange follow-up to coincide with when the test needs to be read (48–72 hours).

Less than 6 months old

Admit all patients <6 months of age with lobar pneumonia and all infants with interstitial pneumonia <2 months of age. Obtain a CBC, blood culture, and chest radiograph, and if the patient appears toxic or is <2 months of age, perform a lumbar puncture and obtain serum electrolytes. Secure an IV if the patient appears toxic or is not taking oral fluids adequately. See pp. 370–373 for the treatment of an infant <8 weeks of age; treat a patient >8 weeks of age with either cefuroxime (150 mg/kg per day div q 8 h, IM or IV) or ceftriaxone (75 mg/kg per day div q 12 h IV). If *C. trachomatis* pneumonitis seems likely, obtain a nasopharyngeal culture and treat with oral erythromycin (40 mg/kg per day div q 6 h) for 14 days or, as an alternative, oral azithromycin (20 mg/kg q day) for 3 days. Treat wheezing with a β_2 agonist (pp. 607–611).

More than 6 months old

Obtain an oxygen saturation (pulse oximetry) if the patient is tachypneic (respiratory rate >60/min <2 years of age; 40–60/min >2 years of age) or has moderate retractions. An ABG is indicated if the patient has poor color and poor breath sounds. Indications for admission include a pO_2 <80 mmHg, oxygen saturation <95%, or pCO_2 > 40 mmHg.

If the pneumonia is lobar, treat with amoxicillin (80 mg/kg per day div bid for 10 days). Give an initial dose of parenteral ceftriaxone (50 mg/kg IM or IV, 500 mg maximum) before oral therapy if the patient is vomiting, although this does not hasten recovery. If the patient is being admitted to the hospital, treat with IV cefuroxime (150 mg/kg per day div q 8 h) or ceftriaxone (50 mg/kg per day div q 12 h). Penicillin G (150,000 units/kg per day div q 6 h IV) is an alternative for a child >5 years of age, depending on the prevalence of penicillin-resistant pneumococcus in the community. Add IV vancomycin (40 mg/kg per day div q 6 h) if MRSA pneumonia is suspected.

Treat a child >5 years of age with erythromycin (40 mg/kg per day div qid, 1 g/day maximum), azithromycin (10 mg/kg, once on day 1, followed by 5 mg/kg q day on days 2–5), or clarithromycin (15 mg/kg div bid, 1 g maximum) for lobar or presumed mycoplasma pneumonia.

If *P. carinii* pneumonia (PCP) is suspected (pp. 378–379), obtain a chest radiograph and LDH. Admit and treat with TMP-SMX (20 mg/kg per day TMP div q 6 h) if the LDH is elevated or the X-ray is consistent with PCP.

Significant pleural effusion is an indication for admission for diagnostic thoracoentesis and parenteral antibiotics.

Follow-up

- Respiratory distress at home: at once
- Lobar pneumonia: 24 hours
- Patient <2 years of age with suspected viral pneumonia: 24–48 hours
- All patients: at the end of treatment or about 2 weeks after presentation to assess for improvement. However, chest X-ray abnormalities can persist for 8–12 weeks after the acute illness, and symptoms (especially cough) can persist for weeks. Therefore, wait at least 8–12 weeks after presentation to consider the need for a follow-up chest X-ray, unless the patient is worsening

Indications for admission

- Patient <2 months of age with pneumonia
- Patient <6 months of age with lobar pneumonia
- Patient with pO_2 <65 mmHg, oxygen saturation <92%, pCO_2 >40 mmHg
- Patient not taking fluids, exhausted, or with parents unable to comply with instructions
- Presence of significant pleural effusion
- Suspicion of PCP

Bibliography

Hausdorff WP, Dagan R: Serotypes and pathogens in paediatric pneumonia. *Vaccine* 2008;26 Suppl 2:B19–23.

Kaplan S: Community-acquired methicillin-resistant *Staphylococcus aureus* infections in children. *Semin Pediatr Infect Dis* 2006;17:113–9.

Ranganathan SC, Sonnappa S: Pneumonia and other respiratory infections. *Pediatr Clin North Am* 2009;56:135–56.

Woods CR: Acute bacterial pneumonia in childhood in the current era. *Pediatr Ann* 2008;37:694–702.

Pulse oximetry

Pulse oximetry is a simple and noninvasive means of measuring the oxygen saturation of hemoglobin. It is based on the principle that deoxygenated blood absorbs more light in the red spectrum, while oxygenated blood absorbs more infrared light. The oximeter measures

Table 21-8. Factors affecting accuracy of pulse oximetry

Condition	Effect on oxygen saturation estimate
Anemia (severe)	False sense of adequate oxygenation
Carboxyhemoglobin	Overestimates
Methemoglobin	Over- and underestimates
Sickle cell anemia	May overestimate (not significantly)
Bilirubin	May underestimate
Dark nail polish	Underestimates
Profound hypoxia (O_2 saturation <80%)	Not reliable
Neonate	Accuracy varies with hemoglobin level

the two different light absorbencies, and then calculates the oxygen saturation. When used appropriately, it provides a reliable assessment of a patient's oxygen status. However, the light source and sensor of the oximetry probe must be placed opposite one another in an accessible area, such as a finger, toe, or earlobe. The pulse rate measured by the oximeter must reflect the patient's actual pulse rate to confirm the reliability of the reading. Verify the oximeter pulse rate reading by correlation with a manually obtained pulse rate. Several factors affect the accuracy of pulse oximetry and may limit its use (see Table 21-8).

Bibliography

Callahan JM: Pulse oximetry in emergency medicine. *Emerg Med Clin North Am* 2008;26:869–79.

Choi J, Claudius I: Decrease in emergency department length of stay as a result of triage pulse oximetry. *Pediatr Emerg Care* 2006;22:412–4.

Lima A, Bakker J: Noninvasive monitoring of peripheral perfusion. *Intensive Care Med* 2005;31:1316–26.

Respiratory distress and failure

Respiratory distress or respiratory failure may be the end point of a multitude of clinical disorders in children, both pulmonary and nonpulmonary in origin. Airway obstruction is the leading cause of life-threatening acute respiratory distress. Causes of upper-airway obstruction include bacterial tracheitis, croup, epiglottitis, and foreign-body aspiration and, rarely, epiglottitis. Asthma or bronchiolitis produce lower-airway obstruction. Other disorders that can culminate in respiratory distress or failure are abnormalities of the neuromuscular control of breathing (seizures, central apnea, meningitis, encephalitis, head trauma), problems with the mechanics of breathing (congenital, acquired, or traumatic chest wall deformities), and alveolar disorders (pneumonia). Nonpulmonary disorders include cardiac disease and heart failure, sepsis, and disorders of oxygen delivery (CO poisoning, methemoglobinemia, severe anemia).

Clinical presentation and diagnosis

Respiratory distress is manifested by difficulty breathing, fatigue, diminished activity and/or feeding, varying degrees of exhaustion, and symptoms associated with the cause. Signs include pallor or cyanosis, tachypnea, retractions, diminished air entry, tachycardia (brady-cardia with severe respiratory failure with hypoxemia), and/or signs of the specific origin of the distress.

Upper-airway obstruction usually presents with stridor. Radiographs may delineate supraglottic disorders such as epiglottitis or a foreign body, although direct visualization of the airway in a controlled setting is the diagnostic and therapeutic procedure of choice.

Lower-airway obstruction presents with hyperinflation, expiratory prolongation, and wheezing. Localized signs are noted more with foreign-body aspiration.

Neurologic diseases lead to depressed level of consciousness, poor respiratory effort or apnea, depressed airway reflexes, and less effective cough.

Mechanical problems present with ineffective chest wall excursion or distorted lung inflation.

Alveolar causes present with general signs of respiratory distress, hypoxemia, and tachypnea. The findings on examination include rales or decreased breath sounds.

Congestive heart failure can present with tachycardia, a gallop, a murmur, diminished heart sounds, venous distention, and sometimes hepatomegaly. Severe anemia presents with pallor and a low hemoglobin.

Nonpulmonary disorders (CO poisoning, methemoglobinemia) require laboratory studies to confirm the diagnosis.

Criteria for respiratory failure

- pO_2 <50 mmHg (oxygen saturation <84%) on 60% FIO_2 (except in cyanotic congenital heart disease)
- pCO_2 >50 mmHg and rising (with pH <7.30) or >40 mmHg with exhaustion
- In neuromuscular and central disorders, central apnea, or decreased vital capacity (<12–15 mL/kg) with exhaustion

ED management

Provide 100% oxygen and perform a rapid cardiopulmonary assessment: assess airway patency, count the respiratory rate, check the stability of the airway (maintainable or unmaintainable), and evaluate color, breath sounds (air entry), heart rate, pulses, capillary refill, and blood pressure. Monitor the oxygen saturation. Ascertain the cause of respiratory failure, and begin immediate therapy.

If the airway is not patent, use the jaw thrust for total airway obstruction and suction for partial obstruction. If respiratory failure is present, continue with 100% O_2 and institute bag-valve-mask ventilation. Intubate patients who are unable to maintain a stable airway for an extended period. Establish IV access and give broad-spectrum antibiotics if infection is likely (cefuroxime 150 mg/kg per day div q 8 h or ceftriaxone 100 mg/kg per day div q 12 h).

Noninvasive positive-pressure ventilation (NPPV)

NPPV is the delivery of positive-pressure ventilation (PPV) through a nasal or oronasal mask. NPPV may reduce the work of breathing and improve gas exchange, without resorting to intubation. It is useful for patients who are alert and able to maintain their own airway, but have evidence of respiratory distress such as retractions, decreased breath sounds, and hypoxia despite 100% oxygen via a nonrebreather mask. Do not use NPPV if the mask does not fit well or the patient is hemodynamically unstable, agitated, unconscious, has facial or neck trauma, or is unable to maintain the airway or handle oral secretions/ongoing emesis.

Compared to traditional positive-pressure ventilation through a tracheal tube, NPPV use reduces the risk of upper-airway trauma, avoids postextubation laryngeal edema and vocal cord dysfunction, decreases the risk of nosocomial respiratory infections, eliminates the need for muscle relaxants, and reduces the need for sedation, and potentially reduces the length of hospitalization.

Continuous positive airway pressure (CPAP)

CPAP delivers uninterrupted pressure support, regardless of the stage of the respiratory cycle. Provide CPAP for infants via nasal prongs. Set the initial positive airway pressure at 4 cmH$_2$O and titrate up to 10 cmH$_2$O, as needed, to reduce the work of breathing.

Bilevel positive airway pressure (BiPAP)

BiPAP provides inspiratory pressure support during inhalation (IPAP) while providing baseline pressure support during exhalation (EPAP). Use BiPAP for older children and adolescents with a well-fitted nasooral mask. Consult with a pediatric pulmonologist to determine whether BiPAP is indicated and the initial settings to be used. Monitor the patient closely for 1 hour following the initiation of BiPAP. Signs of improvement include decreased respiratory rate and work of breathing and improved oxygenation. Lack of improvement suggests the need for intubation.

Mechanical ventilation

Less than 10 kg

Use a pressure-limited ventilator. Adjust inspiratory pressure (IP) to obtain adequate chest movement and audible breath sounds. In disorders with minimal alteration of lung compliance, start with an IP of 20 cm and a rate of 30–40 breaths per minute (bpm). Higher pressures are required in more restrictive (less compliant) disorders.

More than 10 kg

Use a volume-preset ventilator set to deliver 8–10 mL/kg of tidal volume (lower in disorders with hyperinflation), a rate of 20–30 bpm (child) or 12–20 bpm (adolescent).

With either ventilator, consider positive-end-expiratory pressure (PEEP; 4–5 cmH$_2$O) to maintain end-expiratory lung volume and thereby minimize atelectasis and intrapulmonary shunting (except in a patient with hyperinflation). Assess the adequacy of ventilation by chest excursions and breath sounds. Check an ABG after 15 minutes, and obtain other laboratory studies as indicated to ascertain a diagnosis (chest radiograph, lateral neck radiograph, serum electrolytes, respiratory cultures, ECG, lumbar puncture, EEG, CT scan). Subsequent laboratory tests and changes in the ventilator settings are guided by the clinical status, pulse oximetry, and ABG results.

Indications for admission

- Respiratory failure requiring mechanical ventilation or intensive monitoring
- Respiratory distress not reversible with definitive therapy

- New oxygen requirements
- Pulmonary infection requiring parenteral antibiotics

Bibliography

Priestley MA, Helfaer MA: Approaches in the management of acute respiratory failure in children. *Curr Opin Pediatr* 2004;**16**:293–8.

Teague WG: Non-invasive positive pressure ventilation: current status in paediatric patients. *Paed Resp Rev* 2005;**6**:52–60.

Turner DA, Arnold JH: Insights in pediatric ventilation: timing of intubation, ventilatory strategies, and weaning. *Curr Opin Crit Care* 2007;**13**:57–63.

Radiology

Dan Barlev, with Robert Acosta

Ordering radiologic examinations

To maximize the value of ED radiographic imaging, adhere to the following guidelines:

- Order a study if the results will alter the care and management of the patient. For example, the clinical diagnosis of sinusitis is evident in a child who has fever, several days of cough, purulent nasal discharge, and tenderness over the maxilla, so that sinus films will not affect the ED management. However, radiographs might confirm (or help eliminate) the diagnosis of acute sinusitis in a patient with frontal headache and infraorbital swelling, but without purulent rhinorrhea or facial tenderness.
- Consult with a member of the radiology department prior to ordering a test, particularly when the patient's presentation is not straightforward. Discuss the child's signs and symptoms to determine, with the radiologist, the best test or sequence of tests to perform. This may vary by institution or time of day, based on the availability of equipment and expertise of the personnel.
- Inform the radiologist, either in person or when ordering the test, of the location of the patient's findings as well as the tentative diagnosis. Never simply write, for example, "rule out pneumonia," when ordering a chest radiograph. Instead, specify the pertinent history and the nature of the physical findings.
- When ordering radiographic studies for children, limiting the amount of radiation exposure is a critical consideration. The younger the patient the less radiation should be used, as the tissue being irradiated has a longer potential cancer risk. Always use a non-ionizing study if it will yield the answer to your question (i.e. think ultrasound before CT).

The natural radiation exposure in one year is 3 mSV or millisieferts, which is the effect of 300 millirads. Among the more common radiographic studies, the exposure is: chest X-ray (PA and lateral), 0.16 mSv; abdominal X-ray, 0.25 mSv; adult abdominal CT, 10 mSv; and neonatal abdominal CT, 20 mSv. Note that with an adult abdominal CT, a neonate's organs will receive twice the amount of radiation.

Table 22-1 contains suggested radiologic examinations when a patient presents with a particular finding or when a particular diagnosis is being considered.

Table 22-1. Suggested radiologic procedures

	Procedure	Findings	Notes
Neurology			
Head trauma	Noncontrast CT of brain	Epidural bleed: convex (lens shaped) density.	Do not give IV contrast
	Skull films	Subdural bleed: crescentic density which could cross suture lines	Acute blood is dense (white) on CT
		Subarachnoid bleed: blood within sulci.	Calvarial fractures easier to see on plain films
		Brain contusion: focal bleed or edema (hypodense)	Basilar fractures easier to see on CT
VP shunt evaluation	Shunt series	Plain films: identify breaks or kinks in shunt	IV contrast not needed for CT
	Noncontrast CT of brain	CT: evaluate ventricular size	Compare CT to prior studies to assess change in ventricular size
	Abdominal ultrasound (AUS)	AUS: identify CSF pseudocyst	
Acute ataxia Acute hemiparesis Non-febrile seizure Headache	CT of brain	CT: quickly assesses for hydrocephalus, cerebral lesions or acute blood	CT and MRI can be done pre/post IV contrast
	MRI of brain	MRI: more sensitive for posterior fossa (cerebellar) lesions	No imaging needed for febrile seizure
ENT			
Orbital cellulitis	CT of orbits	CT: distinguish preseptal from postseptal disease	IV contrast allows easier abscess identification
		CT: orbital abscess easily seen	
Mastoiditis	CT of temporal bones and mastoids	Opacification of mastoid air cells may be seen	IV contrast not usually necessary, but may be administered if epidural abscess suspected
		Coalescence of air cells represents bony septal destruction	
Sinusitis	Sinus films	Plain films: opacification of sinus or air–fluid level	Limited CT is sufficient (coronal images only, one slice through each sinus)

Table 22-1. (cont.)

	Procedure	Findings	Notes
	Sinus CT	CT: more sensitive in select cases	IV contrast not needed
Retropharyngeal abscess	Soft-tissue neck film	Abnormal retropharyngeal soft-tissue swelling with/ without gas bubbles	Obtain CT only if there is no clinical improvement on IV antibiotics.
	CT of neck	CT: low density center may be seen (IV contrast: ring enhancement)	
Epiglottitis	Clinical diagnosis	Edematous epiglottis and aryepiglottic folds	Do not leave patient unattended
	Soft-tissue neck film only if diagnosis unlikely	Pharyngeal distension	Emergent intubation/ tracheostomy may be needed
Croup	Airway films (usually not necessary)	Steeple sign on frontal view	
Peritonsillar abscess	Imaging not indicated	Infraglottic edema on lateral view	
Cervical adenitis	Imaging usually not indicated		Consider ultrasound if node is enlarging or resistant to antibiotic therapy
Pulmonary			
Foreign-body aspiration	Chest X-rays in inspiration and expiration	Airway obstruction could cause atelectasis, hyperinflation or hyperlucency	Forced exhalation using careful abdominal pressure with a lead-gloved hand may be more useful than decubitus films in a young child
Pneumonia	Chest X-rays	Bacterial (pneumococcal) pneumonia presents as a unifocal pleural- based opacity (usually)	Decubitus views useful in evaluating for pleural effusion
Asthma bronchiolitis	Imaging usually not indicated		
Tuberculosis	Chest X-rays	Lung opacities	
		Hilar and mediastinal adenopathy	
Cardiology			
Congestive failure	Chest X-rays	Large heart and increased central pulmonary blood volume with indistinct vessels	

Table 22-1. (*cont.*)

	Procedure	Findings	Notes
Endocarditis	Chest X-ray	May be normal	
Pericarditis	Chest X-ray	May be normal	
Abdomen			
Appendicitis	Abdomen film	Plain film may be normal Presence of appendicolith associated with perforation	No imaging necessary if clinically positive
	Abdominal ultrasound (AUS)	AUS: blind-ending noncompressable structure >6 mm	
	CT of abdomen	CT: nonfilling of appendix (with oral or rectal contrast), >6 mm in diameter, with thickened wall.	CT done with either: rectal contrast (with/without IV contrast) or PO and IV contrast
Intussusception	Abdominal films	Plain films:crescent or target sign and lack of gas in transverse colon	Hydrate patient prior to reduction attempt
	Abdominal ultrasound (AUS)	AUS: target or pseudokidney sign	
	Contrast/air enema for therapy	Enema for reduction	Hydrostatic reduction contraindicated if peritoneal signs are present
Malrotation/ volvulus	Abdominal films	Plain films may be normal.	
	Abdominal ultrasound (AUS)	AUS: may show reversal of SMA and SMV or whirlpool sign	
	Upper GI series (UGI)	UGI: may show corkscrew sign with dilatation of duodenum	UGI always done through a nasogastric tube
Pyloric stenosis	Abdominal ultrasound (AUS)	Pyloric muscle thickness >3 mm Pyloric channel length >16 mm	Not an emergency study, can wait until the next morning if presentation is in the middle of the night
Meckel's diverticulum	Meckel's scan	Gastric mucosa takes up radiotracer	Findings can be easily obscured by previous barium studies
Cholecystitis	Abdominal ultrasound (AUS)	AUS: stones or thickened GB wall	

Table 22-1. (cont.)

	Procedure	Findings	Notes
	HIDA scan	HIDA scan: cystic duct obstruction	
Gynecology			
Ectopic pregnancy	Transvaginal ultrasound	Extrauterine gestation	Study can confirm an intrauterine pregnancy
		Fluid in cul-de-sac	Twin ectopic pregnancy is very unlikely
Ovarian torsion	Pelvic ultrasound	Enlarged ovary with peripheral follicles	Blood flow may be seen, since ovaries have a dual blood supply
Genitourinary			
Testicular torsion	Scrotal ultrasound (US)	US: absent or decreased flow (especially diastolic flow) on Doppler evaluation	If diagnosis is clear, do not delay surgery to obtain imaging studies
	Testicular (nuclear) scan	Nuclear scan: absent uptake, but a missed torsion may appear as a doughnut sign	
Epididymitis	Scrotal ultrasound (US)	US: enlarged epididymis with increased color Doppler flow	
Trauma			
Cervical spine	Lateral neck X-ray Neck CT	Interruption of anterior vertebral, posterior vertebral, or spinal-laminal lines	Lateral neck: must see C1–C7 and top of T1
		Prevertebral soft-tissue swelling	Once lateral neck is normal, obtain AP, open-mouth views
		Widening of space between dens and anterior arch of C1	Pseudosubluxation seen at C2–3 and C3–4
			Normal films do not exclude major injury
Abdomen	Abdominal film	May see free air or loss of normal fat stripes on plain film	Do not obtain a CT if the patient is unstable
	Abdominal CT	CT with IV contrast (no PO contrast) is very sensitive for visceral organ injury	
Pericardial tamponade	Chest X-ray	Enlarged heart may be seen on plain film	
	Echocardiogram	Echocardiogram can better evaluate size of fluid collection	

Table 22-1. (cont.)

	Procedure	Findings	Notes
Chest	Chest X-ray	Pneumothorax, pulmonary contusion, rib fractures, pleural effusion, pneumomediastinum	CT is contraindicated if the patient is unstable
	Chest CT	CT can better delineate injury seen on plain films	
Renal	CT with contrast	Renal laceration, fracture or pedicle avulsion	Consider delayed scans or delayed abdominal film (after IV contrast injection) to assess bladder (Foley must be clamped beforehand)
Soft-tissue foreign body	Plain films Ultrasound		Most glass is radio-opaque and will be seen on X-ray
Orthopedics			
Osteomyelitis	Plain films	Plain film: periosteal elevation, bone destruction	Plain films not positive for 10+ days
	Bone scan	Bone scan: hot focus	Nuclear scan positive in 24–48 hours
SCFE	AP and frog lateral hip X-rays	Widening of the proximal femoral growth plate with irregularity of the metaphysis may be the earliest sign of the entity (pre-slip slip)	Always image the contralateral side for comparison and since SCFE can be bilateral

Renal emergencies

Sandra J. Cunningham and Preeti Venkataraman, with Beatrice Goilav

Acute glomerulonephritis

Acute glomerulonephritis (AGN) is a clinical syndrome caused by an immune-mediated injury to the glomerulus. Clinical features are reduction in glomerular filtration rate (GFR), oliguria or anuria, azotemia, proteinuria (possibly into the nephrotic range), gross hematuria with RBC casts, pyuria, and evidence of volume overload (hypertension, peripheral edema, vascular congestion). The degree of renal dysfunction and azotemia can range from very mild (subclinical) to severe.

Most cases of AGN result from deposition of preformed immune complexes in glomerular structures (systemic lupus erythematosus) or *in situ* fixation of complement and specific antibody with antigen trapped within glomeruli (postinfectious glomerulonephritis). Other forms of AGN are caused by activation of the classic or alternative complement pathway (membranoproliferative glomerulonephritis), direct antibody-mediated injury (Goodpasture's syndrome), or damage from infiltrated inflammatory cells (Wegener's granulomatosis).

Although hereditary nephritis (Alport syndrome) is considered a form of nephritis, it is caused by a genetic mutation resulting in a structural abnormality of the glomerular basement membrane with subsequent glomerular dysfunction. In IgA nephropathy (Berger's disease), deposition of IgA in the glomerular tuft leads to secondary inflammation. Systemic etiologies that can cause secondary renal injury, but are not a form of glomerulonephritis by definition, include Henoch-Schönlein purpura (vasculitis), hemolytic uremic syndrome (thrombotic microangiopathy), subacute bacterial endocarditis, and shunt (ventriculoatrial) nephritis.

Clinical presentation

As the GFR falls, oliguria/anuria ensues, leading to the clinical symptoms that are the hallmark of AGN: edema (particularly periorbital), weight gain, hypertension (both systolic and diastolic), decreased urine output, and dark green to coca-cola colored urine due to gross hematuria (80% of patients). There may be constitutional symptoms, such as back or abdominal pain, and nausea and vomiting, in addition to the clinical features of the underlying disease. CNS symptoms such as lethargy, irritability, headache, mental status changes, and seizures may occur with a minimal elevation in the blood pressure. Water and salt retention can lead to congestive heart failure, causing dyspnea and orthopnea in association with a systolic murmur, gallop, rales, and a pleural effusion.

Postinfectious glomerulonephritis

The most common etiology of postinfectious glomerulonephritis is group A beta-hemolytic *Streptococcus*. The disease is most common in school-age males and typically starts 1–3 weeks after a sore throat. Impetigo can precede nephritis by up to 6 weeks and is most common in preschool-aged children during the summer months. Onset of AGN that is synchronous with pharyngitis is suggestive of IgA nephropathy. For other infections there may be symptoms of a URI, a mononucleosis-like syndrome, or hepatitis. The onset of the AGN is abrupt, with microscopic/macroscopic hematuria, periorbital edema, and mild-moderate hypertension. More than 90% of children with postinfectious AGN will have a full recovery.

Systemic lupus erythematosos (SLE)

AGN with or without nephrotic syndrome can be the initial presentation of SLE; however, other manifestations of the disease are also usually present, including a butterfly rash, polyserositis, or arthritis.

Henoch-Schönlein purpura

HSP may present with a purpuric rash, abdominal pain, and hematochezia (see pp. 655–656).

Membranoproliferative glomerulonephritis (MPGN)

At the onset of the disease and when there is no clear history of a preceding throat infection, MPGN causes an illness that may be indistinguishable from postinfectious AGN. However, it is more common in older children and adolescent girls and is characterized by persistent (>6 weeks) hypocomplementemia.

Subacute bacterial endocarditis (SBE)

SBE presents with persistent fever, splenomegaly, Roth's spots, Osler's nodes, splinter hemorrhages, and positive blood cultures.

Alport's syndrome

Alport's syndrome, characterized by sensorineural and ocular disorders, can present with gross hematuria and can cause an acute decline in renal function during an intercurrent URI.

Diagnosis

Obtain a careful history, including whether there is a family history of hematuria, hearing loss, or kidney failure. On physical examination, check the blood pressure, note the presence of edema, examine the fundi, skin, heart, lungs, and joints, and assess hearing, mental status, and neurologic function.

If AGN is suspected, order a urinalysis. In glomerular disease, regardless of the etiology, dysmorphic RBCs and RBC casts are almost always present and are diagnostic of this disorder. In renal diseases associated with nonglomerular hematuria, such as nephrolithiasis, trauma, or a bleeding diathesis, the RBCs are eumorphic and RBC casts are not seen. If there is gross hematuria, examine an unspun urine specimen. WBCs may predominate over RBCs early in the course of the disease, suggesting the diagnosis of a urinary tract infection. Proteinuria >2+ on a dipstick is virtually always present. Also obtain a CBC, platelet count, ESR, CRP, serum electrolytes, calcium, BUN, creatinine, total protein, albumin, cholesterol, triglycerides, and complement (C3, C4, C50). Hypocomplementemic forms of AGN include postinfectious, SLE, membranoproliferative glomerulonephritis, shunt nephritis, and embolic renal disease.

If the clinical picture is compatible with poststreptococcal AGN, obtain an ASLO or streptozyme or a skin culture if there is impetigo. If SLE is a consideration, obtain an ANA and anti-dsDNA antibody titer. Obtain serial blood cultures and a cardiac echo to rule out SBE in a patient with persistent fever and no obvious source. If there are any signs of a bleeding diathesis, obtain a PT and PTT.

ED management

Consult a nephrologist for all patients with AGN. Immediate priorities include management of hypertension and hyperkalemia. Because hypertensive encephalopathy can occur at a minimally increased blood pressure, especially in poststreptococcal AGN, treat hypertension promptly and aggressively. For an asymptomatic patient, use oral nifedipine (0.25 mg/kg, 10 mg maximum). The onset of action of nifedipine is immediate after the patient bites the capsule and swallows its contents. For a slower reduction in BP, give amlodipine (0.1 mg/kg per dose), or if the child does not have a history of asthma, oral labetalol (2 mg/kg per dose). These two latter drugs have no significant metabolic effects and the patient can be safely discharged while taking them.

For a patient with acute neurologic symptoms (headache, seizures, altered mental status), treat with IV nicardipine or labetalol (contraindicated in asthma and pulmonary edema) (see Hypertension, pp. 656–658). The goal of the initial antihypertensive therapy is a 20% reduction in the mean blood pressure (diastolic BP + 1/3 [systolic BP–diastolic BP]).

The cornerstone of medical management is fluid and sodium restriction (see acute kidney injury, pp. 647–650). Restrict fluids to insensible losses plus urine output, regardless of whether the patient is oliguric. Withhold potassium until the patient voids and eukalemia is documented (see Hyperkalemia, pp. 176–177). When the child can eat, limit the sodium to 2 g/day.

Conservative medical therapy is the rule, with renal replacement therapy reserved for severe volume overload with pulmonary edema, life-threatening hyperkalemia ($\geq$7 mEq/L), intractable acidosis, intractable hypocalcemia with seizures, or symptomatic uremia (pleuritis, pericarditis, GI bleeding, encephalopathy).

Follow-up

- AGN with asymptomatic hypertension, mild edema, and normal urine output: the next day for a BP check. Ongoing follow-up is needed until the blood pressure and complements normalize and proteinuria resolves

Indication for admission

- AGN with pulmonary edema, hypertension, or oliguria

Bibliography

Ahn SY, Ingulli E: Acute poststreptococcal glomerulonephritis: an update. *Curr Opin Pediatr* 2008;20:157–62.

Beck LH Jr: Glomerular and tubulointerstitial diseases. *Prim Care* 2008;35:265–96.

Rodriguez-Iturbe B, Musser JM: The current state of glomerulonephritis. *J Am Soc Nephrol* 2008;10:1855–64.

Acute kidney injury

Acute kidney injury (AKI; formerly acute renal failure) is characterized by a decrease in the glomerular filtration rate (GFR), associated with increases in blood urea nitrogen and serum creatinine concentrations (azotemia). Oliguria ($\leq$0.5 mL/kg per hr) is a frequent, but not invariable, finding.

The causes of AKI can be divided into three pathophysiologic categories: prerenal, postrenal, and renal parenchymal disease (Table 23-1). Prerenal azotemia reflects a decline in renal function in the absence of primary structural injury. It is a consequence of inadequate kidney perfusion secondary to hypovolemia (dehydration or blood loss), hypotension, or ischemia/hypoxia. The GFR is rapidly restored to normal when renal blood flow is increased; however, severe renal hypoperfusion may lead to acute tubular necrosis (ATN). Postrenal azotemia is secondary to urinary tract obstruction. Renal parenchymal disease can result from glomerular diseases (AGN, hemolytic-uremic syndrome), or tubular injury secondary to nephrotoxins, rhabdomyolysis, or tubular ischemia, as well as acute interstitial nephritis.

Clinical presentation

The clinical presentation of AKI is varied. There may be findings secondary to renal dysfunction such as fluid overload (peripheral edema, weight gain, pleural effusions), hypertension, nausea and vomiting, hypocalcemic tetany, and neurologic symptoms (coma, seizures). Alternatively, the presentation may reflect the primary pathologic process, such as loss of peripheral pulses, prolonged capillary refill time or hypotension (hypovolemic shock); difficulty voiding and an abnormal urinary stream (obstruction); lethargy and fever (sepsis); cutaneous burns, bleeding, or jaundice (hemoglobinuria); myonecrosis due to trauma or heat illness (myoglobinuria); pallor and bloody diarrhea (HUS); rash, abdominal pain and arthralgias (HSP); or gross hematuria in the context of an antecedent sore throat or URI (postinfectious AGN).

Diagnosis

Make a rapid assessment of the patient's volume status, looking for clinical signs of dehydration (orthostatic vital sign changes, poor capillary refill, weak peripheral pulses, hypotension) or volume overload (edema, rales, palpable liver, cardiac gallop). It is essential to identify the cause of oliguria as quickly as possible and to institute immediate treatment. Prerenal azotemia is a reversible condition early in its course; failure to recognize a prerenal etiology (hypovolemia) can lead to ATN.

Estimate the GFR by using the Schwartz formula:

$$GFR = (\text{the patient's height in cm} \times 0.5)/\text{serum Cr in mg/dL}$$

An increase in creatinine of 0.3 from baseline raises suspicion of kidney injury, despite a serum creatinine level that is still within the range of normal.

If the patient is unable or unwilling to void spontaneously, insert a Foley catheter to obtain urine and monitor the urine output. To differentiate among the causes of oliguria, obtain urine for specific gravity, sodium and creatinine, and microscopy. Look for blood, protein, and RBC casts (AGN) or pyuria >5 WBC/hpf (pyelonephritis, ATN). Concentrated urine with a high specific gravity is a feature of prerenal AKI, while isosthenuric urine with a specific gravity $\leq$1.010 and few or no cells or proteinuria is seen in interstitial

Table 23-1. Classification of acute kidney injury

Prerenal	Postrenal	Renal
Mechanism		
Hypovolemia	Obstruction	Nephrotoxin
Hypotension		Ischemia
Hypoxia		Glomerulonephritis
Etiologies		
Dehydration	Urolithiasis	ATN from renal cause not treated expeditiously
Sepsis	Posterior urethral valves	
Hemorrhage	Intraabdominal tumor	Myo- or hemoglobinuria
Anaphylaxis	Neurogenic (herpes, MS, spina bifida)	Antibiotics (gentamicin, amphotericin, vancomycin)
Burn	Renal vein thrombosis	Acute pyelonephritis
Cardiogenic		Heavy metals
Hyperthermia		Cardiopulmonary arrest
Antihypertensives		Acute interstitial nephritis

Table 23-2. Laboratory findings in acute kidney injury

Diagnosis	U_{SG}	U_{NA} (mEq/L)	BUN/Cr	FE_{NA} (%)	U/A
Prerenal azotemia	>1.020	<20	>20	<1	Nonspecific
Acute glomerulonephritis (early)	>1.020	<20	>20	<1	RBC casts, dysmorphic RBCs
Acute tubular necrosis	1.008–1.012	>40	<20	>1	Tubular epithelial cells
Postrenal	1.008–1.012	>40	<20	>1	Nonspecific

Notes: U_{SG}, urine specific gravity; U_{Na}, urine sodium concentration; BUN/Cr, ratio of BUN to creatinine; FE_{Na}, fractional excretion of sodium; $(U_{Na} \times P_{Cr})/(P_{Na} \times U_{Cr})$; U/A, typical urinalysis finding.

nephritis. Hematuria on dipstick examination, but without RBCs seen on microscopy, is consistent with myoglobinuria or hemoglobinuria.

Obtain blood for electrolytes, BUN, and creatinine (see Table 23-2). Calculate the fractional excretion of sodium (FE_{Na}):

(urineNa/plasmaNa)/(urineCr/plasmaCr)

When urine is unavailable or the urinary findings are pending, but there is no evidence of volume overload and obstruction has been ruled-out (sonogram), attempt to discriminate intrarenal AKI from prerenal azotemia by rapidly infusing 20 mL/kg of an isotonic solution (normal saline, Ringer's lactate). If the oliguria persists and there are no signs of volume overload, repeat the bolus until it is clear that the patient is not volume-depleted (based on vital signs and capillary refill). If there is no diuresis, give one dose of IV furosemide (1–2 mg/kg). If oliguria continues, the diagnosis of intrinsic renal disease (frequently ATN) is probable. If urine output increases with these measures, the patient has prerenal insufficiency, which will return to normal provided adequate maintenance fluid therapy is given. If a sonogram cannot be obtained immediately, a distended bladder suggests a postrenal problem.

ED management

Prerenal AKI

See above.

Intrarenal AKI

Fluid

Give a fluid bolus of 20 mL/kg of isotonic solution as quickly as possible to patients with hemodynamic instability and oliguria, especially if there are signs of sepsis. Multiple boluses may be necessary until blood pressure and pulse normalize.

If a hemodynamically stable patient remains oliguric, fluid restriction is required: limit fluids to insensible losses plus urine output. Estimate insensible losses to be 400 mL/m^2 per day; losses are higher with fever and burns and lower with mechanical ventilation.

Sodium

If the patient is hyponatremic, the goal is to correct the sodium to at least 125 mEq/L. In patients with sodium >120 mEq/L, restore the deficit slowly, (2–4 mEq/L q 4 h) using the following calculation:

$$(125 - \text{patient's sodium}) \times (\text{weight in kg}) \times (0.6) = \text{mEq Na}$$

Initiate a rapid correction for patients who are seizing, or are symptomatic and have a sodium <120 mEq/L. Administer hypertonic (3%) saline, which contains 513 mEq/L of Na (every 2 mL contains 1 mEq Na). Calculate the amount of 3% NaCl as follows:

$$3\% \text{ NaCl (mEq/L)} = (125 - \text{measured Na}) \times \text{body weight (kg)} \times 0.6$$

Multiply this result by 2 to determine the volume in mL.

Potassium

Hyperkalemia is often present in AKI as a result of renal dysfunction and an acidosis-induced shift of potassium to the extracellular space. Dietary restriction (1 g/day) is sufficient if the potassium is <6 mEq/L. If the potassium is ≥6.0 mEq/L, immediately obtain an ECG to identify cardiac conduction abnormalities such as peaked T waves (T wave ≥ one-half the R or S wave) and a shortened QT interval. Later changes include lengthening of the PR interval and QRS duration.

The treatment of hyperkalemia primarily entails enhancing potassium excretion or increasing the movement of potassium into cells as a temporary measure, as well as minimizing cardiac effects. Aggressive IV therapy is necessary for patients who are symptomatic (muscle weakness or cramps/tetany) or have ECG changes. Give 0.5–1 g/kg of glucose (2–4 mL/kg of a 25% dextrose solution) over 30 minutes concurrently with regular insulin (1 unit per 5 g of glucose given). The potassium-lowering effect occurs in 10–20 minutes, but carefully monitor the serum glucose for both hyper- and hypoglycemia. Nebulized β agonists, such as albuterol, are also effective at shifting potassium into the cells, but are less predictable than other therapies. The peak effect is 40–80 minutes after administration. The dose is 10–20 mg in 4 mL normal saline (4–8 times the dose used for the treatment of asthma).

In the absence of peaked T waves, treat with polystyrene sulfonate (Kayexalate), 1 g/kg dissolved in 4 mL of water, with sorbitol (PO or PR). This dose lowers the serum potassium by 0.5–1 mEq/L by enhancing GI excretion, but the onset is slow and duration is variable. In a patient who is not anuric, give furosemide (1–2 mg/kg). The onset of action is within one hour, and the dose may be repeated every 6 hours.

Calcium

Calcium will stabilize the myocardium without affecting the serum potassium level. If there is a cardiac arrhythmia, give IV 10% calcium gluconate solution (100 mg/kg). Do not exceed a rate of 100 mg/minute. The cardiac membrane stabilizing effects are seen in 1–3 minutes. Complications include hypercalcemia and bradycardia; continuously monitor the ECG, and stop the calcium if the patient becomes bradycardic. Use the same regimen to treat hypocalcemia causing tetany, laryngospasm, arrhythmias, or seizures. When the symptoms have resolved, add maintenance calcium to the IV solution (100 mg elemental calcium/kg per day).

Bicarbonate

Sodium bicarbonate may be helpful for severe acidosis, but its use is not recommended to lower serum potassium levels. To correct acidosis, use the following equation:

$$\text{mEq bicarbonate} = (\text{desired} - \text{observed bicarbonate}) \times \text{kg} \times 0.5$$

Dialysis

Absolute indications for dialysis include life-threatening hyperkalemia (serum potassium ≥7 mEq/L) not responsive to pharmacologic treatment or in an anuric patient, intractable acidosis, symptomatic volume overload (CHF, pulmonary edema), and symptomatic uremia (pleuritis, pericarditis, encephalopathy, GI bleeding).

Hypertension

Hypertension is frequent in AKI and may be mild and asymptomatic or life-threatening. Treat mild hypertension with salt restriction and oral antihypertensives, but more severe hypertension requires IV medication and dialysis when secondary to fluid overload.

Postrenal AKI

Immediately consult with a urologist to determine the appropriate therapy.

Indication for admission

- Acute kidney injury

Bibliography

Andreoli SP: Acute kidney injury in children. *Pediatr Nephrol* 2009;24:253–63.

Andreoli SP: Management of acute kidney injury in children: a guide for pediatricians. *Paediatr Drugs* 2008;10:379–90.

Whyte DA, Fine RN: Acute renal failure in children. *Pediatr Rev* 2008;29:299–307.

Hematuria

Hematuria is defined as ≥5 RBCs/hpf of unspun urine or >2–5 RBCs/hpf in a centrifuged specimen. Up to 5% of school-age children have microscopic hematuria on a single specimen, and 1–2% have this finding subsequently confirmed. The incidence increases with age and is greater in girls. Gross hematuria reflects RBCs in the urine that are visible upon inspection.

Hematuria can be classified as either traumatic or nontraumatic in origin. Nontraumatic hematuria can be divided into upper and lower genitourinary tract; upper tract bleeding may be further subdivided into glomerular and non-glomerular causes.

Clinical presentation
Traumatic bleeding
See Renal and genitourinary trauma, pp. 285–286.

Nontraumatic bleeding
Lower genitourinary tract
Lower urinary tract bleeding is most often caused by a urinary tract infection and is accompanied by suprapubic pain and dysuria. A bacterial UTI presents with urgency, frequency, pyuria, and bacteriuria, although these signs and symptoms may be absent in the infant or young child. Viral cystitis (adenovirus, BK virus in immunocompromised individuals) can occur in association with URI symptoms and is accompanied by fever, suprapubic tenderness, and gross hematuria. Urine cultures will be negative, and the hematuria resolves within 5–7 days without any specific treatment. Schistosomiasis is a parasitic cause of terminal microscopic and gross hematuria in recent immigrants or travelers to endemic areas (a stool sample is needed to detect characteristic eggs).

A urethral foreign body presents with dysuria in an afebrile toddler. Urolithiasis can present with microscopic or gross hematuria and intense renal colic. Often the patient has a history of urinary tract abnormalities or infections. Some drugs (cyclophosphamide) are toxic to the bladder and can cause hemorrhagic cystitis.

Upper genitourinary tract – glomerular
Hallmarks of glomerular bleeding, which may be microscopic or gross, include RBC casts and dysmorphic RBCs, with or without proteinuria. In addition, edema, hypertension, and oliguria can occur (see AKI, pp. 647–650). There may be a history of a sore throat or impetigo in the previous 2 weeks (poststreptococcal glomerulonephritis, pp. 644–646) or 1–2 days (IgA nephropathy). A family history of early deafness and renal disease predominantly in males defines X-linked Alport's syndrome (hereditary nephritis). Palpable purpura of the lower extremities, abdominal pain, hematochezia, and arthralgias occur with HSP (pp. 655–656). A history of a URI or diarrhea, followed by weakness, pallor, and CNS

symptoms, is seen in HUS (pp. 242–243). Hematuria can be the presenting sign of SLE (pp. 679–681), although generally there are associated findings (butterfly rash, polyserositis, arthritis, hematologic abnormalities).

Upper genitourinary tract – nonglomerular

Urinary RBCs will be eumorphic and RBC casts will be absent. Sickle cell trait is associated with gross or microscopic hematuria without other obvious manifestations of renal disease. Wilms' tumor can cause gross hematuria in children <6 years of age. However, hematuria is the presenting symptom in only 10% of cases, as most present with an abdominal mass.

Congenital and anatomic abnormalities such as polycystic kidney disease, renal hemangioma, and hydronephrosis can also present with hematuria after minor blunt abdominal trauma. Nutcracker syndrome, compression of the left renal vein between the aorta and the proximal superior mesenteric artery, can cause asymptomatic hematuria or left flank pain. Idiopathic hypercalciuria, in the absence of urolithiasis, is a common cause of nonglomerular painless hematuria, which can be microscopic or gross. There is often a positive family history of urolithiasis.

Diagnosis

Hematuria must be confirmed by microscopic examination of the urine, since not all red urine and not all dipstick-positive urine contains RBCs. Foodstuffs such as beets, red dyes, and drugs such as rifampin and phenazopyridine can give the urine a red tint. In infants, urate crystals may stain the diaper pink. A urine dipstick will also detect hemoglobin and myoglobin. In addition, hematuria may be incorrectly diagnosed when a menstruating female provides a voided urine specimen.

Gross hematuria can be bright red, brown, or dark green. The urine sample from a patient with gross hematuria is always turbid, due to the presence of RBCs. This is in contrast to pigmenturia, in which the urine is wine-colored but transparent. Pigmenturia due to myoglobin or hemoglobin can be differentiated by centrifugation of a sample of serum; a pink tinge is found with hemoglobin, whereas the serum is clear with myoglobin.

A careful urinalysis is critical for locating the source of the bleeding. With nonglomerular hematuria, the RBCs appear eumorphic. Gross nonglomerular hematuria is usually red and may be associated with clots. With glomerular hematuria there usually are RBC casts, and the RBCs are dysmorphic. In gross hematuria of glomerular origin, the urine is cloudy and dark brown (cola- or tea-colored) and never associated with clots.

Idiopathic hypercalciuria is suggested by a spot urine Ca:Cr ratio >0.20 in children >2 years of age, with slightly higher normal ratios in younger infants. However, confirmation requires a 24-hour urine collection with a calcium excretion >4 mg/kg per day.

Microscopic hematuria that occurs only with fever or exercise is usually transient and does not indicate underlying pathology.

ED management

Obtain a thorough history, including current symptoms (fever, dysuria, suprapubic pain, URI, pharyngitis, gastroenteritis, joint pain), recent genitourinary trauma, medication use, previous episodes of hematuria or sickle cell trait or disease, recent weight gain and family history of renal disease or deafness (hereditary nephritis [Alport's syndrome] accounts for nearly 40% of patients with microscopic hematuria of glomerular origin).

Priorities on the physical examination include measuring the blood pressure and evaluating the patient for rash or purpura, abdominal mass, signs of a bleeding disorder, edema, and arthritis.

Traumatic hematuria

See Genitourinary trauma, pp. 285–286.

Nontraumatic hematuria

In the absence of edema, hypertension, an abdominal mass, proteinuria, or oliguria, the work-up of nontraumatic hematuria can be performed on an outpatient basis. If the bleeding is nonglomerular, obtain a urine culture, sickle prep, and measurement of urinary calcium excretion. Order an ultrasound if there is gross hematuria. When there is isolated hematuria (no proteinuria) of glomerular origin, minimal testing is warranted. Obtain a BUN, creatinine, and C3 and C4 levels if there is a history of hematuria for >6 months.

Admit patients with acute glomerulonephritis and fluid overload, hypertension, elevated BUN/Creatinine, or oliguria. In addition to the initial workup outlined above, further evaluation includes urine protein to Cr ratio, serum protein and albumin, serology (ANA, ASLO, VDRL), and consultation with a nephrologist. The management of acute kidney injury is detailed elsewhere (pp. 647–650).

Follow-up

- Nontraumatic hematuria (< 50 RBC/hpf) with a normal physical examination and without signs of glomerulonephritis or renal dysfunction: primary care or nephrology follow-up in 2–4 weeks

Indications for admission

- Acute glomerulonephritis with edema, hypertension or oliguria
- Acute kidney injury
- Hematuria associated with an abdominal mass

Bibliography

Bergstein J, Leiser J, Andreoli S: The clinical significance of asymptomatic gross and microscopic hematuria in children. *Arch Pediatr Adolesc Med* 2005;159:353–5.

Massengill, SF: Hematuria. *Pediatr Rev* 2008;29:342–8.

Pan CG: Evaluation of gross hematuria. *Pediatr Clin North Am* 2006;53:401–12.

Hemolytic uremic syndrome

The hemolytic uremic syndrome (HUS), the most common cause of AKI in children, is characterized by the triad of microangiopathic hemolytic anemia, thrombocytopenia, and AKI. Although the mortality from renal failure has decreased, renal sequelae occur in approximately 40% of patients. Late renal deterioration, with hypertension, proteinuria, and reduced renal function, can occur after apparent resolution of the disease. HUS is divided into two subtypes: diarrhea-associated or typical and non-diarrheal or atypical.

The diarrheal form accounts for the majority of cases (>90%) and generally affects previously healthy children who have ingested foods contaminated with *E. coli* O157:H7 that produce a Shiga toxin. *Shigella, Salmonella, Yersinia, Campylobacter,* and *S. pneumoniae* also have been implicated. Common associated foods include hamburger meat, and unpasteurized dairy products and cider. The peak incidence is from 6 months to 4 years of age, and there is a seasonal pattern, with most cases occurring between April and October.

Non-epidemic HUS accounts for fewer than 10% of cases and can occur at any age, with no seasonal predilection. There is no diarrheal prodrome, although an antecedent URI is often reported. Unlike epidemic HUS, the onset is slow and progressive.

Clinical presentation

A generalized, toxin-mediated, thrombotic microangiopathy occurs, presenting as a diffuse colitis with abdominal pain and hematochezia or bloody diarrhea. The diarrhea prodrome lasts for 1 to 15 days, followed by the abrupt onset of pallor and/or jaundice. Fever is generally absent. Renal impairment is manifested by hematuria, proteinuria, and oliguria/anuria, but gross hematuria is rare. Electrolyte disturbances are common and include metabolic acidosis, hyperkalemia, hyponatremia, and hypophosphatemia. There may also be neurologic symptoms secondary to the microangiopathy, uremia, hypertensive encephalopathy (coma, seizures, personality changes), as well as manifestations of fluid overload (edema, hypertension, congestive heart failure). Petechiae may be present.

Diagnosis

Obtain a CBC with peripheral smear, PT/PTT, Coombs test, LDH, haptoglobin, electrolytes, bilirubin, BUN/Cr, urinalysis, and stool for antigen studies specific for *E. coli* O157: H7 (routine stool cultures will not detect *E. coli* O157:H7). Consistent laboratory features include a peripheral blood smear that shows microangiopathic changes, including schistocytes, burr cells, and helmet cells. Anemia can be severe with hemoglobin as low as 5 g/dL. Thrombocytopenia (generally $<60,000/mm^3$) is a consistent finding. The Coombs test is negative, and the PT, PTT, and coagulation factors are normal. LDH and bilirubin may be elevated and the haptoglobin decreased, indicating intravascular hemolysis. BUN/Cr are elevated and the urinalysis is positive for blood and protein.

ED management

Management is supportive and specific to the patient's presentation. Transfuse packed RBCs for patients with a Hgb <6 g/dL, to a conservative goal of 9 g/dL. Transfuse slowly to avoid further fluid overload and resulting cardiac compromise. Platelet transfusions are not routinely needed and are reserved for patients with significant bleeding. Manage fluid and electrolyte disturbances as for AKI. The treatment of hypertension (pp. 656–658) and seizures (pp. 519–523) is detailed elsewhere. Indications for dialysis include life-threatening signs/symptoms that are refractory to medical therapy, such as severe hyperkalemia or acidosis, cardiopulmonary compromise from fluid overload, azotemia with BUN >80 mg/dL, uremia, or oliguria >24 hours.

Indication for admission

- HUS

Bibliography

Fiorino EK, Raffaelli RM: Hemolytic-uremic syndrome. *Pediatr Rev* 2006;27:398–9.

Iijima K, Kamioka I, Nozu K: Management of diarrhea-associated hemolytic uremic

syndrome in children. *Clin Exp Nephrol* 2008;12:16–19.

Tarr PI, Gordon CA, Carter JE: Shiga-toxin-producing Escherichia coli and haemolytic uraemic syndrome. *Lancet* 2005;365:1073–86.

Henoch-Schönlein purpura

Henoch-Schönlein purpura (HSP) is an immune-mediated small vessel vasculitis associated with IgA deposition. Ninety percent of cases occur in children 3–17 years of age (peak incidence at 4–6 years of age). Patients present with one or more of the following: a purpuric rash on the extensor surfaces of the lower extremities and buttocks, abdominal pain, hematochezia, and arthritis/arthralgias of the large joints, although not all of these features are present at the same time. There is often a history of a preceding URI. Etiologies include group A *Streptococcus*, parvovirus, adenovirus, and mycoplasma. Renal involvement may be the initial manifestation of HSP; alternatively, the nephritis can develop after other features of the disease have resolved.

Clinical presentation

The clinical symptoms are a consequence of the small vessel damage occurring in the skin, GI tract, and kidneys. The rash may initially be urticarial. It then evolves into a palpable purpura that occurs in crops on the lower extremities, especially the buttocks and extensor surfaces. Colicky abdominal pain and hematochezia may also be present. The most common GI complication of HSP is intussusception, most often ileoileal.

Arthralgias usually occur in the large joints of the lower extremities (knees, hips, ankles), although the upper extremities are sometimes affected as well. There may be significant limited range of motion with swelling and tenderness but generally without warmth, erythema, or joint effusion. The joint involvement may precede the skin manifestations by a few days. Scrotal edema or pain may also occur.

Renal involvement occurs in 25–50% of children within 4 weeks of presentation. It can range from isolated microscopic or gross hematuria with or without low-grade proteinuria to nephrotic syndrome.

Diagnosis

The rash as described above is characteristic. However, before the classic purpuric rash evolves, the diagnosis may be confused with other diseases that present with the similar symptom complex of rash, edema, arthralgias, abdominal complaints, and renal findings.

In Wegener's granulomatosis the majority of patients present with upper airway complaints such as persistent rhinorrhea, purulent nasal discharge, or sinus pain. In SLE about one-third of patients present with the classic malar rash and hematologic abnormalities are common, including anemia or thrombocytopenia.

Obtain a CBC, ESR, CRP, PT/PTT, IgA, complement levels, BUN and creatinine, and a throat culture. Complement levels, platelet count, and PT/PTT will be normal in HSP. Also obtain a urine for RBC, WBC, casts, and urinary protein to creatinine ratio (abnormal if >0.2).

ED management

Fluid management and the treatment of hypertension are similar to that for AGN and require consultation with a nephrologist. Treat scrotal pain and edema with elevation and cool compresses. An evaluation for testicular torsion (pp. 293–294) may be necessary if the classic signs of HSP are not present. See pp. 249–250 for the evaluation and management of a possible intussusception.

Follow-up

- Every 2–3 days until the blood pressure is normal and the hematuria and arthralgias are resolving (if present)

Indications for admission

- GI hemorrhage or compromise, protein-losing enteropathy, decreased GFR, or hypertension

Bibliography

Chang WL, Yang YH, Wang LC, et al: Renal manifestations in children with Henoch-Schönlein purpura: a 10-year clinical study. *Pediatr Nephrol* 2005;20:1269–72.

Dedeoglu F, Sundel RP: Vasculitis in children. *Pediatr Clin North Am* 2005;52:547–75.

Saulsbury FT: Clinical update: Henoch-Schönlein Purpura. *Lancet* 2007;369:976–8.

Hypertension

Hypertension is estimated to occur in up to 4.5% of children between the ages of 8 and 17 years of age. This represents an increase from 1.1% in the 1980s, probably secondary to the increase in the prevalence of childhood obesity. An identifiable cause of hypertension (mostly renal) is more common in children younger than 10 years of age, whereas in older patients essential hypertension is the leading cause.

The evaluation of blood pressure in children is dependent on the individual's age, gender, and height. Use age-specific blood pressure tables adjusted for height (e.g. the *Harriet Lane Handbook*) to confirm the normal ranges of blood pressure in children.

Classification of blood pressure in children is based on normative data (Table 23-3).

In the ED, hypertension is often an incidental finding and the elevation is generally mild. Further diagnostic testing can usually be deferred to a primary care setting. Hypertensive crises, however, require immediate intervention. Hypertensive crises can be divided into urgent hypertension or emergency hypertension, depending on whether there is end-organ dysfunction (i.e. seizures) as determined by the history, physical examination, or laboratory tests, rather than the absolute increase in the blood pressure. Emergency hypertension in children is unusual; the most common causes are renal parenchymal disorders, renal vascular lesions, pheochromocytoma, and drugs.

Clinical presentation

The clinical presentation of hypertension varies from asymptomatic to hypertensive encephalopathy and evidence of end-organ dysfunction. The patient with emergency

Table 23-3. Classification of systolic and diastolic blood pressures

Normortensive	<90th percentile
Prehypertensive	between 90th and 95th percentiles or >120/80 regardless of percentile
Hypertensive	≥95th percentile on at least 3 occasions
Stage 1	between 95th and 99th percentiles plus 5 mmHg
Stage 2	>99th percentile plus 5 mmHg

hypertension has symptoms (disorientation, seizures) that can be ascribed to the increase in blood pressure, the blood pressure exceeds the 99th percentile in both upper extremities on at least three successive readings by two examiners over 10 minutes, or the primary disease demands emergency treatment (increased intracranial pressure, renal failure). Patients may present with headache, dizziness, vomiting, visual changes, ataxia, or obtundation. Hypertensive infants may present with nonspecific symptoms such as crying, irritability or respiratory distress or in congestive heart failure.

Diagnosis

It is imperative to choose the correct blood pressure cuff size; a cuff that is too narrow gives a falsely high reading. The bladder width should be 40% of the circumference of the arm at midpoint between the acromion and the olecranon, and the bladder length should cover 80–100% of the circumference of the arm. When the choice of cuff size is between one that is too small versus one that is too large, select the larger size cuff. If using an automated blood pressure device, repeat by auscultation using a manual device when the blood pressure measurement is >90th percentile.

Obtain a hypertension-oriented history: neonatal history (prematurity, umbilical line catheterization), congenital anomalies, medication use (sympathomimetics, oral contraceptives), illicit drug (cocaine) or alcohol use, cardiac or renal disease (especially hematuria or history of urinary tract infections), history of pregnancy, the nature of any previous hypertensive episodes (particularly if episodic), and a family history of hypertension, renal, cardiovascular or endocrine disease, as well as stroke.

Useful physical examination findings include height, weight, and differential blood pressure and pulses between upper and lower extremities. Look for evidence of neurologic dysfunction, AV nicking, hemorrhages or papilledema on fundoscopy, heart murmur or pulmonary findings (rales) of CHF, abdominal mass/bruits, skin lesions (purpura in HSP) or virilization. When the heart rate as well as the blood pressure is elevated, consider hyperthyroidism, neuroblastoma, or pheochromocytoma.

If a secondary cause of the hypertension is suspected (young children, significantly elevated blood pressure, physical examination abnormalities, or contributory family history), obtain a urinalysis, serum electrolytes, glucose, BUN and creatinine, chest X-ray, and ECG, and schedule a renal ultrasound. If an adrenal cause is suspected (virilization, cushingoid appearance), obtain a serum cortisol and 17-hydroxyprogesterone. If there are symptoms suggestive of a pheochromocytoma (headache, sweating, nausea, vomiting, flushing), obtain a serum metanephrine level and a 24-hour urine collection for catecholamine excretion.

In general, defer the diagnostic evaluation of asymptomatic mild to moderate hypertension to a primary care setting where further testing can be done if sustained hypertension is confirmed by repeated measurements.

ED management

Hypertensive emergencies

See Table 23-4. Immediate parenteral therapy is required for severe hypertension associated with end-organ damage (seizures, encephalopathy, pulmonary edema). The goal of acute antihypertensive therapy in a hypertensive emergency is to lower the BP by 25% over the first hour to prevent ongoing end-organ damage. The BP should then be brought to normal within 8 hours. Lowering the BP too fast can potentially result in ischemic target-organ damage (cerebral ischemia), although this is more common in adults with preexisting cardiovascular disease. A continuous IV infusion with meticulous monitoring is the safest way to lower the blood pressure. Alternatively, IV boluses may be used; however, these may lead to BP fluctuations, which may worsen end-organ damage. Establish IV access, institute continuous cardiac monitoring, and measure urine output. Nicardipine (see Table 23-4) is an appropriate drug for hypertensive emergencies, especially when the patient's medical history is unknown (e.g. asthma).

Hypertensive urgencies

Patients with BP >99th percentile who are asymptomatic and without a history, physical examination, or laboratory evidence of end-organ damage require a slower reduction in blood pressure with the use of oral antihypertensives. In patients with hypertensive urgency and no evidence of end-organ dysfunction, hospitalization may not be required. If a patient with known hypertension presents with severe hypertension, they may be monitored in the ED for 4–6 hours after administration of an oral antihypertensive. The use of a long-acting antihypertensive is warranted, because short-acting drugs could lead to profound hypotension and cerebral or myocardial ischemia. The goal is reduction of the blood pressure to the targeted normal in three steps, with the first occurring within the first 4–6 hours. Adequate follow-up must be in place to ensure that the patient's blood pressure is reduced by another 1/3 in 24–36 hours, and the final 1/3 by 96 hours.

Follow-up

- Asymptomatic or mild to moderate hypertension: primary care follow-up in 1–2 weeks
- Hypertensive urgency after BP control attained and with assurance of good follow-up: pediatric nephrologist in 1–3 days for BP check and further diagnostic work-up

Indications for admission

- Hypertensive emergency
- Symptomatic or severe hypertension (sustained systolic and/or diastolic >99th percentile for age)
- Hypertension of any degree associated with acute glomerulonephritis, chronic renal failure, or any other urgent underlying condition

Table 23-4. Antihypertensive treatment for emergency hypertension (IV) and urgent hypertension (oral)

Drug	Class	Route/dose	Comments
IV infusions for emergency hypertension			
Nicardipine	Ca^{2+} channel blocker	0.5 mcg/kg per min	Useful when etiology or history unknown (asthma)
		Titrate to 2 mcg/kg per min	Onset 2–5 min
		3 mcg/kg per min maximum	Can cause ↑HR
Labetalol	α and β blocker	0.4–1 mg/kg per hr	Contraindicated in asthma, CHF, pulmonary edema
		3 mg/kg per hr maximum	May start with 0.2–1 mg/kg bolus (20 mg maximum)
			Onset 2–5 min
Nitroprusside	Vasodilator	0.3–0.5 mcg/kg per min	Monitor cyanide levels if > 48 hrs
		Titrate to maximum rate of 10 mcg/kg per min	Protect from light with aluminum foil on tubing
			Immediate onset of action
IV bolus for emergency hypertension			
Hydralazine	Vasodilator	0.1–0.2 mg/kg q 4 hr	Can cause ↑ or extended hypotension
		20 mg/dose maximum	Onset 5–20 min
Oral for urgent hypertension			
Amlodipine	Ca^{2+} channel blocker	0.1–0.3 mg/kg per dose q day or bid	Long acting
			May require dose adjustments every 7 days
Nifedipine	Ca^{2+} channel blocker	0.25 mg/kg q 4–6 h prn maximum 10 mg or 3 mg/kg per day	Short acting with rapid onset
			Capsule must be swallowed to be effective
			Contraindicated in CHF, acute CNS injury, aortic stenosis
Enalapril	ACE-inhibitor	0.2 mg/kg per dose q day or bid	May cause cough and hyperkalemia
			Check electrolytes after 1 week
			Contraindicated in pregnancy
Captopril	ACE-inhibitor	Neonate 0.025–0.1 mg/kg per dose	Rapid onset of action, short acting except infants

Table 23-4. (cont.)

Drug	Class	Route/dose	Comments
		Infant 0.15–0.3 mg/kg per dose	Contraindicated in pregnancy
		Child 0.3–0.5 mg/kg per dose	
Labetalol	α and β blocker	1–1.5 mg/kg per dose bid	Weak alpha blockade in oral formulation
Hydrochloro-thiazide	Thiazide diuretic	0.5–1 mg/kg per dose q day or bid	Monitor electrolytes and triglycerides
Atenolol	β antagonist	0.25–0.5 mg/kg per dose q day or bid	Cardioselective
			Can cause bradycardia
Clonidine	Central α agonist	2.5–5 mcg/kg per dose bid or tid	May initially cause sedation
			Reflex hypertension with abrupt discontinuation
Prazosin	Peripheral α antagonist	0.05–0.1 mg/kg per day div bid or tid	Orthostatic hypotension common at beginning
Minoxidil	Vasodilator	0.1–0.2 mg/kg q day 5 mg/ dose maximum	Contraindicated in pheochromocytoma
			Onset 30 min; long acting
			Hypertrichosis common

Bibliography

American Academy of Pediatrics: The fourth report on the diagnosis, evaluation, and treatment of high blood pressure in children and adolescents. *Pediatrics* 2004; 114;555–76.

Custer JW, Rau RE: *Johns Hopkins: Harriet Lane Handbook*, 18th ed. St. Louis: Mosby-Year Book, 2009, pp. 176–9.

Empar L, Cifkovac R, Kennedy Cruikshark J, et al: Management of high blood pressure in children and adolescents: recommendations of the European Society of Hypertension, 2009; 27:1719–42.

Mitsnefes MM: Hypertension in children and adolescents. *Pediatr Clin North Am* 2006;53:493–512.

Seikaly MG: Hypertension in children: an update on treatment strategies. *Curr Opin Pediatr* 2007;19:170–7.

Nephrolithiasis

Nephrolithiasis in childhood primarily affects Caucasians, with a slightly higher incidence in boys. The etiology may be either metabolic or structural. The most common metabolic causes of stones are hypocitraturia and hypercalciuria (calcium excretion >4 mg/kg per day), which is frequently idiopathic and results in the formation of calcium oxalate stones. Urinary tract abnormalities and, rarely, infection are other etiologies. Stones composed of uric acid, struvite, and cystine are less common.

Clinical presentation

The typical adult presentation of flank pain and hematuria is less common in children, although adolescents may present similarly with intermittent severe pain, nausea, and vomiting. Younger children may present with vomiting, urinary symptoms (dysuria, hematuria or frequency), or colicky abdominal pain. Infants may be misdiagnosed as colic due to nonspecific symptoms. Up to 90% of children in all age groups will have microscopic or gross hematuria.

Diagnosis

Elicit a detailed history, including dietary intake and a family history of nephrolithiasis and renal or metabolic abnormalities. Ask about the onset, duration, and location of the pain, oral intake, medication use, and intake of calcium. Useful physical examination findings include abdominal tenderness or mass and costovertebral angle tenderness. The presence of hypertension or edema with hematuria suggests an alternate diagnosis, such as glomerular disease.

Obtain a urinalysis (hematuria) and urine culture. Microscopy may be particularly helpful if crystals or stones are visualized. Also send a spot urine calcium/creatinine ratio, which is normally <0.2 in children >2 years of age, but may be up to three-fold higher in younger infants. Confirmation requires a 24-hour urine collection with calcium excretion of > 4 mg/kg per day.

Calcium oxalate stones can be identified on plain radiographs, but other types of stones are generally not seen. A sonogram can identify most stones >5 mm, including those that are radiolucent on plain film. The finding of unilateral hydronephrosis on a sonogram may also suggest a stone, but a non-contrast CT scan is the most sensitive imaging study and will identify very small stones (1 mm).

ED management

Hydration and analgesia are the priorities, regardless of the etiology. Give morphine (0.1–0.2 mg/kg, 15 mg maximum) and ketorolac (0.5 mg/kg, 30 mg maximum), either alone or in combination, and hydrate the patient, placing an IV if there is nausea, vomiting, or severe pain. Consult a urologist for urinary obstruction or stones >5 mm to determine whether urologic stone removal is necessary, via shock wave lithotripsy, percutaneous nephrolithotomy, or ureteroscopy. Discontinue the ketorolac 3 days prior to a urologic procedure to minimize the risk of bleeding. Stones <5 mm often pass spontaneously; instruct the patient and family to collect or filter the urine. Arrange urology follow-up so that the stone can be analyzed. If the stone passes unnoticed, a 24-hour urine collection can reveal the etiology of stone formation.

Follow-up

- Urology referral within 1–2 weeks. At that time a 24-hour urine collection will be helpful to evaluate for an underlying metabolic cause of stone formation if no anatomical abnormality can be identified

Indications for admission

- Inability to tolerate oral hydration or pain medications
- Severe pain recalcitrant to pain medications in the ED
- Urinary obstruction or infection
- Surgical stone removal required

Bibliography

Gillespie RS, Stapleton SB: Nephrolithiasis in children. *Pediatr Rev* 2004;25:131–8.

Nicoletta JA, Lande MB: Medical evaluation and treatment of urolithiasis. *Pediatr Clin North Am* 2006;53:479–91.

Palmer JS, Donaher ER, O'Riordan MA, et al: Diagnosis of pediatric urolithiasis: role of ultrasound and computed tomography. *J Urol* 2005;174:1413–6.

Proteinuria

Normal urine can contain small amounts of protein ($<100\,mg/m^2$), while proteinuria in excess of this is considered abnormal. Qualitative proteinuria is prevalent (5–15% of normal individuals), since the urine dipstick is very sensitive to albumin (but not to low molecular weight proteins) and detects protein concentrations as low as 10–15 mg/dL. Transient proteinuria can be found incidentally in an otherwise healthy child with stress, fever, highly concentrated (specific gravity >1.025) or alkaline (pH >8.0) urine, or after vigorous exercise. Orthostatic proteinuria is also a common finding in children. In contrast, false negative results on urine dipstick can occur with very dilute urine.

Significant proteinuria ($>2+$ on dipstick), defined as:

$$\text{urinary protein(mg/dL)/urinary creatinine(mg/dL)} > 0.2$$

in an early-morning specimen, occurs in only 1–2% of these patients. When proteinuria is $\geq 1+$ by dipstick on several occasions, further investigation is warranted.

Clinical presentation

Although fever can induce transient proteinuria, most often proteinuria is an unexpected finding in a child being examined for an intercurrent illness. Edema, hypoalbuminemia (<3 g/dL), hypercholesterolemia, apparent hypocalcemia (secondary to the decreased albumin), and ascites are findings in the nephrotic syndrome. These patients are at increased risk for spontaneous bacterial peritonitis, usually caused by *Streptococcus pneumoniae*. In patients with isolated proteinuria or nephrotic syndrome, the blood pressure and renal function are generally normal, although urine output may be decreased. With renal disease such as glomerulonephritis, there may be edema, hypertension, oliguria, or associated microscopic hematuria. Orthostatic proteinuria can be found in a urine sample collected later in the day, after the patient has been in an upright position for a prolonged period of time. This is a variant of normal and is often found in children and adolescents.

Nephrotic syndrome

The nephrotic syndrome is defined as edema, hypoalbuminemia (<3 g/dL), hyperlipidemia, and heavy proteinuria with a urinary protein/creatinine ratio >2. A glomerular protein leak is the primary disturbance in this syndrome. The edema, which can become generalized, usually begins in the periorbital region and may be the primary complaint. In contrast to AGN, the GFR is usually normal. However, children with nephrotic syndrome are at risk for electrolyte disturbances, infections (cellulitis, spontaneous bacterial peritonitis), pleural effusions, and thromboembolism.

The nephrotic syndrome is classified as primary (no systemic disease) or secondary (associated with a systemic disease or another glomerular injury, such as postinfectious AGN, SLE). Although there are numerous causes of nephrotic syndrome, minimal change disease (MCD) causes 75% of cases in childhood, with a peak incidence at 2–5 years of age. Most patients with MCD are normotensive, have normal complement levels, no hematuria, and will respond to glucocorticoid therapy. Other primary causes are focal segmental glomerulosclerosis (often associated with hypertension), membranoproliferative glomerulonephritis, and membranous nephropathy.

Secondary causes include systemic disorders such as HSP, SLE and sickle cell disease, chronic infections (syphilis, HIV, hepatitis B, diabetes), and medications (captopril, penicillamine, nonsteroidal anti-inflammatories).

Diagnosis

Since very few patients with dipstick proteinuria truly have renal disease, in the absence of edema, hypertension, oliguria, or associated hematuria merely repeat the urinalysis in 2–4 weeks. Examine urine obtained when the patient is in both the recumbent and upright positions. If the proteinuria persists, test the first voided morning specimen in the recumbent position for protein to creatinine ratio and proteinuria on dipstick examination. In orthostatic proteinuria the protein:creatinine ratio is normal and the dipstick is negative.

The most expeditious method of measuring urinary protein excretion is a determination of the protein:creatinine ratio in an early-morning (first void) specimen. This determination correlates well with the 24-hour urinary protein excretion. Moreover, it simplifies the diagnosis of orthostatic proteinuria and eliminates the need for a cumbersome 24-hour collection. Normally, this ratio is < 0.2; with nephrotic-range proteinuria, it is >2.

Consider causes other than minimal change disease if the child is <1 year or >10 years of age, or if there are associated clinical findings, such as fever, rash, or arthralgias. A patient with associated microscopic hematuria is more likely to have glomerular disease, but up to 30% of children with minimal change disease may have microscopic hematuria.

Although edema is a cardinal feature of the nephrotic syndrome, extrarenal causes of edema include cirrhosis, congestive heart failure, and protein-losing enteropathy. Significant proteinuria is absent in these conditions.

ED management

Patients with edema, hypertension, oliguria, or associated gross hematuria require an immediate and more complete evaluation, including serum electrolytes, BUN, calcium, creatinine and creatinine clearance, cholesterol, total protein and albumin, complement (C3, C4), ANA, ASLO, VDRL, and serology for hepatitis B and C, and HIV testing (if indicated).

Follow a patient with isolated proteinuria (urinary protein:creatinine ratio of 0.2–1) for about 6–12 months. If there is no resolution by 1 year or if there is worsening of the ratio, a renal biopsy is warranted.

Nephrotic syndrome

Admit patients with nephrotic syndrome who have moderate edema with hypertension or severe edema with inability to tolerate oral medications, or complications associated with nephrotic syndrome (peritonitis), and consult with a pediatric nephrologist to initiate therapy. For patients who can be discharged, instruct the parents to restrict salt intake by excluding high-sodium prepared foods and by eliminating salt in food preparation and at the table.

Follow-up

- Nonnephrotic proteinuria: primary care follow-up in 2–4 weeks

Indications for admission

- Proteinuria in association with signs or symptoms of renal disease (severe edema, hypertension, oliguria, electrolyte disturbances, infection, thromboembolism)
- Infants with nephrotic syndrome

Bibliography

Hodsen EM, Alexander SI: Evaluation and management of steroid-sensitive nephrotic syndrome. *Curr Opin Pediatr* 2008; 20:145–50.

Hogg RJ: Adolescents with proteinuria and/or the nephrotic syndrome. *Adolesc Med Clin* 2005;16:163–72.

Quigley R: Evaluation of hematuria and proteinuria: how should a pediatrician proceed? *Curr Opin Pediatr* 2008;20: 140–4.

Urinary tract infections

Overall, urinary tract infections (UTIs) occur in approximately 2–3% of children annually. Uncircumcised boys <1 year of age have a higher incidence of UTIs than girls; in all other age groups, girls have a higher incidence. Uncircumcised boys <6 months of age have a 10–12-fold relative risk of having a UTI compared to circumcised boys. The two most common types of infection are cystitis (infection confined to the bladder) and pyelonephritis (infection in the renal parenchyma). The most frequent etiology is *E. coli*; other causative organisms include *Klebsiella*, *Pseudomonas*, *Enterococcus*, *Staphylococcus saprophyticus*, and *S. epidermidis*, which is not a contaminant if cultured repeatedly, particularly in adolescent girls. *Proteus* is an important pathogen in uncircumcised boys, but in girls it is less common and may be a contaminant. In addition, UTIs due to group B *Streptococci* can occur in neonates.

Clinical presentation

The presentation in infancy is nonspecific and includes poor feeding, vomiting, diarrhea, irritability, jaundice, and seizures. From 1 month to 2 years, fever is more common, and some urologic symptoms (change in voiding pattern, foul-smelling urine) occur. Preschool and school-age children usually have specific urologic complaints, such as frequency, urgency, dysuria, suprapubic pain, and enuresis. However, less specific symptoms, such as abdominal pain and vomiting, may be seen in this age group as well. Higher fever (>38.5°C; 101.3°F), flank (CVA) tenderness, and systemic toxicity are consistent with pyelonephritis.

Diagnosis

Traditionally, the amount of bacterial growth required for the diagnosis of UTI is >10^5 CFU/mL in a midstream clean-catch urine, and >10^4 in a catheterized specimen. Any growth in a urine culture obtained by suprapubic bladder tap is considered significant. However, the concept of "significant bacteriuria" is a statistical one indicating an 80% chance of true infection; two consecutive positive cultures increase the likelihood of infection to 95%. In fact, a culture with a pure growth of $>10^2$ CFU/mL from a catheterized or voided specimen, in the context of symptoms associated with UTI, may be indicative of infection. Prompt plating of the specimen is as important as compulsive cleaning of the perineum and urethral meatus for reducing the frequency of false-positive urine cultures. If the urine specimen cannot be plated immediately, refrigerate at 4°C (39.2°F) to prevent overgrowth of contaminating bacteria. A bagged urine specimen is unreliable unless the culture demonstrates no growth.

Urinalysis findings are not sufficient for a definitive diagnosis; however, the urinalysis is a useful screening test in the ED. If a complete urinalysis is normal (including dipstick testing for leukocyte esterase and nitrite, and microscopic examination for bacteriuria), the likelihood that the patient does not have a UTI exceeds 95%. The presence of bacteriuria and pyuria (>10 WBC/hpf) has a positive predictive value over 84%. However, in some culture-proven UTIs, pyuria may be absent. Alternatively, only 50% of patients with WBCs in the urine have a culture-proven UTI, as pyuria can occur with infections near but outside the urinary tract. With a UTI, proteinuria and hematuria are often present, and the leukocyte esterase is generally positive on dipstick testing.

The dipstick nitrite test has a low sensitivity in infants and young children who void frequently; urine must remain in the bladder for at least 4 hours for bacteria to produce nitrite. Also, Gram-positive organisms do not reduce nitrates to nitrites so the dipstick will be negative.

The presence of any organisms on Gram's stain of an uncentrifuged urine correlates with a colony count $>10^5$/mL, and is presumptive evidence of a UTI, with higher sensitivity, specificity, and positive predictive value than urinalysis and dipstick. However, the urine culture remains the definitive diagnostic test.

WBC casts (not clumps) are usually diagnostic of pyelonephritis. Other laboratory findings with pyelonephritis are leukocytosis (WBC $>15,000$/mm^3) and an elevated sedimentation rate (>30 mm/h) on CRP. A DMSA scan can differentiate cystitis from pyelonephritis; there is patchy uptake of the radionuclide during acute pyelonephritis.

Symptoms of a UTI are not sufficient for a definitive diagnosis. Dysuria, frequency, and urgency among patients with suprapubic tenderness and gross hematuria without pyuria or bacteriuria suggest viral cystitis or idiopathic hypercalciuria. The same findings in a patient with pyuria but no hematuria are compatible with the dysuria-pyuria (acute urethral) syndrome. The symptoms of vaginitis and balanitis can mimic a UTI. Negative urine cultures are necessary to confirm these diagnoses.

The co-existence of another source for fever, such as a URI, does not exclude the possibility of a UTI. Consider this diagnosis for all children <2 years of age with fever.

ED management

Inspect the external genitalia for signs of inflammation or infection (epididymitis, epididymoorchitis, vaginitis), and measure the blood pressure. Examine the sacral region for abnormalities such as a dimple or pit, which may indicate a neurogenic bladder. Obtain a catheterized or suprapubic urine specimen for culture from a patient who lacks bladder control, has evidence of vaginitis, or is unable to provide an adequate midstream specimen. A bagged specimen can be used for a screening urinalysis if the clinical condition of the child does not warrant immediate antimicrobial therapy. If the urinalysis suggests an infection, obtain a suprapubic or catheterized urine specimen for culture. In an older child or adolescent, when a midstream specimen is used, collect samples from two separate voids to increase the likelihood of a noncontaminated culture. A large number of epithelial cells in the specimen suggests contamination.

After urine cultures are obtained, treat a nontoxic patient with signs or symptoms and microscopy results consistent with a urinary tract infection on an outpatient basis if the patient has adequate fluid intake, is not vomiting, and reliable follow-up can be assured. Give the first dose of antibiotics in the ED in order to assess the patient's ability to tolerate the medication. Base empiric treatment on the most likely uropathogen and the prevailing local resistance patterns. There are increasing rates of E. coli resistance to trimethoprim-sulfamethoxazole, amoxicillin, ampicillin, and first-generation cephalosporins (cephalexin). Amoxicillin-clavulanate (45 mg/kg per day div q 12 h) is useful first-line therapy, although resistance is increasing. Other empiric therapeutic agents include cefixime (16 mg/kg per day div q 12 h on day 1, followed by 8 mg/kg per day div q 24 h, 400 mg/day maximum) or cefdinir (14 mg/kg per day div q 12–24 h, 600 mg/day maximum). Treat for a 10-day course.

Treat an afebrile, nonpregnant adolescent girl with an uncomplicated lower-tract infection (symptoms for <3 days) and a normal urinary tract, with ciprofloxacin 250 mg bid for 3 days. This therapy may be especially useful when compliance with a 10-day oral regimen is not assured. However, 3-day treatment is inadequate for infants and children. Treat pregnant adolescents >12 years of age with nitrofurantoin (100 mg bid × 7 days). Tailor subsequent antibiotic therapy according to culture and sensitivity results when available. Repeat urine cultures are not necessary when the patient has the expected response to the appropriate therapy.

Prescribe phenazopyridine (Pyridium) for short-term use (<2 days) in children >6 years to treat symptoms of burning, urgency, and frequency. Give 4 mg/kg per dose PO tid with food. Inform the patient that the urine may become orange and the drug may discolor contact lenses.

Indications for admission and IV antibiotics include toxic appearance, inability to tolerate oral intake (including antibiotics), dehydration, immunocompromise, or adherence to treatment and/or follow-up seems unlikely. Also admit an infant <3 months old, regardless of clinical appearance. Treat as follows.

Less than 4 weeks of age

Since a young infant with a UTI is at risk for sepsis, treat with ampicillin (<1 week of age: 100 mg/kg per day, div q 12 h; >1 week of age: 200 mg/kg per day, div q 6 h) and cefotaxime (<1 week: 100 mg/kg per day, div q 12 h; 1–4 weeks: 150 mg/kg per day, div q 8 h).

Greater than 4 weeks of age

Treat with ceftriaxone 100 mg/kg per day div q 12 h.

Continue parenteral therapy until the patient is afebrile and the urine culture is sterile (usually 2–3 days), at which point coverage may be switched to an oral agent. Obtain a follow-up urine culture after 48 hours if the patient does not have the expected clinical response to the appropriate antibiotic or the sensitivities of the organism are not available.

Radiological evaluation

It is important to determine whether there is anatomic or functional uropathology, particularly vesicoureteral reflux (VUR). The presence of an abnormality may increase a child's risk for renal dysfunction and scarring. Radiographic evaluation is indicated for the following: all male patients with their first UTI, children <5 years old with a febrile UTI, UTI in a girl <3 years of age, after two or more episodes in a girl >3 years of age, a patient who does not respond appropriately to antibiotic therapy, and any patient after an episode of pyelonephritis or an atypical UTI with hypertension or a flank mass.

Less than 3 years of age

For children <3 years of age, obtain an ultrasound to evaluate urinary tract anatomy and a voiding cystourethrogram (VCUG) under fluoroscopy to detect VUR. Although ultrasonography may be performed at any time after a UTI is diagnosed, a sterile urine culture must be obtained before the VCUG is performed. If a renal sonogram demonstrates hydronephrosis, assume that the patient has VUR and initiate prophylactic antibiotics. The antibiotics can be discontinued, if the VCUG is negative. If VUR grade 3 or higher is found or there is evidence of parenchymal abnormality on sonogram, a DMSA scan is necessary. In children with VUR or suspected pyelonephritis, a DMSA scan is indicated 2–4 months after resolution of the UTI. The delay is necessary to distinguish acute, reversible changes related to the episode of pyelonephritis from permanent renal parenchymal scarring. With the widespread use of radionuclide scans, an IVP is rarely needed to visualize the kidneys after a UTI.

Over 3 years of age

For children >3 years of age, ultrasonography is sufficient. Obtain a VCUG if there are findings suggestive of reflux. Siblings of patients with VUR require urinary tract imaging, as this can be a heritable abnormality.

Recurrences are common in children with abnormal urinary tracts; 80% occur in the first year after a UTI. Patients must have follow-up cultures monthly for 3 months, then every 3 months for a year, and then every 6 months for 2 years. Routine surveillance cultures are unnecessary in children with a normal urinary tract.

Follow-up

- Children with persistent symptoms on appropriate antibiotic therapy: within 2 days to repeat a urine culture
- For children requiring imaging studies for evaluation of the urinary tract: at the completion of antibiotic therapy to assess the need for prophylaxis

Indications for admission

- UTI in patients <3 months of age
- Any age: toxic-appearing, dehydrated, inability to tolerate oral intake, immunocompromised, at risk for nonadherence to treatment/follow-up
- UTI with fever in a patient at risk for decreased renal function (decreased GFR, single kidney)

Bibliography

Azzarone G, Liewehr S, O'Connor K: Cystitis. *Pediatr Rev* 2007;28:474–6.

Bauer R, Kogan BA: New developments in the diagnosis and management of

pediatric UTIs. *Urol Clin North Am* 2008; 35:47–58.

Chang SL, Shortliffe LD: Pediatric urinary tract infections. *Pediatr Clin North Am* 2006;53:379–400.

Chapter 24

Rheumatologic emergencies

Michael Gorn and Svetlana Lvovich

Acute rheumatic fever

Acute rheumatic fever (ARF) is a nonsuppurative sequela of group A streptococcus (GAS) pharyngitis that can affect the heart, joints, subcutaneous tissue, and central nervous system. The underlying cause of ARF remains elusive, although "specific rheumatogenic" strains of the bacteria and an "abnormal immune response" by the host have been suggested. ARF occurs primarily between 5 and 15 years of age and is rare in children <3 years. The estimated incidence is 1–3% in patients who receive inadequate treatment of a GAS pharyngitis; it is uncommon when appropriate treatment is given. In addition, groups C and G streptococcus have been implicated as causes of ARF in underdeveloped countries.

Clinical presentation and diagnosis

ARF typically presents several weeks after an acute infection with GAS, which can sometimes be asymptomatic. There is no single test for the condition and the diagnosis is based on clinical features embodied in the Jones criteria. Evidence of a recent GAS pharyngitis and the presence of two major, or one major and two minor features, is required for diagnosis. The criteria are described in Table 24-1.

Recent advances in echocardiography have made the detection of subclinical carditis (valvular damage detected only on ECHO) readily available. However, the use of ECHO for the diagnosis of ARF in a patient who has no clinically audible murmur is still controversial. Auscultatory findings remain the basis for the diagnosis of carditis.

Joint involvement is both a major and a minor criterion. Since migratory polyarthritis (major criterion) often resolves with the use of NSAIDs, corticosteroids, or aspirin, only arthralgia (minor criterion) may be evident. Therefore, delay symptomatic treatment if a definite diagnosis of ARF has not been established. In patients presenting with arthritis, other etiologies must be ruled out (see pp. 671–675), especially septic arthritis.

The World Health Organization's revised Jones criteria include several exceptions to these rules:

- Recurrent attack of rheumatic fever (RF): two minor features and evidence of recent GAS infection in a patient with established rheumatic heart disease
- Rheumatic chorea or insidious onset of rheumatic carditis: evidence of GAS infection is not required
- Chronic valvular lesions of rheumatic heart disease: no other criteria are required.

Post-streptococcal reactive arthritis (PSRA) occurs in patients who have arthritis and evidence of a preceding GAS infection, but do not fulfill the Jones criteria. It is a known entity, although it is not clear whether it is truly separate from ARF. In contrast to ARF, the arthritis typically

Table 24-1. Jones criteria and the diagnosis of acute rheumatic fever

Evidence of GAS	Throat culture and rapid strep test are positive in 25% of cases
	Streptococcal Ab (ASLO, anti-DNAse B, streptokinase, antihyaluronidase) is more sensitive
Major criteria	
Carditis	Endocarditis is most common; also peri-, epi-, and myocarditis
	Chest pain, friction rub, aortic and mitral regurgitation murmurs
Polyarthritis	Pain, erythema and swelling of large joints that "migrates" from one joint to the next
	Persists for up to 1 week in each joint
disproportionate	Pain is disproportionate ($\uparrow\uparrow$ severe) to the physical findings
Chorea	Abrupt, purposeless, involuntary movements
	Associated with weakness and emotional lability
Erythema marginatum	Non-pruritic, evanescent, macular serpiginous rash with raised erythematous borders
	Central part of each lesion returns to normal as the rash spreads or resolves
	Typically on the trunk and inner thighs, upper arms
Subcutaneous nodules	Firm, symmetric, 1–2 cm, painless nodules
	Located over bony prominences or tendons, most commonly in the elbow
Minor criteria	
Arthralgia	Significant pain in a single joint with minimal findings of inflammation on exam
	Cannot use as a minor criterion in the presence of polyarthritis as a major
Fever	
Prolonged P-R interval	
Elevated acute-phase reactants: ESR, CRP, WBC	

does not respond dramatically to aspirin or NSAIDs, and patients do not present with carditis. Nonetheless, recommend ARF prophylaxis for one year after the diagnosis of PSRA.

ED management

Since the diagnosis depends on the Jones criteria, obtain a CBC, CRP, ESR, chest radiograph, ECG, throat culture, rapid streptococcus swab, ASLO, and anti-DNAse B antibodies. The throat culture and rapid strep tests may be negative as the GAS pharyngitis can resolve, even

Table 24-2. Primary prevention of rheumatic fever

Antibiotic[a]	Dose
Penicillin G benzathine	≥27 kg: 1 200,000 units IM × 1
	< 27 kg: 600,000 units IM × 1
Penicillin VK	250 mg tid or qid or 500 mg bid PO × 10 days
Amoxicillin	25 mg/kg per day tid PO × 10 days
First-generation cephalosporin	20 mg/kg per day PO × 10 days (dosing frequency varies)
Erythromycin ethylsuccinate	40 mg/kg per day PO div bid or tid × 10 days

Note: [a] Trimethoprim, sulfonamides, and tetracyclines are not effective for eradicating GAS infections.

Table 24-3. Secondary prophylaxis of rheumatic fever

Antibiotic	Dose
Penicillin G benzathine IM	1.2 million units IM q 4 weeks
Penicillin V	250 mg bid PO
Sulfadiazine or sulfisoxazole	<27 kg: 0.5 g/day PO
	≥27 kg: 1 g/day PO
If penicillin-allergic	Erythromycin 250 mg bid PO

without antibiotic treatment. However, when the ASLO and anti-DNAse B are performed simultaneously, evidence of a preceding GAS infection can be found in >90% of patients.

Once the diagnosis is certain, treat migratory polyarthritis with aspirin 50–75 mg/kg per day div tid or qid or naproxen 17.5 mg/kg per day div bid for 2–4 weeks. Arthritis in ARF is exquisitely sensitive to NSAIDs and resolves shortly after institution of therapy.

Treat mild to moderate carditis with aspirin 80–100 mg/kg per day div qid for 4–8 weeks, depending on response, then gradually discontinue. Give prednisone (2 mg/kg per day) for severe carditis and congestive heart failure and consult a pediatric cardiologist for further recommendations.

Chorea resolves spontaneously over 2–3 weeks and most patients do not need to be medicated. Treat severe symptoms with haloperidol, but consult a pediatric neurologist prior to instituting this therapy.

Once the diagnosis is established, the eradication of any existing streptococcal infection or carriage is necessary (Table 24-2). Secondary prophylaxis is critical for preventing disease recurrences (Table 24-3). Carditis is the single most important prognostic factor for ARF, but only valvulitis leads to permanent damage. Therefore, patient age and the presence of valvulitis determine the length of prophylaxis.

Follow-up
- Pediatric rheumatologist within 1 week
- Other pediatric specialists (cardiologist, neurologist) based upon symptomatology

Indications for admission

- Suspected acute rheumatic fever
- Recurrent episode of rheumatic fever

Bibliography

Carapetis JR, McDonald M, Wilson NJ: Acute rheumatic fever. *Lancet* 2005;366:155–68.

Cassidy JT, Petty RE: *Textbook of Pediatric Rheumatology*, 5th ed. Philadelphia: W.B. Saunders, 2006, pp. 614–29.

Hashkes PJ, Tauber T, Somekh E, et al: Naproxen as an alternative to aspirin for the treatment of arthritis of rheumatic fever: a randomized trial. *J Pediatr* 2003;143:399–401.

Arthritis

Arthritis results from synovial inflammation due to infectious and noninfectious causes (Table 24-4). In contrast, arthralgia is pain or tenderness without swelling.

Clinical presentation

The hallmarks of arthritis are joint swelling, pain, and limitation of motion. The patient may limp or refuse to use the affected extremity, which will have a decreased range of motion as the patient holds it in the position that maximizes the volume of the joint. The hip will be flexed, abducted, and slightly externally rotated; the knee and elbow flexed; and the ankle held in plantar flexion.

Diagnosis

A detailed history helps to guide the initial approach to a child with arthritis. Inquire about antecedent or recurrent trauma, history of similar episodes in the past, fever, recent immunizations or illnesses, pharyngitis or gastroenteritis, medication use, travel, tick exposure, weight loss, or fatigue. Ascertain the location of the pain, the number of joints involved, timing and severity of the pain, and any associated swelling, warmth, or limitation in range of motion. In the review of systems ask about ocular symptoms, oral ulcers, rashes (Table 24-5), history of pulmonary disease, endocarditis, hematologic disorders, vasculitis, sexually transmitted infections, infectious or inflammatory gastroenteritis, hepatitis, and psychiatric and renal diseases.

On examination, document that arthritis is present, as opposed to arthralgias, myalgias, sprains, or bruises, and whether it is monoarticular or polyarticular. It is critical to distinguish joint pain from that originating from muscle, tendon, bursa, bone, soft tissue, or nerve. Compare the affected joint(s) to the contralateral side to confirm the presence of joint fluid. Finally, look for evidence of systemic illness, such as lymphadenopathy, hepatosplenomegaly, murmur, or edema. Since most patients will have an infectious, postinfectious, or traumatic etiology for the arthritis, a limited evaluation is usually sufficient to make a presumptive diagnosis. In the ED it is prudent to involve the primary care physician, orthopedist and/or rheumatologist if a more involved work-up seems necessary, so that proper follow-up can be arranged.

Monoarticular arthritis

Consider monoarticular arthritis to be infectious until proven otherwise. Obtain a CBC with differential, ESR or CRP, and blood culture. Obtain a Lyme titer if the evaluation is

Table 24-4. Common etiologies of arthritis in children

Diagnosis	Differentiating features
Traumatic arthritis	Acute or chronic onset of intermittent pain that is worse with activity
	Typically one joint is involved (elbow, shoulder, knee, hip)
	May have an associated fracture, ligamentous injury, bursitis, or tenovitis
Septic arthritis	Most common at 1–3 years of age in one large joint (knee, hip)
	Abrupt onset of painful, persistent, and progressive arthritis
	Presents with erythema, warmth, swelling, pain, and decreased range of motion (especially infants)
	Absence of joint effusion on ultrasound has a high negative predictive value for septic arthritis
Toxic synovitis	Occurs in as many as 3% of 2–10 year-olds
	Good response to NSAIDs
	Can last for 2 weeks, but resolves without complications
Gonococcal arthritis	Subacute onset
	Initially, pauciarticular and often migratory; can be monoarticular
	Adolescents may have tenosynovitis and papular or vesiculopustular rash
Lyme disease	Acute onset of swelling and tenderness without warmth or erythema, most often involving the knee
	Mostly monoarticular, sometimes migratory, rarely polyarticular
	Can persist for weeks to months and recur
ARF	Pain is out of proportion to physical exam findings
	Classic migratory polyarthritis involves knees, ankles, elbows, and wrists
Postinfectious	Subacute onset 2–3 weeks after an illness (URI or gastroenteritis); duration <6 weeks
	Mono or asymmetric oligoarthritis commonly in knees and ankles
	Moderate pain, minimal swelling, no erythema, low-grade or no fever
Serum sickness	Arthralgia/arthritis of the knees, ankles, shoulders, wrists, spine, and temporomandibular joint
	Associated with myalgias, urticaria, angioedema, and hematuria
Kawasaki disease	Subacute-onset polyarthritis involving the small joints of the hands and feet
SLE	Subacute onset of symmetric polyarthritis involving peripheral joints of the hands or feet
	Large joints may be involved during disease exacerbation
	Despite severe pain, arthritis is nondestructive and may be persistent or intermittent

Table 24-4. (cont.)

Diagnosis	Differentiating features
JIA	Arthritis lasting >6 weeks in a child <16 years old
	Typically less painful than swelling suggests
	Worse in the morning with associated stiffness
HSP	Typically a painful monoarticular arthritis of a knee or an ankle
	Distinctive rash may be present
Malignancies	Gradual onset of a persistent mono-, poly-, or migratory arthritis
	Pain out of proportion to physical findings and may be worse at night
	Can be associated with fever, weight loss, and anemia
Dermatomyositis	Frequently involves the small joints of the hands
IBD	Acute onset of a persistent oligoarthritis involving large joints, including hips

Table 24-5. Rashes associated with arthritic diseases

Diagnosis	Skin manifestations
Acute rheumatic fever	Erythema marginatum
Systemic lupus erythematosus	Malar and discoid rashes
Juvenile idiopathic arthritis	Evanescent salmon-pink macular rash
Inflammatory bowel disease	Erythema nodosum
Dermatomyositis	Heliotrope rash and Gottron papules
Lyme disease	Erythema migrans
Gonococcal arthritis	Erythematous, hemorrhagic, papular, or vesiculopustular lesions
Serum sickness	Urticaria, angioedema
Henoch-Schönlein purpura	Palpable purpura and petechiae, usually below the waist

highly suggestive (joint is not erythematous, history of rash consistent with erythema migrans). Occasionally, a migratory or polyarticular arthritis may initially present with single joint involvement. Therefore, also keep two additional red-top tubes in the event that septic arthritis is ruled out.

If a joint effusion is suspected, obtain an X-ray of the affected joint, and arrange for immediate arthrocentesis. The only exceptions to performing arthrocentesis are a traumatic effusion (unless indicated for pain relief), probable Lyme disease, an obvious case of HSP (see pp. 675–677), or a known autoimmune disorder. Culture of the joint fluid is critical; inoculate the specimen into a blood culture bottle. A Gram's stain and cell count of the joint fluid are also necessary, but crystal analysis is rarely helpful in children. The interpretation of joint fluid analysis is summarized in Table 24-6.

Table 24-6. Synovial fluid findings

Diagnosis	Color	Clarity	Viscosity	Mucin clot	WBC/mm^3	% Polys
Normal	Straw	Transparent	High	Good	<200	<25
Traumatic arthritis	Straw to bloody to xanthochromic	Transparent to turbid	High	Good	<2,000 (RBCs predominate)	<25
Rheumatic fever	Yellow	Slightly cloudy	Low	Good	10,000–12,000	50
Rheumatoid arthritis	Yellow to greenish	Cloudy	Low	Poor	15,000–20,000	75
Tuberculosis arthritis	Yellow	Cloudy	Low	Poor	25,000	50–60
Septic arthritis	Grayish or bloody	Turbid or purulent	Low	Poor	80,000–200,000	75

Source: Adapted with permission from Holander JL, McCarthy DJ: *Arthritis and Allied Conditions*, 8th ed. Philadelphia: Lea & Febiger, 1972, p. 72.

Admit the patient for further investigations, which may include a technetium bone scan, MRI, and a bone or synovial biopsy to help identify conditions such as osteomyelitis, myositis, or tuberculosis.

The Kocher criteria employ four elements to assess the risk of septic arthritis of the hip in a patient with a painful limp: non-weightbearing, fever, ESR > 40 mm/h, and WBC >12,000/mm^3. The probability of a septic hip is 99% if all criteria are present, 93% with three criteria, 40% with two, and 3% with one criterion. The criteria are less reliable in younger patients.

Consider toxic synovitis in a well-appearing patient who can partially bear weight and responds to NSAIDs (p. 568) and osteomyelitis (pp. 571–573) in a patient with apparent arthritis, but a negative joint aspiration.

Polyarticular arthritis

Obtain a CBC with differential, ESR or CRP, LDH, ANA, complement (C3, C4, CH50), and urinalysis, as well as tests for group A streptococcal infection (rapid strep test, ASLO titer).

If ARF is suspected, obtain a chest X-ray and an ECG to look for evidence of carditis, including cardiomegaly or a prolonged PR interval. Do not obtain a "rheumatology panel" for a patient with a low probability of having a rheumatologic condition, as this will probably yield false-positive results and create undue stress for the patient and family. Therefore, order specialized tests (HLA-B27, anti-SM antibody, rheumatoid factor, etc.) only after consultation with a rheumatologist.

Suspect that an adolescent with mono- or pauciarticular arthritis associated with tenosynovitis, pustules, or necrotic lesions has gonococcal arthritis. Obtain genital, rectal, and pharyngeal cultures for gonorrhea in addition to cultures already mentioned.

ED management

Septic arthritis is an emergency, since significant joint destruction may occur in a short time; immediately consult an orthopedist. Unless it can be reliably ruled out, joint drainage is necessary to remove the organism's debris and enzymes, which can damage the articular cartilage and underlying bone. After arthrocentesis and blood cultures are performed, start IV antibiotics. Use nafcillin (150 mg/kg per day div q 6 h), cephalexin (100 mg/kg per day div q 6 h), or clindamycin 40 mg/kg per day div q 6 h), but add vancomycin (40 mg/kg per day div q 6 h) if there is any concern about MRSA. If gonococcal infection is likely, use IV or IM ceftriaxone 50 mg/kg q day (1 g/day maximum) or cefotaxime (100 mg/kg per day IV div q 8 h, 1 g/day maximum) for 7 days, along with nafcillin, cephalexin, or clindamycin (as above) until the diagnosis is confirmed.

After the appropriate studies have been obtained, afebrile, well-appearing patients with good follow-up may be discharged for further outpatient management. Admit patients with suspected septic arthritis or malignancy, as well as those with arthritis associated with weight loss, systemic toxicity, or severe pain. The treatment of Lyme disease is discussed on pp. 400–401.

Follow-up

- Afebrile patient with nonmigratory polyarthritis: primary care follow-up within 1 week

Indications for admission

- Septic arthritis
- Suspected acute rheumatic fever or migratory polyarthritis
- Suspected malignancy
- Inability to bear weight

Bibliography

Ravelli A, Martini A: Juvenile idiopathic arthritis. *Lancet* 2007;**369**:767–78.

Taekema HC, Landham PR, Maconochie I: Towards evidence based medicine for paediatricians. Distinguishing between transient synovitis and septic arthritis in the limping child: how useful are clinical prediction tools? *Arch Dis Child* 2009;**94**:167–8.

Thompson A, Mannix R, Bachur R: Acute pediatric monoarticular arthritis: distinguishing lyme arthritis from other etiologies. *Pediatrics* 2009;**123**: 959–65.

Wagner-Weiner L: Pediatric rheumatology for the adult rheumatologist. *J Clin Rheumatol* 2008;**14**:109–19.

Henoch-Schönlein purpura (HSP)

Henoch-Schönlein purpura is the most common form of vasculitis in children. Although the exact cause is unknown, IgA_1 appears to be involved in the mechanism, as it is found in the affected tissues.

Clinical presentation

HSP most commonly occurs after a minor viral illness during the fall to spring seasons. The average age is 6 years and males are affected more frequently.

Table 24-7. Clinical features of HSP

Clinical feature	Presentation
Rash	2–10 mm palpable purpura with associated petechiae and ecchymoses
	Mostly on the buttocks and lower extremities
Arthritis	Occurs in 75% of patients; primarily knees and ankles
	Pain is moderate to severe
Renal	Microscopic hematuria and proteinuria in 40–50% of patients
	May have gross hematuria, but proteinuria alone is rare
	Hypertension may occur upon presentation or may be delayed
Gastrointestinal	Colicky abdominal pain, vomiting, hematochezia
	Occult bleeding is more common than gross blood
	Ileoileal intussusception in up to 5% of patients
Orchitis	Uncommon; acute onset, may mimic torsion
Neurologic	Rare; altered mental status, seizures, ataxia, peripheral neuropathy

HSP usually presents with some combination of palpable purpura of the buttocks and extensor surfaces of the lower extremities. Initially, the rash may be macular or urticarial, and it may occur in successive crops. Other features include arthritis, abdominal pain (which may be secondary to intussusception), scrotal and scalp edema, hematuria, and hematochezia (Table 24-7). Arthritis and abdominal pain may precede the rash by 1–2 weeks so that patients may be misdiagnosed with other conditions. Conversely, the onset of nephritis can be delayed up to 1–3 months after the onset of the rash.

The disease is less common but milder in children <2 years of age and more severe in adults. HSP is most often a self-limiting illness lasting for up to a month.

Acute hemorrhagic edema of infancy (AHEI)

AHEI, or "mild HSP," occurs in patients 4–24 months of age. It is not clear whether the two conditions are related or are separate entities. Following a viral illness, medication use, or a vaccination, patients present with mild fever and a progressive purpuric rash. Characteristically, large annular or target-like purpuric lesions appear on the face, scalp, extremities, and sometimes the torso. Symmetric edema of the hands and feet then develops over 24–48 hours after the onset of the eruption. While the rash and edema can be dramatic, the patients are typically well-appearing. In contrast to HSP, joint, renal or abdominal manifestations are rare. AHEI typically resolves in 2–3 weeks.

Diagnosis

The rash is the hallmark feature and a mandatory criterion for diagnosing HSP, although initially it may not be purpuric. At least one of the following is also required for diagnosis:

diffuse abdominal pain, arthritis or arthralgia, pathologic urinalysis, or a biopsy specimen (usually skin or kidney) showing predominantly IgA deposition. Depending on the presenting symptoms, a high index of suspicion may be necessary to consider the diagnosis. However, the priority in any patient presenting with fever and palpable purpura is to rule out bacterial sepsis.

Ask about rashes, joint pain, headaches, abdominal pain, leg swelling, and urine output and color. On physical examination, look for the Koebner phenomenon (rash at pressure points), especially along the sock band. Check for evidence of arthritis, nephritis, hypertension, and edema.

Laboratory data are nonspecific, but may help to exclude conditions that mimic HSP. Obtain a CBC, electrolytes, liver and pancreatic enzymes, coagulation studies, urinalysis, and a stool guaiac.

ED management

There is no specific therapy for HSP. Monitor the blood pressure and check the urinalysis for hematuria. Reserve the use of corticosteroids for patients with severe symptoms, after consultation with a rheumatologist or nephrologist. Steroids do not prevent nephritis but may shorten the duration of gastrointestinal and joint symptoms. Use prednisone, 1 mg/kg per day for 2 weeks, tapered over an additional 2 weeks.

Follow-up

- Weekly, for blood pressure and urinalysis monitoring in the first month

Indications for admission

- Severe arthritis preventing ambulation
- Moderate–severe nephritis (hypertension, gross hematuria)
- Severe abdominal pain
- Intussusception

Bibliography

Ozen S, Ruperto N, Dillon MJ, et al: EULAR/ PReS endorsed consensus criteria for the classification of childhood vasculitides. *Ann Rheum Dis* 2006;65:936–41.

Trapani S, Micheli A, Grisolia F, et al: Henoch-Schönlein purpura in childhood: epidemiological and clinical analysis of 150 cases over a 5-year period and review of literature. *Semin Arthritis Rheum* 2005;35:143–53.

Weiss PF, Feinstein JA, Luan X, Burnham JM, Feudtner C: Effects of corticosteroid on Henoch-Schönlein purpura: a systematic review. *Pediatrics* 2007;120:1079–87.

Juvenile dermatomyositis

Juvenile dermatomyositis (JDM), also known as idiopathic inflammatory myopathy, is a rare autoimmune disease affecting the skin and muscles. The pathophysiology is unknown, but most studies implicate cell-mediated immunity to muscle antigens and immune complex formation that leads to an autoimmune angiopathy. In children, unlike adults, dermatomyositis is not a risk factor for malignancies.

Clinical presentation

JDM is more common in girls, with a peak age of 5–10 years. It has an insidious onset, with skin involvement of exposed areas being the typical initial complaint. Lesions are often photosensitive and severe pruritus may occur. The major cutaneous manifestations are:

- heliotrope rash: a violaceous, symmetrical eruption involving the upper eyelids with or without associated edema
- Gottron's sign: violaceous papules and plaques found over bony prominences of the finger joints, elbows, knees, and/or feet
- calcinosis cutis: cutaneous deposits of calcium crystals, commonly seen over the joints, while sparing the digits
- other: periungual telangiectasias, alopecia, lipodystrophy, panniculitis, urticaria, and hyperkeratosis of the palms.

Muscle disease may precede or follow skin disease by weeks to years. Systemic manifestations also occur and include non-erosive/deforming arthritis, arthralgia, pulmonary fibrosis/pneumonitis, cardiac arrhythmias, dysphagia, and dysphonia. Approximately 25% of patients are ANA positive.

A visceral vasculopathy is an uncommon complication. It presents with diffuse abdominal pain, melena, hematemesis, and, sometimes, acute mesenteric infarction. Free intraperitoneal air can occur with hollow viscus perforation.

Diagnosis

The initial diagnosis requires a high clinical suspicion. Inquire about skin nodules, weakness, voice changes, joint pain, dyspnea, and dysphagia. Specific diagnostic criteria for JDM have been established:

- characteristic cutaneous changes
- symmetric proximal muscle weakness
- elevated muscle enzymes (CPK, LDH, aldolase, transaminases)
- inflammatory myopathy based on characteristic histopathology
- inflammatory myopathy based on electromyographic and MRI findings.

The diagnosis of JDM can be made if the patient has a typical rash and three of the four other criteria. With the rash and two additional criteria present, the diagnosis is probable, and with the rash and just one it is possible.

ED management

If JDM is suspected, obtain a CBC, comprehensive metabolic panel, CPK, LDH, aldolase chest X-ray, and ECG. Consult a rheumatologist regarding further evaluation (EMG and MRI, muscle biopsy) and treatment.

Immunosuppression with corticosteroids is the initial mainstay therapy for JDM, while physical therapy is important for controlling the myositis and preventing contractures.

Follow-up

- Rheumatology consult within 1–2 weeks

Indication for admission

- Significant disability or severe systemic illness

Bibliography

Feldman BM, Rider LG, Reed AM, Pachman LM: Juvenile dermatomyositis and other idiopathic inflammatory myopathies of childhood. *Lancet* 2008;371:2201–12.

McCann LJ, Juggins AD, Maillard SM, et al: The Juvenile Dermatomyositis National Registry and Repository (UK and Ireland)– clinical characteristics of children recruited within the first 5 yr. *Rheumatology (Oxford)* 2006;45:1255–60.

Rennebohm R: Juvenile dermatomyositis. *Pediatr Ann* 2002;31:426–33.

Systemic lupus erythematosus

Systemic lupus erythematosus (SLE) is a chronic autoimmune inflammatory disorder that is manifested by multisystem involvement and a variable clinical course. The hallmark of the disease is the presence of antinuclear antibodies (ANA) and antibodies to native DNA (dsDNA).

Although the majority of patients are adults, up to 20% of cases involve children over 5 years of age. The female to male ratio is 5–10:1, but this difference is less dramatic in pre-pubertal patients. Overall, African-American females are at the highest risk of developing SLE.

Clinical presentation

Patients with SLE may present to the ED with arthritis, edema or complications of renal disease, hypertensive crises, chest pain or shortness of breath, or infection with fever. There are a number of potential findings and complications in patients with SLE.

- Renal disease is typically present at diagnosis or develops within the first 2 years of disease onset. Hypertension, proteinuria, and red cell casts may be seen.
- Patients on immunosuppressive therapy, particularly if neutropenic (absolute neutrophil count<1,000/mm^3), are at increased risk of developing viral, fungal, or other opportunistic infections. However, it can be difficult to distinguish between a lupus flare and a systemic infection.
- Anemia may be normochromic/normocytic, as in anemia of chronic disease; microcytic/hypochromic suggestive of occult blood loss (gastritis, GI vasculitis); or hemolytic/autoimmune.
- Thrombocytopenia is most commonly a mild autoimmune process. Rarely, it is sign of ensuing thrombotic thrombocytopenic purpura (TTP) with microangiopathic hemolytic anemia, rapidly declining renal function, and CNS dysfunction.
- Antiphospholipid antibody syndrome with arterial and venous thrombosis, livedo reticularis, and the presence of lupus anticoagulant.
- Pulmonary manifestations include pleurisy, pleural effusion or hemorrhage. Suspect hemorrhage in patients with hemoptysis, declining hemoglobin, and shifting pulmonary infiltrates.
- GI manifestations include gastritis, sterile peritonitis, enteritis, or pancreatitis. GI bleeding may be secondary to medications (NSAIDs), gastritis, mesenteric vasculitis (small intestine), or thrombocytopenia.
- Cardiac complications include pericarditis, myocarditis, and valvulitis. Pericardial effusions can occur, but tamponade is rare.

Table 24-8. 1997 SLE classification criteria

Malar rash
Discoid rash
Photosensitivity
Oral or nasal mucocutaneous ulcerations
Nonerosive arthritis
Renal disorder: proteinuria >0.5 g/day; cellular casts
Neurologic disorder: seizures, psychosis
Serositis: pleuritis or pericarditis
Hematologic disorder: hemolytic anemia; leukopenia; lymphopenia; thrombocytopenia
Positive immunoserology: antibodies to dsDNA; antibodies to Sm nuclear antigen; positive finding of antiphospholipid antibodies
Positive antinuclear antibody test

Source: Reproduced with permission from Hochberg MC: Updating the American College of Rheumatology revised criteria for the classification of systemic lupus erythematosus. *Arthritis Rheum* 1997;40:1725.

- Raynaud's phenomenon is a triphasic change in color of the digits in response to cold or stress. Fingers or toes first turn pale then blue, then red upon rewarming. Recurrent vasospasm predisposes to digital ulcers that can lead to superinfection or autoamputation of digits.

Diagnosis

Many of the features of SLE are not specific; therefore maintain a high index of suspicion to consider SLE in the differential diagnosis. Determine whether the patient has constitutional symptoms such as fever, weight loss, or fatigue. Ask about rashes, arthritis, renal manifestations (edema, hematuria, proteinuria), chest pain, and seizures. Explore any family history of SLE or other immune-mediated disorders. On physical examination look for evidence of systemic involvement, including edema, pleurisy, pericardial or pulmonary effusions, ascites, arthritis, and occult infections.

The diagnosis of SLE is made based on American College of Rheumatology classification criteria revised in 1997 (Table 24-8). The patient must meet 4, of the 11 criteria, either simultaneously or at anytime during follow-up. However, these are classification criteria and not diagnostic criteria, so patients may have SLE and not fulfill the criteria, or conversely may meet the criteria but have another illness.

ED management

The management of SLE depends on presenting symptoms and severity of the disease. When the initial diagnosis of SLE is suspected, consult a pediatric rheumatologist to guide further work-up and therapy. Other consultants may include a nephrologist and cardiologist, depending on the presentation. Obtain a CBC with differential, ESR, CRP (usually normal in an uninfected child with SLE), comprehensive metabolic panel, C3 and C4 (complement levels usually are low), ANA with an ENA panel, dsDNA, a urinalysis, and urine protein:creatinine ratio.

If a patient with known SLE is ill-appearing or neutropenic, obtain blood and urine cultures, a chest X-ray, and a lumbar puncture, if clinically appropriate. Initiate broad-spectrum antibiotics if a serious infection cannot be excluded.

Obtain a Coombs test, LDH, haptoglobin, and stool guaiac for patients with significant anemia. Patients with cardiac or pulmonary disease may need an ECG, echocardiogram, or CT of the chest. Management of a hypertensive crisis is discussed elsewhere (pp. 658–660).

There is no specific treatment algorithm for SLE. As outpatients, most patients with lupus receive maintenance hydroxychloroquin, which reduces lupus flares. Treat mild disease manifested by arthritis with NSAIDs (naproxen 17.5 mg/kg per day div bid). Severe systemic disease is an indication for hospitalization and IV methylprednisolone pulses (30 mg/kg per day, 1,000 mg maximum) and other immunosuppressive therapy. Consult a rheumatologist.

Treat Raynaud's by avoidance of the cold, although severe Raynaud's may require nitroglycerin ointment to the webs of the fingers or volar surfaces of the wrists (do not apply for more then 10 hours to prevent tachyphylaxis) and calcium channel blockers.

Follow-up

- Suspected new-onset SLE: pediatric rheumatologist and/or nephrologist within 1 week

Indications for admission

- New-onset SLE
- Worsening renal disease in a known lupus patient
- CNS manifestations (seizures, psychosis, chorea)
- Serositis (pericarditis, pleuritis)
- Serious infection

Bibliography

Gamboa DG, Sugarman JL: An update on selected connective tissue diseases in adolescents. *Curr Opin Pediatr* 2008;20:413–8.

Macdermott EJ, Adams A, Lehman TJ: Systemic lupus erythematosus in children:

current and emerging therapies. *Lupus* 2007; 16:677–83.

Tucker LB: Making the diagnosis of systemic lupus erythematosus in children and adolescents. *Lupus* 2007; 16:546–9.

Sedation and analgesia

Sandra J. Cunningham

Contributing author
Katherine J. Chou: Regional anesthesia

The recognition, assessment, and management of pain in children can be challenging, given the wide range of developmental stages and the difficulty in differentiating pain from anxiety. Therefore, provision of analgesia to younger patients is suboptimal. Furthermore, there is no evidence that relieving pain will obscure the diagnosis and, in fact, making the child more comfortable can facilitate the physical examination and required diagnostic testing. This includes patients with abdominal pain and trauma victims, including those with headache.

The goals of sedation are to provide optimal patient comfort during a procedure while maintaining patient safety. Adhere to strict protocols when administering procedural sedation in order to minimize adverse effects. Persons involved in the sedation process must be experienced in resuscitation in the case of an untoward event. Most importantly, ensure that the provider(s) administering the sedation and monitoring the status of the child is not the same person who is performing the procedure.

Procedural sedation and analgesia (PSA)

PSA employs sedatives or dissociative agents, which are administered at dosages and rates that allow the patient to maintain airway control, protective reflexes, and cardiorespiratory function. However, be prepared to intervene to support airway and ventilation if necessary.

The only acceptable candidates for PSA in the ED are patients who are American Society of Anesthesiology (ASA) Physical Status Classification Classes I, II, or III (see Table 25-1). Perform the assessments for PSA pre-sedation, intra-sedation and post-sedation.

Pre-sedation

When choosing a medication, take into account the physical status of the patient, including age, vital signs, current medical condition, past medical and sedation history, other medications given at home or in the ED, allergies, last oral intake of fluids or solids, and psychological state. Also consider the procedure being performed, including expected level of pain and length of time likely to be required.

The recent intake of solids or liquids is not an absolute contraindication for PSA. Determine the risks and benefits of immediately performing versus delaying the procedure. Data on aspiration risk have been extrapolated from anesthesia literature where the airway is being manipulated (e.g. endotracheal intubation). By definition, with appropriate PSA the patient will maintain airway control and protective reflexes. See Table 25-2 for the American Academy of Pediatrics and the ASA preferred pre-procedural fasting guidelines.

Anticipate both common and uncommon complications. These include vomiting or aspiration, allergic reactions, paradoxical reactions, anaphylaxis, abnormal movements or seizures, airway compromise, respiratory depression and hypoxia, apnea, and

Table 25-1. American Society of Anesthesiology (ASA) Physical Status Classification System

ASA class	Patient description
I	Healthy, no underlying organic disease
II	Mild or moderate systemic disease that does not interfere with daily routines (e.g. well-controlled asthma, essential hypertension)
III	Organic disease with definite functional impairment (e.g. severe steroid -dependent asthma, insulin-dependent diabetes, uncorrected congenital heart disease)
IV	Severe disease that is life-threatening (e.g. head trauma with increased intracranial pressure)
V	Moribund patient, not expected to survive
E (suffix)	Physical status classification appended with an "E" connotes a procedure undertaken as an emergency (e.g. an otherwise healthy patient presenting for fracture reduction is classified as ASA physical status 1E)

Table 25-2. Pre-procedural fasting AAP/ASA guidelines

Age	Solids (includes milk)	Clears
<6 months	4–6 hours	2 hours
6–36 months	6 hours	2 hours
>36 months	6–8 hours	2 hours

cardiorespiratory arrest. Complications generally result from errors in medication dosing, inadequate monitoring, inadequate skill level of the provider, use of multiple agents (three or more), premature discharge of the patient, or higher levels of ASA categorization. Patients are at the greatest risk of complications about 5 minutes after administration of PSA and then after the procedure is completed, when the stimulus has been removed.

PSA equipment

When administering medications with the potential for compromise of ventilation or circulation, monitor the patient continuously with a cardiorespiratory monitor and pulse oximeter. Equipment that must be immediately available at the patient's bedside include bag-mask apparatus with a proper-sized mask, suction with a large diameter suction catheter, an oxygen source, and the correct size nonrebreather face mask (Table 25-3).

Other resuscitation equipment, such as laryngoscopes, endotracheal tubes, and resuscitation medications, must be rapidly available if needed.

Consent

Once the PSA medication has been chosen, explain to parents the nature of the procedure and the expected effect of the drug, including possible side effects. Hospitals differ on whether a separate informed consent for PSA is required. However, there is no evidence

Table 25-3. PSA equipment

Cardiac monitor	Bag-valve-mask apparatus
Oxygen source	Laryngoscope
Pulse oximeter	Endotracheal tubes and stylets
Blood pressure cuffs and sphygmomanometer	Oral/nasal airways
Specific antidotes	Large-bore suction device
Epinephrine (allergic reactions)	
Resuscitation medications (atropine, epinephrine)	

that a separate consent form enhances patient or parental satisfaction, and it is not required by the Joint Commission on Accreditation of Healthcare Organizations (JCAHO).

Intra-sedation

During PSA, continually monitor airway, breathing, and circulation status, with written documentation at specified intervals (5–15 minutes). The provider performing the procedure cannot also monitor the patient.

Post-sedation

Continue to monitor airway, breathing, and circulation status until the patient is awake and no longer at risk for cardiorespiratory compromise. Before discharge from the ED, the patient must return to a baseline level of alertness and motor ability and be able to tolerate oral fluids. Give the parent appropriate discharge instructions with a contact number for the ED.

Medication administration

Medications can be given by a variety of routes, including intranasal, inhalational, intramuscular, intravenous, oral, and rectal. The intravenous (IV) route provides the most reliable and predictable sedation. Many drugs can be titrated to accommodate the level of sedation needed and the length of the procedure. However, rapid administration can lead to hypotension and cardiorespiratory compromise. Always infuse medications at an IV port close to the catheter hub to ensure that the drug reaches the vascular system immediately. When medications are given more distally in the IV tubing while fluids are running, there is a potential for a rapid bolus of the drug.

The intramuscular (IM) route can provide deep sedation without the need for an IV, but drugs cannot be titrated and this route lacks the precise control of the IV route. Oral (PO), intranasal (IN), inhalational, and rectal (PR) routes are generally appropriate for less painful procedures, or procedures in which a local anesthetic will also be used, or as sedation for diagnostic procedures, such as a CT scan. The inhalation route (nitrous oxide) is appropriate for cooperative children who are able to follow directions.

Before administration of the medication, use relaxation techniques such as guided imagery or hypnosis and attempt to create a calm atmosphere (e.g. dim lighting, noise elimination). Insert an intravenous line if needed and place the child on a cardiorespiratory monitor, which includes continuous pulse oximetry. Pulse oximetry provides an early warning of desaturation, since visible cyanosis does not occur until 4.5 g/dL of hemoglobin are desaturated (generally at an oxygen saturation <70%). Although an oxygen source must be immediately available, the routine administration of oxygen during PSA will limit the provider's ability to detect hypoventilation when the pulse oximeter displays a decreasing oxygen saturation.

PSA medications (see Table 25-4)

Opioids

Opioids are potent analgesics that elevate the pain threshold, causing analgesia, euphoria, and respiratory depression. An advantage of opioids is that they are reversible with the pure antagonist, naloxone (Table 25-4). However, the serum half-life of naloxone is approximately 60 minutes, so the effects of the opioid may outlast the naloxone. For patients who require a prolonged course of naloxone, infuse a drip that delivers, per hour, two-thirds of the dose that was required to achieve the desired response initially.

Morphine

Morphine is the principal alkaloid of opium. It has minimal hemodynamic effects in the euvolemic patient when used in appropriate doses. Use morphine for procedures such as burn debridement and hydrotherapy, abscess incision and drainage, and control of pain in patients with burns or sickle cell vasoocclusive crisis.

Fentanyl

Fentanyl is a synthetic opioid that is 25–100 times more potent than morphine. Use fentanyl for painful procedures of short duration such as fracture reduction or incision and drainage of an abscess or pilonidal cyst.

Fentanyl combined with midazolam (see benzodiazepines) provides potent analgesia for short, painful procedures. Administer the midazolam first, followed by fentanyl. Generally, with this combination, the total dose of fentanyl can be decreased by about 50%.

Benzodiazepines

Benzodiazepines possess sedative-hypnotic, anxiolytic, and antegrade amnestic effects. When used as a single agent, they have a low risk of complications, although they are often combined with other drugs, such as opioids, for painful procedures. Untoward effects of benzodiazepines are reversible with the antagonist flumazenil (Table 25-4), which is appropriate for iatrogenic or known overdose of benzodiazepines. However, do not use flumazenil routinely to reverse the known effects of benzodiazepines. Monitor the patient for resedation since the half-life of the benzodiazepine may outlast that of flumazenil.

Midazolam

Indications for use include anxiety-provoking or non-painful procedures such as CT scan or gynecologic examination, or procedures in which a local anesthetic will be used, e.g. laceration repair. Use midazolam in combination with an opioid to augment sedation for painful procedures.

Table 25-4. PSA and pain medications

Drug	Route	Dose	Onset	Duration	Maximum dose	Side effects	Comments
Etomidate	IV	0.15–0.2 mg/kg	<1 min	<12 min	20 mg	Pain at injection site, vomiting	Slow IV push over 1 minute
						$\downarrow$O$_2$ sat, $\downarrow$BP	May require a second dose
						Respiratory depression (with opioids)	
						Myoclonus (not assoc. with EEG changes)	
						Adrenal insufficiency (multiple doses)	
Propofol	IV	1.0 mg/kg	<1 min	<15 min		Pain at injection site	Slow IVP over 1 minute Follow by 0.5 mg/kg every 3–5 min PRN
						Apnea, $\downarrow$BP	Additional dose: 0.5 mg/kg
						Lactic acidosis (continuous infusion)	
Nitrous oxide		See text					
Ketamine	IM	3 mg/kg	1–2 min	30–60 min	150 mg	Vomiting, laryngospasm, $\downarrow$O$_2$ sat	Slow IVP over 1 minute
	IV	1.5 mg/kg	1–2 min	30–60 min	75 mg	Emergence reaction, post-procedure ataxia	Additional doses: 0.5 mg/kg
						$\uparrow$ oral and airway secretions	Use with IM or IV atropine:
						$\uparrow$ sympathomimetic activity	0.01 mg/kg (0.3 mg maximum)
						$\uparrow$ intraocular and intracranial pressure	
Morphine	IM/IV/SC	0.1–0.2 mg/kg	1–2 min	2–4 h	15 mg	Respiratory depression (especially when used with other agents)	Slow IVP over 1 minute

Drug	Route	Dose	Onset	Duration	Maximum dose	Adverse effects	Comments
Fentanyl	IV	1–5 mcg/kg	1–2 min	30 min	0.5 mcg/kg/min to maximum of 25 mcg/min	↓BP in hypovolemic patients Nausea, vomiting, histamine release Respiratory depression and hypoxia (can occur with appropriate dose and IV rate) Facial pruritus early sign of sedation Chest wall rigidity with rapid bolus	Use in combination with midazolam Antidote: naloxone (see below) Chest wall rigidity may require ↑naloxone dose
Midazolam	IV/IM	0.1 mg/kg	5–10 min	30–60 min	IV/IM: 5 mg	↓pulse, ↓BP, nausea, vomiting ↓complications used as a single agent ↓respirations in combination with opioids	Administer before other agents Antidote: flumazenil (see below)
	PO	0.5–1 mg/kg			PO: 20 mg		
	PR	0.5 mg/kg					
Methohexital	PR	25 mg/kg	<10 min	60–90 min	1 gram	Minimal adverse effects at low doses ↓O₂ sat, hiccups, cough, ↑salivation	Effects are dose-dependent and range from mild sedation to coma No analgesic effects
Pentobarbital	PO	2–6 mg/kg	Up to 45 min	2–4 h	PO: 150 mg	Prolonged period to arousal Agitation	Most success in children <8 yrs Limited use due to onset and duration
	PR	2 mg/kg (minimum 30 mg)			PR: 60 mg		

Table 25-4. (cont.)

Drug	Route	Dose	Onset	Duration	Maximum dose	Side effects	Comments
Ketorolac	IM/IV	0.5 mg/kg	0.5–1 hr	6 h	30 mg	Nausea, gastritis, drowsiness	5-day course maximum
						Interstitial nephritis	Do not use in renal or hepatic failure
							Use for sickle cell pain and renal colic
Oxycodone	PO	0.05–0.15 mg/kg	0.5–1 h	6 h	5 mg	Nausea, vomiting, constipation, gastritis	Useful in sickle cell pain crisis
Codeine/acetaminophen	PO	0.5–1.0 mg/kg as codeine	0.5–1 h	4–6 h	30 mg	Nausea, vomiting, constipation	Useful in sickle cell pain crisis
						Abdominal pain	Various formulations available or dose codeine and acetaminophen separately
Acetaminophen	PO	15 mg/kg	0.5–1 h	4 h	650 mg		No anti-inflammatory effect
	PR						
Ibuprofen	PO	10 mg/kg		0.5–1 hr	800 mg	Gastritis, inhibits platelet aggregation.	Has anti-inflammatory effects
							↓ GI distress with food or milk
							Do not use with renal insufficiency

Antidotes

Drug	Route	Dose/kg	Duration	Onset	Max dose	Side effects	Notes
Naloxone (for opioids)	IV,IM, SC,ETT	0.1 mg/kg	60 min	< 1 min	2.0 mg first dose	Seizure risk if opioid-dependent, including newborns of drug-addicted mother	Have at bedside when using fentanyl Smaller doses (0.01 mg/kg/dose) may reverse respiratory depression but maintain analgesic effects Narcotic effects may outlast naloxone
Flumazenil	IV	0.02 mg/kg		1–3 min	1 mg	Crying, agitation	Administer via 0.2 mg increments over 15 sec Repeat dose in 60 s, to 1 mg maximum Useful for iatrogenic/known overdose Not for reversal of known side effects Benzodiazepine may outlast flumazenil

Etomidate

Etomidate is a non-barbiturate sedative hypnotic that has been used as an induction agent in the operating room for several decades. Initially in EDs it was used as a pre-intubation induction agent, but has subsequently gained favor as a PSA medication. It has no analgesic properties, so patients undergoing a painful procedure will need additional medication, such as lidocaine or an opioid. Etomidate produces amnesia for the event in the majority of patients. Use etomidate for procedures of very short duration such as a CT scan of the head, reduction of a dislocation, foreign-body removal, abscess incision and drainage, and lumbar puncture.

Propofol

Propofol is a potent sedative hypnotic agent that has no analgesic or amnestic effects. It can be used alone for painful procedures. Use propofol for painful procedures of short duration such as fracture reduction, and incision and drainage of an abscess or pilonidal cyst.

Nitrous oxide

Nitrous oxide is a sedative hypnotic that has no anesthetic qualities but causes a detached feeling in the patient. In the ED, it is delivered as a mixture of 50% oxygen and 50% nitrous oxide via a two-tank system. Attach a scavenger device from the nitrous oxide tank to wall suction to eliminate the potential for leakage of nitrous oxide into the atmosphere. Prepare an additional suction device in case the patient vomits, which is an indication for discontinuing the nitrous oxide.

The patient must be able to cooperate and follow directions since nitrous oxide is patient-controlled sedation. The patient holds the mask firmly over the nose and mouth and breathes normally, until sleepy or very relaxed, at which time the face mask will be dropped. As a safety measure, the nitrous oxide delivery stops if the oxygen becomes diminished. Discontinue the nitrous oxide if there is no effect after 2–3 minutes; 10% of the population does not respond. Nitrous oxide is contraindicated in patients with head trauma or impaired mental status, abdominal distention or obstruction, pneumothorax, respiratory depression, and pregnancy.

Ketamine

Ketamine is a phencyclidine derivative that provides potent sedation and analgesia and dissociates the central nervous system from outside stimuli such as pain, sight, and sound. Use ketamine for painful procedures of short or moderate duration such as fracture reduction, incision and drainage, or wound repair.

Historically, ketamine was administered with midazolam to prevent emergence reactions. However, there is no evidence to support this. There is no spectrum of dissociation; it is either present or absent, so additional increments of the drug will not increase the level of dissociation. Titrate the drug to achieve the dissociated state over the length of the procedure. Although there is some dispute about the benefit, atropine is usually added as an antisialagogue.

Ketamine is contraindicated in children <3 months of age, patients with cardiovascular disease, respiratory disease (e.g. active asthma), or head injury, any state in which increased intracranial or intraocular pressure is suspected, hyperthyroidism, psychosis, or when there is a history of a previous adverse reaction. Perform meticulous oral suctioning if using for intra oral procedures to avoid pooling of secretions.

Barbiturates

Barbiturates are sedative hypnotics that can provide mild to deep sedation, depending on the dose. They have no analgesic qualities. Use barbiturates for anxiety-provoking procedures such as CT scan or procedures in which a local anesthetic will be used (e.g. laceration repair).

Methohexital

Methohexital is an ultra-short-acting barbiturate that is given rectally, avoiding the need for an IV catheter.

Pentobarbital

This is a short-acting barbiturate. However, the onset of action may be delayed when given by the rectal or oral routes.

Bibliography

Godwin SA, Caro DA, Wolf SJ, et al: Clinical policy: procedural sedation and analgesia in the emergency department. *Ann Emerg Med* 2005;45:77–196.

Gozal D, Gozal Y: Pediatric sedation/anesthesia outside the operating room. *Curr Opin Anaesthesiol* 2008;21:494–8.

MacLean S, Obispo J, Young KD: The gap between pediatric emergency department procedural pain management treatments available and actual practice. *Pediatr Emerg Care* 2007;23:87–93.

Roback MG, Wathen JE, Bajaj L, Bothner JP: Adverse events associated with procedural sedation and analgesia in a pediatric emergency department: a comparison of common parenteral drugs. *Acad Emerg Med* 2005;12:508–13.

Local anesthesia

Lidocaine

Lidocaine is a local anesthetic routinely used in the ED, most commonly for laceration repair. Lidocaine is available as either a 1% (10 mg/mL) or 2% (20 mg/mL) solution, with and without epinephrine. Epinephrine is contraindicated in areas with end arteries (the fingers, toes, penis, nose, or ear).

Dose

With epinephrine: 4.5 mg/kg; without epinephrine: 7 mg/kg.

Administration

In order to decrease the pain of administration, administer slowly with a 27-gauge 1.5 inch needle, warm the solution to 40°C (104°F), and buffer with sodium bicarbonate in a 1:10 ratio, which will give the solution a pH of 7.2. For intact skin, infiltrate subcutaneously until a bleb is apparent. For open wounds, put a few drops directly into the wound, then infiltrate subcutaneously around the wound edge. In areas of large arteries, aspirate before infiltrating to check for blood. Advance the needle slowly with constant infiltration of lidocaine. Withdraw and continue around the wound sequentially, placing the needle in the already anesthetized portion of the subdermis. Ensure that the area is anesthetized by applying the needle to the skin out of view of the child. Anesthesia occurs in approximately 5 minutes.

Table 25-5. Dose and application of EMLA

Age	Weight	Max dose	Max duration	Max area (cm^2)
1–3 months	< 5 kg	1 g	1 h	10
4–12 months	5–10 kg	2 g	4 h	20
1–6 years	> 10 kg	10 g	4 h	100
7–12 years	> 20 kg	20 g	4 h	200

Topical anesthesia

LET

Lidocaine (4%), epinephrine (1%) and tetracaine (0.5%) is available in gel or liquid form and is used for laceration repair.

Dose

1–3 mL.

Administration

Place half of the solution on the wound and half on a cotton swab. Do not use gauze as this will pull the LET away from the wound. Hold the cotton firmly in place for 30–45 minutes; use an elastic bandage on suitable areas such as scalp or extremity lacerations. Otherwise, secure the cotton with firmly placed tape or have an adult hold it in place with pressure. Supplemental local lidocaine is generally required.

EMLA (eutectic mixture of local anesthesia)

EMLA contains 2.5% lidocaine and 2.5% prilocaine. Use it on intact skin for IV placement, phlebotomy, and injections or minor procedures such as incision and drainage of a paronychia. It can be used on mucous membranes of the groin and on compromised skin (e.g. dermatitis). The major adverse event is the potential for methemoglobinemia, especially in infants with G6PD or children receiving other methemoglobinemia-inducing agents such as sulfa drugs.

Administration

Apply a thick layer to the area and cover with an occlusive dressing (Table 25-5), for a minimum of 60 minutes. The effects are maximal at 2–3 hours and may persist up to 2 hours after removal of the cream. The depth of anesthesia is 3 mm after 1 hour and 5 mm after 2 hours.

LMX$_4$ (4% liposomal lidocaine)

Use LMX$_4$ on intact skin (not mucous membranes) for procedures as listed above under EMLA. The onset of anesthesia is 30 minutes. Because it does not contain prilocaine, there is no risk of methemoglobinemia as with EMLA.

Administration

Apply a thick layer to the area. An occlusive dressing will enhance absorption and keep the medication in place, but is not required.

Iontophoresis (Numby stuff)

Numby stuff is 2% ionized lidocaine and epinephrine 1:100,000. It involves the transfer of charged particles through the skin by low-voltage electrical current and therefore requires a specialized iontophoretic drug delivery unit and electrodes. It can be used on intact skin in children >1 year of age. The advantage of iontophoresis is a rapid onset of action in 10–20 minutes. However, the equipment can be cumbersome and many children will not tolerate the accompanying burning, tingling, or itching of the skin. There is also a risk of superficial burns.

Ethyl chloride

Ethyl chloride is a vapocoolant and not a local anesthetic. It transiently lowers the local temperature of the skin to –10°C (14°F) to –20°C (–4°F). The nerves are then desensitized for a brief period. Indications include IV placement, phlebotomy, injections, and incision and drainage of a paronychia or small abscess.

Procedure

Hold the can about 6 inches from the application site. Spray the desired area only until the skin appears white, which will be the point of maximal anesthesia. Perform the procedure immediately since the cooling effect is brief.

Hurricaine spray (benzocaine 20%)

Use Hurricaine spray to anesthetize mucous membranes before draining a peritonsillar abscess or repairing intraoral lacerations. The onset of anesthesia is about 1 minute and the duration is 12–15 minutes. If swallowed, it may suppress the gag reflex. There is a potential risk of methemoglobinemia.

Procedure

Spray 1–2 inches from the intended site for 1 second.

Sucrose 12% solution

The combination of sucrose and sucking can provide an analgesic effect in infants 0–3 months of age. Give 1.5–2.0 mL PO over 2 minutes through a nipple or on a gloved finger. Wait 2 minutes before starting the procedure. The effect lasts up to 8 minutes.

Regional anesthesia

In certain circumstances, use of local infiltration of anesthesia is undesirable. Examples include wounds in areas with little surrounding subcutaneous tissue where local infiltration will significantly distort the tissue architecture, large wounds where the amount of lidocaine needed to achieve anesthesia is excessive, and wounds in areas that are difficult and extremely painful to fully anesthetize, such as fingertips, toes, nailbeds, palms, soles, and the penis. Regional anesthesia provides effective anesthesia in these cases.

Equipment

- 1% lidocaine solution, without epinephrine
- Sodium bicarbonate, if desired (ratio of 10 parts lidocaine to 1 part sodium bicarbonate)
- 25- or 27-gauge hypodermic needle, 0.5–1 inch in length
- Syringe (3–5 mL is usually sufficient)
- Antiseptic solution for the skin
- Sterile gauze

General procedure

Assess for sensory deficits secondary to trauma before performing the nerve block. Cleanse the skin with antiseptic solution for percutaneous nerve blocks. No antiseptic is necessary with intraoral approaches. After inserting the needle, draw back on the syringe slightly before injecting lidocaine to ensure that the needle is not within a blood vessel. If insertion of the needle elicits paresthesias or a sharp jolt of pain in the nerve distribution, withdraw the needle slightly before injecting lidocaine to avoid infiltration directly into the nerve. Although anesthesia may be achieved within several minutes, 10–20 minutes may be needed for maximal effect to occur. Gently massage the area where the lidocaine is deposited to hasten the distribution of the anesthetic in the region of the nerve.

Supraorbital and supratrochlear nerve blocks

Area of effect

Forehead and frontal scalp.

Anatomy

The supraorbital nerve exits the supraorbital foramen at the orbital rim in the midpupillary line. The supratrochlear nerve exits the foramen just medial to the supraorbital nerve (see Figure 25-1).

Technique

Locate the supraorbital foramen and insert the needle subcutaneously just lateral to the foramen. Direct the needle medially and advance it to the hub in a direction both parallel and adjacent to the superior orbital rim (see Figure 25-1B). Lay a track of 2–3 mL lidocaine along this line as the needle is slowly withdrawn.

Infraorbital nerve block

Area of effect

Medial cheek to the nasal ala, upper lip, and lower eyelid.

Anatomy

The infraorbital nerve exits the infraorbital foramen approximately 1.5 cm below the inferior orbital rim, in the midpupillary line.

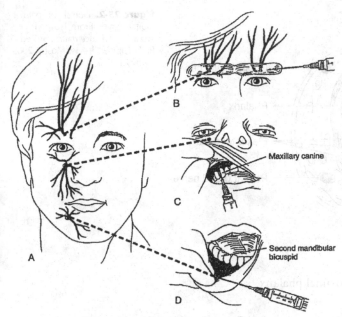

Figure 25-1. Supraorbital and supratrochlear nerve blocks. From Trott AT: *Wounds and Lacerations*, 3rd ed. Philadelphia: Elsevier Mosby, 2005, with permission.

Technique

The intraoral approach is less painful and preferable to the percutaneous approach (see Figure 25-1C). Retract the upper lip. Using a cotton swab, apply a topical anesthetic (2% viscous lidocaine) for several minutes to the oral mucosa of the gingival-buccal sulcus at the level of the maxillary canine tooth. Insert the needle at this location and direct it superiorly towards the infraorbital foramen. Advance the needle subcutaneously approximately 1–2 cm until the tip of the needle is at the level of the infraorbital foramen, then inject 1–2 mL of lidocaine.

Mental nerve block
Area of effect
Lower lip and chin.

Anatomy
The mental nerve exits the mental foramen midway between the upper and lower borders of the mandible, in the midpupillary line, approximately 2–2.5 cm from the midline of the jaw.

Technique
The intraoral approach is less painful and preferable to the percutaneous approach (see Figure 25-1D). Pretreat the injection site with 2% viscous lidocaine (as above). Retract the lower lip. Insert the needle in the gingival-buccal sulcus at the 2nd bicuspid, and advance the needle inferiorly towards the mental foramen. When the tip of the needle is at the level of the mental foramen, inject 1–2 mL of lidocaine.

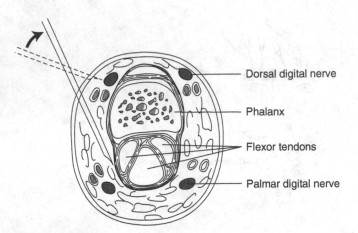

Figure 25-2. Dorsal and palmar digital nerves. From Trott AT: *Wounds and Lacerations*, 3rd ed. Philadelphia: Elsevier Mosby, 2005, with permission.

Digital nerve block

Area of effect

Finger or toe distal to the proximal phalanx.

Anatomy

Each digit is supplied by four nerves, two dorsal and two palmar. On a cross-section of the digit, the dorsal nerves are located at 2 o'clock and 10 o'clock; the palmar nerves are located at 4 o'clock and 8 o'clock. The nerves run adjacent to the phalanges (see Figure 25-2).

Technique

Insert the needle into the web space at the dorsolateral aspect of the proximal phalanx of the digit. Advance the needle until it touches the bone, then withdraw the needle slightly and inject 0.5–1 mL lidocaine. Redirect the needle towards the palmar nerve and advance adjacent to the bone. When the tip of the needle is at the level of the palmar nerve, inject 0.5–1.0 mL lidocaine. Repeat the entire process on the opposite side of the digit (see Figure 25-3).

To properly anesthetize the great toe, instill lidocaine circumferentially. After injecting lidocaine on either side of the great toe as described above, redirect the needle across the dorsal surface of the toe and advance the needle to the opposite side. Lay a track of lidocaine as the needle is slowly withdrawn. Repeat the process on the plantar surface of the toe (see Figure 25-4).

Median nerve block

Area of effect

The palmar surface of the thumb; 2nd, 3rd, and lateral aspect of the 4th fingers; lateral aspect of the hand; and the dorsal surface of the tips of the thumb, 2nd, 3rd and lateral aspect of the 4th fingers (see Figure 25-5).

Anatomy

The median nerve lies between and below the palmaris longus and flexor carpi radialis tendons. For patients who do not have a palmaris longus tendon (up to 20% of the population), the median nerve is just medial to the flexor carpi radialis (see Figure 25-6).

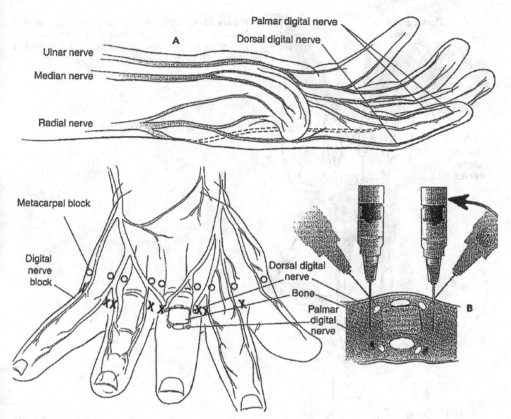

Figure 25-3. Digital nerve block. From King C, Henretig F (eds), *Textbook of Pediatric Emergency Procedures*, 2nd ed. Philadelphia: Lippincott Williams and Wilkins, 2008, with permission.

Technique

Insert the needle between the palmaris longus and flexor carpi radialis tendons at the level of the proximal wrist crease. Insert the needle at the same level, just medial to the flexor carpi radialis for patients who do not have a palmaris longus tendon (see Figure 25-7). Advance the needle approximately 1 cm. A "popping" sensation may be felt as the needle passes through the flexor retinaculum. If paresthesias are elicited, withdraw the needle slightly, and inject 2–3 mL of lidocaine. If no paresthesias are elicited, inject 3–5 mL of lidocaine as the needle is slowly withdrawn.

Ulnar nerve block

Area of effect

Dorsal and palmar surfaces of the 4th and 5th fingers, medial aspect of the hand, and dorsal surface of the medial aspect of the 3rd finger.

Anatomy

The ulnar nerve divides into the palmar and dorsal cutaneous branches several centimeters proximal to the wrist. The ulnar nerve lies beneath the flexor carpi ulnaris tendon at the

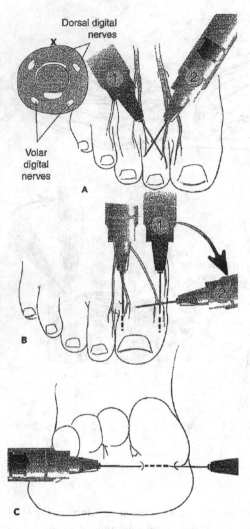

Dorsal digital nerves

X

Volar digital nerves

A

B

C

Figure 25-4. Digital nerve block of great toe. From King C, Henretig F (eds), *Textbook of Pediatric Emergency Procedures*, 2nd ed. Philadelphia: Lippincott Williams and Wilkins, 2008, with permission.

level of the wrist, and runs adjacent to the ulnar artery. Both palmar and dorsal cutaneous branches must be blocked to achieve full anesthesia.

Technique

To block the palmar branch of the ulnar nerve, insert the needle just lateral to the flexor carpi ulnaris tendon at the level of the proximal wrist crease. Advance the needle approximately 1 cm. Check that the needle has not entered the ulnar artery by drawing back on the syringe, then inject 2–3 mL lidocaine. Block the dorsal branch of the ulnar artery by injecting 1–2 mL lidocaine subcutaneously at the dorsal aspect of the wrist just distal to the ulnar styloid.

Alternatively, insert the needle at the medial aspect of the wrist at the level of the proximal crease, just dorsal to the flexor carpi ulnaris tendon. Advance the needle laterally approximately 1 cm, then inject 2–3 mL lidocaine. Withdraw the needle and redirect it towards the distal end of the ulnar styloid. Inject 1–2 mL lidocaine superficially in this area. This approach will block both the dorsal and palmar branches of the ulnar nerve.

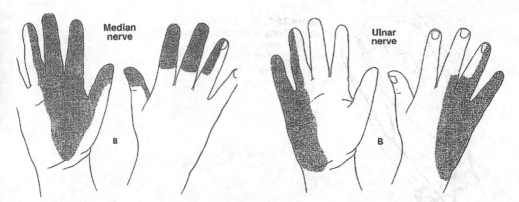

Figure 25-5. Sensory distribution of median and ulnar nerves. From McCreight A, Stephan M: Local and regional anesthesia. In King C, Henretig F (eds), *Textbook of Pediatric Emergency Procedures*, 2nd ed. Philadelphia: Lippincott Williams and Wilkins, 2008, pp. 450–1, with permission.

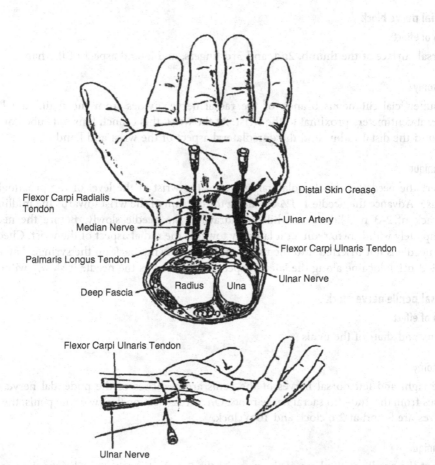

Figure 25-6. Median and ulnar nerve blocks. From Roberts JR, Hedges JR (eds), *Clinical Procedures in Emergency Medicine*, 3rd ed. Philadelphia: W.B. Saunders, 1998, with permission.

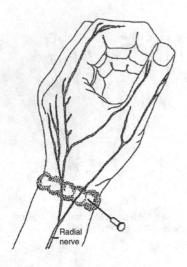

Figure 25-7. Radial nerve block. From Roberts JR, Hedges JR (eds), *Clinical Procedures in Emergency Medicine*, 3rd ed. Philadelphia: W.B. Saunders, 1998, with permission.

Radial nerve block

Area of effect

Dorsal surface of the thumb, 2nd, and 3rd fingers, and lateral aspect of the hand.

Anatomy

A superficial cutaneous branch of the radial nerve divides from the main radial nerve several centimeters proximal to the wrist. At the wrist, this branch fans out subcutaneously around the distal radius and the dorsolateral aspect of the wrist and hand.

Technique

Insert the needle at the dorsolateral aspect of the wrist at the level of the proximal wrist crease. Advance the needle 1–1½ cm along the dorsum of the wrist towards the midline. Lay a track of 2–3 mL lidocaine while withdrawing the needle slowly. Before the needle is completely withdrawn, redirect it laterally towards the radial aspect of the wrist. Check that the needle is not inserted into the radial artery by drawing back on the syringe. Lay a track of 2–3 mL lidocaine along the lateral aspect of the wrist as the needle is slowly withdrawn.

Dorsal penile nerve block

Area of effect

Glans and shaft of the penis.

Anatomy

The right and left dorsal nerves of the penis are branches of the pudendal nerve, which arises from the 2nd–4th sacral nerve roots. On a cross-sectional view of the penis, the dorsal nerves are found at 2 o'clock and 10 o'clock.

Technique

Insert the needle at the base of the penis at the 2 o'clock position. Advance the needle no more than 3–5 mm beneath the skin, just inside Buck's fascia. A "pop" may be felt as

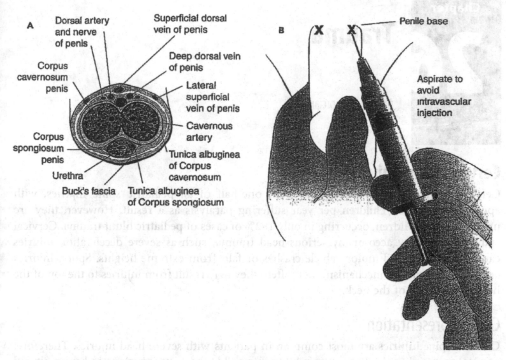

Figure 25-8. Penile nerve block. From King C, Henretig F (eds), *Textbook of Pediatric Emergency Procedures*, 2nd ed. Philadelphia: Lippincott Williams and Wilkins, 2008, with permission.

the needle passes through Buck's fascia. Inject 1–5 mL lidocaine, depending on the size of the child. Repeat the procedure at the 10 o'clock position.

Alternatively, a single midline injection can also be used. Feel for the inferior edge of the symphysis pubis. Insert the needle perpendicular to the skin at the base of the penis in the midline (see Figure 25-8). Advance the needle adjacent to the edge of the symphysis pubis to a depth of 3–5 mm beyond the symphysis pubis into Buck's fascia. A "pop" may be felt as the needle passes through Buck's fascia. Inject 1–5 mL lidocaine, which will anesthetize both dorsal nerves as the lidocaine diffuses through Buck's fascia.

A superficial ring block can be performed to augment the dorsal penile nerve block. Inject a subcutaneous ring of lidocaine circumferentially around the base of the penis. Two injection sites are generally sufficient, one on the ventral surface of the penis, and the other on the dorsal side. Direct and advance the needle both medially and laterally at each injection site. Inject the lidocaine subcutaneously as the needle is slowly withdrawn.

Bibliography

Amsterdam JT: Regional anesthesia of the head and neck. In Roberts JR, Hedges JR (eds), *Clinical Procedures in Emergency Medicine*, 3rd ed. Philadelphia: WB Saunders, 1998, pp. 497–510.

Dean E, Orlinsky M: Nerve blocks of the thorax and extremities. In Roberts JR, Hedges JR (eds), *Clinical Procedures in Emergency Medicine*, 3rd ed. Philadelphia: WB Saunders, 1998, pp. 473–96.

McCreight A, Stephan M: Local and regional anesthesia. In King C, Henretig F (eds), *Textbook of Pediatric Emergency Procedures*, 2nd ed. Philadelphia: Lippincott Williams and Wilkins, 2008, pp. 449–60.

Trott AT: *Wounds and Lacerations*, 3rd ed. Philadelphia: Elsevier Mosby, 2005.

Chapter 26

Trauma

Anthony J. Ciorciari

Cervical spine injuries

Cervical spine injuries account for about one-half of all pediatric spine injuries, with approximately 1000 children per year suffering paralysis as a result. However, they are uncommon in children, occurring in only 1–2% of cases of pediatric blunt trauma. Cervical spine injuries may accompany serious head trauma, such as severe deceleration injuries caused by high-speed motor vehicle crashes or falls from extreme heights. Sports injuries are another common mechanism. Less often, they may result from injuries to the top of the head or the back of the neck.

Clinical presentation

Cervical spine injuries are most common in patients with severe head injuries. Therefore, cervical spine injury is always a possibility in a child who is unconscious or has an altered mental status after head trauma. This is especially true in younger children, whose horizontally aligned facet joints and more elastic intervertebral ligaments can predispose them to subluxation without bony injury. This occurs when the angular momentum resulting from forceful impact levers the proportionately larger head on the fulcrum of the upper cervical spine. The result is a condition known as spinal cord injury without radiographic abnormality (SCIWORA), which predisposes the victim to paraplegia and neurogenic shock or respiratory arrest. Approximately 20% of all pediatric spinal injuries are SCIWORA.

In the alert patient the most common finding is midline cervical tenderness. Less often, there is weakness, pain, or paresthesias along the affected nerve roots. In the unconscious patient with high-grade partial or complete cord transection, common findings include spinal shock (flaccidity and areflexia instead of spasticity, hyperreflexia, and Babinski's sign) and neurogenic ("warm") shock (hypotension that is poorly responsive to volume resuscitation but is paradoxically associated with bradycardia, "normal" urine output, and warm extremities).

Diagnosis

Assume that a cervical spine injury may have occurred in a patient who is unconscious or has an altered mental status after head trauma. Spinal cord injury is sometimes overlooked during the initial evaluation of a comatose patient with severe traumatic brain injury.

See pp. 710–718 for the general approach to the patient with multiple trauma and pp. 716–717 for the general approach to the patient with head trauma.

Often, an awake, alert patient arrives in the ED immobilized on a backboard, in a semirigid extrication collar. Ask about the presence of pain at the top of the head (C2–3) or back of the neck, and about paresthesias of the hands, arms, or legs. If none of these are present, without moving the patient, carefully remove the cervical restraint while maintaining in-line stabilization of the neck. Palpate the spinous processes for local tenderness, associated interspinous muscle spasm, or obvious deformity. The first spinous process that can be palpated is C2; C6 and C7 are the largest. Ask the patient to move the fingers and hands, feet and toes, and to raise the arms and legs. If there is no tenderness, hyperesthesia or paresthesias in the extremities, or evidence of trauma, and the patient moves all extremities easily, ask him or her to move the neck gently from side to side, then up and down. Do not attempt to move the patient's neck yourself; insist that the patient stop immediately if any movement causes pain.

Suspect a cervical spine injury in a patient with any of the following: unresponsiveness after head trauma, paresthesias or weakness, hyperesthesia, limitation of neck motion, inability to cooperate with the examination, pain on top of the head, neck trauma, or injury above the clavicles. Assume that there is a cervical spine injury, until proven otherwise, in a patient who is intoxicated or has a distracting injury that interferes with response to pain.

ED management

Begin by performing an assessment of the ABCs, the initial component of the primary survey (see Resuscitation, pp. 1–28). Immediately stabilize the head and neck of every patient suspected of having a cervical spine injury, if temporary immobilization was not accomplished earlier in the field. The preferred method is with an appropriate-size semi-rigid extrication collar and head immobilizer. A thin layer of padding placed beneath the torso from shoulders to hips is required for a young child to ensure maintenance of a neutral position, as the prominent occiput predisposes the neck to slight flexion unless this precaution is taken. A soft collar, sandbags, or large IV bags placed on both sides of the patient's head (despite being well-secured with tape across the forehead) do not provide adequate immobilization of the head and neck. Finally, because ventilation may be impaired by the very techniques required to achieve adequate immobilization, monitor the patient carefully for signs of respiratory compromise.

If intubation is necessary, apply bimanual in-line stabilization to the sides of the head and remove the extrication collar, if one is present. Have an assistant apply slight downward pressure over the larynx (the Sellick maneuver), if necessary, to bring the vocal cords into view. Avoid hyperextending or flexing the neck during the procedure. Never delay intubation, when indicated, because a cross-table lateral cervical spine X-ray has not been obtained or interpreted.

Once the airway has been secured and the head and neck have been properly immobilized, order a cross-table lateral X-ray of the cervical spine. The base of the skull, all seven cervical vertebrae, and the top of the first thoracic vertebra must be visualized. Continuity of the normal lordotic curves of the cervical spine and important anatomic measurements (Table 26-1) must be confirmed by a physician experienced in interpretation of pediatric cervical spine radiographs. Be aware of certain anatomic features of young children that mimic vertebral injuries, including unfused epiphyses (particularly at the base of the dens), widening of the prevertebral soft-tissue spaces on forced expiration (crying), and hypermobility of the upper cervical spine (resulting in the slight forward shifting of C2 on C3 and C3 on C4, known as pseudosubluxation). Suspect that the cervical spine is unstable in a child

Table 26-1. Normal cervical spine measurements

Measurement	<8 years	≥8 years
Predental space	4–5 mm	3 mm
C2-3 override (flexion)	<4.5 mm	<3.5 mm
Prevertebral space	½–⅔ thickness of C2	5–7 mm at level of C2
Spinal cord area	Varies with age	10–13 mm
Most commonly injured	C1–4	C5–7

<8 years of age if >4.5 mm of subluxation is present at C2–3 or C3–4 or, in an older patient, if >3.5 mm of subluxation is noted at any level.

However, a lateral cervical spine radiograph alone can miss certain vertebral fractures. Thus, once this film is obtained and interpreted as normal, transport a patient with stable vital signs to the X-ray suite, for AP and open-mouth views. An open-mouth view permits visualization of the odontoid process (dens) of the axis (C2) and the ring of the atlas (C1). Obtain a CT of the cervical spine when it is impossible to obtain a full radiographic series, if there is a suggestion of fracture on radiograph without the actual fracture being seen (e.g. increased prevertebral soft tissue), or to look for additional fractures despite a fracture already having been identified on X-ray.

There is no immediate need to ascertain the integrity of the cervical spine in the comatose patient. Normal X-rays cannot definitely exclude spinal cord injury because of SCIWORA, while the patient's inability to relate symptoms compromises the reliability of the physical exam. Thus, it is safest to presume that spinal cord injury may be present, maintain full spinal immobilization, and defer comprehensive evaluation of the cervical spine to a later time. SCIWORA can be evaluated with an MRI; findings include spinal cord transection or hemorrhage, or ligamentous or disc injury.

When a cervical spine injury is diagnosed clinically or radiographically, immediately call the appropriate surgical specialist (neurosurgeon, orthopedist) to assist in further management (e.g. application of Gardner-Wells tongs). Admit any patient in whom cervical spine injury cannot be definitively ruled out in the ED.

Indications for admission

- Cervical spine fracture
- Focal neurologic deficit
- Inability to exclude cervical spine injury

Bibliography

Anderson RC, Scaife ER, Fenton SJ, et al: Cervical spine clearance after trauma in children. *J Neurosurg* 2006;**105** (5 Suppl):361–4.

Klimo P Jr, Ware ML, Gupta N, Brockmeyer D: Cervical spine trauma in the pediatric patient. *Neurosurg Clin N Am* 2007;**18**:599–620.

McCall T, Fassett D, Brockmeyer D: Cervical spine trauma in children: a review. *Neurosurg Focus* 2006;**20**:e5.

Hand injuries

The injured hand requires a thorough evaluation, as improper management may lead to permanent disability. A systematic approach is essential to avoid overlooking subtle injuries.

Clinical presentation

Lacerations

Hand lacerations may affect the skin only or may be deep and involve underlying structures. Active extension of a digit is possible despite partial laceration of the extensor tendon. A dorsal hand laceration associated with pain on extension of the digit against resistance suggests a partial tendon injury.

Bites

Bites (pp. 724–726) are actually lacerations combined with crush injuries. Suspect that an irregular laceration over the metacarpophalangeal (MCP) joint is a human bite sustained by punching another person in the mouth. This is a serious injury, as oral flora can be inoculated into the MCP joint.

Fractures and dislocations

Phalangeal fractures

These fractures are common but not serious unless they are malrotated or the joint, volar plate, or collateral ligament is affected.

Wrist fractures

Wrist fractures are less common in children than in adults. The most commonly fractured carpal bone is the scaphoid. Key findings include tenderness on deep palpation in the anatomic snuff box area (between the extensor pollicus longus, extensor pollicus brevis, the prominent edge of the base of the first metacarpal and the styloid process of the radius); pain with longitudinal pressure placed on thumb; pain on pronation followed by ulnar deviation of the wrist; pain in the snuff box with resisted pronation or supination (ask the patient to "shake hands" with you while resisting your efforts to twist the wrist).

Metacarpophalangeal (MCP) joint dislocations

MCP dislocations are rare. They usually involve the thumb and index and fifth fingers. Most of these dislocations can only be detected on lateral radiographs.

Proximal and distal interphalangeal (PIP and DIP) joint dislocations

PIP and DIP joint dislocations present with obvious deformity, unless already reduced at the scene by the patient or an onlooker.

Tendon injuries

Gamekeeper's (skier's) thumb

Gamekeeper's thumb is caused by acute radial deviation of the thumb at the MCP joint that tears the ulnar collateral ligament. Typically the injury occurs when a patient falls with the thumb abducted. On examination, there is tenderness along the ulnar aspect of the first

MCP joint, associated with >15 degrees of joint laxity on passive radial abduction (performed under local anesthesia) when compared to the unaffected thumb.

Mallet (baseball) finger

A mallet finger results from a direct blow to the tip of an extended digit, rupturing the DIP extensor tendon or avulsing it from the base of the distal phalanx (a Salter I, II, III, or IV fracture). The finger is flexed at the DIP joint. Radiographs, which must contain a view of the PIP joint, may reveal an avulsed bone chip remaining attached to the extensor tendon.

Boutonnière (buttonhole) deformity

A boutonnière deformity follows violent flexion of the PIP joint. It presents with PIP flexion and DIP hyperextension. The lateral bands of the intrinsic muscles are pulled volar to the PIP axis, such that the lateral bands become PIP flexors while hyperextending the DIP. As a result, the PIP "buttonholes" through the torn extensor hood.

Nailbed injuries

Blunt trauma to the nail can cause a subungual hematoma, bleeding between the nail and the nailbed. A very tender nail with blue-black subungual discoloration is seen.

Infections

Paronychia

A paronychia is an infection of the soft tissues around the fingernail. It usually begins as a hangnail and is more common in patients with a history of finger sucking or nail biting. There is exquisite tenderness to palpation of the nail as well as erythematous swelling along the nail margin. There may also be a purulent collection or discharge and/or an associated felon (see below).

Felon

A felon is a serious distal pulp space infection. Tense, tender, erythematous swelling of the volar surface of the distal phalanx is seen.

Purulent tenosynovitis

This infection of the flexor tendon sheath is a true surgical emergency. There is usually a history of penetrating trauma. Kanavel's four cardinal signs of tenosynovitis are (1) symmetric swelling, (2) slight flexion of the finger, (3) tenderness over the flexor tendon sheath, and (4) increased pain on passive finger extension. Tenosynovitis may progress to a palmer space infection.

Palmar space infection

A palmar space infection presents with tense, tender, erythematous swelling of the palmar surface with pain and decreased mobility of the third and fourth fingers (midpalmar space) or thumb (thenar space). In certain circumstances, the dorsum of the hand may be more swollen than the palmar surface. These infections can spread to the flexor tendon sheaths. Associated signs may include fever, lymphangitis, and lymphadenitis.

Ganglion

A ganglion is a benign, well-defined, smooth, cystic lesion of synovial origin. It is fixed to the deep tissues, typically tendon sheaths, or, less commonly, herniated joint lining. Usually less than 3 cm in diameter, it is most often found on the volar or dorsal surface of the wrist or on the palmar surface at the base of a digit.

Traumatic amputations

Most traumatic amputations involve the distal fingertip only. Loss of the entire nail bed results in a more significant injury. However, children have remarkable regenerative ability, so consider reimplantation of virtually any amputated part.

Diagnosis

The evaluation begins with a careful history, including hand dominance, tetanus immunization status, and description of any previous hand injuries. Inquire about the mechanism of injury, including the hand position at the time of injury, the time elapsed since injury, and whether the trauma occurred in a clean or dirty environment.

Expose and inspect the entire upper extremity. Note any discrepancy between active and passive mobility of upper-extremity joints. Inspect the hand and evaluate the vascular status. Look for an alteration in the usual resting cascade of the digits, suggestive of a tendon or nerve injury. Check the color and temperature of the injured digit, and assess capillary refill.

Before anesthetizing the hand in preparation for a surgical procedure, assess sensory function by evaluating two-point discrimination with two points of a paper clip. Apply both points to the radial side of each digit. Then move the points closer together until the patient can no longer distinguish between them. Use an uninjured digit as a control. Repeat the exam on the ulnar side. Then, evaluate the median (volar index fingertip), radial (dorsal web space between the thumb and index finger), and ulnar (volar fifth fingertip) sensory nerves. The "immersion test" can substitute when an adequate two-point discrimination test cannot be obtained. Failure of the skin to wrinkle after 5–10 minutes in water suggests sensory nerve injury.

Motor (nerve, muscle, and tendon) function must be evaluated in a systematic manner. First, test the extrinsic flexors: the IP joint of the thumb (flexor pollicis longus), the DIP joints of the fingers while the PIP joints are held in extension (flexor digitorum profundus), and then the PIP joints of each finger while the other fingers are held completely extended (flexor digitorum superficialis). Next, have the patient flex the wrist against resistance, and palpate the three tendons (flexor carpi ulnaris, palmaris longus, and flexor carpi radialis, from medial to lateral) at the base of the wrist. The palmaris longus is best seen by flexing the wrist against resistance with the thumb and fifth finger opposed; however, it is absent in approximately 15–20% of children.

Evaluate the thenar muscles and median motor function by opposing the pulp of the thumb with that of the other four fingers. Test thumb adduction (adductor pollicis) and ulnar nerve function by having the patient grasp a piece of paper between the thumb and radial surface of the proximal index finger. Weakness is indicated by Froment's paper sign, contraction of the flexor pollicis longus with flexion of the IP thumb joint. To check the hypothenar muscles, ask the patient to abduct the small finger. Evaluate the interosseus muscles (ulnar nerve) by having the patient spread the fingers apart. Test the lumbricals (median and ulnar nerves) by asking the patient to flex the digits at the MCP joints while keeping the PIP and DIP joints extended. Assess motor function of the radial nerve by having the patient extend the wrist against resistance.

ED management

Manage profuse bleeding with elevation and pressure. Never use clamps for hemostasis, as the nerves traveling with the blood vessels can be damaged.

Palpate for localized bony tenderness or soft-tissue swelling, and examine for obvious deformities, ecchymoses, and functional deficits. Obtain X-rays if any of these findings are present over the wrist or hand. Radiographs of the fingers are indicated for gross deformities, lacerations in association with crush injuries, or loss of IP joint mobility.

Instill local anesthesia for surgical procedures only after a satisfactory sensory examination has been completed. If a digital block is required, allow the skin to dry after preparing it with povidone iodine. Use a 25- or 27-gauge needle to inject 2–4 mL of 2% lidocaine without epinephrine into both medial and lateral sides of the digit at the level of the metacarpal head. The maximum allowable dose of lidocaine is 4–5 mg/kg (without epinephrine). Before administration, be sure to inquire about personal or family history of previous reactions to local anesthetics.

Lacerations and bites

Carefully debride and irrigate these wounds after administration of local anesthesia (see pp. 691–693). Close with 5–0 or 6–0 nylon, using simple sutures that are left in place for 7 days. Avoid the use of deep sutures due to the risk of infection. A drain may be needed if the laceration is large. Carefully evaluate human bite wounds adjacent to MCP joints for evidence that the joint capsule has been violated. Open irrigation in the operating room is necessary if the wound has penetrated the capsule.

All deep lacerations and bite injuries of the hand require prophylactic antibiotics for 7 days. Treat human and animal bite wounds with an IV dose of ampicillin/sulbactam (45 mg/kg). Follow this with amoxicillin/clavulanate alone (875/125 formulation, 45 mg/kg per day of amoxicillin div bid). Alternatively, give penicillin VK (50 mg/kg per day div qid) plus 40 mg/kg per day of either cephalexin (div qid) or cefadroxil (div bid) for 5 days. For other deep or potentially contaminated lacerations, discharge the patient with cephalexin or cefadroxil, as above. Administer tetanus toxoid to all tetanus-prone wounds as well as tetanus immune globulin if the patient's tetanus immunization status is incomplete or is unknown.

Fractures and dislocations

Refer patients with fractures (except distal tuft), MCP dislocations, or non-radiographic suspicion of a scaphoid fracture to an appropriate surgical specialist (orthopedic, plastic, or hand surgeon). Treat distal tuft phalangeal fractures with a hairpin splint or bulky dressing.

A PIP dislocation can be reduced with traction and splinted after X-rays rule out an associated avulsion fracture. To reduce a dorsal (most common) PIP joint dislocation, first anesthetize the finger with a digital block. Hold the finger proximal to the injury, then use a distracting force to hyperextend at the PIP joint to bring it back to its normal anatomic position. If successful, repeat the examination of active and passive range of motion and immobilize the joint for 3 weeks. If abnormal, or reduction was unsuccessful, consult with a hand specialist. A dorsal DIP joint dislocation can also be reduced using distracting force at the involved joint.

Tendon injuries

Refer a patient with a gamekeeper's thumb or boutonnière deformity to an appropriate surgical specialist. Treat a mallet finger with a short dorsal splint, ensuring mild DIP joint hyperextension with free PIP joint mobility, for 6–8 weeks. A paper clip or tongue blade wrapped in tape can serve as a temporary splint for a mallet finger.

Nail bed injuries

To drain a subungual hematoma, first soak the digit in warm water for 20 minutes. Then, "screw" through the nail with an 18-gauge needle. After several holes are made, soak the digit in warm water to permit blood to escape. Remove the nail only if there is disruption of the nail or nail margin. Repair lacerations of the nailbed with 6.0 absorbable sutures to prevent abnormal growth of the new nail. If the nail is present, suture or glue (Dermabond®, LiquiBand®) it in place to act as a dressing and splint. With crush injuries, however, it may be necessary to remove the nail in order to identify and repair occult lacerations to the nailbed. If the nail cannot be used as a splint, insert petrolatum gauze into the eponychial fold until the wound heals and the nail begins to grow.

Infections

Treat a paronychia without fluctuance with warm soaks q 2–3 h, elevation, and 40 mg/kg per day of cephalexin (div qid), cefadroxil (div bid), or if MRSA is a concern, clindamycin (div q 6 h), for 3–5 days. If fluctuance is present, soak the digit, then lift the edge of the eponychial fold with a No. 15 scalpel blade in order to remove pus from the eponychium. If is not clear whether all of the pus was removed, place a wick under the eponychium. Warm soaks and elevation are also necessary. If pus extends under the nail, partial nail removal is indicated.

Refer a patient with a felon to an appropriate surgical specialist (orthopedic, plastic, or hand surgeon) for immediate drainage. Admit patients with purulent tenosynovitis (culture for gonococcus) and palmar space infections for IV ampicillin/sulbactam (200 mg/kg div qid) or, if allergic to beta-lactams, IV clindamycin (40 mg/kg per day div q 6 h). Immediately consult with an appropriate surgical specialist.

Ganglion

Elective surgical removal is indicated if the lesion is painful or very disfiguring.

Traumatic amputations

Rinse the amputated part gently in saline, wrap it in saline-soaked (but not dripping) gauze, and place it in a sealed plastic bag immersed in ice (do not allow direct contact with the ice). Distal fingertip amputations may require wrapping in petrolatum gauze. For more serious injuries, obtain a CBC and type and cross-match, start an IV line with maintenance fluids, treat pain with morphine sulfate (0.1–0.15 mg/kg IV or IM), and give IV ampicillin/sulbactam (200 mg/kg of ampicillin div qid). Gently cleanse the wound and cover it with petrolatum gauze or saline-soaked gauze until the patient can be taken to the operating room. Obtain an X-ray if there is suspicion of a crush injury to the distal phalanx.

Follow-up

- Bite wound or laceration being treated with prophylactic antibiotics: 2–3 days
- Drained subungual hematoma: 2 days
- Paronychia with wick in eponychial fold: 1–2 days; without wick: 3–5 days

Indications for admission

- Felon, purulent tenosynovitis, or palmar space infection
- Any fracture requiring open reduction in the operating room
- Intraarticular fracture (>25% articular surface) or MCP dislocation
- Amputations other than distal fingertip
- Extensor tendon laceration that requires operative repair
- Flexor tendon laceration

Bibliography

Elhassan BT, Shin AY: Scaphoid fracture in children. *Hand Clin* 2006;22:31–41.

Kozin SH: Fractures and dislocations along the pediatric thumb ray. *Hand Clin* 2006;22:19–29.

Lindley SG, Rulewicz G: Hand fractures and dislocations in the developing skeleton. *Hand Clin* 2006;22:253–68.

Multiple trauma

Trauma is the leading cause of death in children 1–14 years of age, exceeding all other causes combined; each year, over 10 000 children die from serious injury. Blunt injuries are most common at all ages, although the incidence of penetrating trauma increases in adolescence. The main factors contributing to early morbidity and mortality are upper-airway compromise and respiratory failure or arrest due to central neuraxis injury (brain and cervical spinal cord). Intracranial and intraabdominal hemorrhages are less common. Late deaths are caused chiefly by traumatic brain injury. Posttraumatic pulmonary insufficiency, respiratory distress syndrome, or "shock lung," and multiple organ system failure are not common.

Children are subject to unique mechanisms of injury that interact with their immature anatomic features and physiologic responses to produce distinct patterns of trauma. Children are struck by cars or fall from heights while playing, are propelled into the windshields or ejected through the windows of moving vehicles in which they ride as unrestrained passengers, and fall while bicycle riding, in-line skating, scooter riding, or skateboarding. Because the head is proportionately larger and heavier in the child than in the adult, it bears the brunt of the forces of injury, even if other body regions are involved. Thus, serious head injury is more common in multiple blunt trauma in childhood, while internal organ injury is less common. It is estimated that at least 80% of multiple injury cases involve the head.

As a result, pediatric trauma is far more often a disorder of airway and breathing than of bleeding and shock. Apnea, hypoventilation, and hypoxia occur five times more often than hypovolemia with hypotension in the seriously injured child. The mortality associated with neuroventilatory derangements (concomitant abnormalities in mental status and respiratory function) approaches 25%. Hypotensive (decompensated) shock is present in <10% of all cases of major pediatric trauma, but mortality in those cases exceeds 50%. Eight percent of all injuries in children involve the chest, and over two-thirds of children with chest injuries have multiple injuries.

Initial management of the injured child must be expeditious, in accordance with consensus protocols with which all participants in the resuscitative effort must be thoroughly familiar. This is best accomplished through the use of an aggressive team approach, with one member serving as team leader who takes responsibility for directing and coordinating the resuscitative effort. Although trauma resuscitation may be initiated in the ED, major trauma is a surgical illness that requires the immediate participation of experienced surgeons. The most common cause of preventable trauma death in children is inadequate initial resuscitation. Other preventable deaths are due to missed internal injuries, both intracranial and intraabdominal. Surgical interventions are ultimately required in more than 50% of major pediatric trauma victims, despite the greater reliance on nonoperative management in children than adults.

Clinical presentation

The presentation usually depends on the extent of central neuraxis injury, respiratory compromise, and blood loss. Head injuries are the most common anatomic findings, followed by axial skeletal injuries; internal organ injuries are least common. Abnormalities in level of consciousness and respiratory status are the most common physiologic findings. While hypotensive shock is uncommon in the pediatric trauma victim, particularly after blunt injury, a child may be in early shock with little or no external evidence (see Shock, pp. 26–27), leading to what may be called the "deceptive" presentation of shock in the child.

Diagnosis and ED management
Primary survey

The first priority is the primary survey, a rapid initial assessment that combines rapid cardiopulmonary assessment (the foundation of pediatric advanced life support) with rapid cranial-truncal examination, to identify life-threatening problems that require immediate intervention (Table 26-2). Note the patient's general condition, and take the following actions (A, B, C, D, E):

1. Assess the *Airway* for patency and maintainability. Confirm spontaneous air movement and listen for gurgling or stridor while protecting the cervical spine from flexion and extension. If needed, use a jaw-thrust maneuver with in-line spinal immobilization to open the airway. Placing a 2-cm-thick layer of padding under the infant's or toddler's torso will preserve this alignment.

2. Check the adequacy of *Breathing* by simultaneously watching chest excursions, listening for breath sounds, and evaluating respiratory effort and rate. Palpate the trachea and ribs, and search for other signs of immediately life-threatening chest injuries.

3. Evaluate the *Circulation* for signs of shock by obtaining the pulse (tachycardia is the earliest measurable response to hypovolemia). In addition, examine the skin for pallor, cyanosis, mottling, and moisture. Check for the presence of active

Table 26-2. Management options for life-threatening conditions

Finding	Problem	Management
Noisy breathing, stridor	Upper-airway obstruction	Jaw thrust/C-spine control, intubation
Difficulty breathing	Respiratory failure	Bag-valve-mask ventilation, intubation
Unconsciousness	Severe traumatic brain injury	Intubation, mild hyperventilation
External bleeding	External wound	Direct pressure
Neck pain, spasm, tenderness; head injury	Possible C-spine fracture	Immobilize neck (semirigid extrication collar, tape, and head immobilizer)
Asymmetric breath sounds and hyperresonant percussion note	Possible tension pneumothorax	Insert over-the-needle plastic catheter (2nd ICS in MCL) or chest tube
Asymmetric breath sounds and dull percussion note	Possible massive hemothorax	Chest X-ray Insert chest tube through separate incision in midaxillary line at level of nipple
Penetrating chest wound with difficulty breathing	Possible sucking chest wound	Apply occlusive dressing. Insert chest tube through separate incision in mid-axillary line at level of nipple
Penetrating chest wound with muffled heart sounds or distended neck veins	Possible pericardial tamponade	Pericardiocentesis (subxiphoid or 4th ICS 1 cm lateral to left sternal border)
Paradoxical chest wall movement	Flail chest	Positive-pressure ventilation for respiratory failure
Orthostasis (pale, cool skin)	Compensated shock	Establish two large-bore IVs. Give up to two 20 mL/kg boluses
Hypotension	Decompensated shock	Transfusion: Emergency: type O (Rh-neg for ♀) Urgent: type-specific
	Transient response to volume resuscitation	
Upper abdominal distension, hyperresonant percussion note	Gastric dilatation	Insert nasogastric tube (use orogastric tube if major orofacial trauma or an infant)

bleeding and delayed capillary refill (>2 seconds). Obtain a core temperature to assess for hypothermia.

4. Estimate the degree of *Disability* by noting the response to verbal and painful stimuli using the "AVPU" score (A = alert, V = responsive to verbal stimuli, P = responsive only to painful stimuli, U = unresponsive). Record pupillary size and reaction to light.
5. Fully *Expose* the patient, taking quick note of all external signs of injury (especially in penetrating trauma) before covering him or her to prevent heat loss.

6. Resuscitation. Trauma resuscitation is conducted concurrently with the primary survey. If life-threatening problems are identified, the team leader must immediately begin treatment, summon surgical assistance, and organize a sequence of therapy, corresponding to the alphabetical order listed below.

A: airway/cervical spine

As described in the section on cardiopulmonary resuscitation (pp. 1–28), establish and maintain a patent airway. Noisy or stridulous breathing suggests airway obstruction, most often due to the tongue falling against the posterior pharyngeal wall. Perform a modified jaw thrust and combine with bimanual in-line stabilization of the cervical spine in a neutral position (as described above). Keep the plane of the midface parallel to the spine board in a neutral position. If the child is A (alert) or V (responsive to verbal stimuli) and is breathing spontaneously, administer humidified 100% oxygen. Use a nonrebreathing mask with a flow rate high enough to keep the nonrebreathing bag inflated throughout the respiratory cycle. If the child is P (responsive only to painful stimuli) or U (unresponsive), insert an oropharyngeal airway and ventilate with humidified 100% oxygen via a bag-valve-mask device. If these measures are unsuccessful in effectively maintaining or immediately restoring spontaneous ventilation and oxygenation, or if the child is comatose as determined by a GCS ≤8, perform orotracheal intubation while continuing to apply bimanual in-line stabilization to the head and neck.

If severe orofacial injuries prevent orotracheal intubation and bag-valve-mask ventilation is unsuccessful, perform needle cricothyroidotomy by inserting a large-bore (16- to 18-gauge) over-the-needle catheter through the cricoid membrane (located between the thyroid cartilage and the cricoid ring). Then attach oxygen tubing containing a side hole or a Y-connector to the hub of the catheter, and insufflate oxygen by intermittently occluding (1 second) and releasing (4 seconds) the open end of the side hole or Y-connector, thereby avoiding chest overexpansion. Alternatively attach the Luer-lock tip of a 3.0 mL syringe from which the plunger has been removed to the hub of the catheter. Administer oxygen by ventilating with a bag-valve device through a no. 7.5 endotracheal tube adaptor inserted into the open end of the barrel of the syringe.

Severe multiple trauma, significant head or neck trauma, neck pain and tenderness, cervical muscle spasm, or a history of a sudden deceleration suggests the possibility of cervical spine and spinal cord injury. Immobilize the neck once the airway has been secured with a semirigid cervical extrication collar and a head immobilizer (soft collar or sandbags or large IV bags and tape are inadequate) until AP, lateral, and open-mouth radiographic views of the cervical spine and a careful neurologic examination rule out an injury (see cervical spine injuries, pp. 702–704). Note that a lateral cervical spine X-ray, by itself, is insufficient to rule out cervical spine injury, due to possible SCIWORA. Therefore, it is neither necessary nor indicated as part of the initial management of the multiply injured child. Despite the importance of early cervical spine control, however, do not sacrifice the airway by efforts to maintain neck immobilization; never delay intubation because a radiologist or neurosurgeon has not reviewed the radiographs and confirmed that the film shows no fracture.

B: breathing/chest injuries

Administer humidified 100% oxygen to all victims of major trauma without waiting for ABG results. Immediately intubate a patient who is unconscious, has decreased breath sounds, or has persistent evidence of respiratory failure after opening the airway.

The mobility of mediastinal structures makes a child more prone to a tension pneumothorax. Look for contralateral tracheal deviation, a hyper-resonant percussion note, subcutaneous emphysema, distended neck veins, and continued respiratory distress after intubation (see pneumothorax, pp. 720–721). If they are found, immediately decompress by inserting a large-bore (16- to 18-gauge) over-the-needle catheter into the second intercostal space, above the third rib, in the midclavicular line on the affected side, without waiting for X-ray confirmation.

Asymmetric breath sounds associated with a hyperresonant percussion note and subcutaneous emphysema but without tracheal deviation or distended neck veins suggest a simple pneumothorax. Asymmetric breath sounds associated with a dull percussion note suggest a simple hemothorax. Tube thoracostomy is indicated for both, after the airway, breathing, and circulation have been adequately addressed.

Hypotension after a penetrating chest wound suggests the possibility of pericardial tamponade. Tachycardia is the most common finding. Muffled heart sounds, distended neck veins, and pulsus paradoxus are variable. Emergency thoracotomy is required, but pericardiocentesis (see pericardial tamponade, pp. 719–720) is indicated if emergency thoracotomy is not initiated in the ED.

Also examine the patient for rib fractures, subcutaneous emphysema, and signs of penetrating chest trauma. A flail chest, though rare in children, can cause paradoxical chest wall movement after blunt chest trauma. Positive-pressure ventilation is required if large flail segments are impairing ventilation. Small flail segments are associated with enough muscle spasm that they rarely impair ventilation. They require supportive treatment only, primarily for the underlying pulmonary contusion that is invariably present. Once the patient is stable, give analgesics as necessary.

Penetrating chest trauma can cause an open pneumothorax (sucking chest wound). Cover penetrating chest wounds completely with petrolatum gauze, and perform tube thoracostomy to prevent the subsequent development of tension pneumothorax.

After securing the airway, obtain a chest radiograph if any of the above abnormalities are found on examination of the chest (except tension pneumothorax, which must be treated immediately). Review the film carefully for intrapleural air (simple or tension pneumothorax), intrapleural fluid (hemothorax), rib fractures, lung densities (pulmonary contusion), mediastinal emphysema, and widened mediastinum and loss of aortic contour (traumatic dissection of the aorta). Do not rely on normal chest radiographs when there is a suspicion of traumatic dissection of the aorta; obtain a CT of the chest.

Obtain an ECG to assess for the possibility of cardiac contusion, although no single finding is pathognomonic. Nonspecific changes, including sinus tachycardia, are present in up to 80% of the ECGs obtained in patients with suspected blunt cardiac injury. Assume that a child has a possible cardiac contusion and consult with a pediatric cardiologist if there are ECG changes such as relative tachycardia, relative bradycardia, conduction delays, or atrial or ventricular dysrhythmias.

C: circulation/bleeding and shock

Cardiopulmonary arrest in a pediatric trauma victim may be an indication for emergency thoracotomy with pericardiotomy in the ED for relief of pericardial tamponade, cross-clamping of the descending aorta, or both, if personnel experienced in these techniques are available. ED thoracotomy is not indicated for victims of blunt trauma but is occasionally successful in victims of penetrating trauma, particularly those who have pericardial tamponade or develop profound hypotension during the course of the resuscitative effort. ED thoracotomy is also indicated for victims of penetrating trauma who have lost pulses en route to the hospital. A patient with penetrating parasternal chest wounds or pericardial tamponade who is not in hypotensive shock should immediately be transported to the operating room for urgent thoracotomy. Summon the surgical team immediately upon the arrival of any such patient, and notify the operating room that the need for surgery may be imminent.

Control external bleeding with direct digital or manual pressure, pressure dressings, or pneumatic splints, but do not use tourniquets or clamps. Secure two large-bore (16- to 18-gauge) peripheral IV lines using over-the-needle catheters. Substitute a tibial intraosseous line, provided the extremity is uninjured, if two attempts at IV access have failed or if venous access is impossible secondary to circulatory collapse. The distal femur (3 cm above the external condyle) can be used if the tibia is fractured. Give 20 mL/kg of warmed isotonic crystalloid (normal saline or Ringer's lactate) as a rapid IV bolus after obtaining blood for type and cross-match and a CBC. Monitor the blood pressure carefully, and repeat the bolus every 5–10 minutes, as needed. If 40 mL/kg does not raise the blood pressure, give another 20 mL/kg bolus and prepare for a transfusion of 10 mL/kg of packed red blood cells. In an emergency, when there is evidence of hypotensive shock, use type O blood, which is available immediately: O positive for males, O negative for females; transfusion reactions are extremely rare. Type-specific blood that is not cross-matched can be available in 10 minutes; it can be used in urgent but not emergency circumstances.

Base ongoing volume resuscitation on the response to the initial fluid challenge. Remember that fewer than 10% of children present in hypotensive shock after major trauma. Also, for most seriously injured children, excessive fluid administration is as detrimental as inadequate fluid administration because of the potential for further increases in the elevated intracranial pressures associated with traumatic brain injury, the most common internal organ injury sustained from pediatric blunt trauma. However, cerebral hypoxia due to inadequate cerebral perfusion is the most common cause of secondary brain injury, and it dramatically worsens cerebral swelling. Thus, never restrict fluid until hemodynamic stability has been completely restored.

Attempt to identify sources of potential or ongoing blood loss. Following a careful physical exam, obtain a chest X-ray to rule out hemothorax and obtain a pelvic X-ray, since a pelvic fracture is a common cause of retroperitoneal hemorrhage. Obtain urine for urinalysis. Hematuria (>50 cells/hpf) may indicate urinary tract injury (see genitourinary trauma, pp. 284–287) or injury to other intraabdominal organs, as 80% of blunt renal injuries are associated with damage to adjacent organs. Although isolated hematuria is rarely a life-threatening problem, expeditious imaging of the urinary tract is indicated.

If the patient remains in shock or has a falling hematocrit, reassess for occult blood loss in the pleural cavities, abdomen, retroperitoneum, and pelvis, repeat diagnostic tests, if indicated, and transport the patient to the operating room.

Diagnostic peritoneal lavage is not routinely employed for injured children with suspected intraabdominal bleeding to determine the need for urgent laparotomy. Conservative, nonoperative management of solid organ (liver, spleen, kidney) injury is standard, so a positive result (>100 RBC/mm^3) does not constitute an automatic indication for surgery. Abdominal CT with IV contrast enhancement is the diagnostic procedure of choice for identifying injuries and bleeding sites in a hemodynamically stable patient. For an unstable patient, use a focused abdominal sonography for trauma (FAST). It is noninvasive and does not interfere with resuscitation. It is accurate for the identification of free abdominal fluid as well as pericardial fluid. Reserve abdominal paracentesis for a patient with unstable vital signs in whom the source of the bleeding is unknown or the abdominal sonogram is suboptimal, and/or the child with stable vital signs who is going immediately to the operating room for treatment of intracranial or musculoskeletal injuries. If necessary, the paracentesis can be performed in the operating room.

D: disability (neurologic)

Once vital signs have been stabilized, direct resuscitative efforts toward the diagnosis and treatment of central neuraxis injuries (see cervical spine injuries, pp. 702–704). Priorities in the neurologic evaluation are accurate determination of the level of consciousness, pupillary size and reactivity, eye movements, and motor, sensory, and reflex responses. Asymmetry in pupillary size and reactivity or in motor, sensory, or reflex responses suggests the possibility of serious intracranial or spinal cord injury.

Request neurosurgical assistance and arrange for an immediate CT scan of the head for any patient with a history of prolonged unconsciousness (>5 minutes) or a seizure occurring >3 seconds after impact, GCS ≤14, focal neurologic signs, or symptoms of increased intracranial pressure, such as nausea, vomiting, or persistent headache or dizziness. Monitor the patient fully (ECG, vital signs, pulse oximetry) throughout the study, and ensure that someone (emergency physician, trauma surgeon, physician-anesthesiologist, nurse-anesthetist) capable of emergency management of the pediatric airway is present. The leading cause of the increased intracranial pressure commonly observed after pediatric closed head injury is not intracranial hematoma, as in adults, but cerebral swelling due to the secondary brain injury that is caused by cerebral hypoxia. For this reason, and because the outcome of traumatic brain injury in children is far better than it is in adults, children with traumatic brain injury who present in coma require aggressive resuscitative efforts.

A number of factors contribute to the development of cerebral hypoxia in the child with severe closed head injury. Normal cerebral blood flow increases to nearly twice that of adult levels by the age of 5, and then decreases. Unconsciousness produces hypotonia in the muscles supporting the soft tissues of the larynx and oropharynx, resulting in passive closure of the upper airway. Both primary brain injury (direct trauma) and secondary brain injury (cerebral hypoxia) can cause temporary paralysis of cerebrovascular autoregulation, resulting in cerebral vasodilatation and cerebral hyperemia, leading to progressive increases in intracranial pressure. These, in turn, decrease cerebral perfusion pressure and disrupt medullary control of breathing, thereby worsening cerebral hypoxia and leading to further increases in intracranial pressure.

Immediate intubation and mild hyperventilation, if instituted promptly, may interrupt this vicious cycle, which otherwise leads to uncal herniation and brain death. Intubation reopens the airway, permitting oxygen to reach the circulation and facilitating hyperventilation. Hyperventilation induces alkalosis, normalizing cerebral blood flow and allowing blood to perfuse the brain. Immediately intubate any child who presents with a GCS ≤8 and initiate mild hyperventilation with tidal volumes of 10 mL/kg, at a rate that lowers the pCO_2 to approximately 35 mmHg. Mild hyperventilation is preferred, due to the potential risk of cerebral ischemia associated with aggressive hyperventilation.

Rapid-sequence intubation is indicated for the head-injured child who presents in coma, and it must be performed only by personnel experienced in emergency intubation of the pediatric patient and familiar with the use of neuromuscular blockers. It is technically more difficult in the trauma patient whose neck must remain in a neutral position throughout the procedure because of the possibility of spinal cord injury. A number of therapeutic regimens are in common use (see Airway management, pp. 5–6).

Treat ongoing seizures with lorazepam (0.05–0.1 mg/kg) or diazepam (0.1–0.3 mg/kg) slowly over 2 minutes, followed by fosphenytoin (20 phenytoin equivalents [PE]/kg, IV over 10–15 min) or phenytoin (20 mg/kg, IV at a rate of 1 mg/kg per min). If cervical or thoracic spinal cord injuries are suspected within 8 hours of the trauma, treat any associated focal neurologic deficits with IV methylprednisolone (30 mg/kg per 15 min loading dose, followed 45 min later by a 5.4 mg/kg per hr constant infusion for 23 hours). Corticosteroids have no established role in the acute management of head injuries. Avoid the use of diuretic agents such as IV mannitol (0.5–1 g/kg) or furosemide (1 mg/kg) unless there is evidence of uncal herniation (unilateral dilated pupil or other lateralizing signs). Carefully document key neurologic findings before rapid-sequence intubation or other treatments that alter neurologic status, but never delay treatment of life-threatening neurotrauma while awaiting arrival of neurologic or neurosurgical consultants.

E: expose (examine)

Expose the patient completely, and perform a rapid but thorough physical exam (including the back, buttocks, and all skin creases), looking for associated injuries. Palpate all bones, including the pelvic and facial bones, and palpate and percuss the teeth. Check the extraocular movements and corneal clarity, and recheck pupillary reactivity and symmetry. Look for signs of depressed (scalp hematoma or laceration with underlying deformity or crepitance) and basilar (hemotympanum, clear rhino- or otorrhea, infraorbital and retro-auricular ecchymoses) skull fractures. Once the exam is completed, cover the patient with a blanket to prevent hypothermia. The diagnosis and management of other traumas is detailed elsewhere: ocular (pp. 535–541), dental (pp. 277–80), orthopedic, genitourinary, and soft tissue (pp. 738–744).

F: Foley catheter

Insert a catheter into the bladder to monitor the urine output closely in all multiple-trauma patients. The sole exception is a patient with suspected urethral disruption, suggested by blood at the urethral meatus, and males with scrotal hematoma or a "high-riding" or "boggy" prostate. These injuries are usually associated with a pelvic fracture, straddle injury, or penetrating wound. Call a urologist immediately to obtain a retrograde urethrogram; urine output can be monitored with a suprapubic catheter if needed. The desired urine output is at least 2 mL/kg per hr in an infant, 1 mL/kg per hr in a child, and 0.5 mL/kg per hr in an adolescent. Gross or significant microscopic (>50 RBC/hpf) hematuria requires radiologic evaluation to rule out renal injury.

G: gastric decompression

Insert a nasogastric tube and attach to intermittent (Levin tube) or continuous (sump tube) suction to prevent aspiration and improve ventilation by reducing gastric dilatation. Use an orogastric tube instead if there is evidence of significant orofacial trauma.

Secondary survey

Once the primary survey has been completed and the resuscitation phase is under way, proceed with the secondary survey: a careful, complete head-to-toe examination of the trauma patient to determine the full extent of tissue injury. If life-threatening problems are not identified during the primary survey, but the mechanism of injury indicates that the patient is potentially at risk for life-threatening problems, secure a large-bore IV, obtain frequent vital signs, arrange for initial blood and X-ray studies, order a urinalysis as a screen for occult intraabdominal injury, and admit for observation.

Obtain a CBC, ABG, and type and cross-match for any patient admitted for observation to a critical care unit. In addition, obtain serum lipase (looking for pancreatic injury) and hepatic transaminases for a patient admitted for evaluation of abdominal trauma. CPK and urine myoglobin are indicated for the child with suspected crush injury, as well as electrolytes, BUN, and creatinine. The last three, as well as serum glucose, are useful as baseline studies in children with severe traumatic brain injury.

Most multiple-trauma victims require X-rays of the chest and pelvis. A lateral cervical spine X-ray is also commonly obtained, although, as discussed previously, it cannot reliably rule out spinal cord injury. Therefore, maintain full spinal immobilization of any patient in whom spinal cord injury has not been or cannot be properly ruled out. If the vital signs are stable but intraabdominal injury is suspected (based on physical signs of internal hemorrhage, such as abdominal tenderness, distention, bruising, or gross hematuria), prepare the patient for a CT scan of the abdomen with IV and oral contrast (to follow CT scan of the head when obtained). For oral contrast, the dose of Gastrografin for a child >10 years of age is 15 mL in 485 mL of water. Give 8–10 mL in 350 mL water to a patient 8–10 years old and 5 mL in 245 mL water to a child 1–5 years of age. Oral contrast is not helpful in children unless the full dose can be given (usually requires a nasogastric tube). If this is not possible, obtain the CT scan with IV contrast, only. Plain X-rays may then be ordered as necessary. Victims of minor trauma with stable vital signs who are awake, alert, and able to ambulate normally require X-rays only if indicated by historical and physical findings.

Indications for admission

- Serious head or neck injury
- Respiratory distress or compromise
- Hypotension or orthostatic vital sign changes
- Suspected intrathoracic or intraabdominal injury
- Serious fracture or soft-tissue injury
- Minor injuries caused by major trauma
- Gunshot or stab wound unless surgical evaluation determines it to be superficial

Bibliography

American College of Surgeons Committee on Trauma: *Advanced Trauma Life Support for Doctors*, 8th ed. Chicago: American College of Surgeons, 2008.

Avarello JT, Cantor RM: Pediatric major trauma: an approach to evaluation and management. *Emerg Med Clin North Am* 2007;25:803–36.

Bixby SD, Callahan MJ, Taylor GA: Imaging in pediatric blunt abdominal trauma. *Semin Roentgenol* 2008;43:72–82.

Eppich WJ, Zonfrillo MR: Emergency department evaluation and management of blunt abdominal trauma in children. *Curr Opin Pediatr* 2007;19:265–9.

Pericardial tamponade

Pericardial tamponade is a life-threatening emergency requiring immediate intervention. The most common cause is penetrating thoracic trauma, when blood accumulates in the pericardial sac and interferes with cardiac filling. Tamponade is rare after blunt thoracic trauma.

Clinical presentation

Suspect pericardial tamponade if there are failing vital signs or pulseless electrical activity after penetrating chest trauma, especially following a poor response to tube thoracostomy. Shock associated with tachypnea, clear lungs with equal breath sounds bilaterally, and neck vein distention (if the patient is not hypovolemic) suggest the diagnosis. The pulse pressure may be narrowed, and pulsus paradoxus (a >10 mmHg drop in the systolic blood pressure on inspiration) may be present but is not necessary to establish the diagnosis. Deterioration can lead to pulseless electrical activity and death.

Diagnosis

See pp. 710–718 for the approach to the multiple-trauma patient. The clinical presentation of pericardial tamponade may resemble that of other life-threatening chest injuries; often, they occur simultaneously. Distended neck veins and pulsus paradoxus can both be seen in a patient with nontraumatic disorders such as congestive heart failure. Pulsus paradoxus may also be noted in a patient with severe asthma (wheezing, poor air movement). Tachypnea and tachycardia are frequent in patients with pneumothorax or hemothorax.

In acute pericardial tamponade, the chest X-ray frequently reveals a normal heart or a waterbag cardiac shadow, but the pericardial effusion is usually evident on the FAST examination.

Insert a right atrial catheter or central venous pressure (CVP) line if the diagnosis is uncertain. The CVP is usually elevated (>15 cmH$_2$O), unless the patient is hypovolemic from other injuries. The ECG in pericardial tamponade may reveal low-voltage and non-specific ST–T-wave changes. Electrical alternans (alternating variations in the height of the QRS complex, due to shifts in the QRS axis from beat to beat as the heart swings to and fro in the pericardial sac) is diagnostic of a pericardial effusion. Also, generalized low voltage (R wave height <1 cm in all leads) may be observed.

ED management

Once the diagnosis is made, immediately consult a surgeon to perform a thoracotomy or pericardiotomy in the operating room. If an experienced surgeon is not available, pericardiocentesis is indicated. Monitor the patient's vital signs and ECG before, during, and after the procedure. Use a large-bore (16- to 18-gauge) over-the-needle catheter, attached by three-way stopcock to a 30 mL syringe and by alligator clip (placed just beyond the hub of the needle) to the chest lead (V$_1$) of an ECG machine. Puncture the skin inferior to the xiphoid process, directing the needle toward the tip of the left scapula, at a 45° angle to the skin. Free flow of nonclotted, nonpulsatile blood suggests that the pericardium has been entered. If the needle touches the epicardial surface, a "current of injury pattern" (ST segment elevation) will be seen on the ECG; withdraw the needle slightly. An improvement in vital signs may follow removal of as little as 10–20 mL of blood. After aspiration is complete, withdraw the needle but leave the catheter in with the stopcock closed in case fluid reaccumulates. A negative pericardiocentesis does not rule out tamponade, since blood in the pericardial sac clots rapidly.

Indications for admission

- Pericardial tamponade
- Pericardial effusion

Bibliography

Balci AE, Kazez A, Eren S, et al: Blunt thoracic trauma in children: review of 137 cases. *Eur J Cardiothorac Surg* 2004;26:387–92.

McGillicuddy D, Rosen P: Diagnostic dilemmas and current controversies in blunt chest trauma. *Emerg Med Clin North Am* 2007;25:695–711.

Sartorelli KH, Vane DW: The diagnosis and management of children with blunt injury of the chest. *Semin Pediatr Surg* 2004;13:98–105.

Westra SJ, Wallace EC: Imaging evaluation of pediatric chest trauma. *Radiol Clin North Am* 2005;43:267–81.

Pneumothorax

Pneumothorax can result from blunt or penetrating thoracic trauma. It can also occur in asthmatics, patients with cystic fibrosis, newborns (pneumothorax occurs most commonly among neonates), and in association with smoking "crack" cocaine or marijuana. Occasionally, a pneumothorax occurs without trauma in an otherwise healthy adolescent.

Clinical presentation

Pneumothorax presents with signs of respiratory distress, including tachypnea, nasal flaring, accessory muscle use, and anxiety or altered mental status. Breath sounds may be decreased or absent on the affected (ipsilateral) side. The percussion note can be tympanitic. Pulsus paradoxus (>10 mmHg drop in the systolic blood pressure on inspiration) may be noted.

Signs of a tension pneumothorax may include all of the above, along with deviation of the trachea away from the affected side and, if severe, may include cyanosis, jugular vein distention (if the patient is not hypovolemic), and deterioration of the vital signs, leading to pulseless electrical activity and death. Pneumomediastinum can occur with or without pneumothorax. Although a pneumomediastinum requires no immediate treatment, its presence suggests the possibility of barotrauma and an associated pneumothorax.

Diagnosis

See pp. 710–718 for the general approach to the patient with multiple trauma. Always be suspicious of the possibility of pneumothorax in a trauma victim. Air can leak from the lung, the tracheobronchial tree, the esophagus, or through a sucking wound in the chest wall. Trauma can produce pneumothorax directly in penetrating injury, or indirectly in blunt injury (by fracturing ribs). However, a pneumothorax can occur in the absence of either.

Table 26-3. Diagnosis of immediately life-threatening chest Injuries

Physical sign	Tension pneumothorax	Massive hemothorax	Cardiac tamponade
Breath sounds	Ipsilateral decrease	Ipsilateral decrease	Normal
Percussion note	Hyperresonant	Dull	Normal
Tracheal location	Contralateral shift	Midline	Midline
Neck veins	Distended	Flat	Distended

Tension pneumothorax may be confused with other immediately life-threatening chest injuries (Table 26-3). In massive hemothorax, breath sounds are decreased on the affected side, as in tension pneumothorax, but the percussion note is dull and the neck veins are flat. In pericardial tamponade, the neck veins may be distended (if the patient is not hypovolemic), but breath sounds are adequate, and ECG monitoring may reveal low voltage. In hypovolemic shock, vital signs will have deteriorated, but breath and heart sounds are usually equal on both sides and the neck veins are flat.

The diagnosis of tension pneumothorax is made on clinical grounds alone. Treat immediately if it is suspected, without waiting for a confirmatory chest X-ray. However, a chest X-ray is indicated to confirm the diagnosis of simple pneumothorax. A pleural effusion in the asthmatic with pneumonia can mimic hemopneumothorax.

ED management
Immediately give humidified 100% oxygen with a flow rate high enough to keep the nonrebreathing bag inflated throughout the respiratory cycle and secure a large-bore (16-to 18-gauge) IV line, unless the patient has severe respiratory distress.

Tension pneumothorax
Decompress immediately, without waiting for X-ray confirmation. Insert a large-bore over-the-needle plastic catheter into the chest above the top of the third rib, in the midclavicular line of the affected side. A rush of air and improvement in the patient's ventilatory status confirm both the diagnosis and the adequacy of the therapy. Remove the needle and leave the catheter in place. Then insert a chest tube in the fifth intercostal space above the sixth rib in the anterior to mid-axillary line, attach it to an underwater seal device once the tube has been properly secured, and remove the over-the-needle catheter used for decompression.

Simple pneumothorax
If the patient is alert, with an oxygen saturation >90% and stable vital signs, provide 100% oxygen via nonrebreather mask and consult with a pediatric surgeon regarding the possible placement of a chest tube. If the clinical condition deteriorates, immediately place a chest tube.

Indication for admission
- Any pneumothorax or hemothorax

Bibliography

Balci AE, Kazez A, Eren S, et al: Blunt thoracic trauma in children: review of 137 cases. *Eur J Cardiothorac Surg* 2004; 26:387–92.

McGillicuddy D, Rosen P: Diagnostic dilemmas and current controversies in blunt chest trauma. *Emerg Med Clin North Am* 2007;25:695–711.

Sartorelli KH, Vane DW: The diagnosis and management of children with blunt injury of the chest. *Semin Pediatr Surg* 2004;13:98–105.

Chapter 27

Wound care and minor trauma

Anthony J. Ciorciari

Abscesses

A cutaneous abscess is a localized collection of pus, usually secondary to disruption of skin integrity. The organisms most often involved are methicillin-sensitive (MSSA) and methicillin-resistant *Staphylococcus aureus* (MRSA) and group A *Streptococcus*.

Clinical presentation and diagnosis

An abscess presents as a discrete, well-circumscribed swelling with central fluctuance. It is tender and is usually associated with erythema and warmth of the overlying skin. Lymphangitis and lymphadenitis are complications that can herald hematogenous dissemination and sepsis.

Cellulitis presents with localized swelling, tenderness, erythema, and warmth, but there is no fluctuance.

ED management

The definitive treatment of an abscess is incision and drainage, which can usually be performed in the ED. However, when the abscess is in immediate proximity to neurovascular structures, first perform either a needle aspiration to confirm purulence or obtain an ultrasound to avoid incising a vascular aneurysm. This precaution specifically applies to abscesses in the neck, supraclavicular fossa, antecubital fossa, popliteal fossa, and inguinal and axillary areas.

Maintain strict aseptic technique to prevent the spread of the infection; prepare the skin with a povidone-iodine solution. Although total anesthesia may be difficult to achieve, use a combination of a regional field block (a ring of 1% lidocaine outside the perimeter of the abscess and erythema) and a linear injection of 1% lidocaine into the roof of the abscess along the planned incision line. The maximum dose of lidocaine is 4–5 mg/kg without epinephrine and 7 mg/kg with epinephrine. If this technique is unsuccessful, provide sedation and analgesia (pp. 682–691).

Make the incision along the natural dynamic skin tension lines to prevent excessive scarring. In view of the increasing incidence of MRSA, after the incision obtain a specimen for culture in case the patient subsequently requires antibiotic therapy. Explore the abscess cavity with a blunt instrument or sterile gloved finger to break up any loculated pockets of purulence. Copiously irrigate the cavity with NS under moderate pressure, pack it loosely with iodoform gauze to promote drainage and ensure hemostasis, and apply a sterile dressing.

Oral antibiotics are of no additional benefit after incision and drainage of uncomplicated abscesses <5 cm in otherwise healthy children; antibiotics are indicated when the abscess is >5 cm or there is an area of surrounding cellulitis. Use cephalexin (40 mg/kg per day div qid), cefadroxil (40 mg/kg per day div bid), amoxicillin-clavulanate (875/125 formulation; 45 mg/kg per day of amoxicillin div bid). If MRSA is a concern, use clindamycin (20 mg/kg per day div qid) alone or add trimethoprim-sulfamethoxazole, which does not reliably cover group A strep, to one of the above regimens (8 mg/kg per day of trimethoprim div bid).

Have the patient return in 24–48 hours to evaluate for complications, remove the packing, and repeat the irrigation. Loosely repack the cavity only if pus is again found. Usually, by 48 hours, the incision remains open without packing while the cavity heals from below. Instruct the family to irrigate the cavity under running warm water or to apply warm wet soaks three times daily at home for 5 days.

Refer breast, perirectal, fingertip (pulp), hand, and deep abscesses of the neck to an experienced surgeon.

Follow-up

- After abscess drainage: daily for 2–3 days

Indications for admission

- Abscess associated with lymphangitis, fever >38.9°C (102°F), or signs of toxicity
- Abscess in an immunocompromised patient

Bibliography

Gorwitz RJ: A review of community-associated methicillin-resistant Staphylococcus aureus skin and soft tissue infections. *Pediatr Infect Dis J* 2008;27:1–7.

Korownyk C, Allan GM: Evidence-based approach to abscess management. *Can Fam Physician* 2007;53:1680–4.

Payne CJ, Walker TW, Karcher AM, et al: Are routine microbiological investigations indicated in the management of non-perianal cutaneous abscesses? *Surgeon* 2008;6:204–6.

Bite wounds

About 1% of all ED visits are for bites, the majority of which are caused by dogs. More than one-half of bite victims are children, most of them toddlers. While a patient may seek medical attention because of cosmetic concerns, bleeding, or fear of rabies, the most common complication is infection. An increased risk of infection occurs with puncture wounds, hand wounds, or when there has been a delay (>24 hours) in seeking medical attention.

Clinical presentation and diagnosis

Usually, the history of an animal bite is readily obtained, so the diagnosis is evident. The three major types of bite wounds are puncture wounds, lacerations, and closed-fist injuries (CFIs). Puncture wounds are of particular concern, as the small break in the skin belies the significant risk of infection. Suspect that a laceration over the metacarpophalangeal joint of an adolescent represents a CFI, sustained when the patient punched another person in the mouth.

ED management

General measures

Thoroughly clean every bite wound with soap and water. Moderate-pressure irrigation in the ED is indicated for lacerations and CFIs, but it is probably ineffective for punctures. Use an 18- or 20-gauge IV catheter attached to a 1 liter bag of NS, around which a blood transfusion cuff is inflated to 300 mmHg. If the irrigation is not tolerated, anesthetize the intact skin margins of the wound with 1% lidocaine and then irrigate. Debride devitalized tissue, which is an excellent culture medium. This is particularly important with dog bites, which are, in part, crush injuries.

Suturing

Dog bites

Do not suture puncture wounds; hand, forearm or foot lacerations; wounds >8 hours old (except the face in children >1 year old); wounds over a joint; crush wounds that cannot be debrided; or if the patient is immunosuppressed. In these circumstances, if the wound appears clean and cosmesis is a concern, close the wound at 96 hours (delayed primary closure). Alternatively, allow the wound to granulate (secondary closure). Low-risk dog bite wounds can be sutured, but avoid deep closure to minimize the possibility of infection.

Cat bites

Because the infection rate is high, leave cat bite wounds open. Exceptions are easily cleaned wounds that are not on the hand, forearm or foot. Once again, avoid deep closure to minimize the possibility of infection.

Human bites

Do not close wounds on the distal extremities. However, suture facial bites <8 hours old that can be cleaned adequately.

Other bites

Consult with a pediatric infectious disease expert to determine the risk of infection.

Antibiotics

Dog and cat bites

Organisms causing infections include *Pasteurella multocida, Staphylococcus aureus*, and *Streptococcus* species. Give antibiotics for puncture wounds, hand and forearm wounds, and lacerations that are sutured. Use amoxicillin-clavulanate (875/125 formulation; 45 mg/kg per day of amoxicillin div bid). Give a penicillin-allergic patient clindamycin (20 mg/kg per day div qid) and trimethoprim-sulfamethoxazole (8 mg/kg per day of trimethoprim div bid). If MRSA is a concern, use clindamycin (20 mg/kg per day div qid) alone or add trimethoprim-sulfamethoxazole, (which does not reliably cover group A strep), to the above regimen (8 mg/kg per day of trimethoprim div bid). For patients requiring parenteral antibiotic therapy, use ampicillin-sulbactam (50 mg/kg per dose of ampicillin every 6 hours, max 2 grams).

Human bites

Etiologies of infections include *Eikenella corrodens, Staphylococcus aureus*, and *Streptococcus* species. Use the same guidelines as for dog and cat bites (above).

Other bites

Consult a pediatrics infectious diseases expert (as above).

Tetanus

Clostridia can be present in the mouths of coprophagic animals. Give tetanus toxoid unless it is certain that a booster was received in the previous 5 years. For patients <7 years of age, use 0.5 mL of DTaP, unless pertussis vaccination is contraindicated, in which case use DT. For patients 7–10 years old, use 0.5 mL of dT. If the patient is ≥11 years old, use 0.5 mL of Tdap.

Rabies

Decisions regarding rabies treatment depend on the prevalence of the disease in the species in the area where the animal lives. See pp. 731–733 for the indications for prophylaxis.

Follow-up

- Bite wound: daily for 2–3 days. Initiate antibiotic therapy if the patient develops fever, increasing pain or erythema, or a purulent discharge

Indications for admission

- Bite wound infections unresponsive to oral antibiotics
- Infected bite wounds in patients who initially seek attention >24 hours after the bite
- Bite wounds in immunocompromised patients

Bibliography

Brook I: Management of human and animal bite wounds: an overview. *Adv Skin Wound Care* 2005;18:197–203.

Dendle C, Looke D: Review article. Animal bites: an update for management with a focus on

infections. *Emerg Med Australas* 2008;20:458–67.

Harrison M: A 4-year review of human bite injuries presenting to emergency medicine and proposed evidence-based guidelines. *Injury* 2009 Jan 31.

Foreign-body removal

Small fragments of wood or pieces of glass are the most common foreign bodies embedded in the skin.

Clinical presentation

A fresh wound is usually tender, and the foreign body is often seen or palpated just below the skin surface. Delayed presentations are associated with induration and tenderness, often with purulent or serosanguinous drainage.

Fishhooks embedded in the skin merit special consideration, as there may be more than one barb. The barb may completely penetrate a finger or earlobe, emerging from the other side, leaving the hook shaft still embedded.

Diagnosis

Radiographs can be helpful in identifying and locating foreign bodies. Use a radioopaque marker, such as a bent paperclip taped to the overlying skin, as a reference point for estimating the exact location of the object. A radiograph is also indicated when the presence of a foreign body cannot be ruled out, as when an old wound does not heal, continues to drain serosanguinous or purulent material, or remains tender. Virtually all glass is radio-opaque, and wooden splinters can occasionally be seen if they are covered with dirt particles. Obtain an ultrasound to locate a nonradioopaque foreign body such as a thorn or piece of plastic.

ED management

Attempt to remove a foreign body in the ED only if it is close enough to the surface to be seen or palpated. Cleanse the skin with povidone-iodine, and anesthetize the area by local infiltration, field block, or regional nerve block. Using the paperclip marker and X-rays for reference, make a stab incision with a no. 11 blade directed at the foreign body. Carefully explore the wound with a small hemostat to find and remove the object. Then gently palpate over the wound with a gloved finger to identify any remaining fragments.

When removal attempts are prolonged or unsuccessful, consult with a surgeon to plan for a definitive operative procedure under fluoroscopic or sonographic guidance. Foreign bodies in the plantar surface of the foot are especially difficult to remove in the ED. Refer patients with foreign bodies in the face or hand to a surgeon, and consult with a surgeon before attempting to remove a foreign body from the neck, unless it is clearly superficial.

When the foreign body is small or cannot be palpated, probing the wound is usually fruitless. If the wound is tender and crusted over, however, unroof it with the point of an 18-gauge needle to facilitate the drainage of any pus; the object may emerge over the next several days. Continue with warm soaks at home, and reevaluate the wound in 48 hours.

To remove a fishhook, advance the barbed end until the skin is tented and anesthetize that area with 1% lidocaine. Then advance the point until the barb leaves the skin, sever the barbed point with wire cutters, and pull the shaft of the hook back out through the original entrance wound. Small-barb hooks may be removed in a retrograde fashion through the original wound site. If the fishhook has several barbs, separate them with wire cutters and remove each one individually. If the barb is already through the skin, cut it off and pull the shaft out without using any anesthetic.

Give tetanus toxoid unless it is certain that a booster was received in the previous 5 years. For patients <7 years of age, use 0.5 mL of DTaP, unless pertussis vaccination is contraindicated, in which case use DT. For patients 7–10 years old, use 0.5 mL of dT. If the patient is ≥11 years old, use 0.5 mL of Tdap.

Follow-up

- Small or nonpalpable foreign body: 48 hours

Bibliography

Blankenship RB, Baker T: Imaging modalities in wounds and superficial skin infections. *Emerg Med Clin North Am* 2007;25:223–34.

Trott AT: *Wounds and Lacerations: Emergency Care and Closure*, 3rd ed. Philadelphia: Elsevier, 2005.

Turkcuer I, Atilia R, Topacoglu H, et al: Do we really need plain and soft-tissue radiographies to detect radiolucent foreign bodies in the ED? *Am J Emerg Med* 2006;24:763–8.

Insect bites and stings

Insect bites and stings usually cause a local reaction. However, systemic anaphylactic reactions occur 1–3% of the time after Hymenoptera stings (honeybees, wasps, hornets, yellow jackets, harvester and fire ants) in susceptible patients.

Clinical presentation

Reactions can be classified as immediate (within 2 hours) or delayed (after 2 hours). Immediate reactions may be local or systemic.

Immediate local reactions

These include local pain, erythema, swelling, tingling, warmth, and pruritus at the sting site. Local reactions usually last 24–48 hours; they can be extensive, although all affected skin is contiguous with the sting site.

Delayed reactions

These can occur after a 1–2 week interval. They present as large local reactions, serum sickness (fever, arthralgia, urticaria, lymphadenopathy), and rarely, peripheral neuritis, vasculitis, nephritis, or encephalitis.

Immediate systemic reactions

The hallmark of a systemic reaction is swelling that occurs at locations not contiguous with the sting site. The reaction may be mild, with itching and urticaria. More severe anaphylactic reactions can occur with hypotension, wheezing, laryngeal edema, and shock. Eighty-five percent of sensitive patients manifest symptoms within 5 minutes; all have symptoms within 1–2 hours.

Diagnosis

The diagnosis is suggested by the history of a sting or by the typical appearance of a local reaction in the warm-weather months. Stings, as opposed to insect bites, are always painful. Cellulitis may look similar, but a bacterial infection usually does not develop abruptly. Also, a cellulitis may be associated with fever, lymphangitic streaking, and local lymphadenopathy.

Consider other causes of systemic allergic reactions, such as drugs (penicillins, sulfonamides, contrast dyes) and foods (shellfish, eggs). Try to ascertain whether the insect was a member of the Hymenoptera order, and inquire about a history of allergies and any previous systemic reactions to insect stings.

ED management

Local reactions

Among the Hymenoptera, only honeybees lose their stingers, which may remain at the sting site. Remove the stinger (if it is still in place), by grasping as close to the puncture site as possible with a small forceps. Cleanse the site, apply ice or cool compresses to the area, and give oral diphenhydramine (5 mg/kg per day div qid, 50 mg/dose maximum) or hydroxyzine (2 mg/kg per day div tid, 50 mg/dose maximum). If the erythema continues to spread during the 24 hours after the bite or sting, consider the wound to be infected (see Cellulitis, pp. 75–76). Treat with 40 mg/ kg per day of cephalexin (div qid) or cefadroxil (div bid), warm compresses every 2 hours, and elevation. If MRSA is a concern, use clindamycin (20 mg/kg per day div qid) alone or add trimethoprim-sulfamethoxazole, (which does not reliably cover group A strep), to one of the above regimens (8 mg/kg per day of trimethoprim div bid).

Systemic reactions

Treat mild reactions (itching, urticaria) with oral diphenhydramine or hydroxyzine. The management of severe systemic reactions is the same as for anaphylaxis (see pp. 30–34). Prescribe an EpiPen and refer the patient to an allergist for evaluation and possible immunotherapy.

Follow-up

* Local reaction: 24 hours, if the erythema is spreading
* Systemic reaction (not anaphylaxis): 2–3 days

Indication for admission

* Systemic anaphylactic reaction

Bibliography

Golden DB: Insect sting anaphylaxis. *Immunol Allergy Clin North Am* 2007;27:261–72.

Graft DF: Insect sting allergy. *Med Clin North Am* 2006;90:211–32.

Järvinen KM: Allergic reactions to stinging and biting insects and arachnids. *Pediatr Ann* 2009;38:199–209.

Marine stings and envenomations

Marine stings and envenomations can be caused by either invertebrates or vertebrates. Invertebrates such as the jellyfish, Portuguese man-of-war, sea anemones, and corals can contain thousands of stinging cells (nematocysts); others contain toxin that can be transmitted by contact (certain sponges, sea urchins).

Envenomation from vertebrates results from contact with toxin on the dorsal spines of the *Scorpaenidae* family (scorpionfish, stonefish, and lionfish) or the spines on the tail of a stingray.

Clinical presentation and diagnosis
Invertebrates

The presentation can vary substantially depending upon the species, the number of nematocysts coming into contact with the skin, the amount and duration of the contact, and the patient's body weight. Signs and symptoms can vary from mild dermatitis with pain, burning, swelling, and erythema at the site of the sting to anaphylactic reactions.

The Portuguese man-of-war produces a single long strap dermatitis, along which are small blisters. There may also be generalized muscular cramps, vomiting, and cardiovascular collapse.

Sponges deposit silica spicules, causing pruritic or irritant dermatitis that can lead to epidermal desquamation.

The barbs of sea urchins can become deeply embedded with venom injection. Local reactions, as well as muscle spasms, shortness of breath, and cardiovascular collapse can ensue.

Vertebrates

Contact with the dorsal spines of scorpionfish, stonefish, and lionfish causes excruciating pain (especially the stonefish), associated with erythema, swelling, and paresthesias of the affected extremity, sometimes followed by vesicle formation. The pain will peak in about an hour and can last for 12 hours if not treated, although milder pain can persist for weeks. Examination usually reveals one or more puncture wounds. The patient may also have GI and respiratory symptoms. Serious envenomations can lead to dyspnea and shock.

The tail of a stingray can cause a severe laceration, without venom release. If venom is released from the tail spines, local pain and burning ensue, followed by muscular cramping, vomiting, diarrhea, diaphoresis, fasciculations, weakness and, on occasion, cardiac arrhythmias and seizures.

ED management

As a rule, the venoms are heat-labile. Soaking the affected area in hot water (43.3–45.0°C; 110–113°F) for 30–90 minutes may greatly reduce the pain. Additional therapy consists of local wound care, analgesia, tetanus prophylaxis (if indicated), antihistamines (hydroxyzine 2 mg/kg per day div tid, 50 mg/dose maximum or diphenhydramine 5 mg/kg per day div qid, 50 mg/dose maximum) for itching, and antibiotics (40 mg/kg per day of cephalexin div qid or cefadroxil div bid) for lacerations.

Invertebrates

Immobilize the limb and inactivate the nematocysts by applying vinegar or acetic acid for 10–15 minutes. Do not apply alcohol or fresh water, which may cause nematocyst discharge. Lift away the tentacles, then shave the area (shaving cream can be used) to remove any remaining nematocysts.

Treat the dermatitis from sponges by removing the stingers and soaking the contact area in dilute acetic acid, vinegar, or isopropyl alcohol.

Remove sea urchin spines carefully, as they are easily broken. If the sea urchin possesses pedicellariae, apply shaving cream and shave the area.

Vertebrates

Immerse the area in hot water for at least 1 hour. Provide local wound care and systemic support as necessary. Surgically remove spines that are in proximity to nerves, vessels, or joints. Radiographs and/or ultrasonography may assist in the identification of retained spines.

Stonefish antivenin is available via the regional poison control center for your area.

Indications for admission

- All marine animal envenomations associated with signs or symptoms of systemic toxicity

Bibliography

Atkinson PR, Boyle A, Hartin D, McAuley D: Is hot water immersion an effective treatment for marine envenomation? *Emerg Med J* 2006;23:503–8.

Isbister GK, Kiernan MC: Neurotoxic marine poisoning. *Lancet Neurol* 2005;4:219–28.

Perkins RA, Morgan SS: Poisoning, envenomation, and trauma from marine creatures. *Am Fam Physician* 2004;69:885–90.

Rabies

Most rabies viruses are transmitted by the bite of infected mammals. While the issue of rabies postexposure prophylaxis is considered most often after domestic animal (dog and cat) bites, wildlife (skunks, raccoons, bats, foxes, ferrets, opossums, weasels, wolves, wood-chucks) now constitute the major reservoir of rabies in the United States. Rodents (squirrels, hamsters, rats, mice) and rabbits can be infected, but they do not secrete the virus in their saliva, so they rarely transmit the disease.

Clinical presentation

The most common scenario in which rabies is considered is when a patient comes to the ED after an unprovoked bite (such as while attempting to feed an animal). On occasion, abnormal behavior (abnormally aggressive, reserved, or withdrawn) on the part of the animal is noted. Exposure can be by bite (any penetration of the skin by the animal's teeth) or by scratch, abrasion, or saliva. Petting alone, contact with blood, urine, or feces, or contact with saliva on truly intact skin does not constitute exposure.

The incubation period of rabies ranges from 4 days to years, with an average of 4–6 weeks. Clinical rabies presents with a nonspecific 2–10 day prodrome of fatigue, anxiety, fever, headache, anorexia, nausea and vomiting, and abdominal pain. Pain, paresthesias, and fasciculations may occur at the site of the injury. This is followed by increasing agitation, incoordination, hyperactivity, hallucinations, seizures, pharyngeal spasm, and hydrophobia. Rabies is virtually universally fatal once the virus becomes established in the CNS.

Diagnosis

The definitive diagnosis is made from examination of the animal's brain. Unfortunately, the specimen is not always available, so management decisions must be based on the likelihood of rabies in that species in the particular locale. The best information will come from the local health authorities. Postexposure prophylaxis for any bat contact is recommended, even if there is no evidence of soft-tissue injury, although the risk of rabies varies with the type of exposure (see Table 27-1).

Clinical rabies can be confused with a variety of neurologic conditions, including poliomyelitis, Guillain-Barré, herpes simplex, brain abscess, vaccine reaction, sepsis, and psychosis.

ED management

Recommend confinement and observation of healthy domestic animals for 10 days. If any signs of rabies develop, the animal must be sacrificed and the head sent to an appropriate laboratory. Contact the local veterinary public health service to arrange for transportation of stray domestic animals to the ASPCA. Because the incubation time is so variable, initiate prophylaxis, if indicated, regardless of the time elapsed since exposure.

Table 27-1. Rabies risk from bats

Exposure unlikely	Exposure reasonably possible
Bat droppings found in sleeping quarters	Bat found in same room of someone sleeping, mentally disturbed, intoxicated, or an unattended child
Patient touches bat, but is certain there is no scratch	Young child touches bat, but may be unaware or unable to communicate about the bite
Bat swoops by patient who does not feel it touch, or there is no contact with bare skin	Bat flies into patient, touching bare skin and unable to determine what contact occurred
Patient has contact with carcass of bat	Patient with bare feet steps on a live bat
Bats are heard or seen in the attic or walls	Patient puts hand in firewood or brush, feels pain, then sees a live bat

Table 27-2. Initiation of rabies postexposure prophylaxis (PEP)

Exposure indicated[a]	No PEP	PEP
Dog, cat, ferret, livestock, or other mammal that is either owned or stray and is available for 10-day observation	X	
Dog, cat, ferret, livestock, other mammal NOT available for 10-day observation		X
Bat, coyote, fox, groundhog, skunk, raccoon available for rabies testing	X	
Bat, coyote, fox, groundhog, skunk, racoon NOT available for rabies testing		X
Rodents, rabbits[b]	X	

Notes: [a] Consider additional factors to help determine the need for PEP, including whether the attack was provoked or not, the incidence of rabies in the community and the species, and the type of exposure. Bites, scratches, and abrasions from the animal or contamination by the animal's saliva of cuts or mucous membranes constitute high or moderate risk. Petting, or contact with the animal's blood, urine, feces or saliva onto the patient's intact skin does not constitute rabies exposure. Consult your local health department for specific questions regarding individual cases.

[b] Bites from squirrels, hamsters, guinea pigs, gerbils, chipmunks, rats, mice, other small rodents, rabbits, and hares almost never require PEP.

Regardless of the nature of the attack, thoroughly clean all wounds. Infiltrate high-risk wounds with 1% lidocaine, then thoroughly irrigate to the depth of the wound. Give prophylactic antibiotics, if indicated (see Bite wounds, pp. 724–726).

The indications for postexposure prophylaxis are summarized in Table 27-2. Use human rabies immune globulin (HRIG) and human diploid cell vaccine (HDCV) at the initial time of presentation day. Give a single dose of 20 units/kg of HRIG. Infiltrate as much of the dose as is anatomically possible in and around the wound, and inject the remainder IM in a site that is distant from the wound. Give 1 mL IM of HDCV, with subsequent doses 3, 7, and 14 days after the first. Use the deltoid area for adolescents and older children; the anterolateral aspect of the thigh may be used in younger children. Do not give the vaccine at the same site as HRIG (may cause prophylaxis failure).

Ideally, give HRIG and HDCV on day 0. Then continue with HDVC on days 3, 7, and 14. Immunocompromised patients will require a 5th dose on day 28. If HDCV is not available, give HRIG and initiate the vaccination series as soon as possible. If HRIG is not available, vaccinate the patient immediately and give HRIG as soon as possible if it becomes available within 7 days of the initial vaccination. Beyond 7 days after the initial vaccination, HRIG is contraindicated.

Follow-up

- Rabies prophylaxis initiated: 3 days
- Immunocompromised patient for documentation of antibody response after series is completed

Indication for admission

- Clinical rabies

Bibliography

Committee on Infectious Diseases, American Academy of Pediatrics: Rabies. In *Red Book 2006: Report of the Committee on Infectious Diseases*, 27th ed. Elk Grove Village, IL: American Academy of Pediatrics, 2006, pp. 552–9.

Leung AK, Davies HD, Hon KL: Rabies: epidemiology, pathogenesis, and prophylaxis. *Adv Ther* 2007;24:1340–7.

Manning SE, Rupprecht CE, Fishbein D, et al: Advisory Committee on Immunization Practices Centers for Disease Control and Prevention (CDC). Human rabies prevention–United States, 2008: recommendations of the Advisory Committee on Immunization Practices. *MMWR Recomm Rep* 2008;57(RR-3):1–28.

Scorpion stings

There are 650 species of scorpions worldwide. However, only one species in the United States, *Centruroides exilixauda*, produces serious toxicity. This scorpion, also known as the "bark scorpion" because it lives in the bark of trees, is found in Arizona and to a lesser extent in other southwestern states. Scorpions are nocturnal and will frequently enter houses to feed on cockroaches.

The scorpion has two claws anteriorly and a tail which ends in a telson, which contains poisonous glands and a stinger. The venom contains a neurotoxin which can lead to autonomic and neuromuscular dysfunction.

Clinical presentation

Systemic symptoms are more likely in children. These include sympathetic (tachycardia, hypertension, diaphoresis, altered mental status), parasympathetic (hypotension, bradycardia, salivation, bronchorrhea, urination), and neuromuscular (extremity jerking) findings.

Diagnosis

In most cases, there is a definite history of a scorpion sting. When the history is lacking, consider a scorpion bite when local pain and numbness are accompanied by autonomic symptoms.

ED management

As soon as the patient arrives in the ED, apply an ice bag to the area of the sting. Immobilize the affected area in a functional position below the level of the heart. Treat anxiety with diazepam (0.05–0.2 mg/kg IV), hypertension with labetalol (0.1 mg/kg IV) or diazoxide (1 mg/kg minibolus IV push), and the parasympathetic effects with atropine (0.01 mg/kg IV). Parenteral analgesics may be required for severe pain and agitation. Monitor IV fluids carefully as these patients are at risk for pulmonary edema and hypertension. Although commercially prepared antivenin is produced in other parts of the world for endemic scorpions, in the United States commercially prepared scorpion antivenin is available only for Arizona.

Indication for admission

- *Centruroides* bite, if the patient is symptomatic after 4 hours of ED observation

Bibliography

Chase P, Boyer-Hassen L, McNally J, et al: Serum levels and urine detection of Centruroides sculpturatus venom in significantly envenomated patients. *Clin Toxicol (Phila)* 2009;47:24–8.

Holve S: Venomous spiders, snakes, and scorpions in the United States. *Pediatr Ann* 2009;38:210–7.

Snakebites

Most snakes in the United States are not venomous. However, snakebites cause approximately 5–15 deaths annually. Poisonous snakes indigenous to the United States include the *Crotalidae* (rattlesnakes, water moccasins, copperheads) and the *Elapidae* (coral snake). Crotalids account for 99% of venomous snakebites occurring in the wild and can be found in virtually any state in the continental United States. The poisonous coral snake (which is the only elapid found in the United States) is found in southeastern and Gulf Coast states as well as Arizona. On occasion, victims will be bitten by exotic snakes that are kept as pets.

Clinical presentation

Crotalid envenomation

The pain usually starts within 1 minute of the bite, although a deep bite or one not on an extremity can cause more rapid symptoms. Crotalid envenomation can affect the following organ systems.

- Skin and soft tissue: local necrosis.
- Cardiovascular: increased capillary permeability leading to progressive edema and local hemorrhage. In the most severe cases, pulmonary edema, hemorrhage and hypotension may occur.
- Hematologic: thrombocytopenia and defibrination may occur. Hemorrhage, hemolysis, and DIC may also develop.
- Renal: acute tubular or cortical necrosis can occur, especially in the presence of marked hemolysis and shock.
- Immune: anaphylactic-like symptoms.
- Neurologic: symptoms are uncommon, although the Mojave rattlesnake may cause neuromuscular blockade. Cranial nerve palsies are often seen as the first manifestation.

Elapid envenomation

- Skin and soft tissue: small amount of local erythema and swelling. However, there is a possibility that the snake will chew the skin, leading to a large laceration
- Neurologic: paresthesias, nausea, emesis, muscle fasciculations, tremors, and bulbar paralysis can occur. Severe cases can lead to respiratory and muscular paralysis.

Diagnosis

The diagnosis of a snakebite is generally clear from the history. The key diagnostic issue is determining the type of snake. The crotalids can be identified by their large triangular heads and heat-sensing pits located above the nostrils. Elapids have red and yellow bands adjacent to each other.

ED management

Nonvenomous

Clean the wound, give tetanus prophylaxis, if necessary, and appropriate pain medication. Prescribe a 5-day course of oral antibiotics, using either amoxicillin/clavulanic acid (875/ 125 formulation; 45 mg/kg per day of amoxicillin div tid) or the combination of penicillin VK (50 mg/kg per day div qid) and cephalexin (40 mg/kg per day div qid). If there is any uncertainty about the identity of the snake, contact the regional poison control center, and observe for venomous symptoms for at least 3–4 hours.

Venomous

In the field, the priority is expedient transfer to a medical facility. Splint the affected extremity and remove jewelry that could cause a tourniquet effect. Do not apply cold packs or tourniquets. Although up to 20% of bites from venomous snakes are "dry" bites and are therefore asymptomatic, emergency medical treatment is needed to clean the wound and evaluate the need for antivenin.

Once the patient arrives in the ED, the decision to use antivenin is based on the type of snake and the duration and progression of symptoms. Contact the regional poison control center to consult with someone experienced in managing snakebites. For all patients, start an IV in the contralateral side and keep the affected extremity at heart-level. Give antibiotics and pain medication as for nonvenomous snakebites, but do not give aspirin or NSAIDs. Obtain blood for CBC, electrolytes, BUN, creatinine, PT, PTT, fibrinogen level, and blood type. Also obtain a urinalysis to look for hematuria and proteinuria.

Most commercially available snake antivenin is produced from horse serum, so be prepared for possible allergic reactions. Skin testing prior to treatment is contraindicated and may sensitize the patient. Pretreat with diphenhydramine (1–2 mg/kg, 50 mg maximum) before starting a continuous infusion of the antivenin diluted in normal saline. Pulse therapy or starting and stopping the infusion can sensitize the patient and lead to an allergic reaction. The volume of antivenin is based on the presumed degree of envenomation (see Table 27-3). During the infusion, reassess the progression or regression of symptoms to determine the need for continued antivenin administration.

A new crotalid antivenin produced from sheep (serum CroFab) has been approved for treatment of mild to moderate crotalid envenomations. It is clearly indicated for patients known to be allergic to horse serum.

Debridement is often necessary after the first 48 hours, but fasciotomy is rarely required for treatment of compartment syndrome. Warn the patient that serum sickness may occur

Table 27-3. Antivenin therapy

Severity	Clinical features	Vials
None	Fang punctures, only	0
Mild	Local swelling (<10 cm), not progressive. No systemic signs or evidence of coagulopathy	0
Moderate	Swelling progressive beyond bite site (10–30 cm). Systemic reaction: coagulopathy, fever, vomiting, weakness	5–10
Severe	Marked progressive swelling. Severe coagulopathy. Proteinuria, hematuria, azotemia, hypertension	15–20

10–14 days after treatment. This presents with a pruritic urticarial rash, which can be associated with fever, nausea, headache, arthralgias, and adenopathy. Admit all symptomatic patients for at least 24 hours, regardless of whether antivenin was given.

Indication for admission

- Snakebite with signs of envenomation or requiring antivenin treatment

Bibliography

Nazim MH, Gupta S, Hashmi S, et al: Retrospective review of snake bite victims. *W V Med J* 2008;104:30–4.

Pizon AF, Riley BD, LoVecchio F, Gill R: Safety and efficacy of Crotalidae polyvalent immune Fab in pediatric crotaline envenomations. *Acad Emerg Med* 2007;14:373–6.

Schmidt JM: Antivenom therapy for snakebites in children: is there evidence? *Curr Opin Pediatr* 2005;17:234–8.

Spider bites

There are 50 species of North American spiders with fangs capable of penetrating human skin. However, only two species (black widow and brown recluse) can cause fatalities.

The black widow (*Latrodectus*) is distinguished by a red hourglass marking on the abdomen. The spiders are found throughout North America, except in Alaska. The female can grow up to 4 centimeters (including leg span), with a male being about one-quarter to one-half smaller.

The brown recluse (*Loxosceles*) is the most common cause of serious spider bites in the United States. They can be up to 3 centimeters in length and are distinguished by a dark-orange violin-shaped marking on the cephalothorax. It generally lives in dark, dry environments such as abandoned houses or vacation homes.

Clinical presentation
Black widow

The bite causes a pinprick sensation with slight local erythema and swelling. Within 10–90 minutes there are systemic symptoms, including muscle cramps, especially in the abdomen after bites of the lower extremities. Agitation and irritability may also be part of the initial presentation. There may be spasms with intense pain, paresthesias (particularly intense in the soles of the feet), headache, dysphagia, dizziness, nausea and vomiting, facial edema, and hypertension (which can be life-threatening). A venom dose that may cause only pain in an adult may lead to respiratory and cardiac arrest in a child.

Brown recluse

The bite of this spider is generally trivial. Within 10 minutes to several hours there is sharp, stinging, or burning type of pain at the bite site, followed by an aching pain and pruritus. The lesion becomes an irregular violaceous blister surrounded by an erythematous halo. In about 50% of cases, over 2–3 days the blister becomes an eschar that later sloughs, leaving an ulcer that is very slow to heal. The larger South American *Loxosceles* genus gives a more pronounced cutaneous picture, with intense pain and accompanying facial edema.

Systemic involvement is rare but can occur in any *Loxosceles* envenomation. The manifestations include fever, chills, nausea, vomiting, malaise, and a confluent scarlatiniform rash. There may be an associated hemolytic anemia presenting as hemoglobinuria, as well as thrombocytopenia and renal failure. The systemic response is usually not seen until 24 hours after the bite, making the diagnosis difficult.

ED management

Assess the ABCs and treat as necessary (see Shock, pp. 26–27). Insert an IV on the contralateral side and infuse D5½NS (use NS if the patient has signs of shock), and obtain a CBC, electrolytes, CPK, calcium, PT, and PTT. Apply ice to the bite site to reduce toxin absorption and decrease the pain.

Black widow

Give diazepam (0.05–0.2 mg/kg IV) and morphine (0.05–0.2 mg/kg) for analgesia, anxiety, and muscle relaxation. For most cases this will be the only treatment needed. Give labetalol (0.1 mg/kg IV) if hypertension is present despite the benzodiazepine and morphine.

For severe envenomations an antivenin is available. Dilute one vial in 100 mL of normal saline and give over 30–60 minutes. Immediate and delayed hypersensitivity reactions may occur.

Brown recluse

Apply repeated ice compresses for 2–3 days; these will reduce pain and the local cutaneous inflammation. There is no demonstrable benefit for any specific treatment for brown recluse bites other than routine wound care. Persistent ulceration may require skin grafting. If hemolysis occurs, ensure a good urine output (at least twice normal).

Follow-up

- Black widow: daily until the patient is asymptomatic
- Brown recluse: daily, until the wound is healing well

Indication for admission

- Systemic symptoms

Bibliography

Furbee RB, Kao LW, Ibrahim D: Brown recluse spider envenomation. *Clin Lab Med* 2006;26:211–26.

Holve S: Venomous spiders, snakes, and scorpions in the United States. *Pediatr Ann* 2009;38:210–7.

Peterson ME: Black widow spider envenomation. *Clin Tech Small Anim Pract* 2006;21:187–90.

Wound management

Most lacerations can be treated in the ED using basic principles of aseptic technique and wound closure. Plastic surgical consultation may occasionally be required for complex wounds, cosmetic concerns, functional deficits, or loss of subcutaneous tissue.

Clinical presentation and ED management

History

Determine the elapsed time since the injury. Most wounds <8–12 hours old may be closed primarily without an increased risk of infection; scalp and face wounds can be sutured up to at least 12–24 hours after injury. Delayed closure of face, head, and neck wounds does not cause an increased rate of wound infection. Knowing the mechanism of injury is helpful in predicting the likelihood of infectious complications: wounds resulting from compressive forces (blunt scalp trauma) often cause stellate lacerations, and may be more susceptible to infection than linear lacerations due to shearing forces (razor). Assess the general health of the patient, and ask about any possible immunocompromise that may increase the risk of an infection, such as underlying chronic illnesses (diabetes, vasculitis), steroid use, or chemotherapy.

Examination

Determine the extent of the injury, and evaluate sensation, general strength, vascular supply, motor function, and range of motion with and without resistance (looking for tendon injuries). This is difficult in an uncooperative young child, but if an extremity is involved, observe that the patient is able to movie it normally through a full range of motion before closing the wound. During the assessment, keep the wound edges moist by applying gauze pads moistened with NS.

Radiology

Radiographs are indicated when the mechanism of injury or physical examination suggests a bony injury or a retained foreign body. Metal fragments and glass can be seen on plain films, and wood fragments are visible if coated with radioopaque particles of dirt. Obtain radiographs of a crush injury to rule out a compound fracture. When possible, irrigate the wound before radiographs are taken to remove superficial debris.

Shaving

Shaving has the potential to increase the risk of infection. Therefore, clip the hair around a wound with scissors only if it interferes with wound closure. Never shave eyebrows, since there is no guarantee that they will grow back.

Anesthesia

Local anesthesia may be required to perform adequate irrigation and debridement. Apply a solution of either LET or LMX$_4$ (see Topical analgesia, pp. 692–693) prior to administering the local anesthetic. Topical anesthesia is especially useful for lacerations of the face and scalp. To prepare the wound for local anesthesia, apply povidone-iodine solution twice to the skin surrounding the wound, allowing it to dry for 4 minutes between applications.

Lidocaine is the usual anesthetic agent. To minimize the possibility of a toxic reaction, use the 1% strength in children, although 2% can be used when only a limited volume of anesthetic is to be injected (small child's finger). Use lidocaine with epinephrine for vascular areas (scalp, face), but epinephrine is contraindicated in areas with end-arteries (digits, pinna, nose). Do not exceed a total dose of 5 mg/kg of lidocaine (7 mg/kg when used with epinephrine). Procaine is the alternative in the patient allergic to lidocaine (extremely rare).

In unquestionably clean wounds, inject the lidocaine through the open wound (less painful), but in wounds likely to be dirty, administer it through the surrounding skin to avoid injecting debris into the deeper tissues.

Debridement and irrigation

After anesthesia has been achieved, debride any devitalized tissue, including fat. Irrigate the wound using a large (35 mL) luer lock syringe attached to a splash shield, which will produce 5–8 psi, an adequate pressure for wound irrigation The solution of choice for irrigation is NS; use copious amounts (at least 100 mL but often >1 L, depending on the wound size). Tap water may be an effective alternative, especially for preliminary cleansing before radiographs are obtained.

Exploration

Examine every wound for foreign substances and any associated trauma to blood vessels, ligaments, tendons, and bone. Remove fragments of hair, pieces of clothing, other debris, and blood clots, which may camouflage other injuries and be a source of infection. For scalp wounds, examine with a sterile gloved finger to determine any disruption of the galea and the outer table of the skull.

Suturing

For skin closure, nonabsorbable suture material is indicated, the least reactive of which is monofilament nylon. For typical outpatient wounds, deep sutures must be absorbable. Synthetics (Dexon) are less reactive than naturally occurring substances (gut). The appropriate suture size for different areas is given in Table 27-4. For areas where there is an increase in tension, such as over joints, choose the next heavier size.

Hemostasis may be accomplished with a simple ligature, a loop of absorbable suture either around the bleeder or tied in a small figure 8 (Figure 27-1). Never use a hemostat to clamp blindly, as a tendon, tendon sheath, or nerve may be clamped and destroyed.

Close deep wounds in two layers to obliterate dead space (Figure 27-2). When using deep sutures, bury the knot (Figure 27-3), except where it will cause friction (fascia, tendon sheaths), and cut the ends fairly short.

Most wounds can be closed with simple interrupted sutures (Figure 27-4). The skin edges must be everted and touching. Inverted edges result in poor healing but can be avoided by ensuring that the suture is at equal depth on both sides of the wound, that the depth is greater than the width (B>C), and that the width at the bottom of the suture (C) is greater than at the top (A). Evenly space the sutures so that the tension is distributed equally.

A vertical mattress (Figure 27-5) is a good method of closing a wound when there are problems with wound edge eversion or tension on the wound edge or when a wound is deep but does not require a two-layer closure. It is also useful in areas of skin laxity, for example, the back of the hand. The area inside the suture has all the tension, leaving the edges with

Table 27-4. Suggested suture size

Site	Suture size
Scalp (consider wounds at the hairline to be facial)	3–0, 4–0
Face, orbit	5–0, 6–0
Neck	
Ventral	5–0, 6–0
Dorsal	4–0, 5–0
Arms, legs, trunk	4–0, 5–0
Hands and fingers	5–0, 6–0
Feet	
Dorsum	4–0, 5–0
Plantar	3–0, 4–0
Toes	5–0, 6–0
Deep (absorbable)	
Hemostasis	4–0, 5–0
Deep closure	3–0, 4–0, 5–0 [a]

Notes: [a] The more superficial the subcutaneous suture, the smaller the size of suture material.

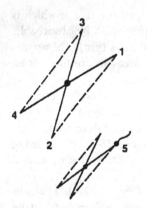

LEGEND

● Bleeding Site
  Point of Clamp
1-Start/Enter
2-Exit
3-Enter
4-Exit
5-Knot

Figure 27-1. Figure-eight suture.

none. The suture must be of equal depth on the two sides of the wound, to prevent a stepping scar.

Employ a horizontal mattress (Figure 27-6) when there are problems with wound edge eversion; do not use it where there will be any tension or to eliminate a two-layer closure. Note that each horizontal mattress takes the space of two sutures, so this is a fast way to close a wound.

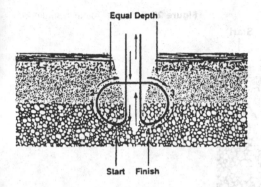

Figure 27-2. Suture for a deep wound.

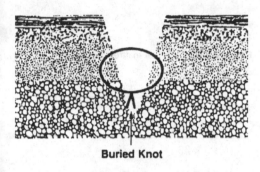

Figure 27-3. Suture for a deep wound burying the ends.

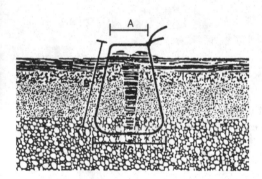

Figure 27-4. Interrupted suture.

The half-horizontal mattress is the best way to handle any sharp corner (Figure 27-7A and B) and can be used for a "v," "y," "t," "z," or stellate type of wound (Figure 27-7C–F).

In wounds of the lip, the first suture must bring together the edges of the vermilion border; otherwise, a noticeable scar results.

Wound adhesives

Cyanoacylates, such as Dermabond, can be used for minor facial lacerations that are small (<5 cm), clean, under minimal tension, with sharp edges. Anesthesia may not be necessary and wound closure time can be decreased by as much as 50%. The adhesive polymerizes in about 1 second; hold the wound margins together with forceps or the wooden ends of swabs

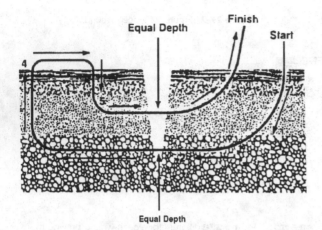

Equal Depth

Finish

Start

Figure 27-5. Vertical mattress suture.

Equal Depth

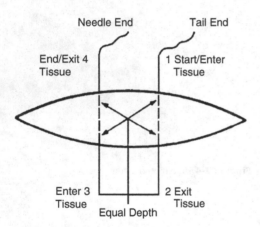

Needle End

Tail End

Figure 27-6. Horizontal mattress suture.

End/Exit 4 Tissue

1 Start/Enter Tissue

Enter 3 Tissue

2 Exit Tissue

Equal Depth

placed about 3–5 mm from the edges. Do not use Dermabond if there is evidence of active infection or on mucosal surface wounds, skin exposed to body fluid regularly, or areas with dense hair.

Referral

Refer complex wounds, in which underlying structural injury is a possibility, to a surgeon. Among these are deep lacerations of the wrist or hand, chest, abdomen, perineum, or anterior neck. Also refer ear and eyelid wounds.

Tetanus

Clean minor wounds require tetanus prophylaxis only if the patient has not had at least three documented previous tetanus toxoid doses or if a previously immunized patient has not had a tetanus dose in at least 10 years. Serious wounds at greater risk for tetanus include contaminated (dirt, feces, saliva) and puncture wounds and wounds with devitalized tissue. With these wounds, give tetanus toxoid to patients who have had three previous doses if >5 years has elapsed since the last dose. For patients with less than three previous doses, use toxoid and tetanus immune globulin (250 to 500 units IM). When tetanus toxoid is

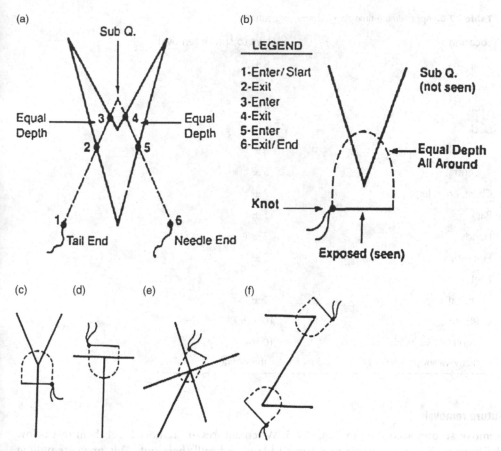

Figure 27-7. A–F: half-buried horizontal mattress sutures.

indicated for patients <7 years of age, use 0.5 mL of DTaP, unless pertussis vaccination is contraindicated, in which case use DT. For patients 7–10 years old, use 0.5 mL of dT. If the patient is ≥11 years old, use 0.5 mL of Tdap.

Other measures

Splint wounds in areas of great mobility (across joints, on the hand) using a thick wrapping of gauze for 2 days, until healing is under way. Advise the patient to avoid getting the wound wet for the first 24 hours; after that, it can be cleaned gently and allowed to air-dry. Give the parents dry bandages to apply in case the original dressing becomes wet.

No antibiotics are necessary for small, uncomplicated wounds that are not a result of an animal or human bite. Give antibiotics for facial wounds >24 hours old; other wounds >12 hours old; contaminated wounds; and wounds in immunosuppressed patients. Use amoxicillin-clavulanate (875/125 formulation; 45 mg/kg per day of amoxicillin div bid). For penicillin-allergic patients, give clindamycin (20 mg/kg per day div tid) or erythromycin (40 mg/kg per day div qid).

Table 27-5. Approximate timetable for removing sutures[a]

Location	Days to suture removal
Scalp	8 ± 2
Face	4 ± 1
Orbit	4 ± 1
Neck	
Dorsal	6 ± 1
Ventral	5 ± 1
Chest, arms, legs	7 ± 1
Back	11 ± 1
Hands	7 ± 1
Fingertips	9 ± 1
Feet	
Dorsal, toes	9 ± 1
Plantar	10 ± 2
Skin over joints	$10–14$

Note: [a]Remove any packing in 24 hours and reevaluate the wound.

Suture removal

Remove sutures according to Table 27-5. When sutures are removed, cut them just below the knot with suture scissors or a curved blade and pull them out. This prevents pulling contaminated material through the tissue. After sutures are removed, apply Steri-Strips to give additional strength for a few days without the risk of infection or foreign-body reaction.

Follow-up

- Immediately for signs of infection (fever, erythema, proximal streaking, induration, purulence). Otherwise, return for suture removal

Bibliography

O'Sullivan R, Oakley E, Starr M: Wound repair in children. *Aust Fam Physician* 2006;35:476–9.

Singer AJ, Dagum AB: Current management of acute cutaneous wounds. *N Engl J Med* 2008;359:1037–46.

Singer AJ, Quinn JV, Hollander JE: The cyanoacrylate topical skin adhesives. *Am J Emerg Med* 2008;26:490–6.

Valente JH, Forti RJ, Freundlich LF, Zandieh SO, Crain EF: Wound irrigation in children: saline solution or tap water? *Ann Emerg Med* 2003;41:609–16.

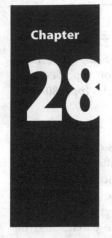

Chapter 28

Special considerations in pediatric emergency care

Contributing authors
David P. Sole: The crying infant
Frank A. Maffei: The critically ill infant
Joshua Vova: Children with special healthcare needs
Kirsten Roberts: Failure to thrive
Loren Yellin: Telephone triage

The crying infant

Regardless of how ideal parents' care-taking practices might be, crying is a normal and expected behavior of infancy. Crying increases steadily from birth through the second to third month of life, so that an infant can be expected to cry approximately 2 hours a day, on average. The crying often has two occurrence spikes during the day, with the first being in the late afternoon and the second later in the evening. Not surprisingly, after trying soothing methods such as cuddling and carrying fail to quiet the infant, the parents or care-taker may become distressed and seek medical evaluation. Persistent crying has also been associated with maternal depression, exposure to tobacco smoke, and infant abuse and neglect.

Clinical presentation

The list of etiologies for infant crying is long, but several diagnoses must be considered. These include colic, viral illness, corneal abrasion, hair tourniquet, gastroesophageal reflux, and constipation.

Colic

No single definition exists for colic (pp. 234–236), although the "rule of threes" is helpful: infants from 3 weeks to approximately 3 months of age with periods of crying lasting 3 hours a day on at least 3 days out of the week.

Viral illness

The incompletely vaccinated or unvaccinated infant presenting for evaluation of crying associated with fever can be challenging. Many institutions have policies requiring a full evaluation for bacterial sepsis in febrile infants (pp. 371–372). A thorough investigation is necessary to identify the source of fever.

Corneal abrasion

Suspect an abrasion (p. 536) if a crying infant has scratches around the eyes. However, a history of eye trauma may not be elicited and obvious physical findings may not be present.

Hair tourniquet

Less commonly, crying may be caused by the strangulation of a digit, the penis, or clitoris by a strand of hair or a piece of thread or fiber, the so-called hair tourniquet. Use a magnification device, such as an ocular loop or ophthalmoscope, during the examination of the digits and genitalia.

Other potential etiologies include gastroesophageal reflux (pp. 274–275), anal fissures (p. 259), urinary tract infection (pp. 664–665), osteomyelitis (pp. 571–572), otitis media (pp. 635–636), thrush (p. 151), meningitis (pp. 401–403, intussusception (pp. 249–250), incarcerated hernia (p. 292), testicular torsion (p. 291), and inflicted injuries (pp. 580–581).

Diagnosis

Assume that a crying infant has a true medical issue; colic is a diagnosis of exclusion.

Obtain a comprehensive history, including feeding and sleeping patterns, medication changes (including those of a breast-feeding mother), recent vaccination(s), and consider the possibility of neonatal withdrawal syndrome. Review the infant's medical record looking for a pattern of encounters that may suggest infant neglect or abuse. While taking the history, pay particular attention to interaction between the parents and the infant.

Perform a thorough physical examination. Document a complete set of vital signs, including weight, and inspect the undressed infant from head to toe. Priorities on the examination include the skin (rashes, abrasions, healing wounds), anterior fontanel (fullness), cardiac auscultation and palpation of distal pulses (unrecognized congenital heart disease), abdomen (hard stool), external genitalia (diaper rash, inguinal hernia, penile hair tourniquet), and extremities (decreased range of motion secondary to trauma, hair tourniquet). If the infant has facial scratches perform fluorescein staining of the cornea looking for an abrasion.

In general, no laboratory testing or imaging studies are needed. However, if the infant appears ill or there is a concern about a serious cause for crying, obtain a CBC, in addition to studies based on the clinical suspicion for specific disorders. A lumbar puncture may be required in a persistently crying febrile young infant in whom no obvious etiology is identified on examination.

ED management

The priority in the ED is to rule out a serious or life-threatening condition. Once that is ensured, tailor the management to the specific diagnosis (refer to the specific sections elsewhere in the text). If the examination and work-up is unremarkable and a period of observation is reassuring, the infant may be discharged with close follow-up. Include in the documentation a review of the medical decision-making and discussion of care-taker counseling points. Review the discharge instructions with the care-takers and answer their questions. Arrange for primary care follow-up within 24–48 hours. However, if the family seems overwhelmed with the infant's crying, respite admission to an inpatient service may be necessary. This admission may reduce the risk of abuse or neglect.

Follow-up

- Primary care in 24–48 hours

Indications for admission

- Surgical emergencies (incarcerated hernia, testicular torsion, intussusception)
- Infectious disease emergencies (sepsis, meningitis, UTI, osteomyelitis)
- Cardiac emergencies (supraventricular tachycardia, anomalous coronary artery)

- Suspected child abuse
- Parents no longer able to cope with crying infant

Bibliography

Akman I: Mother's postpartum psychological adjustment and infantile colic. *Arch Dis Child* 2006;91:417–19.

Freedman SB, Al-Harthy N, Thull-Freedman J: The crying infant: diagnostic testing and frequency of serious underlying disease. *Pediatrics* 2009;123:841–8.

Herman M: The crying infant. *Emerg Med Clin North Am* 2007; 25:1137–59.

The critically ill infant

The ongoing maturation of the young infant creates a unique state of physiologic transition. The infant may develop signs of severe illness due to a congenital disorder that was not initially apparent or become ill due to environmental forces or infectious agents that produce severe disease. Establishing the correct diagnosis is challenging owing to the variety of pathologic processes that can cause rapid deterioration in the young infant. Additionally, the initial stabilization can be difficult and requires expertise in airway, respiratory, circulatory, and neurological support. The approach to the critically ill-appearing infant demands simultaneous initiation of diagnostic and therapeutic measures.

Clinical presentation

The clinical presentation of the critically ill infant depends upon the patient's previous health, the primary organ system affected, and when in the course of the illness the infant is brought to medical attention. Often, with severe disease, the infant may present with derangements in respiratory, cardiovascular, and/or neurological function. A meticulous and ordered examination can quickly narrow the diagnostic possibilities and allow the timely initiation of specific therapies. While stabilization is the priority, begin gathering data simultaneously with the initial therapeutic measures. Physical examination findings are summarized in Table 28-1.

Diagnosis and ED management

A basic tenet when dealing with any critically ill infant is to assume sepsis (pp. 370–371) and administer antibiotics quickly. Obtain blood and urine cultures, preferably before antibiotics are given, but defer a lumbar puncture until the patient is stabilized (but initiate the antibiotics). For any critically ill infant obtain a CBC, electrolytes, liver function tests, coagulation profile, and a urinalysis. Also send cultures, rapid antigen testing, and PCR (if available) for viral pathogens if a serious viral infection is clinically suspected (respiratory syncitial virus, herpes simplex virus, enterovirus). Other laboratory tests to consider include an ABG (assess acid–base and ventilatory status); methemoglobin level (unexplained cyanosis); blood lactate, pyruvate, ammonia and amino acids, as well as urine for amino and organic acids (inborn error of metabolism), cortisol and 17-hydroxyprogesterone (adrenal insufficiency); blood and urine for toxicological testing (accidental or intentional ingestion); and imaging studies as indicated by the clinical presentation (chest and/or abdominal radiographs, head CT, skeletal survey, echocardiogram).

Table 28-1. Physical examination findings in the critically ill-appearing infant

Organ system	Examination finding	Diagnoses
General appearance	Cyanosis	Congenital heart disease, respiratory failure, sepsis, methemoglobinemia
	Dehydration/emesis	Gastroenteritis, insufficient intake, volvulus, congenital adrenal hyperplasia
	Hypotonia	Sepsis, botulism
HEENT	Bulging fontanelle	Meningitis, shaken baby syndrome, ↑ICP, inborn error of metabolism
	Miosis	Toxic ingestion
	Ptosis/mydriasis	Botulism
	Retinal hemorrhages	Shaken baby syndrome
Cardiovascular	Bradycardia	↑ICP (meningitis, shaken baby syndrome), sepsis, toxic ingestion
	Poor perfusion	Hypovolemia, sepsis, congenital heart disease, tachyarrhythmia, myocarditis
	Tachycardia	Hypovolemia, sepsis, SVT, myocarditis, toxic ingestion
Respiratory	Apnea	Bronchiolitis, sepsis, ↑ICP
	Wheeze/rales	Bronchiolitis, congenital heart disease, myocarditis
Gastrointestinal	Distention/tenderness	Hirschsprung's enterocolitis, volvulus, necrotizing enterocolitis,
	Hepatomegaly	Congenital heart disease, myocarditis, inborn error of metabolism
	Mass	Pyloric stenosis, intussusception
Skin	Purpura	Sepsis, inflicted trauma
	Vesicles	Herpes simplex
Neurologic	Bulbar findings	Botulism
	Irritability/lethargy	Meningitis, shaken baby syndrome, inborn error of metabolism

Proceed with stabilization in a systematic manner (see Resuscitation, pp. 1–22). Following an expanded "ABCDs" format will aid in stabilization and early initiation of life-saving therapies, but keep in mind several unique attributes of young infants, as follows.

Airway

The small infant has a proportionately larger tongue and a smaller, more compliant subglottic airway than an older child or adult. As a result they are at greater risk for upper-airway obstruction.

Breathing

If there is evidence of respiratory failure or insufficiency, begin bag-mask ventilation with 100% oxygen and prepare for endotracheal intubation (see Respiratory failure, pp. 634–636). If there is coexisting hemodynamic compromise, provide volume expansion while preparing for intubation, as positive-pressure ventilation may impede venous return.

Circulation

To help differentiate a primary pulmonary process versus congenital heart disease with restriction of pulmonary blood flow, obtain an ABG after hyperoxygenation with 100% O_2 for 10 minutes (see cyanosis, pp. 60–61). With a pulmonary process the PaO_2 is above 150 mmHg, while in CHD it remains <50 mmHg. Consider a left-sided heart lesion with ductal-dependent systemic blood flow (i.e. coarctation of the aorta, critical aortic stenosis, hypoplastic left heart syndrome) in an infant with poor to absent distal pulses, a gallop rhythm, enlarged liver, abnormal chest radiograph, and acidosis. In contrast, right-sided lesions with ductal-dependent pulmonary blood flow (i.e. pulmonary stenosis/atresia, tricuspid atresia) often present shortly after birth with cyanosis as the primary abnormality. Start a prostaglandin E_1 infusion (0.05–0.1 mcg/kg per min) early and consult with a pediatric cardiologist. Continuous cardiopulmonary monitoring is essential during prostaglandin infusion as apnea is a known side effect.

A rapid (>220 bpm), regular, narrow complex tachycardia is suggestive of supraventricular tachycardia (pp. 42–43). The P waves may be normal, inverted or absent. In a hemodynamically stable infant, attempt vagal maneuvers.

Disability

An infant with meningitis, intracranial injury (shaken baby syndrome), or certain metabolic disorders (Reye's syndrome, inborn error producing hyperammonemia) may have progressively increased ICP. Perform a rapid neurologic assessment, looking for associated signs (i.e. altered mental status, hypertension, bradycardia, bulging fontanel). See pp. 517–518 for the treatment.

Dextrose

Obtain a rapid glucose determination promptly in every critically ill infant. Treat hypoglycemia (pp. 185–186) with 0.5–1 gm/kg of dextrose (2–4 mL/kg of D_{25} or 1–2 mL /kg of D_{50}). Inadequate intake, limited glycogen stores, and an increase in glucose utilization during stress states (gastroenteritis, pneumonia, sepsis) can lead to clinically significant hypoglycemia. A primary endocrine or metabolic abnormality (congenital adrenal hyperplasia, fatty acid oxidation disorders) may also lead to hypoglycemia.

Drugs

Inquire about medications given to the infant, and those taken by a breast-feeding mother. Also, consider specific medications needed for further stabilization (i.e. antibiotics, intubation medications, prostaglandin, inotropes and/or pressors).

Environment/equipment

Due to a relatively large surface area, reduced subcutaneous fat stores, and immature thermoregulatory mechanisms, a young infant is at risk for significant heat loss.

Hypothermia leads to increased oxygen consumption and pulmonary and systemic vasoconstriction, and it impedes effective resuscitation. However, perform rewarming slowly. Avoid active rewarming in the post-cardiac arrest situation and in cases where severe neurological injury exists, as this may promote tissue reperfusion injury. In such cases, allowing the infant to remain hypothermic and while permitting passive rewarming may be beneficial.

Check equipment for proper functioning. An acute decompensation during stabilization may be secondary to equipment failure, rather than a true physiologic change. Assume that any decompensation after endotracheal intubation is the result of the ETT, until proven otherwise.

Foley

A bladder catheter is necessary to assess urinary output during volume resuscitation.

Gastric tube

If the airway is secured, insert a gastric tube and decompress the stomach. This is especially important if prolonged bag-mask ventilation was employed prior to intubation.

Hematology/hydrocortisone

Consider the need for packed red blood cell infusion in infants with ongoing blood loss or the need for surgery (see Transfusion therapy, pp. 341–342). Check for the possibility of congenital or acquired coagulopathy and treat with fresh frozen plasma if needed. Consider the need for steroid replacement in an infant with suspected adrenal insufficiency (i.e. congenital adrenal hyperplasia, hypopituitarism, adrenal hemorrhage from overwhelming infection).

Specific diagnostic considerations
Neonatal sepsis (sepsis neonatorum)
Group B streptococcal disease (GBS)

GBS is a major cause of systemic and focal infections in infants and accounts for 70% of all early-onset sepsis, although the incidence has fallen dramatically. Early-onset disease usually occurs within the first 24 hours of life (range 0–6 days). There is often a history of maternal perinatal complications, such as prolonged rupture of membranes, premature birth, or chorioamnionitis. It may present as fulminant sepsis, pneumonia, and occasionally, meningitis. Pulmonary disease often mimics hyaline membrane disease and may be further complicated by severe pulmonary hypertension.

In contrast, an infant with late-onset disease (7-90 days) often presents with fever, sometimes associated with bacteremia. Meningitis occurs in 25% of cases and focal infections, such as septic arthritis, osteomyelitis, adenitis, may occur. In contrast to early-onset disease, these infants do not usually have multisystem involvement.

Herpes simplex virus

Most infants are infected at the time of delivery and become symptomatic at 7–16 days of life, although with in utero transmission the patient is symptomatic at birth. In addition, infection can be horizontally acquired, from close contacts with fever blisters, whitlows, or other skin infections. Neonatal herpes presents in three forms: disseminated disease, localized CNS disease, and disease localized to skin, eyes, and mucosa (pp. xx–yy).

Consider the diagnosis of HSV infection in any septic-appearing infant <4 weeks of age, regardless of the presence or absence of cutaneous lesions. Infection can be confirmed by isolation of virus in tissue culture from lesions, mucosa, and cerebrospinal fluid or antigen identification techniques, such as ELISA and DFA. Polymerase chain reaction provides rapid detection of HSV in cerebrospinal fluid.

Cardiac disease

There are two important milestones during the transition from neonatal to postnatal circulation that may "unmask" congenital heart disease: the closure of the ductus arteriosus (2 days to 3 weeks of age) and the progressive decline in pulmonary vascular resistance (first 18 weeks of life). Infants with congenital heart disease may present with subtle symptoms such as poor feeding, failure to thrive, or irritability. Alternatively, severe congenital heart disease may present with obvious cyanosis (right-sided lesions with right to left shunting), circulatory shock (left-sided lesions with obstruction), and signs of congestive heart failure (lesions producing large left to right shunting).

Cyanotic infant

Lesions where pulmonary blood flow is ductal-dependent often present in the first few hours after birth. Clinically, these conditions are characterized by minimal respiratory distress, fair to good distal perfusion, variable presence of a murmur, a failed hyperoxia test, an abnormal chest X-ray (decreased pulmonary vascular markings, abnormal cardiac contour), and minimal metabolic acidosis. While definitive treatment is surgical, preoperative management includes restoration of pulmonary blood flow via the ductus arteriosus with the institution of prostaglandin E_1. Due to prostaglandin's propensity to induce apnea and its potent vasoactive affects, careful attention to respiratory mechanics, gas exchange, and hemodynamics is essential.

Cardiogenic shock

Lesions which obstruct systemic blood flow increase in severity and become apparent with closure of the ductus arteriosus. As such, infants may present after newborn discharge with acute onset of cardiogenic shock. Clinically, obstructive left-sided lesions often present with signs of cardiogenic shock, including poor distal perfusion, ashen to mildly cyanotic color, respiratory distress, severe metabolic acidosis, variable hepatomegaly, variable murmur, and a chest X-ray with pulmonary venous congestion and cardiomegaly. The diagnosis requires a high index of suspicion in infants <4 months of age, as sepsis, myocarditis, and the shaken baby syndrome can also produce profound circulatory changes. The early use of prostaglandin (PGE_1) to reestablish systemic blood flow may be life-saving, while an inotrope infusion is often required for myocardial support.

Congestive heart failure

Lesions in which the natural fall in pulmonary vascular resistance leads to pulmonary over-circulation (pulmonary edema) may present in a delayed and/or indolent fashion. Clinically, infants with significant left to right shunts may present with subtle complaints (FTT, poor feeding, diaphoresis). moderate respiratory distress, hyperdynamic precordium usually with murmur, hepatomegaly, chest X-ray with cardiomegaly and increased pulmonary vascular markings, and right ventricular hypertrophy on ECG. See pp. 58–59 for the treatment of CHF.

Neurologic conditions

Infantile botulism

Infantile botulism (pp. 362–363) usually occurs in infants <6 months of age. The initial symptom is often constipation, followed by signs of a descending paralysis beginning with the cranial nerves. Bulbar findings include a weak cry, poor suck, and bilateral ptosis. Loss of airway reflexes coupled with progressive muscular hypotonia often leads to respiratory failure. Treatment remains mainly supportive, although human-derived botulism immune globulin is effective when started early in the course. Avoid giving drugs known to impede neuromuscular transmission (i.e. aminoglycosides).

Shaken baby syndrome

Physical abuse (pp. 580–581) is the leading cause of serious head injury in infants. The classic triad is seen in shaken infants: retinal hemorrhages, subdural hematomas and little, if any, sign of external trauma. Although, an infant who has been shaken can present with subtle symptoms, such as irritability and vomiting, the abused infant often presents with profound neurological dysfunction due to rising intracranial pressure. Respiratory failure and hemodynamic compromise are usually concomitant in such cases. If abusive head injury is suspected, obtain a complete skeletal survey and arrange for a dilated fundoscopic examination by a pediatric ophthalmologist, although these can be deferred until the patient is stable. However, on the first day, obtain photographs of any external injury, for the use in any future legal proceedings, and notify social services.

Hematologic disorders

Methemoglobinemia

Methemoglobin (MH) is produced when normal ferrous (2+) hemoglobin is oxidized to the ferric (3+) form. This leads to profound tissue hypoxia and acidosis because MH has a low affinity for O_2 and it causes a left shift in the oxyhemoglobin dissociation curve. Methemoglobinemia can be congenital due to deficiencies in MH reduction enzymes or from abnormal hemoglobin structure (Hgb M). More commonly, the disease is acquired due to an oxidant stress from an endogenous or exogenous source. Alteration in gut flora during a diarrheal illness in an infant may lead to overproduction of nitrite that may act as an oxidant stress. Exogenous oxidant stressors include analgesics (benzocaine), aniline derivatives (dyes, inks, polishes), sulfonamides, dapsone, and nitrite/nitrate-containing compounds (well water, nitroprusside, nitroglycerin, bismuth subnitrate).

Clinical manifestations vary according to the percent methemoglobin present, ranging from fatigue with brown mucous membranes (10–30%) to cyanosis, dyspnea, tachycardia, dizziness, and headache (30–50%), then profound acidosis, stupor, and seizures (50–70%). A concentration above 70% is fatal.

Suspect methemoglobinemia when evaluating a cyanotic infant without obvious cardiac or respiratory pathology (the infant will appear more cyanotic than pulse oximetry would predict). Cooximetry, which calculates the oxyhemoglobin saturation in the context of both reduced and abnormal hemoglobins (methemoglobin, carboxyhemoglobin), provides a more accurate saturation. There is a minimal response to oxygen therapy and the blood may appear brown in color. Blood gas analysis reveals a higher than expected pO_2, normal to low pCO_2, and profound metabolic acidosis. An elevated methemoglobin level confirms the diagnosis.

Start methylene blue (1-2 mg/kg of 1% solution) therapy if the MH level is >30% or the infant is progressively symptomatic. When possible, obtain a G6PD screen prior to initiating methylene blue, as in G6PD-deficient infants methylene blue may not be effective. Ascorbic acid (300 mg PO tid) is the treatment of choice in patients with G6PD deficiency.

Metabolic disorders

A metabolic crisis secondary to an inborn error of metabolism (IEM) is a rare, but serious, cause of a critically ill infant. Suspect an IEM in all such who present without an obvious etiology, especially if there is a positive family history of an IEM, sudden infant death, or consanguinity. The infant with an IEM may present with a history of poor feeding, vomiting, failure to thrive, tachypnea or hyperpnea without obvious pulmonary pathology, temperature instability, cardiomyopathy, or what seems to be a primary neurological disorder (lethargy, encephalopathy, seizures, hypo/hypertonia) or sepsis.

If an IEM is suspected, obtain blood for a CBC, glucose, electrolytes (calculate the anion gap), liver enzymes, simultaneous arterial pyruvate and lactate, ammonia, serum amino acids, and an ABG. Also send urine for ketones, reducing substances, and amino acids. Consult with a pediatric endocrinologist as treatment of a suspected IEM must commence prior to a definitive diagnosis. Initial management consists of correction of metabolic derangements (hypoglycemia, acidosis, electrolyte abnormalities) and prevention of further catabolism by providing adequate glucose and limiting protein intake.

Indication for admission

- Critically ill infant, generally to a pediatric intensive care unit unless the primary process was easily identified and stabilized in the emergency department

Bibliography

Brooks PA, Penny DJ: Management of the sick neonate with suspected heart disease. *Early Hum Dev* 2008;84:155-9.

Gerber P, Coffman K: Nonaccidental head trauma in infants. *Childs Nerv Syst* 2007;23:499-507.

Jeena PM, Adhikari M, Carlin JB, et al: Clinical profile and predictors of severe illness in young South African infants (<60 days). *S Afr Med J* 2008;98:883-8.

Kamboj M: Clinical approach to the diagnoses of inborn errors of metabolism. *Pediatr Clin North Am* 2008;55:1113-27.

Children with special healthcare needs (CSHCN)

Although only 13-18% of children have special healthcare needs, they are responsible for approximately 80% of pediatric healthcare costs. The complexity of their care often results in ED visits, and they are four times as likely to be hospitalized as children without disabilities. In addition, approximately 1 in 1000 CSHCN requires technology assistive care, and complications from these devices are often the reasons for ED visits.

DARES model for the evaluation of the child with special healthcare needs

Caring for CSHCN can be difficult for the ED physician, who must determine whether the chief complaint is a manifestation of the underlining diagnosis or a new acute problem. In addition, there are over 800 congenital syndromes responsible for childhood disability, so it is impossible for any one physician to be familiar with every aspect of a given disease. It is therefore critical for the ED physician to communicate effectively with parents, while obvious inexperience with a CSHCN may make a parent less trusting. The American Academy of Pediatrics advocates using the "DARES" model for communicating with families of CSHCN patients:

D: Describe

Allow the parent to describe what is wrong with their child and what prompted the ED visit. The patient's medical baseline may be much different than a normal healthy child, while the parents may have extensive knowledge about and experience with their child's medical care and disease process. They may have previously encountered the current problem and have unorthodox solutions. A physician who has no prior knowledge of this child may inadvertently attempt "standard care" without considering previous successful treatment.

Also, communication with the child who has special needs is an important part of the ED evaluation, but many CSHCN have neuromuscular or expressive disorders. It is essential for the ED physician to recognize this and communicate with the child in a manner that is appropriate for age and disability.

A: Avoid arguing

The family may be frustrated with their caregivers or angry about traveling to the ED. They may have had unsatisfactory previous experiences in the ED or received misinformation about the disease. Also, they may have a special relationship with their primary physician and may be reluctant to trust others.

R: Roll with resistance

Be patient when families are in stressful situations, as they may not be very receptive to ideas, suggestions, or treatment plans.

E: Express empathy

Acknowledge the family's feeling of frustration and reassure them that you have their child's best interests in mind.

S: Social services

While in the DARES model "S" is for "support self-efficacy," here it is used to mean "social services." The ED social worker may be able to identify external sources of support that can assist in some of the needs for the child. Remember that children with chronic disabilities are at increased risk for neglect, physical abuse, and sexual abuse. Often the care of these children is so overwhelming for a caregiver that any neglect is unintentional.

Review of systems

For CSHCN, perform a more extensive review of systems, including a functional history. This may provide valuable information as to possible causes of the acute problem.

Constitutional

Is there weight loss, weight gain, chills, or fever? At baseline, does your child have an unusually high or low temperature?

FEN

How does your child eat, orally or through a gastrostomy/jejunostomy tube? If so what is the feeding schedule, how much time is needed for a feeding, and have there been any changes in appetite? Does the child cough or choke after eating? Is the child gaining weight?

Respiratory

Are there any changes in breathing patterns? When did this occur? Has your child ever had a pneumonia, and if so, how often?

Sleep

Does your child sleep through the night? If not, how often does he or she awaken? Does your child have frequent nightmares or awaken with headaches? Does he or she awaken well rested?

Gastrointestinal

What is his or her usual bowel regimen and stooling pattern and have there been any recent changes?

Neurology

Have there been any changes in muscle tone, range of motion, strength, sensation, or seizure pattern?

Functional history

Since your child has been ill, has he or she lost the ability to perform any actions or participate in activities?

Equipment

What equipment does your child have at home (wheelchair, car seat, bath chair, etc.)? How old are they and are they in good condition?

Mobility

How does your child move around the house, school, or community?

Hygiene

Who bathes your child and how is it performed? Are there any ulcers or areas of skin breakdown?

Medications

Many CSHCN receive multiple medications, prescribed by different providers, with very little coordination. When taking a medication history, be sure to include the following:

- Have any medications recently been added or discontinued and if so, why?
- What is the current dosage of the medications and have there been any recent changes?
- Is your child currently able to take all his or her medications?
- Have you recently exhausted the supply of any of the medications?
- Is your child taking any vitamin supplements, herbal supplements, or over-the-counter medications?

Enterostomy tubes

Many CSHCN require an enterostomy tube because of oral motor problems, dysphagia, inadequate calorie intake, unpalatable medications, or severe aspiration. Tubes are classified as gastrostomy, gastrojejunostomy or jejunostomy, depending upon the location of the distal end. Advise the parents to keep a detailed record of their child's current tube size and type in order to facilitate any future replacements.

Dislodgement

Dislodgement is the most common reason a family will visit the ED for a GT or JT. This may occur due to trauma, tension on the tube, rupture of the balloon, or unintentional balloon deflation. A feeding tube may also malfunction due to deterioration over time or obstruction. If an excessive time has elapsed prior to the family seeking medical attention, the stoma may have constricted. To avoid this, do not delay replacement while seeking the correct size replacement tube. If the proper-size feeding tube is unavailable, insert a Foley catheter to stent the stoma until a replacement can be obtained. Or, if the stoma is partially closed, use a series of progressively larger Foleys in order to dilate it.

Early dislodgement

Dislodgement in the first 4 weeks after insertion is the most common complication of feeding tubes. A tract for the tube will begin to mature within 7–10 days, although it may not be complete for up to 3 months. However, if a tube dislodges within the first 2–4 weeks, there is a risk that the stomach may separate from the anterior abdominal wall, so that blindly reinserting a new feeding tube may result in placing it within the peritoneal cavity. Using aseptic technique, stent the site with a replacement tube, then contact the service that originally inserted the feeding tube (i.e. GI, pediatric surgery, interventional radiology). Do not use the feeding tube at this point. Instead, place an NG tube while awaiting consultation.

Later dislodgement

If the dislodged tube was from an older stoma, immediately replace it with either a Foley catheter or an appropriate-sized replacement tube. Lubricate the distal end with petroleum jelly using aseptic technique. Reinsert the tube carefully to avoid placing it into the peritoneal cavity through a false tract.

After a GT has been reinserted, check for proper placement by first aspirating the tube to obtain gastric fluid, then injecting 10–15 mL of air while listening over the stomach for borborygmi. The tube is ready to be used if both of these maneuvers are positive; inflate the balloon with sterile water (not saline). Otherwise, obtain an abdominal film with water-soluble contrast to confirm the location of the tube. Abdominal pain upon balloon inflation is an indication of improper position; remove the tube and retry. Apply an abdominal binder or a loose-fitting ace bandage wrap to secure the enterostomy tube flush against the stomach and to reduce the risk of recurrent dislodgement. A dislodged JT must be replaced by either interventional radiology or surgery, as there is a risk of subsequent ischemia and bowel necrosis.

Removing a GT

Generally, there is no reason to remove a GT in the emergency department. If it is necessary, use a 20 mL syringe to deflate the balloon prior to removing the tube. Some tubes have an internal bumper. In order to determine whether or not the child has an internal bumper or a balloon, inspect the outer ports. If the port is meant for inflating a balloon it is typically white and labeled with the volume of fluid needed to maintain the balloon. If the situation remains uncertain, use a syringe and aspirate the contents of the port.

Other complications

Skin irritation

A frequent complaint is redness or bleeding around the tube site due to leakage, tape sensitivity, infection, or granulation tissue. If the tube is not properly secured against the skin, the stoma may become widened over time and gastric contents can leak around the tube. It is important to determine whether leakage is caused from a defect in the tube itself, or from gastric contents refluxing around the tube. Shield the skin from leaking gastric contents with a plastic barrier (i.e. Tegaderm), or a barrier agent, such as sucrulfate, hydrocolloid agents, or zinc oxide. Add an antacid to the feeding regimen to increase the pH of the leaking gastric contents, and refer the patient to the primary physician for further care.

Occlusion

Gastrostomy tube occlusion may occur in up to 45% of patients, secondary to kinking or obstruction of the lumen by the accumulation of formula or medications. The usual complaint is an inability to flush the tube or infuse liquid into it. Attempt to flush the tube with sterile water using a 30 mL, or larger, syringe to avoid excessive pressure. Use 20–30 mL of warm water to unclog PEG tubes. If conservative measures fail, replace the gastrostomy tube or use a Foley catheter of equal size. However, as noted above, newly placed gastrostomy tubes, as well as jejunostomy tubes, and nasoenteric tubes may be difficult to replace. In these cases, consult the appropriate subspecialist and do not remove the tube.

Granulation tissue

Granulation formation around the tube is a common complaint. While these areas are usually painless and only rarely become infected or cause obstruction of the stoma, on occasion they may bleed. Apply warm saline compresses and cauterize with silver nitrate. Then apply a topical antibiotic cream and dress with sterile gauze.

Vomiting

Although vomiting is a common problem in children, it is rarely related to an enterostomy tube. However, vomiting may be secondary to balloon migration causing duodenal obstruction.

Local infection

Approximately 20% of patients will experience a local infection after placement of an enterostomy tube. Although most infections are minor, there is a small risk of progression to a necrotizing fasciitis. See Cellulitis (pp. 99–100) for the treatment of a local infection in a nontoxic-appearing patient.

Buried bumper

Buried bumper syndrome occurs when the internal bumper erodes through the stomach wall with subsequent reepithelialization which covers or buries the bumper. Often this is a result of excess traction on the enterostomy tube. It usually presents as resistance to flow or vomiting and/or abdominal pain during feedings. Suspect a buried bumper if the tube cannot be freely rotated. Consult a surgeon or gastroenterologist to plan removal and replacement of the tube.

Tracheostomy

Tracheostomy tubes are sized according to three dimensions: the inner diameter, the outer diameter, and the length. Regardless of the manufacturer, the inner diameter is consistent among manufacturers and it is always imprinted on the flange. In contrast, outer diameters and lengths are not consistent and may or may not be printed on the tube. If a patient requires a tracheostomy change, use a tube with similar dimensions. If the replacement does not fit in the stoma it may be a consequence of the outer dimensions, so it may be necessary to select a smaller size tube. Before replacing a tracheostomy, have a smaller-size back-up available in case you are unable to successfully reinsert the original.

The proper tube diameter optimizes airway resistance and limits the risk of aspiration, without irritating the mucosa or damaging the airway wall. Typically, the outer diameter is <2/3 of the tracheal diameter and the end of the tube is >2 cm beyond the stoma, but no closer than 1–2 cm from the carina. To prevent esophageal obstruction, tracheo-esophageal fistula, or a tracheo-innominate artery fistula, use a curved tube to ensure that the distal end is concentric and parallel to the trachea. The standard pediatric tracheostomy tube has a 15 mm connector at the proximal end that allows for a connection to a bag mask or a ventilator. However, a metal tube does not have this adapter.

A tracheostomy tube may be cuffed or uncuffed. Limited indications for a cuffed tube in the pediatric population include chronic aspiration or a child who requires high positive pressure for ventilation. The patient cannot speak with the cuff inflated.

The tracheal lumen may be fenestrated or nonfenestrated. A fenestrated tracheostomy tube is usually reserved for patients who are able to speak and may require intermittent mechanical ventilation.

Complications

Bleeding

Any bleeding from the tracheostomy site requires an endoscopic evaluation of the airway. If the tip of the tracheostomy tube rests against the tracheal wall it may cause irritation, inflammation, and ulceration with bleeding. This tends to be more common in patients receiving mechanical ventilation. If the erosion occurs on the anterior tracheal wall it has the potential of causing a hemorrhage of the innominate artery, which typically lies 9–12 rings below the cricoid cartilage. This is a potentially life-threatening event and a surgical emergency which presents with a pulsating tracheostomy tube, bleeding around the tracheostomy site, or massive hemoptysis. If an innominate artery hemorrhage is suspected, do not remove the tracheostomy, as it may be the only way to ensure an adequate airway. If the patient does have a cuffed tracheostomy, overinflating the cuff may help to tamponade the bleeding.

Infection

Patients with a tracheostomy, especially those requiring ventilatory support, are at high risk for infections involving the stoma and lower respiratory tract. A patient with a neuromuscular disease is at particularly high risk. In general, a tracheostomy is usually colonized with potential pathogens including *Pseudomonas aeruginosa, Streptococcus* species, *Staphylococcus aureus, Haemophilus influenza,* and *Candida albicans.* Signs of an acute infection include a change from the baseline respiratory status, fever, tachypnea, increased oxygen requirement, changes in tracheal secretions, cough, or accessory muscle use. Minor bleeding may also be a sign of infection if accompanied by other symptoms.

Tracheoesophageal fistula

A tracheo-esophageal fistula can occur when the posterior wall of the trachea is exposed to chronic pressure from the tip of the tracheostomy. This is potentially life-threatening because of bacterial contamination of the tracheobronchial airway. Symptoms include more copious secretions, new or increased aspiration of food contents, dyspnea, cuff leak, or gastric distention. The diagnosis can be made with a CT scan or barium esophagography. Treatment is usually surgical.

Granuloma formation

This is the most frequent complication of a tracheostomy and can be caused by frictional trauma from the tube, inflammation from stasis of secretions, infection, poor tube position, or traumatic suction technique. Granulomas are most common just superior to the internal stoma site on the anterior tracheal wall, but may also be seen along the posterior tracheal wall. Up to 80% of pediatric tracheostomies develop suprastomal granulation tissue, but the majority are small and asymptomatic and require no intervention. Large granulomas may cause bleeding and may delay decannulation or pose an obstruction for recannulation after accidental decannulation. Treat granulation tissue along the external stoma with silver nitrate.

Stenosis

Stenotic lesions are classified according to their anatomical sites, including suprastomal, stomal, cuff, and at the tip of the cannula. Most patients with tracheal stenosis remain asymptomatic until the original tracheal lumen diameter is reduced by 50–75% or the actual diameter is <5 mm. Symptoms include cough, inability to clear secretions, and dyspnea.

Skin breakdown and ulcers

Pressure ulcers are common in patients who are immobilized, wheelchair-dependent, or have insensate skin. Other predisposing factors are fecal or urinary incontinence, chronic steroid use, muscle atrophy, elevated tissue temperatures, chronic malnutrition, and improper transfer techniques. In addition, many CSHCN are malnourished due to oral motor control issues, predisposing them to pressure ulcers. The most affected areas are bony prominences, such as the sacrum, greater trochanter, and ischial tuberosity. Younger children are also at risk for developing skin ulcers over the occipital region. Ulcers can lead to sepsis and osteomyelitis. Use the Shea Classification to assess skin breakdown (Table 28-2).

When evaluating skin breakdown, document the anatomical location, Shea stage, length, width, depth, type of tissue present at the wound base and its color, presence of exudate (none, minimum, moderate, large amount), and odor. Note whether there is undermining (destruction beneath intact tissue) or tunneling at the wound base, which can create dead space and lead to abscess formation. Several factors may interfere with an accurate

Table 28-2. Shea Classification of skin ulcers

Grade	Findings
I	Involve the superficial epidermis and dermal layers
	Nonblanchable erythema with edema, warmth, induration, or discoloration
	Red discoloration in lighter skin; blue or purple in darker skin
II	Partial thickness epidermal or skin loss that extends through the epidermis and upper dermis
	May appear as a blister, abrasion, or superficial ulceration
III	Full thickness deficit with extension into the subcutaneous tissue
	Does not extend into the fascia
IV	Wound extends to the muscle, tendon, bone and/or joint structures
	Complications include osteomyelitis, dislocations or fractures
	Also assess for undermining

assessment, including the presence of either an eschar or copious necrotic material. Necrosis may begin deeper within the tissue at the bony prominence. Also, multiple ulcers within a limited area may be indicative of interconnecting fistula tracts.

Clean the wound to remove the necrotic, devitalized tissue and exudate while minimizing trauma to the wound bed. First, irrigate with a 30–35 mL syringe attached to an 18- or 19- gauge needle (delivers 8 pounds per square inch). Use normal saline, but do not add an antiseptic solution, which may be cytotoxic. Debridement is then necessary if there is a fibrinous exudate. Use either mechanical debridement, with wet to dry dressings, or enzymatic debridement, with a topical medication containing collegenase (i.e. Santyl). Use calcium alginate, foam, or hydrogel dressing (Table 28-3) for exudative wounds.

Wound cultures are not useful, as most wounds above Stage I are colonized with bacteria. Arrange for daily cleansing and dressing changes to help control colonization as wound healing will not occur if the bacterial count is too high. Give antibiotics only if there is a cellulitis (erythema and warmth) or the patient has signs of a systemic infection (fever, chills, toxicity). If a wound infection is suspected, consult a burn specialist or dermatologist to perform a wound biopsy or obtain fluid via needle aspiration. A bacterial count $>10^5$/gram of tissue indicates an infection. Prescribe topical mupirocin, bacitracin, or polymixin, all of which are effective against Gram-negative and Gram-positive organisms.

Dressing selection

Wounds heal better in a moist environment, which enhances cell migration, granulation tissue formation, and WBC effectiveness. Select a dressing (Table 28-3) which provides an appropriate environment while managing the amount of exudate that the wound is producing. Use these guidelines as a framework to provide temporary care measures until the patient can be evaluated by a wound management expert. All pressure ulcers require close follow-up, as superficial-appearing wounds may reflect a deeper injury.

For Stage I and II ulcers, use transparent film, hydrocolloid, or foam. For Stage III and IV wounds, use calcium alginate, foam, or hydrogel, but obtain surgical consultation to

Table 28-3. Wound dressings

Dressing type	Properties	Brand names
Hydrocolloid	Forms occlusive gel by interacting with wound barrier	Duoderm
	Provides barrier to external contaminates	Replicare
	Use with low to moderate exudates	Tegasorb
	Provides autolytic debridement	Duoderm gel
	Do not use with infected wounds	
Hydrogel	Use with minimal to moderate exudates	Solosite
	Promotes autolytic debridement of devitalized tissue/eschar	Vigilion
	Maintains moist environment	
	May ease pain and inflammation	
Film dressing	Use on skin tears	Bio Occlusive
	Use on wounds with little or no drainage	Tegaderm
	Allows water and oxygen into wound, keeps bacteria out	
	If too much exudates in wound it will interfere with evaporation and oxygen diffusion and cause maceration	
Foam dressing	Absorbs moderate to heavy exudates	Polymem
	Nonadherent	Allevyn
Calcium alginates	Fibers absorb exudates and convert into a gel, providing moisture for healing	Kaltostat
	Absorbs moderate to heavy drainage	
	Controls minor bleeding	
	Provides a moist healing environment	
	Use under a dressing (ABD pad, gauze or transparent film)	
Enzymatic debriding agents	Will chemically lyse necrotic tissue	Santyl
	Must use within moist environment	Biozyme
	Reassess frequently to ensure healthy tissue is intact	

determine whether inpatient management is needed. When applying a dressing leave at least a 1–1½ inch margin around the wound. Also, remove the weight load from the injured area. Limit the use of an orthotic device that may be causing pressure and refer the patient to the orthotist to modify or fabricate a new orthosis. If the ulcer is in an area of pressure, use a hydrocolloid dressing (i.e. duoderm) to protect the skin. Review with the parents the proper techniques for preventing wounds, including recognizing potential skin hazards such as radiators, car heaters, hair dryers, and hot plates placed in laps. In the summer, warn parents about hot sidewalks, metal storm drains, and hot sand. Teach proper positioning, including weight shifts every 15–20 minutes for 30 seconds while sitting, and bed turns every 2 hours. Encourage the patient to participate in wound checks and arrange for the patient to see either the primary care provider or a local skin specialist (i.e. physiatrist, plastic surgeon) the next day.

Neurogenic bladder

A child with a spinal cord injury or spina bifida with resultant neurogenic bladder is at increased risk of developing a urinary tract infection due to incomplete voiding, elevated intravesical pressure, and catheter use. An indwelling catheter is the most important risk factor, while repeated antibiotic exposure increases the likelihood of resistant organisms.

For patients with neurogenic bladders, significant bacteriuria is defined as $>10^2$ CFU/mL for catheter specimens from patients with intermittent catheterization; $>10^4$ CFU/mL for clean void specimens from catheter-free males using condom catheter devices; or any detectable growth from patients with indwelling catheters or from a suprapubic aspirate. Patients often reuse their catheters, which may become colonized with bacteria and then yield confusing results. Therefore, use a clean catheter to obtain culture specimens. If the patient has an indwelling catheter replace it before collecting a specimen. Since chronic catheterization may cause pyuria in the absence of a UTI, use 50 WBC/hpf in an unspun urine to suggest a UTI.

Signs and symptoms suggestive of a urinary tract infection (pp. 664–665) include fever, pain over the bladder or kidney, urinary incontinence, increase in spasticity, cloudy urine with increased odor, malaise, lethargy, feelings of anxiety, or autonomic dysreflexia.

Autonomic dysreflexia

Autonomic dysreflexia is a life-threatening syndrome characterized by excessive uncontrolled sympathetic output below the level of a spinal cord injury, particularly in patients whose injury level is above T6. A noxious stimulus causes an afferent impulse along an intact spinal reflex mechanism below the level of injury, leading to hypertension. Above the level of lesion there is an excess of parasympathetic output that results in peripheral vasodilatation that often results in the symptoms that are used to characterize this condition. The most common causes of autonmomic dysreflexia include bladder distention, fecal impaction, pressure sores, infection (UTI most common), ingrown toenails, fractures, hemorrhoids, heterotopic ossification, and hip dislocation. Less common triggrs include menstruation, appendicitis, gallstones, urinary stones, delivery, syringomyelia, testicular torsion, DVTs, and pulmomary emboli. Medications such as nasal decongestants, methylphenidate, or illicit drugs such as cocaine may also produce these symptoms.

Clinical presentation

The presenting symptoms include hypertension, pounding headache, sweating above the level of injury, bradycardia or tachycardia, piloerection, blurred vision, and anxiety. In the infant or young child there may be sleepiness or irritability. If unrecognized, the hypertensive episodes can lead to retinal hemorrhage, stroke, subarachnoid hemorrhages, seizures, and cardiac arrhythmias (including atrial fibrillation).

When evaluating a child or young adult with a spinal cord injury it is important to recognize that resting blood pressure is lower due to decreased tone below the level of the injury. The median systolic blood pressure for a patient with a spinal cord injury is (90 + [age in years $\times$ 2]). A systolic blood pressure of 150 mmHg or 20–40 mmHg above baseline is consistent with autonomic dysreflexia.

ED management

Obtain IV access and place the patient on a cardiac monitor. Sitting the patient upright, with the legs dangling off the stretcher, will cause an othostatic decrease in blood pressure. Loosen the patient's clothing and remove TED hose or abdominal binder, if present. Catheterize the bladder, but first apply lidocaine jelly. If there is an indwelling catheter check for obstructions and either irrigate it or replace it. If the blood pressure is labile, apply 2% nitropaste ½–1 inch above the level of the injury. If the above measures do not decrease the blood pressure, add nifedipine (0.25–0.5 mg/kg, maximum 10 mg), using the bite and swallow method rather than sublingually, which can cause rebound hypotension. If symptoms persist, manually disimpact the bowel, but use lidocaine jelly first. Consult with a neurologist and admit the patient if symptoms persist and no precipitant is found that can be successfully addressed in the ED.

Spina bifida

Spina bifida is the second most common disability in children. It results from incomplete closure of the neural tube during fetal development, and is often associated with other abnormalities of the brain, spinal cord, and other mesodermal structures (such as the bones and kidneys). These are typically the precipitating cause for an ED visit.

Hydrocephalus

Hydrocephalus occurs in approximately 90% of children with spina bifida, usually secondary to an Arnold Chiari type II malformation. The clinical presentation is usually obvious with mental status changes, seizures, or vocal cord paralysis with stridor. However, sometimes signs can be more subtle with changes in school performance, chronic cough, sleep apnea, periodic breathing, or aspiration.

Tethered cord

Most children who have spina bifida will have a tethered cord, which refers to an abnormal attachment of the spinal cord at its distal end, below the normal L1–L2 anatomic position. In the majority of cases this is asymptomatic and will not require treatment. However, in some children, growth is associated with increased tension on the cord. This can cause back pain radiating to the legs, especially with neck flexion. There may also be functional deficits, such as changes in lower extremity strength and function, upper extremity strength, bowel or bladder function, or muscle tone and/or spasticity. Other symptoms include paresthesias and rapid progression of scoliosis. If a tethered cord is suspected, consult with neurosurgery and order an MRI. Emergency release may be needed for severe symptoms, such as bowel or bladder changes, sensory changes, loss of function, or a marked increase in scoliosis.

Syringomyelia

Syringomyelia is a tubular cavitation that can occur anywhere in the spinal cord, often in the cervical area, but also in the medulla or pons. Early signs include rapidly progressive scoliosis and unexplained vertebral abnormalities. It is also correlated with progressive upper motor and lower motor neuron defects, loss of upper extremity function, wasting of hand intrinsic muscles, and sensory dysfunction. Arrange for an MRI and consult with neurosurgery.

Latex allergy

Approximately 60% of children with spina bifida have a latex allergy. Therefore, assume that the patient is allergic until proven otherwise, and avoid contact with medical supplies that contain latex. In addition, there can be cross-reactions after a sensitized child eats bananas, avocados, or water chestnuts, which can then cause anaphylaxis of unknown etiology in children with spina bifida.

Neurogenic bladder

Nearly all children with spina bifida have a neurogenic bladder, either an upper motor neuron bladder (spastic) which is large with a strong urinary stream, or a lower motor neuron bladder (hypotonic) which is associated with a history of dribbling. The resultant urinary retention places them at increased risk of UTIs.

Bibliography

Eber E, Oberwaldner B: Tracheostomy care in the hospital. *Paediatr Respir Rev* 2006; 7:175–84.

Goldson E, Louch G, Washington K, Scheu H: Guidelines for the care of the child with special health care needs. *Adv Pediatr* 2006;53:165–82.

Rowe DE, Jadhav AL: Care of the adolescent with spina bifida. *Pediatr Clin North Am* 2008;55:1359–74.

Srivastava R, Stone BL, Murphy NA: Hospitalist care of the medically complex child. *Pediatr Clin North Am* 2005;52:1165–87.

Failure to thrive

Failure to thrive (FTT) represents an inability to maintain appropriate growth for age. It is essentially a sign of undernutrition, and not a diagnosis per se. By definition, a patient <2 years of age is found to have a weight that is <3rd percentile for age (or <80% of the ideal weight for age) or has a history of crossing two major percentiles (90th, 75th, 50th, 25th, 10th, and 5th) downward on a standardized growth chart. While weight is the usual concern, in severe cases height and head circumference can also be affected. The possible etiologies of FTT can be divided into four major categories (Table 28-4), although a patient may have more than one problem contributing to growth failure.

Clinical presentation
Inadequate caloric intake
Lack of appetite

This usually occurs in the toddler age group. The parents report a refusal of foods and frustration with their inability to get their child to eat. Psychosocial stressors, including lack of food/resources, domestic violence, and parental mental illness can play an important

Table 28-4. Differential diagnosis of failure to thrive

Diagnosis	Possible etiologies
Inadequate caloric intake	
Lack of appetite	Anemia
	Psychosocial
	Chronic infection
Unavailability of calories	Insufficient food
	Inappropriate feeding
	Withholding of food
Difficulty ingesting calories	Craniofacial anomaly
	CNS disorder, cerebral palsy, mental retardation
	Tracheoesophageal fistula
	Oral motor dysfunction
Vomiting	CNS pathology
	Gastrointestinal obstruction
	Gastroesophageal reflux
Inadequate calorie absorption	
Malabsorption	Celiac disease
	Food allergies
Diarrhea	Infection
Increased calorie requirements	
Increased metabolism	Chronic infection
	Malignancy
	Endocrine disease
	Toxins (lead)
	Cardiopulmonary disease
Inefficient use of calories	Metabolic disorder
	Diabetes mellitus
	Renal tubular acidosis

role. Anemia, lead poisoning, and chronic infections (recurrent otitis media) may also contribute to poor appetite.

Difficulty ingesting

Infants with congenital anomalies, such as cleft palate or choanal atresia, as well as toddlers with poor dentition or severe tonsillar hypertrophy may have difficulty ingesting adequate calories. Dyspnea due to congestive heart failure or bronchopulmonary dysplasia can interfere with oral intake. The parents may report that the patient seems to be exhausted during feeds and needs to rest frequently. Neurodevelopmental problems such as cerebral palsy and oral motor dysfunction are some of the most common causes of FTT. In such a case, growth may be adequate the first 6–8 months, then FTT develops after solid foods are introduced. The child often has difficulty with textures, and finds solid foods aversive, thereby making eating an unpleasant experience. The parents report prolonged mealtimes and a preference for liquids. The patient commonly also presents with speech and language delays. An infant who was critically ill and therefore not given oral feeds during the first months of life may have difficulty acquiring oral feeding skills.

Recurrent vomiting

Gastroesophageal reflux with subsequent esophagitis can lead to refusal to eat because of pain upon swallowing. The parents may report irritability and grimacing with feeds, but there may not be a history of frank vomiting. Increased ICP of any etiology can cause recurrent vomiting leading to inadequate intake. Gastrointestinal obstruction in an infant (pyloric stenosis, malrotation) can present as poor weight gain and recurrent vomiting. The infant typically appears very hungry since appetite is unaffected.

Lack of available calories

Inadequate availability of calories is a common cause of FTT, and may be due to economic problems, stresses within the family, mental health problems (maternal depression leading to neglect), and intentional abuse. Improper breast-feeding technique or mixing of formula and feeding primarily foods that are nutritionally empty ('junk food') can result in inadequate calorie intake.

Inadequate calorie absorption

Once ingested, foods may be inadequately digested, malabsorbed, or eliminated too rapidly. Malabsorption generally presents with a history of failure to grow accompanied by chronic diarrhea. Enzyme deficiencies, severe food allergies, and celiac disease are possible etiologies. The parents may be able to correlate onset of symptoms with introduction of specific foods. Cystic fibrosis can cause malabsorption, usually in association with other manifestations of the disease, but FTT may be the initial presentation. Inflammatory bowel disease can also lead to chronic malnutrition through malabsorption. Diarrhea due to bacterial or parasitic infection can interfere with nutritional uptake by shortening transit time as well as consumption of nutrients by the parasites. Hepatic dysfunction secondary to biliary atresia, cirrhosis, or hepatitis can also result in malabsorption of nutrients.

Increased calorie requirements

Conditions that cause increased metabolic rate or inefficient use of calories resulting in FTT typically are secondary to a disorder that is not difficult to diagnose. Chronic infection with TB or HIV, malignancy, hyperthyroidism, chronic cardiac or pulmonary disease, metabolic diseases, renal tubular acidosis, and diabetes mellitus can all cause defective or inefficient use of calories and subsequent FTT.

Diagnosis

Obtain a complete, detailed history, including a feeding history: adequacy of breast-feeding, formula preparation, amounts consumed, feeding techniques, child's feeding behaviors, what types of food the child can and cannot tolerate, timing of solid foods, introduction, and any parentally imposed dietary restrictions such as no sugar, no fat, or vegan diet. Ask about the perinatal and developmental history (prematurity, delayed oral feeds, IUGR, congenital infections, developmental milestones, child's temperament), psychosocial history (ability to buy food, household stresses such as illness or domestic violence, history of abuse or neglect, environmental exposure to lead or other toxins, and travel to areas with high rates of intestinal parasites, TB, or hepatitis). Ask about the details of the FTT, including the age of onset and rate of growth deceleration, and history of diarrhea, vomiting, food intolerance, and recurrent infections.

On physical examination, observe a feeding to assess the quality of child and caregiver interaction, the quality of suck/swallow, abnormal use of tongue and lips, aversion to oral stimulation, and any evidence of pain during or after feeding. Plot the weight, height, and head circumference on an appropriate, gender-specific growth chart. Whenever possible, include previous measurements to assess changes in growth velocity. Examine an infant for dysmorphic features and congenital facial anomalies. Check the oral cavity of a toddler, looking for dental caries and tonsillar hypertrophy. Other priorities on physical examination are the cardiopulmonary (tachypnea, cyanosis, murmur, rales, hepatosplenomegaly), gastrointestinal (hepatomegaly, jaundice), neurologic (micro- or macrocephaly, asymmetry) examinations as well as signs of abuse or neglect (unexplained bruises or burns, poor hygiene, inappropriate behavior).

Laboratory testing is very unlikely to establish a diagnosis in the absence of specific abnormalities noted on history or physical examination. If no probable diagnosis is suggested, obtain a limited battery of routine laboratory tests (CBC, urinalysis, urine culture, serum electrolytes, and a TB skin test) to reassure the family that there is no immediate life-threatening pathology. Further tests, such as a sweat test, chest radiograph, or stool analysis, are indicated only if history or physical examination suggest a particular diagnosis.

The majority of cases of FTT in infants and toddlers represent "failure to feed," secondary to the provision of inadequate food (quantity or quality) or improper feeding technique. In such a case, the best diagnostic test is hospital admission, with feeding supervised or performed by the nursing staff. Appropriate weight gain while under close supervision confirms the diagnosis; however, this may require up to 7–10 days.

ED management

The goal of ED management is to rule out the presence of an immediately life-threatening condition, assess the severity of the malnutrition, and ensure that adequate outpatient services (medical subspecialist, speech or occupational therapist, nutritionist, family support services) and follow-up with a primary provider are arranged. As noted above, the results of a thorough history and physical usually indicate the diagnostic and therapeutic course to follow.

Follow-up

- Primary care or subspecialty follow-up in 3–5 days

Indications for admission

- Infant <4 months with FTT
- Severe malnutrition or ill appearance
- Underlying disease which requires hospitalization
- Suspicion of abuse or neglect in a child with moderate or severe malnutrition
- Poor response to outpatient evaluation and therapy

Bibliography

Bergman P, Graham J: An approach to "failure to thrive". *Aust Fam Physician* 2005;34:725–9.

Olsen EM: Failure to thrive: still a problem of definition. *Clin Pediatr(Phila)* 2006;45:1–6.

Stephens MB, Gentry BC, Michener MD, Kendall SK, Gauer R: Clinical inquiries. What is the clinical workup for failure to thrive? *J Fam Pract* 2008;57:264–6.

Telephone triage

Parents and caregivers may call the ED to obtain information and advice regarding an acute or chronic illness, clarify prior explanations or instructions, review medication-related issues, and ask questions about primary care. Skillful triage can prevent unnecessary visits while ensuring ill patients receive appropriate and timely care.

Priorities

Calls must be prioritized, with possible life-threatening situations handled immediately by activation of the 911 system. In particular, keep an acutely suicidal or intoxicated caller on the line while help is summoned. Handle urgent calls (e.g. fever in a young infant) next, followed by non-urgent calls to be returned in the order received.

Protocols

As telephone triage duties are often delegated by the physician to other medical staff, the use of established protocols enables the triager to give targeted advice, while minimizing variability among personnel. Selecting the appropriate protocol is a critical step in the telephone triage process. Employing an incorrect protocol can lead to serious errors in evaluation and disposition. Telephone protocols are symptom-driven. Therefore, to use the protocols properly, the main concern of the caller must be identified expeditiously. When there are multiple complaints, it is useful to focus on the one with the highest likelihood of requiring an office or ED visit. Ask the caller which symptom or complaint is of most concern, then use the most specific protocol available. Inquire about each symptom, from the most serious or significant to the least urgent, as well as any associated complaints (for example, is diarrhea associated with decreased urine output?). A positive response to one of the protocol questions may place the patient into a specific triage category and expedite the patient's care.

Demographic and basic information

When conducting a telephone interview, obtain demographic information: patient's name, caller's name and relationship to the patient (is this the mother of the child or the babysitter, who may be unaware of past medical history?), patient's age and approximate weight (for medication advice), and callback number. Past medical history or birth history (for a newborn) is vital, as it may change the advice and triage disposition.

Interview technique

When conducting a telephone interview, it is helpful to have a quiet area, so the triager can concentrate and the caller is not asked to repeat information. Callers are often stressed, and differences in educational level and cultural idiosyncrasies affect the ability of the triager to give, and the caller to understand, telephone advice. Telephone triage is a subtle balance of listening and inquiring, with the triager guiding the caller to serve as the "eyes and ears" in order to focus the interview and reach a timely conclusion. Ask the caller to measure a lesion or compare it to a known object (such as a coin) or to gently touch a painful or injured area to elicit the child's response. If there is cough, noisy breathing, or respiratory distress, have the caller hold the phone in front of the patient for 30–60 seconds. However, do not accept the caller's suggested diagnosis (i.e. croup, streptococcal pharyngitis) unless it clearly meets diagnostic criteria.

In addition to the fact that the typical visual clues used to assess severity of illness are not available, there may be a language or cultural barrier or an evasive or uninformed caller. Therefore, pay special attention to aural cues, such as tone of voice, rapidity of speech, and the manner in which questions are answered. With experience, the triager can become adept at sensing that "something doesn't sound right." In such a case, request that the caller bring the patient to the ED.

Disposition

By interviewing the caller, using protocols as guidelines to ask focused, selected questions, and evaluating the information obtained, the triager can establish a working diagnosis. The triager can then place the patient into a disposition category, thus directing the child to the level of care best suited to the current need. Depending on the practice setting and the acuity and severity of the complaints, these categories include immediate activation of the 911 emergency response system, seeing the patient immediately, referring the patient to the primary care setting later that day, giving an appointment for a future time, or giving home care advice. However, both the triager and the caller can elect to move a patient to a more urgent disposition, advising or requesting that a child be seen despite negative responses to "be seen" indicators. Examples include symptoms in a very young infant, a patient with multiple or vague complaints, significant past medical history, multiple previous telephone calls for the same illness, or if no protocol can be found that pertains to the patient. "Up-triaging" is medically harmless. In contrast, be cautious about "down-triaging" a patient to a less urgent disposition (i.e. agreeing with a caller that an ill child can remain home despite the triager's medical judgment that the symptoms warrant a visit) and ensure that a clear follow-up plan is in place.

Home care

Home care can be arranged for patients not needing a visit or who will be seen at a later time. Ask about any treatments or remedies the caller may have already tried and how they are working; if appropriate, encourage the caller to continue. Change or add to the home treatments if they are incomplete or inadequate based on the recommendations in the protocol. When the treatment or remedy being used is potentially harmful, be nonjudgmental but firm in recommending a change. A phrase such as "I suggest you do not do that; try this instead," is useful.

It is helpful to have the caller write down the information, especially if medication dosages will be given. Give three or four instructions or recommendations consisting of two or three sentences each. Be clear when moving from one instruction to another. The triager may need to recap the conversation, particularly medication advice, as communication errors with numbers are common. After giving advice, ask whether the caller has any questions, then have him or her repeat the instructions. If there is any question as to the caller's ability to understand the instructions, recommend that the patient be seen. End each telephone triage encounter with call back instructions: advise a call back if the symptoms worsen or do not improve within a finite time, as dictated by the symptom complex. Assess the caller's comfort level with the plan; if the caller is not comfortable, arrange for a call back or for the patient to be seen. Give reassurance that the problem can be handled at home. This is helpful in calming stressed or nervous callers.

Documentation

A documentation system for all telephone triage calls helps both ongoing quality improvement review and record-keeping for medical-legal purposes. A preprinted sheet is extremely useful in allowing the triager to document as the conversation is taking place, as delayed documentation leads to errors and omissions. At a minimum, the sheet should include space for demographic information, chief complaint, protocol used for assessment, disposition category, and medication dosages. Check boxes are useful for indicating the caller's understanding of the recommendations and callback instructions and agreement with the plan discussed, with space to elaborate reasons for deviation from the protocol, if applicable. Sign, date, and time the form. It is also helpful to have space for documentation of a follow-up phone call, if needed.

Summary

The goal of the telephone triager is to be an interviewer and communicator who, by collecting focused data, quickly and competently triages ill patients into an appropriate disposition category. Recognition of serious, sometimes subtle symptoms is critical, but it is also important to manage high frequency, non-urgent symptoms such as nasal discharge.

Bibliography

Belman S, Chandramouli V, Schmitt BD, et al: An assessment of pediatric after-hours telephone care: a 1-year experience. *Arch Pediatr Adolesc Med* 2005;**159**:145–9.

Schmitt BD: Telephone triage liability: protecting your patients and your practice from harm. *Adv Pediatr* 2008; **55**:29–42.

Sutton D, Stanley P, Babl FE, Phillips F: Preventing or accelerating emergency care for children with complex healthcare needs. *Arch Dis Child* 2008;**93**:17–22.

Index

abandonment 594–595

ABCDE assessment *see* primary survey

abdominal imaging 224, 226, 249, 445, 641–642, 643, 715, 718

abdominal pain 219–222, 312, 582
  appendicitis 225
  cholecystitis 245
  dysmenorrhea 308–310
  intussusception 248
  pancreatitis 223
  pneumonia 630
  RUQ 247, 319, 356

abdominal signs of poisoning 442

abdominal thrust maneuver (Heimlich maneuver) 6

abdominal trauma 715–716, 718

abortion (miscarriage) 311, 313–314

abscesses 723–724
  brain 507
  breast 301, 302, 303
  dental 75, 76, 378
  epidural 548
  hepatic 411
  orbital 153
  peritonsillar 153–154
  retropharyngeal 156–157, 621, 623, 640

acanthosis nigricans 174

ACE inhibitors 659

acetaminophen 688
  overdose 256, 448–450, 466

acetylsalicylic acid *see* aspirin

achondroplasia 278

acidosis
  bicarbonate therapy 62, 650
  DKA 168–173, 174
  poisoning 444, 482, 483

acids
  in the eye 537, 538, 540
  ingestion of 461, 462

acne vulgaris 91–93
  neonatal 91, 124

acrodermatitis chronica atrophicans 399

acrodermatitis enteropathica 105

acromioclavicular joint 557

activated charcoal 446, 448

acute alternating hemiplegia of childhood 491

acute disseminated ence-phalomyelitis (ADEM) 487

acute hemorrhagic edema of infancy (AHEI) 676

acute kidney injury (AKI) 647–650

acute lymphoblastic leukemia (ALL) 345, 346

acute necrotizing ulcerative gingivostomatitis (ANUG) 82, 85

acute rheumatic fever (ARF) 668–671, 672, 674

Addisonian crisis 161, 162, 163–164, 165

Addison's disease 161–162, 163, 164

adenitis
  clinical presentation 139, 347, 424
  diagnosis 140, 392, 426
  management 141, 350, 408, 427

adenopathy
  see lymphadenopathy

adenosine 21, 44

ADH *see* antidiuretic hormone

adhesives, for wound closure 741

adipsic hypernatremia 177, 180

adolescents
  acne 91–93
  breast disorders 300, 301, 302, 303
  hyperventilation 54, 70, 180
  menstrual problems 310
  poisoning in 433
  psychosis 597, 598
  resuscitation 7, 17
  sexual abuse/assault 585, 591
  substance abuse 56, 469–471, 475, 598
  UTIs 666
  vaginitis 317, 325, 327–328, 328–329, 330–331
  see also pregnancy; sexually transmitted diseases

adrenal insufficiency 161–165, 750

adrenaline *see* epinephrine

adverse reactions to drugs 350
  cutaneous 107–110
  gastrointestinal 376
  gingival hyperplasia 84, 86
  hepatic 255
  hyponatremia 186
  renal 376

air emboli 207, 210

airway management
  anaphylaxis 31–32
  assessment of patency 3, 15, 711, 748
  foreign bodies
    diagnosis 614, 621, 623, 624–625, 627, 631, 640
    management 6–8, 626
  resuscitation 5–8, 626, 635, 713
  see also asthma; croup; epiglottitis

AKI (acute kidney injury) 647–650

albuterol 33, 607, 615

alcohols *see* ethanol; ethylene glycol; isopropanol; methanol

aldosterone
  hyperaldosteronism 178, 180
  hypoaldosteronism 161,
    162, 163

"Alice in Wonderland"
  syndrome 387

alkalis
  in the eye 537, 538, 540
  ingestion of 461–462

allergy
  anaphylaxis 24, 27, 30–34,
    728
  angioedema 34
  asthma 606–612, 614, 630
  conjunctivitis 544
  dermatitis 96–97, 102, 104,
    105
  insect bites and stings
    728–729
  to latex 764
  to milk protein 234, 242, 260
  urticaria 36–38, 107, 115

alopecia 93–95, 129, 130, 131

alopecia areata 94, 95

Alport syndrome 644, 645

amebiasis 410, 411, 412

amiloride 168

aminophylline 611

amiodarone 21, 41, 49

amlodipine 659

amniotocele 531, 532

amoxicillin 107

amphetamine 450, 469

ampicillin 107

amylase (elevated) 224

anal fissure 259, 260

anal warts 322
  see also genital warts

analgesia see pain relief

anaphylaxis 24, 27, 30–34, 728,
  see also angioedema;
    urticaria

anaplasmosis 399

anemia 332–336, 341
  in DUB 304, 307
  in HUS 653, 654

in sickle cell disease 354–355,
    357–358
  transfusion of RBC 335,
    341–342

anesthesia
  local (by injection) 691,
    738–739
  regional 693–701, 708, 723
  topical 692–693, 738
  see also pain relief

angioedema 34

angular cheilitis 83, 85, 101

anion gap, increased 444,
  482, 483

ankle injuries 555, 564–565,
  577

ankylosing spondylitis 549

anogenital warts 322
  see also genital warts

antibiotics
  abscesses 76, 154, 156, 723
  acne 92, 93
  adenitis 141, 350
  adverse reactions to 107
  ANUG 85
  appendicitis 228
  balanoposthitis 283
  bites 725
  burns 196
  cat scratch disease 364
  cellulitis 76, 152, 153, 543, 729
  endocarditis 65
  febrile patients 371, 372, 377
  gastroenteritis 244, 379, 380
  hand infections 708, 709
  immunodeficient patients
    344, 353, 377
  lacrimal sac infection 532
  leptospirosis 397
  Lyme disease 401
  mastitis 303
  mastoiditis 146
  meningitis 404, 405
  meningococcemia 394
  neck masses 141, 148
  omphalitis 268
  osteomyelitis 573
  otitis media 137
  parotitis 151, 378
  pericarditis 68
  pertussis 416
  pharyngitis 155

pneumonia 378–379, 406,
    632
  rheumatic fever 670
  rickettsial infections 420
  septic arthritis 675
  septic shock 27
  sickle cell disease 358
  sinusitis 137
  skin infections 97, 99–100,
    106
  STDs 298, 320–324, 329, 330
  toxic shock syndrome 423
  tuberculosis 426–427
  UTIs 666
  wounds 725, 743

anticholinergics
  for asthma 610
  overdose 443, 451–452,
    485–486

anticonvulsants 444, 520, 522,
  523, 717

antidepressants, overdose
  452–454, 485–486

antidiabetic agents, overdose
  466–467

antidiuretic hormone (ADH)
  diabetes insipidus 165–167
    hypernatremia 177, 178,
      179
  SIADH 186, 187, 188, 189,
    404

antidotes 446, 447
  antivenins 730, 734,
    735–736, 737
  flumazenil 470, 685, 689
  Lilly Cyanide Antidote Kit
    214
  NAC 256, 449
  naloxone 440, 451, 464,
    470, 685, 688

antiemetics 274, 307

antifungal agents
  skin infections 101–102,
    106, 131
  vaginitis 330

antihistamines 33,
  H_1 blockers 35, 37, 103, 489
  H_2 blockers 38, 224, 256
  overdose 465

antihypertensives 659–660

antileukotrienes 38

antiprotozoal agents 330, 412

antipsychotics, overdose 454–455

antipyretics 192

antivenins 730, 734, 735–736, 737

antiviral agents
for HIV 376, 384
for HSV 117, 322
for varicella 378, 393

anxiolytics see sedation

AOE (acute otitis externa) 149–150

AOM (acute otitis media) 135–138, 146, 503

aortic dissection 55

aphthous ulcers 83, 84

aplastic crises in sickle cell disease 354, 357

appendicitis 225–228, 263, 569, 641

appendix testis, torsion 291, 293, 294

appetite, lack of 764

arc burns 202

ARF (acute rheumatic fever) 668–671, 672, 674

arm see hand; upper limb injuries

arrhythmias 39, 55
atrial fibrillation 22, 39–40
atrial flutter 40–41
AV block 50–52, 69
in electrical injuries 201, 202
in hypothermia 211, 212
implant malfunction 53
long QT syndrome 69
in poisoning/overdose 445, 456, 467, 468, 486
resuscitation 21–23, 27
ST 41–42, 43
SVT 21, 22, 27, 42–46, 749
syncope and 69, 70
VF 21, 22–23, 27, 50, 211
VPC 47–48
VT 21, 27, 43, 48–49, 69

arterial ischemic stroke 491, 493

arthritis 569, 671–675
Lyme disease 399, 567, 672
reactive 668, 672
rheumatic fever 668, 674
septic 566, 570, 672, 674, 675
viral infections 567

arthrocentesis 673

ASA Physical Status Classification System 683

ascariasis (roundworm) 409, 411, 412

aspirin 393, 670
overdose 481–483

asthma 606–612, 614, 630

asystole see cardiac arrest

ataxia, acute 487–490, 639
see also paralysis

atenolol 660

athlete's foot (tinea pedis) 130, 131

atopic dermatitis 96–97, 105

atrial fibrillation 22, 39–40

atrial flutter 40–41

atrioventricular (AV) block 50–52

atropine 20, 463

attention deficit hyperactivity disorder, overdose of medications for 450–451, 464

automatic external defibrillators 22

autonomic dysreflexia 762–763

autopsies 596

avian influenza (H5N1) 428

AVPU (assessment of consciousness) 4, 712

babesiosis 400

babies see infants; neonates

back pain 547–552

bacterial meningitis score (BMS) 403
see also meningitis, bacterial

bacterial tracheitis 613–614, 621, 623

bacterial vaginosis 327, 328, 325, 330

bag masks 8–9, 749

balanoposthitis 283

baldness (alopecia) 93–95, 129, 130, 131

barbiturates 522, 687, 691
overdose 469

barotrauma 209

baseball finger 579, 706, 709

bats, rabies risk 732

batteries, swallowed 144, 145, 473

Beckwith-Wiedemann syndrome 278

bee stings 728

Bell's palsy 503

benzene 474

benzocaine 693

benzodiazepines
overdose 469, 470, 685, 689
in PSA 685, 687
for seizures 521

benzoyl peroxide 92, 93

bereavement 596–597

beta agonists
for anaphylaxis 32–33
for asthma
in the ED 607–609, 610
home use 612
for bronchiolitis 615
for cardiac stimulation 19–20
for croup 621
overdose 456

beta blockers
anaphylaxis treatment and 30, 33
for hypertension 659, 660
for hyperthyroidism 192
overdose 456

bicarbonate 21, 62, 172, 357, 486, 650

biguanides 466

bilevel positive airway pressure (BiPAP) 12, 636

biliary colic 245

bilious emesis 274

bilirubin 250, 251
see also jaundice

Biobrane 196

BiPAP (bilevel positive airway
pressure) 12, 636

bird 'flu (H5N1) 428

bisphosphonates 177

bites 708, 724–726
human 725,
in child abuse 590
on the hand 705, 708, 724
HIV exposure and 383
insects 728–729
mammals 725, 726
see also rabies
snakes 734–736
spiders 736–737

black widow spiders 736, 737

bladder (urinary)
catheterization 717, 750
neurogenic 762, 764
trauma 284, 285, 286

bleeding
epistaxis 142–144
GI tract
lower 257–260, 263
upper 260–263
hand injuries 708
intracranial 491, 510
intraocular 536, 538, 539
in major trauma 715
retrobulbar 537, 540
sutures 739
tracheostomy complication
758
transfusion therapy 335, 341
vaginal (DUB) 304–308

bleeding disorders 339
diagnosis 143, 306, 337
in HIV-positive patients
376, 380
management 256, 337–339,
342
warfarin and 337, 480–481

blepharitis 533, 534

blisters (burns) 196

blood pressure
measurement 657

normal 4
see also hypertension;
hypotension

Boas' sign 245

body louse 120, 121

boils (furunculosis) 98, 99

bone infections (osteomyelitis)
356, 548, 566, 571–573

bone pain 356, 569, 572

bone tumors 569

Bordatella pertussis 346,
414–416, 630

Borrelia burgdorferi see Lyme
disease

botulism 362–363, 495, 752

boutonnière deformity 579,
706, 709

bowel irrigation 446, 477

bowel obstruction 248–249, 263

bowel perforation 263, 352, 353

bradycardia
in overdose/poisoning, 441,
457, 459, 468
treatment in resuscitation 20

brain
acute ataxia 487–490, 639
ADEM 487
encephalitis 364, 366–369,
405, 488
encephalopathy
see encephalopathy
HIV-positive patients 377,
380
mass lesions
abscesses 507
causing coma 499, 500,
501
causing headache 507
tumors 489, 507
stroke 491, 493
trauma 515, 639, 710, 712,
716–717, 718
see also intracranial pressure,
raised

branchial cleft cyst 147, 148

breast 300–304
developmental abnormalities
300–301, 301–302, 302–303
gynecomastia 301, 302, 303

infections 301, 302, 303
masses 301, 302, 303

breath sounds 3
in cardiac disorders 57, 58,
61
in chest trauma 714
in pneumonia 630
in poisoning 442
see also stridor; wheezing

breathholding spells 70, 498

breathing
hyperpnea 60
management *see* intubation;
ventilation
normal rates by age 99
in the primary survey 3, 711
tachypnea 23, 57, 60, 441,
615–616

bretylium 49

bronchial foreign bodies 625,

bronchiectasis 379, 626

bronchiolitis 58, 379, 614–616

bronchodilators
in asthma 33, 607–609, 610,
611, 612
in bronchiolitis 615
in drowning 199

Broselow tapes 10

brown recluse spiders 736, 737

brucellosis 428

Brudzinski's sign 402

bruising, in child abuse 580,
582

buckle fractures 553

bullous impetigo 98

bupropion overdose 450, 453

buried bumper syndrome 757

burns 194–198
first-degree 194, 195, 198
second-degree 194, 195–196,
198
third-degree 195, 196, 197,
198
fourth-degree 195
chemical 461–462, 537,
538, 540
in child abuse 194, 195,
197, 590

electrical 194, 203
inhalation injuries 212, 214
lightning 217
ocular 537, 538, 540
transfer to burns unit 198
treatment 195–198, 462,
540

BURP maneuver 15

caffeine overdose 458

CAH (congenital adrenal
hyperplasia) 162, 164

calcinosis cutis 678

calcitonin 176

calcium
in AKI 650
hypercalcemia 174–177
hypocalcemia 180–182,
353, 650
in resuscitation 21

calcium channel blockers
for arrhythmias 40, 44
for hypertension 659
overdose 458–460

calculi
gallstones 244, 245–247
urinary system 376,
660–661

camphor poisoning 478

Campylobacter gastroenteritis
241, 242, 379

cancer 350–354
see also specific sites

candidiasis 100
cutaneous 101–102
diaper 101, 104, 106
oral 83, 85, 101, 102
vulvovaginitis, 325, 326,
327, 328, 330

cannabis 469

captopril 659

carbamates 462–463

carbamazepine 444

carbon monoxide poisoning
208–210, 212, 213, 214,
460–461

carboxyhemoglobin 444, 460

cardiac arrest 1
resuscitation 16, 18, 20, 21

cardiac arrhythmias
see arrhythmias

cardiac contusion 714

cardiac disease, congenital 65,
749, 751
cyanosis 60–62, 751

cardiac failure (CHF) 19, 27,
56–59, 631, 751
in HIV-positive patients
375, 379

cardiac implants
pacemakers and
defibrillators 52, 53
prosthetic valves 65

cardiac ischemia 55, 395

cardiac murmurs 58, 61, 62–64

cardiogenic shock 19, 25,
27, 751
vasoactive infusions 19–20,
27

cardiomegaly 58

cardiopulmonary resuscitation
see resuscitation

cardioversion, synchronous
22–23
atrial flutter 41
SVT 44–45
VT 49
see also defibrillation

caries 74–75, 76

carotenemia 251

carotid artery massage 44

carpal fractures 560, 705

casts (splints) 556, 573–579

cat bites 725

cat scratch disease 139, 141,
363–364

catheters
bladder 717, 750
for suctioning airways 5

caustic substances
in the eye 537, 538, 540
ingestion of 461–462

cellulitis 99, 728, 729
head/neck 75, 76
orbital/periorbital 151–153,
541–542, 543, 639

central nervous system
see brain; spine, spinal
cord conditions

central pontine myelinolysis
188

cerebellar ataxia, acute 487, 490

cerebral contusion 510

cerebral edema, in DKA 173

cerebral hypoxia 69, 715, 716

cerebrospinal fluid (CSF)
encephalitis 369
leakage in head trauma 511,
515
meningitis 400, 403, 404
see also intracranial pressure,
raised

cerebrovascular accidents
(stroke) 489, 491, 493

cerumen, removal of 136

cervical (neck) imaging 640,
642, 703–704

cervical (neck) masses see neck
masses

cervical (neck) trauma 11, 642,
702–704, 713, 717

cervical warts 322
see also genital warts

cervicitis 315, 318, 323

Chadwick's sign 311

chalazion 533, 534

chancre 317, 320

chancroid 317, 320, 323, 325

charcoal 446, 448

chelation therapy
for iron 477
for lead 216

chemical burns 461–462, 537,
538, 540

chemotherapy, complications
of 350

chest compressions 16–17

chest imaging 630, 640–641,
642, 714, 719

chest pain 54–56, 66, 356

chest trauma 714–715

chest trauma (*cont.*)
see also pericardial tamponade; pneumothorax

CHF see congestive heart failure

chicken pox see varicella

child abuse 580–595
abandonment/neglect 589, 594–595
diagnosis 580–581, 584–585, 594
documentation 585, 587–591, 593–594
failure to thrive 766
management 581, 585–586, 594–595
Munchausen syndrome by proxy 602–603
physical 126, 510, 537, 580–581, 752
burns 194, 195, 197, 590
fractures 555, 562, 580, 581, 582
reporting 581, 585, 590, 594
sexual 583–586
presentation 132, 285, 297, 326, 328, 584
testifying in court 591–594

child protection services (CPS) 581, 594

children with special healthcare needs (CSHCN) 753–764

chin lift maneuver 5

Chlamydia pneumoniae 630

Chlamydia trachomatis 298, 315–316, 318–319, 321
lymphogranuloma venereum 317, 320, 323
neonatal infections
eye 542, 544
pneumonia 630
in prepubertal females 326, 329
vaginal discharge 326, 327, 329

chloral hydrate overdose 469

choking see foreign bodies, in the airways

cholecystitis 244–247, 642

cholinergics, poisoning 443, 462–463

chondromalacia patellae 568, 571

Chvostek sign 180

circulation
in the primary survey 4–5, 711
resuscitation treatment 16–23, 714–716, 749

clavicular injuries 557

clonidine 660
overdose 450, 464

closed fist injuries 705, 708, 724

Clostridium botulinum 362–363, 495, 752

Clostridium difficile 242, 380

coagulopathy see bleeding disorders

coated tongue 84, 86

cocaine 56, 469, 470

codeine 688

cold caloric stimulation test 501

cold injuries see frostbite; hypothermia

cold medicines, overdose 465–466

cold sores (herpes labialis) 82, 115, 117, 391

colic 234–235, 745

colitis
C. difficile 242, 380
GI bleeding 258,

coma 256, 499–501

common cold 159–160
overdose of cold medications 465–466

communication, during telephone triage 768–770

computed tomography (CT)
abdomen 226, 641, 642, 643, 718
chest 643
head 509, 639, 716
neck 640, 642, 704

concussion 510

conduct disorders 597, 599

condylomata acuminata (genital warts) 132, 133, 316, 320, 322, 324

congenital diseases, genetic 278
CAH 162, 164

congenital heart disease 65, 749, 751
cyanosis 60–62, 751

congenital muscular torticollis 147, 148

congenital syphilis 105

congenital tuberculosis 425

congestive heart failure (CHF) 19, 27, 56–59, 631, 751
in HIV-positive patients 375, 379

conjunctiva
anatomy 528
conjunctivitis 542, 543–544
herpetic infections 116, 117, 118, 534
red eye 151–153, 541–545
trauma 536, 538

consciousness
assessment
AVPU 4, 712
GCS 512, 513
loss of; see unconscious patients

consent
for examination in cases of sexual abuse 584, 591
for PSA 683

constipation 235–239
differential diagnosis 219, 226, 237

contact dermatitis 96, 102–103, 104
caused by sponge spicules 730,

contact vaginitis 327, 330

continuous positive airway pressure (CPAP) 12, 636

contraceptives
for DUB 307
emergency 585

convulsions see seizures

coral snake bites 734, 735–736

cornea

keratitis 116, 117, 118, 542, 544
trauma 536, 538, 539, 745
coronary artery disease 55
corticosteroids
adrenal insufficiency and 161, 162, 163, 164–165, 750
for anaphylaxis 33, 35
for asthma 609–610, 612
for Bell's palsy 503
for burns 195
for dermatitis 97, 103, 104
for hypercalcemia 175
for sinusitis 158
for spinal conditions 497, 717
cortisol 161, 163
costochondritis 54, 56
coughs 606, 616–619, 620
whooping cough 346, 414–416, 630
see also hemoptysis
Coxsackie viruses 388–389
CPAP (continuous positive airway pressure) 12, 636
crab louse *see* pubic louse
cranial nerve palsies 502–503
craniosynostosis syndromes 278
cricoid pressure 9, 15
cricothyroidotomy 713
Crotalidae bites 734, 735–736
croup 620–622, 623
crying infants 745–747
colic 234–235, 745
cryptococcal meningitis 380
cryptorchidism 295–296
Cryptosporidium gastroenteritis 376
CSF *see* cerebrospinal fluid
CSHCN (children with special healthcare needs) 753–764
culdocentesis 313
Cullen sign 223
Cushing's triad 511
cutis marmorata 123

cyanide poisoning 197, 212, 213, 214
cyanosis 60–61, 751
Tet spells 61–62
cystic hygroma 147, 149
cystosarcoma phyllodes 301
dacryocystitis 531, 532
dacryostenosis 531, 532
Dance's sign 248
DARES model for evaluation of CSHCN 753–754
deafness 138, 157
death
in the ED 28, 596–597
and hypothermia 212
SIDS 600
suicide 601
decompression sickness 208, 209
decubitus ulcers 759–762
deep vein thrombosis 340, 341
deferoxamine 477
defibrillation 22–23, 49, 50, 211
see also cardioversion, synchronous
defibrillators, implantable 53
dehydration 228–233, 582
DI 166
DKA 169, 171
hypernatremic 177, 178, 179, 232
delirium tremens 472
dengue 365–366, 389
dental anatomy 72
dental caries 74–75, 76
dental discoloration 80
dental eruption 72–74
dental infections 74, 75–76, 378, 506
dental trauma 77, 80
depression 597–598, 604
Dermabond 741
dermatitis
atopic 96–97, 105

contact 96, 102–103, 104
caused by sponge spicules 730,
diaper 101, 103–106
seborrheic 105, 124, 125, 533, 534
dermatomyositis, juvenile 677–679
dermoid cyst 148, 149
desmopressin (DDAVP) 167
Destot's sign 561
developmental dysplasia of the hip 568
dexamethasone 192, 621
dextromethorphan 465
dextrose 21, 172, 466
diabetes insipidus (DI) 165–168
hypernatremia 166, 177, 178, 179
diabetes mellitus (DM) 173–174, 183, 187
diabetic drug overdoses 466–467
diabetic ketoacidosis (DKA) 168–173, 174
dialysis
for hypothermia (peritoneal) 211
for renal conditions 650, 654
for salicylate poisoning 483
diaper rashes 101, 103–106
diarrhea 239–244
bloody 239, 242, 258
dehydration 229, 230, 234, 242
HIV-associated 376, 379–380
dietary recommendations
in colic 234
in constipation 236
in diarrhea 230, 234, 242
in hypoglycemia 185
in vomiting 230, 233–234
diffuse axonal injury 511
digital nerve block 696, 697, 698, 708
digitalis *see* digoxin
digits *see* fingers; nails; toes

digoxin
  for CHF 59
  poisoning/overdose 444,
    467–468
  for tachycardias 40, 41, 44

DIP (distal interphalangeal)
  joint 579, 705, 706, 709

diphenhydramine 33, 35,
  103, 489

diphtheria 495

disability (primary survey)
  712, 716–717, 749

disks see intervertebral disks

dislocations 554, 555, 556
  clavicle 557
  elbow 559–560
  finger 561, 705, 708
  hip 562
  patella 563
  shoulder 557
  tarsometatarsal joint 565

distal interphalangeal (DIP)
  joint 705, 706, 709

distributive shock 24–25, 27, 32
  septic 19, 24, 26, 27

diuretics
  for CHF 58, 59
  for hypertension 660
  for nephrogenic DI 168

diving reflex 44

DKA (diabetic ketoacidosis)
  168–173, 174

dobutamine 19

documentation
  child abuse 585, 587–591,
    593–594
  legal access to medical
    records 604
  telephone triage 770

dog bites 725

doll's-eyes maneuver 500

dopamine 19

DOPE (assessment of
  intubation) 12

Down syndrome 279

doxycycline 420

dreams (nightmares) 524, 525

dressings 760–761

drowning 199–200

drug abuse see substance abuse

drug reaction with eosinophilia
  and systemic symptoms
  (DRESS) 107, 108

drugs (medications)
  administration routes 18,
    20, 684
  adverse reactions see adverse
    reactions to drugs
  history-taking in CSHCN
    755
  overdose
    signs of 441, 443, 487
    treatment of 444
  toxicity of 438, 439
  see also individual drugs

dynamic splinting 577

dysfunctional uterine bleeding
  (DUB) 304–308

dysmenorrhea 308–310

dystonia, antipsychotic
  overdose 454, 455

E. coli 0157:H7 242, 653
  see also Escherichia coli

E-C clamp technique 9

ear
  acute otitis externa 149–150
  acute otitis media 135–138,
    146, 503
  earache 136, 138
  foreign bodies in 144
  lightning injuries 218
  serous otitis media 157
  tumors 148

Earle's sign 561

early childhood caries (ECC) 75

earwax, removal of 136

eating problems 764–766, 767

ECGs see electrocardiograms

echocardiograms 55, 56, 59

echovirus 9, 389

'Ecstasy' (MDMA) 469, 470

ectodermal dysplasias 279

ectopic pregnancy 311–312,
  312–313, 314, 642

eczema see dermatitis

eczema herpeticum 96, 116, 118

EEGs (electroencephalograms)
  523

ehrlichiosis 399, 416, 417–418,
  419–420

Elapidae (coral snake) bites
  734, 735–736

elbow injuries 558–560, 575,
  576

electrical injuries 200–203
  burns 194, 200, 201, 202
  high-voltage 200, 203
  lightning 218
  low-voltage 200, 203

electrocardiograms (ECGs)
  atrial fibrillation 39, 40
  atrial flutter 40, 41
  AV block 51, 52
  cardiac contusion 714
  hypocalcemia 181
  hypothermia 210
  pacemaker spikes 53
  pericardial tamponade 719
  pericarditis 67
  in poisoning/overdose 445,
    456, 485
  potassium ion abnormalities
    171, 649
  SVT 42, 43, 44
  VF 50
  VPC 47
  VT 49

electroencephalograms
  (EEGs) 523

electrolyte imbalances
  adrenal insufficiency 162,
    163
  AKI 649–650
  DKA 170, 171, 172, 173
  hyperkalemia 353, 468,
    649–650
  hypernatremia 166, 177–180,
    232, 233
  hypokalemia 163, 171
  hyponatremia 186–189,
    231–232, 232–233,
    522, 649
  pyloric stenosis 265

Ellis classification of dental
  fractures 78

EM *see* erythema migrans; erythema multiforme

embolism
air 207
pulmonary 25, 27, 340

EMLA (eutectic mixture of local anesthesia) 692

EN (erythema nodosum) 112–113

enalapril 659

encephalitis 364, 366–369, 405, 488
acute disseminated encephalomyelitis 487

encephalopathy
hepatic 254–256, 257
lead poisoning 215, 216
pertussis and 415
postinfectious glomerulonephritis 646

endocarditis
infective 64–65, 376, 645
in rheumatic fever 668, 670

endotracheal tubes (ETT) 5, 10, 20
see also intubation

enema
for constipation 236
for intussusception 249

Entamoeba histolytica 410, 411, 412

enterostomy tubes 756–758

enteroviruses
encephalitis 368, 369
exanthems 388–389, 392
herpangina 82, 388
meningitis 389, 403
poliomyelitis 495

EOM (extra ocular movements) 500

ephedrine 469

epididymoorchitis
prepubertal 292, 293, 294
sexually transmitted 315, 318, 321, 324

epidural abscess 548

epidural hematoma 506, 510

epiglottitis 620, 622–624, 640

epilepsy 70, 520, 523
status epilepticus 519, 521–523

epinephrine
for anaphylaxis 32–33
for asthma 609
for cardiac stimulation 19–20
for croup 621
in local anesthetics 691, 692

epiphyseal injuries 554, 555, 559, 564

epistaxis 142–144

Epstein-Barr virus
encephalitis 367
infectious mononucleosis 386, 387

eruption of teeth 72–74

erysipelas 99, 100

erythema annulare 111

erythema infectiosum 390, 392

erythema marginatum 111

erythema migrans (EM) 115, 398, 399

erythema multiforme (EM) 107, 111–112, 115
conjunctival 543, 544

erythema nodosum (EN) 112–113

erythema toxicum neonatorum 123, 125

erythrocytes
appearance of, in diagnosis of anemia 332–334
transfusion 335, 341–342, 357, 715

erythromycin 92, 416

Escherichia coli
diarrhea 241
HUS (with *E. coli* 0157:H7) 242, 243, 653
vaginitis 326

esophagus
caustic injuries 461–462
foreign bodies in 144, 145, 473, 625
reflux disease 54, 615, 619, 766
tracheoesophageal fistula 759

ethanol
intoxication 471–472
treatment of methanol/ethylene glycol poisoning 484–485

ethmoid sinusitis 158

ethyl chloride 693

ethylene glycol 445, 483, 484–485

etomidate 686, 690

ETT (endotracheal tubes) 5, 10, 20
see also intubation

euthyroid hyperthyroxinemia 189

euvolemic hyponatremia 186, 187, 188, 189

exanthematous cutaneous eruptions
drug-induced 107
infectious causes 388–394, 417

expert witnesses 592

exposure (primary survey) 712, 717

eye
anatomy 528
caustic substances in 537, 538, 540
decontamination 445
examination 528–529, 538, 545
in differential diagnosis of coma 500–501
foreign bodies in 532, 536, 538, 539
Graves' ophthalmopathy 190, 193
herpetic infections 116, 117, 118, 534
heterophoria 506
lightning injuries 218
pain due to facial nerve palsy 503
poisoning, signs of 440, 441
red 151–153, 541–545
reduced vision 529–530
tearing, excessive 530–533
trauma 532, 535–541, 745

eyebrow, shaving 738

eyelashes, lice in 121, 534, 535

eyelid
cellulitis 151–153, 541–542, 543
inflammation 533–535
lacerations 535, 539

Fab antibody fragments, for digoxin poisoning 468

facial anesthesia 694–695

facial trauma 79–80
dental injuries 77, 80
fractures 77–79,
orbital 537, 538, 540
soft tissue injuries 77, 80

facial weakness 502–503

failure to thrive 582, 589, 764–768

fainting (syncope) 68–71, 518

Fallot's tetralogy 61, 62, 69
Tet spells 61–62

families
bereaved 28, 596–597
present during resuscitation 28, 596

fasting guidelines (pre-sedation) 683

febrile children 370–373
febrile seizures 519–520, 523
with HIV 374, 377
with sickle cell disease 357, 358

fecal impaction 236, 297

felon 706, 709

femur
aseptic necrosis of the femoral head 357
fractures 562
osteochondrosis 568, 571
SCFE 568, 570, 643

fentanyl 685, 687

fetal death (missed abortion) 311

fever see febrile children

fibromatosis colli 147, 148

fibromyalgia 549

fibula, fractures 564

fifth disease 390, 392

figure eight suture 740

fingers
infections 116, 117, 118
injuries 561, 705–706, 708–709
nerve block 696, 697, 708
splinting 577–579, 709
traumatic amputation 707, 709
see also nails

fire injuries see burns; inhalation injuries

first-degree AV block 51, 52

fishhooks 726, 727

Fitz-Hugh-Curtis syndrome 319, 324

fixed drug eruptions 107

flail chest 714

flea-borne diseases 418, 429

Fleets enema 236

fluid therapy
adrenal crisis 163
AKI 648–649
asthma 610
burns 197
DI 167
DKA 171, 172, 173
drowning 200
electrical injuries 202
gastrointestinal disorders 230–233
heat stroke 207
HHS 174
hypercalcemia 175
hypernatremia 178–180
hyponatremia 188
major trauma 715
resuscitation 18–19, 26
sickle cell disease 356

flumazenil 470, 685, 689

Foley catheters 717, 750

folliculitis 98, 99

fomepizole 484

foot
injuries 565, 573
nail conditions 128, 130, 131, 706, 709
plantar warts 132, 133, 134
tinea pedis 130, 131

Fordyce granules 84, 85

forearm fractures 560, 575

foreign bodies 144
in the airway
diagnosis 614, 621, 623, 624–625, 627, 631, 640
management 6–8, 626
in the ear 144
in the eye 532, 536, 538, 539
in the nose 144, 145
in the skin/soft tissues 643, 726–727
swallowed 144, 145, 473, 625
urethral 298
vaginal 326, 327, 328, 330

fosphenytoin 522

fractures 552–554, 555–556, 565
in child abuse 555, 562, 580, 581, 582
see also specific sites

Francisella tularensis 431

Froment's sign 707

frostbite 203–205
see also hypothermia

fructose intolerance 184

furunculosis 98, 99

gallbladder 244–247, 642

gamekeeper's thumb 705, 709

gamma-hydroxybutyrate (GHB), overdose 469

ganglion 707, 709

gastric decompression 9, 717, 750

gastric lavage 446, 459, 474

gastroenteritis
dehydration 229–230, 242
diarrhea 239–244
HIV-associated 376, 379–380
vomiting 273–274

gastroesophageal reflux 54, 615, 619, 766

gastrointestinal bleeding
lower 257–260, 263
upper 260–263

gastrointestinal causes of abdominal pain 220

gastrointestinal
decontamination 445–446,
459, 474, 477

gastrostomy tubes 756–758

GBS (group B streptococcal
disease) 750

GBS (Guillain-Barré syndrome)
489, 494, 497

GCS (Glasgow Coma Scale)
512, 513

genetic diseases 278
CAH 162, 164
hereditary angioedema
34, 35

genital examination
in cases of suspected abuse
584–585, 589
in female adolescents 306,
328
in prepubertal girls 328,
584

genital herpes
clinical presentation 116,
316, 326, 391
diagnosis 117, 319
management 117, 322, 324

genital warts (condylomata
acuminata) 132, 133, 316,
320, 322, 324

geographic tongue 84, 86

Ghon complex (TB) 424

Giardia lamblia 410, 412

Gilbert's syndrome 251

gingival hyperplasia 84, 86

gingivitis 73, 84, 86

gingivostomatitis
ANUG 82, 85
herpetic 82, 115, 117, 391

Glasgow Coma Scale (GCS)
512, 513

glaucoma, congenital 531, 532

glitazones 466

glomerular filtration rate
(GFR) 647

glomerulonephritis 644–646,
648, 651, 652, 653

glucagon 33, 185, 457, 467

glucose
high see hyperglycemia
low see hypoglycemia
in resuscitation 21, 200

glucose-6-dehydrogenase
deficiency (G6PD) 336, 753
naphthalene poisoning 478,
479

glue ear (serous otitis media)
157

goiter see Graves' disease

gonorrhea 315–316, 318–319,
321
gonococcal arthritis 672, 674
neonatal eye infections 542,
544
in prepubertal females 326,
329
vaginal discharge/vaginitis
326, 327, 329

Gottron's sign 678

granuloma
associated with tubes 757,
759
umbilical 267, 268

granuloma annulare (GA)
113–115

Graves' disease 190, 191–192
neonatal 189, 190
ophthalmopathy 190, 193

greenstick fractures 553

Grey-Turner sign 223

grief, parental 596–597

griseofulvin 131

groin
inguinal hernia 292, 293,
294
tinea cruris 129, 130, 131
see also scrotum; testis

Guillain-Barré syndrome (GBS)
489, 494, 497

guttate psoriasis 128

gutter splints 575

gynecological causes of
abdominal pain 221

gynecomastia 301, 302, 303

hair loss (alopecia) 93–95,
129, 130, 131

hair tourniquet 287, 745

hairy tongue 84, 86

half-horizontal mattress
sutures 741, 743

hallucinogens 469

hand
burns 196
injuries 560–561, 575–576,
577–579, 705–710, 724
nail conditions 128, 130,
131, 706, 709
regional anesthesia 696–700

hand-foot-mouth disease 82,
117, 389

HBOT (hyperbaric oxygen
therapy) 207–208, 214, 460

hCG (human chorionic
gonadotropin), in
pregnancy 312

head louse 120, 121

head tilt–chin lift maneuver 5

head trauma 515, 639, 710, 718
imaging 79, 512, 639, 716
posttraumatic headache 506
resuscitation 716–717
see also facial trauma

headache 337, 504–509, 517
migraine 70, 489, 504–505,
508–509
ventriculoperitoneal shunt
overdrains 526

hearing loss 138, 157

hearsay evidence in child
abuse 587–588

heart conditions
arrhythmias see arrhythmias
congestive heart failure 19,
27, 56–59, 631, 751
in HIV-positive patients
375, 379
heart block 50–52
heart murmurs 58, 61,
62–64
see also entries at cardiac

heart valves, prosthetic 65

heat-excess syndromes
205–207
heat cramps 205, 206
heat exhaustion 205, 206

heat-excess syndromes
(*cont.*)
heat stroke 206, 441, 470

heat rash (miliaria) 123, 125

Hegar's sign 310

Heimlich maneuver 6

heliox 12, 611

hemangioma 148, 149

hematemesis 260, 261

hematocele 293, 295

hematochezia 257, 260

hematoma, epidural/subdural
506, 510

hematuria 284, 285, 651–653,
715
glomerular 644, 645, 651,
652, 653

hemiparesis, acute 491–493,
639

hemodialysis 483, 650, 654

hemolysis 334, 355, 478

hemolytic anemia 334, 336
autoimmune 335, 341
see also sickle cell disease

hemolytic uremic syndrome
(HUS) 242, 243, 258,
653–654

hemophilia 336, 337

hemoptysis 626–628

hemorrhage *see* bleeding

hemorrhagic fever (dengue)
365–366

hemostatic disorders 339

hemothorax 714, 721

Henoch-Schönlein purpura
(HSP) 126, 645, 655–656,
675–677

hepatic conditions *see* hepatitis;
liver

hepatitis 251
HAV 269, 271, 272
HBV 269, 271–272, 273
HCV 269, 271, 273
toxins 252

hepatomegaly 58, 185, 248

hereditary angioedema 34, 35

hernia
inguinal 292, 293, 294
umbilical 267, 268

herpangina 82, 388

herpes simplex virus (HSV)
115–118, 391, 394
eczema herpeticum 96, 116,
118
encephalitis/meningitis 367,
369, 403
eye/eyelid 116, 117, 118, 534
genital *see* genital herpes
neonatal 116, 117, 118, 124,
125, 367, 369, 750
oral 82, 115, 117
whitlow 116, 117, 118

herpes zoster 375, 391, 393

heterophile antibodies 142,
348, 387

heterophoria 506

HHS (hyperosmolar
hyperglycemic state) 174

hip
injuries 561
limps 357, 567–568, 570–571
SCFE 568, 570, 643
septic arthritis 566, 674

histiocytosis X 105

HIV (human
immunodeficiency virus)
374–384, 585
clinical presentation 343,
374–377
diagnostic tests 384
management 377–380
opportunistic infections 101,
105
PEP 381–384
safety precautions 381

hives (urticaria) 36–38, 107,
115

Hodgkin's disease 148, 345

Holiday-Segar method for
calculation of fluid
therapy 231

home care 612, 769–770

hookworm 409, 411, 412

hordeolum (stye) 533, 534

horizontal mattress sutures
740, 742

household items with limited
toxicity 434, 436

HPV (human papillomavirus)
315
see also genital warts

HSV *see* herpes simplex virus

human chorionic gonadotropin
(hCG), in pregnancy 312

human granulocytotrophic
anaplasmosis (HGA) 417,
see also ehrlichiosis

human immunodeficiency
virus *see* HIV

human monocytotrophic
ehrlichiosis (HME) 417,
see also ehrlichiosis

human papillomavirus (HPV)
315
see also genital warts

humerus, injuries 557–559

Hurricaine spray 693

HUS (hemolytic uremic
syndrome) 242, 243, 258,
653–654

hydralazine 659

hydrocarbons, ingested
474–475

hydrocele 292, 294

hydrocephalus 763

hydrochlorothiazide 168, 660

hydrocortisone 104, 163,
164–165

hydrops of the gallbladder 245,
246

hyperaldosteronism 178, 180

hyperbaric oxygen
therapy (HBOT) 207–208,
214, 460

hyperbilirubinemia (jaundice)
249–253, 269

hypercalcemia 174–177

hyperglycemia
in DKA 169, 171–172,
in DM type II 174

in hypernatremia 179
during stress 173

hyperhemolytic crises in sickle cell disease 355

hyperinsulinism 184, 185

hyperkalemia 353, 468, 649–650

hypernatremia 177–180, 232, 233
DI 166, 177, 178, 179

hyperosmolar hyperglycemic state (HHS) 174

hyperpigmentation 162

hyperpnea 60

hypersensitivity see allergy

hypertension 180, 656–658
in autonomic dysreflexia 762–763
management 453, 522, 646, 650, 658
in poisoning/overdose 441, 453

hyperthermia 206, 207, 441, 470

hyperthyroidism see thyroid disease

hyperuricemia 353

hyperventilation 54, 70, 182
in hypocalcemia 181, 182
in resuscitation 716

hypervolemic hyponatremia 186, 187, 189

hyphema 536, 538, 539

hypoaldosteronism 161, 162, 163

hypocalcemia 180–182, 353, 650

hypoglycemia 182–186, 749
in adrenal crisis 163
in poisoning/overdose 457, 466–467
in syncope 70

hypokalemia 163, 171

hyponatremia 186–189, 231–232, 232–233, 522, 649

hypopigmented skin lesions 118–120

hypotension
in head trauma 511, 513
in poisoning/overdose 441, 453
postural 69
see also shock

hypothermia 199, 200, 210–212, 441, 750
see also frostbite

hypothyroidism, neonatal 189, 193

hypovolemic hyponatremia 186, 187, 188

hypovolemic shock 18–19, 24, 163, 261

hypoxemia 60–61, 751
acute (Tet spells) 61–62

hypoxia, cerebral 69, 715, 716

hysterical fainting 70

ibuprofen 688
overdose 479–480

ICP see intracranial pressure

icterus see jaundice

IgA nephropathy 644, 645

imaging see radiology

immunization
hepatitis 269, 272–273
pertussis 416
pneumococcus 355, 401
rabies (postexposure) 732
tetanus (postexposure) 197, 726, 727, 742
varicella (postexposure) 353, 378, 393

immunodeficiency
infections 101, 102, 343–345, 352, 353, 402
transfusion therapy 341
see also HIV

impetigo 98, 99

implants
cardiac 52, 53
for neurologic disorders 515–516

IMSOPP (resuscitation equipment) 3, 10

inborn error of metabolism (IEM) 753

indomethacin 168

infants
botulism 362, 363, 495, 752
cardiac disease 52, 751
colic 234–235, 745
constipation 235, 236
coughs 415, 416, 618
critically ill 747–753
crying 745–747
diarrhea 242, 244
febrile 370, 371–373, 745
foreign bodies in the airway 6
GBS 750
GCS 513
GI bleeding 260, 262
HSP 676
increased ICP 517, 749
inguinal hernia 292, 293, 294
intussusception 248–249, 263
jaundice 250–251, 253
meningitis 402
methemoglobinemia 752–753
milk protein allergy 234, 242, 260
osteomyelitis 572
otitis media 138
pneumonia 629, 630, 632
poisoning in 433
pyloric stenosis 264–266, 641
regurgitation 274
resuscitation 7, 20, 748–750
chest compressions 16
post-resuscitation care 28
ventilation 8, 16, 749
seizures 518, 519
shaken baby syndrome 510, 752
SIDS 600
skin conditions 101, 103–106
tearing, excessive 531, 532
teething 72
umbilical lesions 267–268
ventriculoperitoneal shunts 525–527
visual acuity testing 529, 530
vital signs 4
see also neonates

infectious colitis 258

infectious mononucleosis 139, 155, 247, 270, 346, 348, 386–388

infective endocarditis (IE) 64–65, 376, 645

infestations *see* parasites

inflammatory bowel disease 242, 260

influenza (H5N1) 428

infraorbital nerve block 694

ingestion difficulties 765

ingestions *see* poisoning

inguinal hernia 292, 293, 294

inhalation injuries 632
  in fires 212–214
  volatile substances 475–476

innocent heart murmurs 62–63

inotropic agents
  for CHF 59
  in resuscitation 19–20, 27
  for tachycardias 40, 41, 44

insect bites and stings 728–729

insecticides
  poisoning 462–463
  for treatment of infestations 121, 122, 323

insulin
  in DKA 171–172, 173
  in DM type II 174,
  hyperinsulinism 184, 185

interrupted sutures 739, 741

intervertebral disks
  diskitis 548, 567, 570
  injured 547, 550

intestinal obstruction 248–249, 263

intestinal perforation 263, 352, 353

intracranial bleeding 491, 510

intracranial complications of cancer 352, 353

intracranial pressure (ICP), raised 256, 508, 511, 516–518, 716, 749
  in DKA 173
  headache 507
  ventriculoperitoneal shunt malfunction 525–527

intraosseous fluid infusion 18

intrathecal baclofen pumps 516

intubation 9–12, 14–16, 713

for asthma 611
for croup 622
for inhalation injuries 214
in patients with cervical spinal injuries 703
RSI 14–15, 518, 716

intussusception 248–249, 263, 641

iodide solution 192

iontophoresis 693

ipecac syrup 446

ipratropium bromide 610

iris
  iritis 531, 532, 537
  trauma 537, 540

iron
  deficiency 334–335,
  poisoning/overdose 476

irrigation of wounds 739

irritation fibroma 84, 85

ischemic stroke 491, 493

isoniazid (INH) 426, 427, 447

isopropanol 445, 483, 484

itching *see* pruritis

Janeway lesions 64

Jarisch-Herxheimer reaction 324, 397

jaundice 249–253, 269

jaw
  fractures 77–79, temporomandibular joint dysfunction 506

jaw thrust maneuver 5

jellyfish stings 729, 730

Jones criteria for diagnosis of rheumatic fever 668, 669

Jones fracture 565

juvenile dermatomyositis (JDM) 677–679

Kaposi's varicelliform eruption (eczema herpeticum) 96, 116, 118

Kawasaki syndrome 55, 395–396, 543, 544, 672

keratitis 116, 117, 118, 542, 544

keratosis pilaris 96

kerion 94

Kernig's sign 402

ketamine 686, 690

ketoacidosis, diabetic 168–173, 174

ketonuria 169

ketorolac 228, 688

ketotic hypoglycemia 184, 185

kidney conditions
  acute kidney injury (AKI) 647–650
  glomerulonephritis 644–646, 648, 651, 652, 653
  HIV-associated 376
  hyponatremia 187, 648, 649
  nephrogenic DI 165, 168
  nephrotic syndrome 662–663
  pyelonephritis 664, 665, 667
  trauma 284, 285–286, 643
  see also hemolytic uremic syndrome

knee injuries 555, 562–564, 568–569, 571

Kocher criteria (septic arthritis of the hip) 674

Koplik's spots 389

kyphosis 547

labetalol 659, 660

lacerations
  eyelid 535, 539
  hand 705, 708
  lip and tongue 77, 80, 741
  management 738–744

Lachman test 563

lacrimal sac disorders 531, 532
  see also nasolacrimal duct obstruction

Langerhans cell histiocytosis 105

laryngeal foreign bodies 624, 625

laryngeal mask airways 13

laryngomalacia 621

laryngoscope blades 10

laryngotracheobronchitis
(croup) 620–622, 623

latex allergy 24, 764

laxatives 236–239

Le Fort fractures 79

lead poisoning 215–217

leg see foot; lower limb

legal issues
autopsies 596
child abuse 581, 583, 584,
585, 587–588, 591
interpersonal violence 604
testifying in court 591–594

Legg-Calvé-Perthes disease
568, 571

leptospirosis 396–397, 429

LET (lidocaine, epinephrine,
tetracaine) 692

lethargy 499, 516

leukemia 345, 346

leukocoria 545

leukorrhea 328, 330

lice see louse

lidocaine
for arrhythmias 22, 41, 50
in EMLA 692
injectable 691, 738–739
in LET 692
LMX₄ 692
for oral ulcers 85, 117
see also regional anesthesia

ligament injuries (sprains) 554,
555, 556
knee 562–563
lumbar spine 548

lightning injuries 218

Lilly Cyanide Antidote Kit 214

limps 357, 566–571, 643, 674

lipase 223

lips
cold sores 82, 115, 117, 391
lacerations 77, 80, 741

lithium 444

Little League elbow 559

liver
abscesses 411

failure 254–257
acetaminophen overdose
448–450
hepatitis see hepatitis
hepatomegaly 58, 185, 248
infarction 356
jaundice 249–253, 269

liver function tests 271, 272

LMX₄ 692

local anesthesia
injectable lidocaine 691,
738–739
topical preparations
692–693, 738
see also regional anesthesia

long QT syndrome 69

louse 120–122, 323, 534, 535
typhus and 418

lower limb
causes of limps 357, 566–571,
643, 674
injuries 555, 561–566, 577
see also foot

LSD (lysergic acid
diethylamide) 469

Ludwig's angina 75

Lugol's solution 192

lumbar punctures 369, 373,
404, 519, 527

lung infections
bronchiolitis 58, 379,
614–616
pneumonia see pneumonia
tuberculosis 423–427, 640

Lyme disease 115, 398–401,
502, 503, 567, 672

lymphadenopathy 138–142,
347–350
adenitis
clinical presentation 139,
347, 424
diagnosis 140, 392, 426
management 141, 350,
408, 427
generalized 139, 140, 142,
347, 348–349
reactive 139, 140, 347, 349,
364
see also infectious
mononucleosis

lymphogranuloma venereum
(LGV) 317, 320, 323

lymphoma 148, 343, 345–346

MAC (Mycobacterium avium
complex) 376, 407

macrocytic anemia 332, 333

magnesium sulfate 610

magnetic resonance imaging
(MRI) 516, 551, 639, 704

magnets, swallowed 473

malabsorption 766

malaria 410–411, 413–414

male pattern baldness 94

Mallampati classification 15

mallet finger 579, 706, 709

mandible, fractures 79

Marfan syndrome 279

marijuana 469

marine organism stings/
envenomations 729–730

masks
bag masks 8–9, 749
laryngeal mask airways 13
for oxygen supplementation 8

mastitis 301, 302, 303

mastoiditis 146, 639

maxilla, fractures 77, 79

McBurney's point 225

McMurray's test 563

MDMA ("Ecstasy") 469, 470

measles 389, 392, 393
encephalitis 367, 368

Meckel's diverticulum 258,
263–264, 641

median nerve block 696–697,
699

mediastinal masses 352, 353

medical records
in child abuse 587–591,
593–594
legal access to 604

medications
administration routes 18,
20, 684

medications (*cont.*)
adverse reactions *see* adverse reactions to drugs
history-taking in CSHCN 755
overdose
signs of 441, 443, 487
treatment of 444
toxicity of 438, 439
see also individual medications

medicolegal issues *see* legal issues

megaloblastic crises in sickle cell disease 355, 358

melena 257, 261

membranoproliferative glomerulonephritis 645

menarche 304

meningitis 401–405
bacterial 402, 403, 404, 405
Lyme disease 400
TB 403, 424, 427
clinical presentation 402–403, 424, 488, 507, 526
diagnosis 400, 403
in immunodeficient patients 377, 380, 402
treatment 404–405, 427, 501
viral 389, 402, 403, 404

meningococcemia 126, 391, 392, 394

meniscal injuries 563

Menser index 332

menstrual toxic shock syndrome 420, 421, 422

menstruation
dysfunctional uterine bleeding 304–308
dysmenorrhea 308–310

mental nerve block 695

mescaline 469

metabolic acidosis
bicarbonate therapy 62, 650
DKA 168–173, 174
poisoning 444, 482, 483

metacarpal fractures 560, 575

metacarpophalangeal (MCP) joint injuries 705, 724

metatarsal injuries 565

metformin 466

methanol 445, 483, 484–485

methemoglobinemia 444, 447, 478, 692, 752–753

methimazole 191

methohexital 687, 691

methylsalicylate 481

metronidazole 330

microcytic anemia 332, 333, 334

midazolam 685, 687

migraine 70, 489, 504–505, 508–509

milia 123, 125

miliaria 123, 125

miliary tuberculosis 424

milk protein allergy 234, 242, 260

Miller-Fisher syndrome 494

mineral oil, as a laxative 239

minoxidil 660

miosis 441

miscarriage 313–314, 311

mite infestations (scabies) 97, 122, 374

mitral valve prolapse 55

Mobitz heart block (type I/II) 51, 52

molluscum contagiosum 132, 133, 134
eyelid 534, 535

Mongolian spots 124, 125

monoamine oxidase (MAO) inhibitors 453
overdose 453

mononucleosis-like illnesses *see* infectious mononucleosis

monosomy X 281

morphine 62, 685, 686

mothballs, poisoning 478–479

mouth *see entries at* dental; oral

MRI (magnetic resonance imaging) 516, 551, 639, 704

MRSA (methicillin-resistant *S. aureus*)
abscesses 156, 724
balanoposthitis 283
bites and stings 725, 729
cellulitis 152, 153, 543
in HIV-positive patients 378
mastitis 303
neck masses, infected 141, 148, 151, 156
osteomyelitis 573
pericarditis 68
pneumonia 629, 630, 633
skin infections 97, 99, 100
toxic shock syndrome 422, 423

mucocele, oral 83, 85

multiple trauma 710–718

Munchausen syndrome by proxy 602–603

Murphy's sign 245

muscle cramps
heat cramps 205, 206
hypocalcemia 180, 182

muscle relaxants 23

myasthenia gravis 494–495, 497

mycobacterial infections, nontuberculous 407–408
cervical lymph nodes 139, 140, 142, 408, 426
Mycobacterium avium complex (MAC) 376, 407

Mycobacterium bovis 423, 427

Mycobacterium tuberculosis see tuberculosis

Mycoplasma pneumoniae 405–407, 630, 633

mydriasis 441

myelitis, transverse 489, 496, 497

myelomeningocele 279

myocardial ischemia/infarction 55, 395

NAC (*N*-acetylcysteine) 256, 449

nails
  bacterial infections 706, 709
  psoriasis 128
  subungual hematoma 706, 709
  tinea unguium 130, 131,

naloxone 440, 451, 464, 470, 685, 688

naphthalene poisoning 478–479

nappy (diaper) rashes 101, 103–106

nasal cannulas 8

nasogastric tubes 9, 717, 750

nasolacrimal duct obstruction 531, 532,

nasopharyngeal airways 6

nasopharyngeal masses 148

natal teeth 74

neck imaging 640, 642, 703–704

neck masses 147–149
  benign tumors 147–148, 149
  congenital 147, 148–149
  goiter 190
  lymphadenopathy 138–142, 348, 408, 424, 426, 427
  malignant 139, 142, 148, 149
  parotitis 150–151

neck trauma 11, 642, 702–704, 713, 717

needle cricothyroidotomy 713

needle stick injuries, HIV exposure and 381, 383

neglect 589, 594–595

Neisseria gonorrhea
  see gonorrhea

nematodes 326, 330, 409–410, 411, 412

neonates
  breast hypertrophy 300, 301, 302
  cardiac disease 60, 751
  clavicular fractures 557
  congenital malformations 278
  conjunctivitis 542, 544
  encephalitis 367, 369

febrile 371
GI bleeding 262
HSV infections 116, 117, 118, 124, 125, 367, 369, 750
hypoglycemia 183,
jaundice 250–251, 253
meningitis 402, 403,
pneumonia 629, 630
poisoning in 433
seizures 518
sepsis 750–751
skin conditions 91, 112, 123–125
teeth 74
thyroid disease
  Graves' 189, 190
  hypothyroidism 189, 193
UTIs 666
ventilation 12, 16
vital signs 4

nephritis
  glomerulonephritis 644–646, 648, 651, 652, 653
  pyelonephritis 664, 665, 667

nephrogenic diabetes insipidus 165, 168

nephrolithiasis 376, 660–661

nephrotic syndrome 662–663

nerve blocks 693–701, 708

neural tube defects 763

neurofibromatosis types I and II 279

neurogenic bladder 762, 764

neurogenic shock 24

neuroleptic drugs, overdose 454–455

neurological injuries in trauma
  limbs 552, 556
    lower 563
    upper 557, 558, 560
  major trauma 712, 713, 716–717
  neck 11, 642, 702–704, 713, 717
  see also head trauma

neutropenia 344,

nicardipine 659

nifedipine 659

night terrors 524, 525

nightmares 524, 525

Nikolsky's sign 99

NIPPV (non-invasive positive-pressure ventilation) 12, 635–636

nitroprusside 659

nitrous oxide 690

nits 120, 121

non-Hodgkin's lymphoma 148, 345

non-invasive positive-pressure ventilation (NIPPV) 12, 635–636

nonspecific vaginitis 326, 329

nonsteroidal anti-inflammatory drugs (NSAIDs) 393, 670
  overdose 479–480, 481–483

Noonan syndrome 280

norepinephrine 19, 20

normocytic anemia 333

norovirus 241

nose, foreign bodies in 144, 145

nosebleeds 142–144

NSAIDs see nonsteroidal anti-inflammatory drugs

numby stuff 693

nummular eczema 115

nursemaid's elbow 559–560

nystatin 85, 102, 106

obstructive shock 25

obtundation 499

octreotide 467

ocular disorders see eye

odontogenic infections 74, 75–76

odors, associated with poisoning 443

oesophagus see esophagus

oliguria 647

omphalitis 267, 268

omphalomesenteric duct 267, 268

onychomycosis (tinea unguium) 130, 131

ophthalmology *see* eye; eyelid

ophthalmoscopic evaluation 529, 538, 545

opioids
in acute cyanosis 62
overdose 440, 469, 470, 685, 688
in PSA 685, 686–687, 688

oral contraceptives
for DUB 307
emergency 585

oral infections 74–76, 82–83, 378, 506
candidiasis 83, 85, 101, 102
herpetic 82, 115, 117, 391
HIV-associated 375

oral soft tissue lesions 82–86
traumatic 77, 80, 83

oral trauma 77–80, 83
electrical burns 201, 202

orbital cellulitis 152, 153, 541–542, 543, 639

orbital fractures 537, 538, 540

orbital septum 151

orchiepididymitis
prepubertal 292, 293, 294
sexually transmitted 315, 318, 321, 324

organophosphates 462–463

oropharyngeal airways 5–6, 713

orthostatic hypotensive syncope 69, 70

Osgood-Schlatter disease 564, 568, 571

Osler nodes 64

osmolality
in DI 165, 166, 167
in HHS 174
in poisoning 445, 484

osteochondritis dissecans 569, 571

osteochondrosis, femoral head 568, 571

osteogenesis imperfecta 280

osteomyelitis 356, 548, 566, 571–573

otalgia 136, 138

otitis externa, acute 149–150

otitis media
acute 135–138, 146, 503
serous 157

ovarian torsion 642

overdose 433–446, 487, 601
see also individual medications

oxycodone 688

oxygen
for asthma attacks 607
hyperbaric therapy 207–208, 214, 460
pulse oximetry 633–634, 685
in resuscitation 8–9, 26, 713
preoxygenation before RSI 14
in sickle cell disease 357, 358
toxicity 209
see also heliox; hypoxemia; hypoxia

pacemakers 52, 53

pain relief 682
appendicitis 228
burns 195, 196
dental abscesses 76
dysmenorrhea 309–310
earache 138
oral ulcers 85
orthopedic injuries 556
pancreatitis 224
PSA 682–691
sickle cell disease 357
teething 72
see also anesthesia

palate, puncture wounds 77, 80

palmar space infections 706, 709

PALS (Pediatric Advanced Life Support) guidelines 27, 45, 46

pancreatitis, acute 223–225

papilloma, oral 83, 85

paracentesis, abdominal 716

paracetamol *see* acetaminophen

paradichlorobenzene 478,

paralysis
acute hemiparesis 491–493, 639

acute weakness 494–497
botulism 362–363, 495, 752
see also ataxia

paranasal sinuses *see* sinusitis

paraphimosis 288–289

parasites 408
lice 120–122, 323, 418, 534, 535
scabies 97, 122, 374

parents
bereaved 596–597
presence during resuscitation 28, 596

paronychia 706, 709

parotitis 150–151, 375, 378

partial thromboplastin time (PTT) 338

parvovirus B19 390, 392

patellar injuries 563, 568, 571

PCP (phencyclidine) 469

PCP (*Pneumocystis carinii* pneumonia) 375, 378–379, 633

peak expiratory flow rate (PEFR) 609

Pediatric Advanced Life Support (PALS) guidelines 27, 45, 46

pediculosis capitis (head louse) 120, 121

pediculosis corporis (body louse) 120, 121

pediculosis pubis (pubic louse) 120, 121, 318, 320, 323
eyelash/eyebrow infestations 121, 534, 535

pelvic examination 306, 309, 310, 319, 328, 584

pelvic fractures 561

pelvic inflammatory disease (PID) 314, 315–316, 318–319, 321, 324, 569

penis
balanoposthitis 283
herpes *see* genital herpes
paraphimosis 288–289
phimosis 283, 289–290

priapism 290–291
  regional anesthesia 700–701
  trauma 285, 287

pentobarbital 691, 687

PEP see postexposure
  prophylaxis

perianal infections 105, 106

pericardial effusion 66, 67

pericardial tamponade 66
  clinical presentation 25, 66
  diagnosis 67, 642, 714, 719,
    721
  management 68, 714,
    719–720

pericarditis 55, 66, 67

pericoronitis 74, 75, 76

perihepatitis (Fitz-Hugh-Curtis
  syndrome) 319, 324

periodontitis 84, 86

periorbital (preseptal) cellulitis
  152–153, 541, 543

peritoneal dialysis 211

peritoneal lavage 715

peritonsillar abscesses 153–154

perlèche (angular cheilitis)
  83, 85, 101

permethrin 121, 122, 323

pertussis 346, 414–416, 630

pesticides
  poisoning 462–463
  for treatment of infestations
    121, 122, 323

phalanges see fingers; nails; toes

pharynx
  peritonsillar abscesses
    153–154
  pharyngitis 154–156, 391
  retropharyngeal abscesses
    156–157, 621, 623, 640

phenobarbital 444, 522

phenothiazine 447

phenylephrine 465, 469

phenytoin 522

phimosis 283, 289–290

photographic evidence in
  suspected child abuse 590

photosensitivity 107

phototherapy 254

physical abuse 126, 510, 537,
  580–581, 752
  burns 194, 195, 197, 590
  documentation 587–591,
    593–594
  fractures 555, 562, 580, 581,
    582
  testifying in court 591–594

physical examination findings
  in critically ill infants 748
  in poisoning 441

physical status classification
  683

physostigmine 452

phytophotodermatitis 102

Pierre-Robin malformation 280

pimecrolimus 97

pinworm 326, 330, 409, 411,
  412

PIP (proximal interphalangeal)
  joint 579, 705, 706, 708

pituitary gland 167, 185, 508

pityriasis alba 118

pityriasis rosea 127–128

pityriasis (tinea) versicolor
  130, 131

plague 429

plants
  household (limited toxicity)
    436
  poisonous 437, 467

Plasmodium species see malaria

platelet disorders
  see thrombocytopenia;
    thrombocytosis

pleural chest pain 54

pleural effusions in TB 426

pneumococcus
  see Streptococcus
    pneumoniae

Pneumocystis jiroveci (carinii)
  pneumonia (PCP) 375,
    378–379, 633

pneumomediastinum 720

pneumonia 356, 358, 373,
  629–633, 640
  antibiotics 378–379, 406, 632
  HIV-associated 375,
    378–379, 633
  M. pneumoniae 405–407,
    630, 633

pneumonitis, aspiration 463,
  474

pneumothorax 208, 720–721
  open 714
  simple 714, 721
  tension 25, 714, 720, 721

poisoning 433–446, 487, 601
  see also individual chemicals
    and drugs

Poland syndrome 300

poliomyelitis 495

polydipsia 166, 177

polyps (bowel) 258, 260

polyuria 166, 171

Portuguese man-of-war stings
  729, 730

posterior arm splints 576

posterior fossa tumors 489, 507

posterior leg splints 577

postexposure prophylaxis
  (PEP)
  hepatitis 272–273
  HIV 381–384
  rabies 732
  tetanus 197, 726, 727, 742
  varicella 353, 378, 393

postinfectious encephalitis 367,
  368

postinfectious
  glomerulonephritis 644, 646

postural hypotension 69

potassium
  in DKA 170, 171
  hyperkalemia 353, 468,
    649–650
  hypokalemia 163, 171

PR interval, prolonged see first-
  degree AV block

Prader-Willi syndrome 280

pralidoxime 463

prazosin 660

pregnancy
  abortion 311, 313–314
  ectopic 311–312, 312–313, 314, 642
  normal 310–311, 312, 314
  tests for 312

Prehn's sign 291

pressure ulcers 759–762

priapism 290–291

prilocaine 692

primary survey 1–5
  in critically ill infants 747–750
  in major trauma 711
  in overdose/poisoning 435–440

procainamide 22

procedural sedation and analgesia (PSA) 682–691

proctitis 316, 319, 324

progesterone 312

propofol 686, 690

propranolol 192, 457

propylthiouracil (PTU) 191, 192

prostaglandin 749, 751

proteinuria 662–664

prothrombin time (PT) 338

proximal interphalangeal (PIP) joint 579, 705, 706, 708

pruritis
  atopic dermatitis 96, 97
  lice 120–122
  pinworm 326, 330, 411
  scabies 122
  urticaria 37

PSA (procedural sedation and analgesia) 682–691

pseudoephedrine 465, 469

pseudomembranous colitis 242, 380

pseudoseizures 519

pseudotumor cerebri 507

psilocybin 469

psittacosis 429

psoriasis 105, 128–129

psychological disorders 597–599
  conduct disorders 597, 599
  depression 597–598, 604
  hysterical fainting 70
  psychogenic chest pain 54
  psychogenic weakness 496
  psychosis 597, 598
  urinary retention 296, 297
  see also suicide

puberty, precocious 300, 302, 303

pubic louse 120, 121, 318, 320, 323
  eyelash/eyebrow infestations 121, 534, 535

pulmonary edema 57, 178, 615

pulmonary embolism 25, 27, 340

pulmonary infections
  bronchiolitis 58, 379, 614–616
  pneumonia see pneumonia
  tuberculosis 423–427, 640

pulmonic ejection murmurs 63

pulse, normal rates by age 4

pulse oximetry 633–634, 685

pulsus alternans 58

pulsus paradoxus 66, 719, 720

pupils
  afferent pupillary defects 541
  fixed 500
  signs of drug toxicity 441
  unequal 517
  white (leukocoria) 545

purpura
  HSP 126, 645, 655–656, 675–677
  palpable 126–127

pustular melanosis 124, 125

pyelonephritis 664, 665, 667

pyloric stenosis 264–266, 641

pyoderma 96, 97, 98–100

pyogenic granuloma 84, 85

pyrethrin 121

pyrexia see febrile children

Q fever 418, 419–420

rabies 368, 369, 726, 733

RACE (primary assessment of breathing) 3

radial nerve block 700,

radiology
  abdomen 224, 226, 249, 445, 641–642, 643, 715, 718
  chest 630, 640–641, 714, 719
  fractures 555
  head 79, 509, 512, 639, 716
  implantable devices 516,
  neck 640, 642, 703–704
  ordering tests 638
  radiation exposures 638
  spine 353, 551, 642
  wounds 726, 738

radius
  fractures 559, 560
  radial head subluxation 559–560

ranitidine 33, 38, 224, 256

ranula 83, 85

rapid-sequence intubation (RSI) 14–15, 518, 716

rashes
  adverse reactions to drugs 107–110
  arthritic diseases associated with 673, 678
  infectious diseases associated with 388–394, 417
  lesion types 87–91, 115, 118
  see also individual disorders

rat-bite fever 430

rat poison (warfarin) 337, 480–481

rattlesnake bites 734, 735–736

Raynaud's phenomenon 680, 681

reactive arthritis 668, 672

recreational drug abuse
  see substance abuse

rectal bleeding 257–260, 263

rectal examinations 226, 236

rectal inflammation (proctitis) 316, 319, 324

rectal prolapse 266

recurrent parotitis of childhood 150, 151

red blood cells (RBC)
appearance of, in diagnosis of anemia 332–334
transfusion 335, 341–342, 357, 715

red eye 151–153, 541–545
herpetic infections 116, 117, 118, 534,

red reflex 538, 545

reflex sympathetic dystrophy (RSD) 549

regional anesthesia 693–701, 708, 723

regurgitation 274

renal conditions see kidney conditions

respiratory distress/failure 3, 634–637
in drowning 199, 199,
in sickle cell disease 356, 358
see also ventilation

respiratory infections
bacterial tracheitis 613–614, 623
bronchiolitis 614–616
croup 620–622, 623
epiglottitis 620, 622–624, 640
HIV-associated 375, 378–379
pertussis 346, 414–416, 630
pneumonia see pneumonia
psittacosis 429
SARS 430
in tracheostomies 758
tuberculosis 423–427, 640
URIs (mild) 159–160, 343

resuscitation 1–28
airway
assessment 3, 15, 711, 748
management 5–8, 626, 635, 713
breathing
assessment 3, 711
management 8, 713, 716
circulation
assessment 4–5, 711
management 16–23, 714–716, 749
in drowning 200

in electrical injuries 203
family presence during 28, 596
in infants 748–750
after major trauma 711, 713–717
in overdose/poisoning 435–440
planning 1, 684
post-resuscitation care 27
shock 23–27
termination 28

retinoic acid 92, 93

retrobulbar hemorrhage 537, 540

retropharyngeal abscesses 156–157, 621, 623, 640

rhabdomyolysis 202

rheumatic fever, acute 668–671, 672, 674

rhinosinusitis 137, 157, 375, 506, 639

rib fractures 627, 714

rickettsial infections 416–420

rifampin 427

ringworm (tinea corporis) 96, 129, 130, 131

risk assessments
head injuries 514
HIV PEP 383
suicide 601

Rocky Mountain spotted fever (RMSF) 416, 418–419, 419–420

roseola infantum 390, 392

rotavirus 241, 274

roundworm 409, 411, 412

Roux's sign 561

Rovsing's sign 225

RSI (rapid-sequence intubation) 14–15, 518, 716

rubella 390, 392, 393

rubeola see measles

rule of nines 194

safety of healthcare staff
HIV risk

PEP 381, 383
treatment of patients 381
pesticide poisoning 463

salicylates 393, 670
overdose 481–483

salivary glands
parotitis 150–151, 375, 378
ranula 83, 85

Salmonella gastroenteritis 241, 242, 376

salpingitis 306

salt poisoning 178, 180

Salter-Harris classification of growth plate injuries 554

SAMPLE history (pre-intubation) 14

SARS (severe acute respiratory syndrome) 430

SBE (subacute bacterial endocarditis) 64–65, 376, 645

scabies 97, 122, 374

scald burns 194

scalp wounds 738, 739

scaphoid fractures 560, 705

scarlet fever 391, 394

SCD see sickle cell disease

SCFE (slipped capital femoral epiphysis) 568, 570, 643

Scheuermann's kyphosis 547

schizophrenia 597, 598

SCIWORA (spinal cord injury without radiographic abnormality) 702, 704

scorpion stings 733–734

scrotum
swellings 291–295
trauma 285, 287

sea urchin barbs 730

seborrheic dermatitis 105, 124, 125, 533, 534

second-degree AV block 51, 52,

secondary survey 441, 717–718

sedation 682
PSA 682–691

sedation (*cont.*)
in psychosis 599
in RSI 14, 17
see also anesthesia

Seidel test 536

seizures
clinical presentation and
diagnosis 70, 489, 518–520
in head trauma 510, 513, 717
in hyponatremia 231, 522
management 521–524
vagus nerve stimulators
515–516

selective serotonin reuptake
inhibitors (SSRIs),
overdose 453

self-harm *see* suicide

Sellick maneuver 9

sepsis
diagnosis and management
in febrile children 370–373
neonatal 750–751
septic shock 19, 24, 26, 27
toxic shock syndrome
420–423

septic arthritis 566, 570, 672,
674, 675

serotonin syndrome 453, 454,
471

serous otitis media (SOM) 157

serum sickness 107, 672, 735

severe acute respiratory
syndrome (SARS) 430

sexual abuse 583–586
clinical presentation 132,
285, 297, 326, 328, 584
documentation 585,
587–591, 593–594
testifying in court 591–594

sexually transmitted diseases
(STDs) 314–325
HIV 381, 383, 585
pubic lice 120, 121, 318,
320, 323
in sexual abuse 326, 585, 590
syphilis 105, 317, 320, 323,
324
urethritis 298, 323
vaginitis 317, 325, 326, 327,
328, 330

*see also Chlamydia
trachomatis*; genital herpes;
genital warts; gonorrhea

shaken baby syndrome 510, 752

shaving, in wound
management 738

Shea classification of skin
ulcers 760

Shigella gastroenteritis 241, 242

shingles (herpes zoster) 375,
391, 393

shock 23
anaphylactic 24, 27, 32
cardiogenic 19, 25, 27, 751
decompensation 5, 23, 711,
750
diagnosis 3, 25–26
hypovolemic 24
neurogenic 24
obstructive 25
septic 19, 24, 26, 27
treatment 26–27
fluids 18–19, 26, 163,
261, 715
vasoactive infusions
19–20, 27

shoulder, dislocation 557

SIADH (syndrome of
inappropriate ADH) 186,
187, 188, 189, 404

sick sinus syndrome 69

sickle cell disease (SCD) 290,
343, 354–359
bone pain 356, 549, 569, 572

SIDS (sudden infant death
syndrome) 600

silver sulfadiazine 196

sinus tachycardia (ST) 41–42,
43

sinusitis 137, 157, 375, 506, 639

SJS *see* Stevens-Johnson
syndrome

skier's thumb 705, 709

skin conditions
adverse reactions to drugs
107–110
in HIV-positive patients
374–375, 378
hyperpigmentation 162

hypopigmentation 118–120
infectious diseases with
exanthems 388–394, 417,
lesion types 87–91, 115, 118
neonatal/infantile 101,
103–106, 112, 123–125
signs of arthritic diseases
678, 673
signs of overdose/poisoning
441
signs of physical abuse 580
see also individual disorders

skull
fractures 511, 512, 515
orbital 537, 538, 540
mastoiditis 146, 639

slapped cheeks syndrome
(erythema infectiosum)
390, 392

SLE (systemic lupus
erythematosus) 112, 645,
679–681, 672

sleep disorders 524

slipped capital femoral
epiphysis (SCFE) 568,
570, 643

smoke inhalation 212, 214

snakebites 734–736

Snellen charts 528

social services 605, 754
child protection services
581, 594

sodium
in AKI 187, 648, 649
in DI 166, 177, 178, 179
in DKA 170, 173
hypernatremia 166, 177–180,
232, 233
hyponatremia 186–189,
231–232, 232–233, 522, 649
isotonic dehydration 231,
232

sodium bicarbonate 21, 62, 172,
357, 486, 650

somnambulism 525

sotalol 456

special healthcare needs
753–764

spider bites 736–737

spina bifida 763

spine
back pain 547–552
diskitis 548, 567, 570
imaging 353, 551, 642
spinal cord conditions
autonomic dysreflexia
762–763
causing acute weakness
489, 496, 497
causing urinary retention
296, 297
compression 352, 353
spina bifida 763–764
trauma 24, 547–548, 642,
702–704, 713, 717
tumors 549

splenomegaly 349, 359–361
in infectious mononucleosis
386, 387
in sickle cell disease 355, 357

splinter hemorrhages 64

splints 556, 573–579

spondylolisthesis 547

spondylolysis 547, 550

sponges (marine) 730

sprains 554, 555, 556
knee 562–563
lumbar spine 548

sputum, in differential
diagnosis of coughing 618

SSRIs (selective serotonin
reuptake inhibitors),
overdose 453

ST (sinus tachycardia) 41–42,
43

staphylococcal infections
pneumonia 630
skin 98, 99
toxic shock syndrome
(SaTSS) 420–423
vagina 326
see also MRSA

staphylococcal scalded skin
syndrome (SSSS) 98, 99

status asthmaticus 612

status epilepticus 519, 521–523

Stenson's duct 151

sternoclavicular joint 557

steroid acne 91, 93

steroids see corticosteroids

Stevens-Johnson syndrome
(SJS) 107, 108
eye involvement 543, 544

Still's murmur 63

Stimpson method for reduction
of shoulder dislocation 557

stingrays 730

stings
insects 728–729
marine organisms 729–730
scorpions 733–734

stomach pumps (gastric lavage)
446, 459, 474

stonefish 730

stones see calculi

stool softeners 239, 239

stools
in infancy 235
testing
diarrhea 241–242
GI bleeds 257, 261
parasitic infections 411

streptococcal infections
neonatal sepsis (GBS) 750
scarlet fever 391, 394
skin 98, 99, 105, 106
throat 155
toxic shock syndrome
(SpTSS) 420–423
vagina 326
see also rheumatic fever

Streptococcus pneumoniae 146,
372, 401, 629

stridor 387, 635
see also bacterial tracheitis;
croup; epiglottitis

stroke 489, 491, 493

strongyloidiasis (threadworm)
409–410, 411, 412

stupor 499

Sturge-Weber syndrome 281

styes (hordeolum) 533, 534

subacute bacterial endocarditis
(SBE) 64–65, 376, 645

subdural hematoma 506, 510

subluxation 554, 555
in the cervical spine 704
nursemaid's elbow 559–560

substance abuse
drugs of abuse 56, 469–471,
598
volatile substances 475–476

subungual hematoma 706, 709

succinylcholine
(suxamethonium) 23

sucrose solution 693

suction catheters 5

sudden infant death syndrome
(SIDS) 600

sugar tong splints 575

suicide 598, 601–602

sulfonylureas 466, 467

sunburn 194, 195

superior vena cava obstruction
352, 353

supraorbital/supratrochlear
nerve block 694, 695

supraventricular tachycardia
(SVT) 21, 22, 27, 42–46,
749

sutures 80, 739–741
removal 744

swimmer's ear (otitis externa)
149–150

sympathomimetic toxidrome
450, 451, 453, 465

syncope 68–71, 518

syndrome of inappropriate
ADH (SIADH) 186, 187,
188, 189, 404

synovial fluid 674

synovitis
toxic 672, 674
transient synovitis of the
hip 568, 570

syphilis 317, 320, 324, 323
congenital 105

syringomyelia 764

systemic lupus erythematosus
(SLE) 112, 645, 672,
679–681

systems review in CSHCN 754–755

tachycardia
 atrial fibrillation 22, 39–40
 atrial flutter 40–41
 in overdose/poisoning 441
 ST 41–42, 43
 SVT 21, 22, 27, 42–46, 749
 syncope and 69, 70
 VF 21, 22–23, 27, 50
 VT 21, 27, 43, 48–49, 69

tachypnea 23, 57, 60, 441
 in bronchiolitis 615–616

tacrolimus 97

tamponade see pericardial tamponade

tarsometatarsal joint dislocation 565

TB see tuberculosis

team management in resuscitation 1

tears, excessive 530–533

teenagers see adolescents

teeth see entries at tooth

teething 72

telephone triage 768–770

telogen effluvium 93, 94, 95

temporomandibular joint dysfunction 506

TEN (toxic epidermal necrolysis) 107, 108

tenosynovitis, purulent 706, 709

Tensilon test 497

tension headache 505, 508

tension pneumothorax 25, 714, 720, 721

terbutaline 609, 610

testis
 epididymoorchitis
  prepubertal 292, 293, 294
  sexually transmitted 315, 318, 321, 324
 torsion 291, 293–294, 642
 tumors 293, 295
 undescended 295–296

Tet spells 61–62

tetanus 197, 726, 727, 742

tetracaine 692

tetralogy of Fallot 61, 62

thelarche
 failure 300, 302, 303
 premature 300, 302, 303

theophylline 444, 611

thermal injuries see burns; frostbite

thiazide diuretics 168, 660

third-degree AV block 51–52

thirst/polydipsia 166, 177

thoracotomy 714

threadworm 409–410, 411, 412

3-3-2 rule 15

throat see pharynx

thrombocytopenia 336, 337, 339, 342
 in HIV-positive patients 376, 380

thrombocytosis 340, 341

thrombophilia 340–341

thrombus, atrial 40

thrush see candidiasis

thumb injuries 705, 707

thumb spica splint 576

thyroglossal duct cyst 147, 148

thyroid disease
 Graves' ophthalmopathy 190, 193
 hyperthyroidism 189–193
 neonatal
  Graves' disease 189, 190
  hypothyroidism 189, 193
 thyroid storm 190, 192
 TPP 191, 192

tibia
 injuries 564, 577
 Osgood-Schlatter disease 564
 site of IO needle insertion 18

tick paralysis 495, 497

ticks 398, 401, 416, 417
 diseases spread by
  see anaplasmosis; ehrlichiosis; Lyme disease;

Rocky Mountain spotted fever
 removal of 400

Tietze's syndrome (costochondritis) 54, 56

tinea capitis 93, 94, 129, 130, 131

tinea corporis 96, 115, 129, 130, 131

tinea cruris 129, 130, 131

tinea pedis 130, 131

tinea unguium 130, 131

tinea versicolor 118, 130, 131

toddler's fracture 564

toes
 fractures 565
 nerve block 696, 698
 see also nails

tongue lesions 84, 86
 lacerations 77, 80

tonsils
 peritonsillar abscesses 153–154
 tonsillitis 154–156

tooth anatomy 72

tooth decay (caries) 74–75, 76

tooth discoloration 80

tooth eruption 72–74

tooth infections 74, 75–76, 378, 506

tooth injuries 77, 80

topical anesthesia 692–693, 738

torsades de pointes 69

torticollis 147, 148

toxic epidermal necrolysis (TEN) 107, 108

toxic shock syndrome 420–423

toxidromes 443

TPP (transient periodic paralysis) 191, 192

trachea
 bacterial tracheitis 613–614, 621, 623
 foreign bodies in 624, 625
 tracheoesophageal fistula 759

tracheal tubes (ETT) 5, 10, 20
  see also intubation
tracheostomy 758–759
traction alopecia 94, 95
transfusion 335, 341–342, 357
  emergency 715
transfusion reactions 341
transient neonatal pustular
  melanosis 124, 125
transient periodic paralysis
  (TPP) 191, 192
transverse myelitis 489, 496,
  497
trauma
  interpersonal violence
    603–605
  multiple injuries 710–718
  in near-drowning 199
  see also physical abuse;
    specific sites
traumatic arthritis 672
trazodone 453
tretinoin 92, 93
trichomoniasis 317, 326, 327,
  328, 330, 325
trichotillomania 94, 95
trichuriasis (whipworm) 410,
  411, 412
tricyclic antidepressants,
  overdose 485–486
trisomy 21 (Down syndrome)
  279
Trousseau sign 180
tuberculin skin tests (TST)
  425–426
tuberculosis (TB) 423–427, 640
  cervical lymph nodes 142,
    424, 426, 427
  meningitis 403, 424, 427
tuberous sclerosis 118, 120,
  133, 281
tularemia 431
tumors 350–354
  see also specific sites
Turner syndrome 281
tympanic membrane 136, 157

tympanocentesis 138
typhus fevers 418, 419–420
Tzanck smear test 116
ulcers 90
  genital 116, 316, 317,
    oral 82–83, 84–85
    pressure 759–762
ulna, fractures 560
ulnar nerve block 697–698, 699
ultrasound 226, 264, 641–642,
  715
umbilical hernia 267, 268
umbilical lesions 267–268
unconscious patients
  coma 256, 499–501
  poisoning in 435–440
  removal of foreign bodies
    from airways 6
  syncope 68–71, 518
  with traumatic injuries 513,
    514, 702, 704, 716–717
upper limb injuries 557–561,
  705–710, 724
  splints 575–577, 577–579
  see also hand
upper respiratory infections
  (URIs) 159–160, 343
urachus 267, 268
ureter, trauma 284, 285, 286
urethra
  meatal stenosis 288
  meatal warts 322
  prolapsed 297, 298
  trauma 284, 285, 287, 561
  urethritis 297–299, 315, 318,
    323
URI (upper respiratory
  infections) 159–160, 343
uric acid 353
urinary retention 288, 296–297
urinary tract infections (UTIs)
  373, 664–667
  in neurogenic bladder 762
urine
  hematuria 284, 285, 644, 645,
    651–653, 715
  oliguria 647
  polyuria 166, 171

proteinuria 662–664
urticaria 36–38, 107, 115
UTI see urinary tract infections
uveitis 542, 544
vaccination see immunization
vaginal bleeding, dysfunctional
  (DUB) 304–308
vaginal examination in
  prepubertal girls 328
  in cases of suspected abuse
    584, 585, 589
vaginal foreign bodies 326, 327,
  328, 330
vaginal herpes see genital
  herpes
vaginal warts 322
  see also genital warts
vaginitis
  prepubertal 325, 326, 328,
    329–330, 331
  pubertal 317, 325, 327–328,
    328–329, 330–331
vagus nerve stimulation 43,
  515–516
valproic acid 444
Valsalva maneuver 44
vancomycin 68, 100, 153, 156,
  344, 380, 423, 573
varicella 390, 392, 393
  encephalitis 367
  eyelid 534, 535
  in immunodeficient patients
    353, 375, 378
  see also herpes zoster
varicocele 292, 294
vascular access, during
  resuscitation 18
vasculitis see Kawasaki
  syndrome; purpura; Rocky
  Mountain spotted fever
vasoocclusive crises in sickle
  cell disease 354, 355–357,
  572
vasopressin (ADH)
  DI 165–167
    hypernatremia 177, 178,
    179

vasopressin (ADH) (*cont.*)
SIADH 186, 187, 188, 189, 404

vasovagal syncope 68

venereal warts (condylomata acuminata) 132, 133, 316, 320, 322, 324

venom
marine organisms 729, 730
scorpions 733–734
snakes 734–736
spiders 736–737

venous hum 63

ventilation
in asthma 611
bag masks 8–9, 749
BiPAP 12, 636
CPAP 12, 636
in drowning 199
in head injuries 513, 518, 716–717
heliox 12, 611
intubation *see* intubation
laryngeal mask airways 13
mechanical ventilator settings 12, 16, 636
NIPPV 12, 635–636
in salicylate poisoning 483
in shock 26

ventricular fibrillation (VF) 21, 22–23, 27, 50, 211

ventricular premature contractions (VPC) 47–48

ventricular tachycardia (VT) 21, 27, 43, 48–49, 69

ventriculoperitoneal shunts 525–527, 639

verapamil 40, 44
overdose 458–460

verrucae (warts) 132–133, 133–134
see also genital warts

vertebral column *see* spine

vertical mattress sutures 739, 742

vertigo 490

vesicoureteral reflux 666–667

VF (ventricular fibrillation) 21, 22–23, 27, 50, 211

Vincent's angina 117

violence, interpersonal 603–605
see also child abuse

vision
assessment of visual acuity 528–529, 538
decreased 529–530

vital signs
normal 4
in overdose/poisoning 441

vitamin K, treatment with 256, 337, 481

vitiligo 120, 118

volar splints 575

volvulus 641

vomiting 273–277, 757, 766
dehydration 229, 230, 233–234, 242
hematemesis 260, 261
HIV-associated 376
pyloric stenosis 264

VPC (ventricular premature contractions) 47–48

VT (ventricular tachycardia) 21, 27, 43, 48–49, 69

vulval herpes *see* genital herpes

vulvovaginitis *see* vaginitis

warfarin, poisoning 337, 480–481

warts (verrucae) 132–133, 133–134
see also genital warts

weakness
acute 489, 494–497
facial 502–503

Weil disease (leptospirosis) 396–397, 429

West Nile virus 367, 389

wheezing 58, 614–615, 635
in HIV-positive patients 379
see also asthma

whipworm 410, 411, 412

white blood cells *see* leukemia

whitlow 116, 117, 118

whole bowel irrigation (WBI) 446, 477

whooping cough (pertussis) 346, 414–416, 630

Williams syndrome 175, 281

Wolff-Parkinson-White syndrome 22, 40, 42

worms 326, 330, 409–410, 411, 412

wounds
management 80, 726, 738–744
skin ulcers 759–762
see also bites; lacerations

wrist fractures 560, 705

X-rays
abdomen 445, 642
chest 630, 640–641, 642, 643, 714
fractures 555
head 512, 639
neck 640, 703–704

Yale Observation Scale (YOS) 370

Yankauer catheters 5

Yersinia enterocolitica 241, 431

Yersinia pestis 429

Yersinia pseudotuberculosis 431

zipper injuries 287

zoonoses 428
see also individual diseases